Introduction to Neurogenic Communication Disorders

Introduction to Neurogenic Communication Disorders

Fifth Edition

Robert H. Brookshire, PhD, CCC/SP

Director, Speech Pathology Section
Neurology Service
Department of Veterans Affairs Medical Center
Professor, Department of Communication Disorders
University of Minnesota
Minneapolis, Minnesota

with 136 illustrations

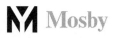

Mosby

St. Louis Baltimore Boston Carlsbad Chicago Naples New York Philadelphia Portland
London Madrid Mexico City Singapore Sydney Tokyo Toronto Wiesbaden

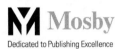
Mosby
Dedicated to Publishing Excellence

FIFTH EDITION
Copyright ©1997 by Mosby—Year Book, Inc.

Previous edition copyrighted 1992

Printed in the United States of America

Mosby-Year Book, Inc.
11830 Westline Industrial Drive
St. Louis, Missouri 63146

Library of Congress Cataloging-in-Publication Data
Brookshire, Robert H.
　　Introduction to neurogenic communication disorders / Robert H.
　Brookshire. — 5th ed.
　　　p.　cm.
　　Includes bibliographical references and index.
　　ISBN 0-8151-1014-6
　　1. Communicative disorders.　2. Speech disorders.　3. Aphasia.
　I. Title.
　　[DNLM:　1. Aphasia.　2. Communicative Disorders.　WL 340.5 B872i
　1997]
　RC423.B74　1997
　616.85´52—dc21
　DNLM/DLC　　　　　　　　　　　　　　　　　　　　　　　96-53118

99 00 01/9 8 7 6 5 4 3 2

For Lisa

The autumn wind touches the mountain _____
The spring leaf falls to earth

Foreword

The remarkable capacity to communicate emerged in a gradual, evolutionary way for our species and today it nearly explodes on the scene during the early years of life. As normal communicators, we benefit from the reliability and adaptability conferred by evolution. We could be reminded daily—if we stopped to think about it—of the crucial roles that speech, language, and communication ability play in our social, emotional, intellectual, and working lives.

Of course, we don't usually stop to think about it. Communication is so much a part of our "selves" that the wonder of it all usually is apparent only when we choose to study and appreciate it. Readers of this book have probably already engaged in such a process. If so, you have a better sense than most of the complexity of the processes that make us normal speakers, listeners, readers, writers, and communicators.

Most of you have now chosen to embark on an effort to learn about what happens when—because of neurologic disease—the ability to communicate becomes impaired. Such impairments sometimes seem to insult and diminish the accomplishments of evolution. Fortunately, neurologic disease doesn't happen to an entire species. Unfortunately, it can happen to people, often in ways that disable, handicap, and devastate. It is one of life's paradoxes that our

language ability permits us to examine the effects of the destruction of that very capacity and then share that knowledge with others. Such study should be conducted with a keen awareness that our "subjects" deserve our commitment to use what we learn from them responsibly and productively.

Don't misinterpret the word *Introduction* in the title of this book. The contents herein represent more than a handshake. The text will provide you with a solid foundation of knowledge about the neurology of communication, as well as the causes, symptoms, diagnosis, and management of the most frequently encountered neurologic communication disorders. Serious students will leave this book prepared to study the disorders in greater depth. Aspiring clinicians will leave it prepared to develop the skills necessary to work with people whose lives are affected by the disorders.

Many texts about neurogenic disorders of communication have come and gone over the years. Some texts became extinct because of limited substance, some because they failed to communicate their content effectively, and some because their content no longer reflected current knowledge, thinking, technology, or practice. This Fifth Edition of *Introduction to Neurogenic Communication Disorders* has survived because it reflects the evolution of several things. First, methods of assessing, diagnosing, understanding, and managing neurogenic communication disorders and their causes have changed in subtle-to-dramatic ways. Those changes are reflected in these pages. Second, the range of communication disorders to which we must attend has broadened. Twenty years ago clinicians were "up to speed" if they knew something about aphasia, dysarthria, and apraxia of speech. We now appreciate, by virtue of their increased prevalence and careful clinical observation and research, that right hemisphere lesions, traumatic brain injury, and dementia can affect communication in ways that often aren't captured by our concepts of aphasia and motor speech disorders. Those changes are also reflected in these pages. Finally, Dr. Brookshire's very special talents as a clinician, researcher, and teacher have evolved. No book reaches a second, let alone a fifth edition, without its author having gotten something right the first time and then building upon it. You can feel confident that this book's con-

tent reflect what a recognized expert believes are the core of facts and concepts necessary to understanding neurogenic communication disorders. You should also know that you will be learning from someone whose clarity of thought and expression have been, for many years, greatly respected and admired by his colleagues.

Be assured that the organization, style, and clarity of this book will meet your needs if you are coming to this complex subject for the first time. I also suspect this book will become a friend and valuable resource to those of you who already have or who will develop a lasting interest in neurogenic communication disorders. It almost certainly will contribute to your own evolution as students, teachers, researchers, or clinicians.

Joseph R. Duffy, PhD
Head, Section of Speech Pathology
Department of Neurology
Mayo Clinic
Rochester, Minnesota

Preface

I have written this book to provide its readers with a general understanding of neurogenic communication disorders—their causes, symptoms, typical course, treatment, and outcome. I have tried to be practical about what I have included in this book. I have tried to include material that I believe to be both important and useful to those who are beginning their study of neurogenic communication disorders. My decisions regarding what to include and what to leave out no doubt reflect my personal biases about who, how, and why we treat. They also reflect my experiences in approximately 25 years of teaching university students about neurogenic communication disorders and my sense of what has seemed important to them.

This book is neither a training manual nor a catalog of techniques. Reading it will not make the reader competent to evaluate, diagnose, or treat patients with neurogenic communication disorders. No book or collection of books can do that. Clinical competence comes from a blending of knowledge acquired from the clinical and scientific literature, supervised clinical training, and independent clinical experience. This book will, I hope, help the student get started on the road to clinical competence by providing a basic understanding of what neurogenic communication disorders are, what the individuals who have them are like, and how they may be measured and treated.

A reviewer of the manuscript for the fourth edition of this book commented:

I was somewhat nonplussed by the opinions Brookshire puts forth as facts. There are many controversies surrounding many of the issues covered in the text, and few of them are specifically targeted as controversial issues.

I included the reviewer's comment in the preface to that edition and responded with the following:

My purpose herein is to provide an overview of neurogenic communication disorders together with basic concepts about their causes, diagnosis, assessment, and treatment. It may be that I have not identified areas of controversy, and it is certain that I have often presented my opinions as "facts." One "fact" is, I think, inescapable—that there are few "facts" in the domain treated by this book. Even such seeming "facts" as the pyramidal system and apraxia of speech are in one sense matters of opinion or convenient fictions. . . . It may be that half (or more) of everything in this book is "wrong" in some sense and it may be that there are few, if any, true and enduring "facts" in it. The content of this book represents my best guess about what is likely to prove true over time, and I hope that I will have guessed right more often than not.

I repeat the reviewer's comment and my response to it in this preface because it seems to me as important now as it was then and no less true now than it was then. It is extremely important, I think, that readers of this book know that much of what passes for "fact" in the scientific and clinical literature about neurogenic communication disorders (and in the literature relating to many other areas of knowledge as well) is in truth opinion, intuition, or someone's best guess about what seems true. It is also extremely important that readers understand that clinical competence comes as much (or more) from one's development of intuitions based on regularities observed in patients than from reading "facts" in the literature. We must all remember that treatment of neurogenic communication disorders remains as much *art* as *science*, and that many empirically verified "facts" may prove trivial or irrelevant to helping the neurologically compromised adult become a better communicator.

Finally, an editorial note. The word "aphasic" is an adjective and not a noun. I strongly believe that using the word "aphasic" as a noun, as in "Wernicke's aphasics," depersonalizes those for whom we provide services in addition to being stylistically deplorable. Therefore readers will not (I trust) find that I refer to "aphasics" in this book, and I trust that readers will, in their own writing, speech, and professional activities, focus on the person and not the condition.

Robert H. Brookshire

Acknowledgments

Few of the ideas in this book are truly my own. The influence of colleagues, students, and the patients I have known and worked with permeates the contents. Without these people, this book would not exist.

My special thanks go to several colleagues:

To Linda E. Nicholas, Research Speech-Language Pathologist, Minneapolis Veterans Affairs Medical Center, for reading, commenting, and correcting throughout the manuscript for this book.

To John Davenport, staff neurologist, Minneapolis Veterans Affairs Medical Center, for reading the parts of this book that deal with neurology and medicine, correcting my factual and conceptual mistakes, and cleaning up my writing style.

To Jack Avery, Meredith Gerdin, Steve Kosek, Martha Manthie, Don MacLennan, Jim Schumacher, and Mary Sullivan, clinical staff of the Speech Pathology Section, Minneapolis Veterans Affairs Medical Center, for my continuing education in assessment and treatment of patients with neurogenic communication disorders.

To Jeanne Robertson, whose drawings illustrate key concepts with elegance and clarity.

To the staff at Mosby–Year Book for their support and encouragement. My special thanks go to Kellie White, Developmental Editor, and Julie Eddy, Production Editor, for shepherding this work through the editorial process with enthusiasm, professionalism, and good humor.

Robert H. Brookshire

Contents

Introduction to Neurogenic Communication Disorders

Neuroanatomy and Neuropathology

Neurogenic communication disorders are one consequence of nervous system damage. The features and severity of neurogenic communication disorders depend on the location and magnitude of the damage. Their course and eventual outcome depend on what causes the damage and how much damage has been done. Consequently, clinicians who wish to understand these communication disorders must have a rudimentary understanding of the human nervous system and what can go wrong with it. This chapter will begin by describing the parts of the nervous system that are likely to be involved when neurogenic communication disorders appear. Some of the major pathologic processes that underlie the most common neurogenic communication disorders will then be described.

Students learning neuroanatomy soon learn three disconcerting facts—(1) there are many different parts in the nervous system, (2) almost every part has several different names, and (3) most of the parts are not really different parts, but inventions by humans to make it easier to

1

describe, analyze, illustrate, and explain the nervous system. The nervous system is exceedingly complex, and one may have to subdivide it to understand how it works, even though the subdivisions may be imaginary.*

The proliferation of names for parts of the nervous system began in the nineteenth century, when many people were studying the nervous system, when communication among investigators was not what it is today, and when there was a tendency for explorers of the nervous system, like explorers of the planet, to name things they discovered after themselves. Eventually, those investigating the nervous system began to call for more descriptive names, because the old names were difficult to remember, and most of the parts of the nervous system had already been named, so the new people couldn't name things after themselves. Unfortunately, there still remained some gratification to be gotten from attaching a name to something, even if that something already had a name. The proliferation of names hasn't completely stopped, although it has slowed to a crawl.

In this chapter, I will give the most common multiple names when identifying a part of the nervous system. Then I will use what I consider the most discriptive (and easy to remember) names.

■ THE HUMAN NERVOUS SYSTEM

Descriptions of the human nervous system have usually divided it into two major parts—the *central nervous system* and the *peripheral nervous system.* The central nervous system (CNS) is hidden inside the skull and vertebrae. It includes the *brain,* the *brain stem,* the *cerebellum,* and the *spinal cord.* The CNS is responsible for perception and discrimination of sensory stimuli, for regulation of processes such as res-

piration and heartbeat, for emotional expression, for organization and regulation of behavior, and for mental processes such as thinking, remembering, and understanding this sentence. The peripheral nervous system mostly lies outside the skull and vertebrae. It can be divided into two functional systems—the *somatic nervous system* and the *autonomic nervous system.* The somatic system is responsible for conscious sensory perception and volitional motor activity. Its two major components are the *cranial nerves* and the *spinal nerves.* The autonomic system is a self-regulating system that controls the glands and the operations of vital functions such as breathing and heartbeat. Although the autonomic nervous system is responsible for many vital life functions, it is not directly concerned with communication. Consequently, it will not get much more attention in this book, and from here on when I use the term *peripheral nervous system,* I will be referring to the *somatic* part.

The central nervous system is fragile, but well protected from injury. Bony enclosures (the skull and spinal column) surround it. Tough membranes anchor the brain and spinal cord to the skull and the vertebrae. An envelope of fluid cushions the brain and spinal cord and provides a buoyant medium to counteract the effects of gravity and to minimize displacement and distortion caused by movement of the head and body.

The *skull* encloses and protects the brain. Human skulls are roughly symmetrical, although one half usually is slightly larger than the other. The human skull is made up of eight plates, joined together to form a continuous surface. The plates of an infant's skull are less firmly joined than those of an adult's, making the infant's skull pliable and elastic (a characteristic for which mothers in childbirth have cause to be thankful). Skull elasticity diminishes across the life span—an 80-year-old's skull is much more rigid and brittle than a 20-year-old's skull. The adult human skull is thin in the front and on the sides (3 mm to 5 mm) and thick in the back (15 mm to 20 mm). The space inside the skull is

---

* Many names for parts of the nervous system seem obscure today and some have lost currency and perhaps should be abandoned. However, many names and the concepts that underlie them are traditional in spite of their scientific faults and need to be understood for purposes of communicating with other clinicians.

called the *cranial vault.* The ceiling and walls of the cranial vault are smooth, but the floor is irregular, with numerous depressions, openings, partitions, and ridges giving it a craggy appearance (Figure 1-1). The large opening in the base of the cranial vault is called the *foramen magnum* (great opening). It is the opening through which the brain stem passes on its way to the spinal cord. (A *foramine* is an aperture or opening in tissue or bones. *Foramen* comes from a Latin word meaning "aperture.")

The *vertebrae* provide the bony structure of the spinal column. There are 33 vertebrae, divided into 5 categories. Seven are *cervical vertebrae,* 12 are *thoracic vertebrae,* 5 are *lumbar vertebrae,* 5 are *sacral vertebrae,* and 4 are *coc-*

cygeal vertebra* (Figure 1-2). The vertebrae are separated from each other by disks of cartilage and are held together and in alignment by strong muscles, tendons, and ligaments. The lower vertebrae are larger than those at the top, reflecting their greater weight-bearing responsibility and their greater exposure to twisting forces. Down the center of each vertebra is a roughly circular opening through which the spinal cord passes. There are notches between the vertebrae through which nerves and blood vessels pass to and from the spinal cord. These notches are called the *intervertebral foramina.* Pathologic changes in the vertebrae or the intervertebral discs may create pressure on these nerves and blood vessels, causing neurologic symptoms (pain, loss of sensation, weakness, or paralysis). Patients with spinal nerve or blood vessel compression make up a significant part of most neurosurgeon's caseloads, and decompression of spinal nerves and blood vessels is a common neurosurgical procedure.

---

* The five sacral and the four coccygeal vertebrae are fused into two larger masses, the *sacrum* and the *coccyx,* respectively. (*Sacrum* comes from Latin and means, roughly, "sacred bone." *Coccyx* comes from Greek, and means "cockoo," or more likely "cuckoo's beak.")

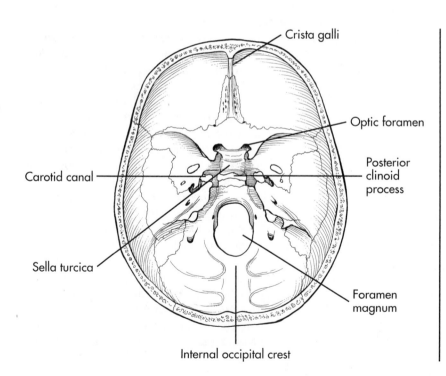

Figure 1-1 ▪ **The floor of the cranial vault. The crista galli, the posterior clinoid process, and the sella turcica are three of several ridges and projections that arise from the floor of the cranial vault.**

Crista galli
Optic foramen
Posterior clinoid process
Carotid canal
Sella turcica
Foramen magnum
Internal occipital crest

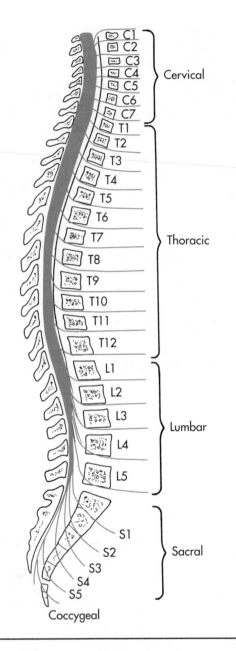

Figure 1-2 ■ The human spine, showing the division of vertebrae into cervical, thoracic, lumbar, sacral, and coccygeal groups.

The Meninges

Three membranes, called *meninges,* enclose the central nervous system (as a peel encloses an orange). The outermost membrane is called the *dura mater,* the middle membrane is called the *arachnoid,* and the innermost membrane is called the *pia mater* (Figure 1-3). Why isn't the arachnoid called the "arachnoid mater"? "Mater" comes from Latin for "mother," and one of its meanings is "that which nourishes and forms." The arachnoid, being web-like, can't be considered to "form" the brain, although it certainly plays a role in its nourishment. Because the meninges help to *cushion* and protect the CNS from injury, the mnemonic *PAD* (for *p*ia, *a*rachnoid, and *d*ura) may help the reader keep them in order.

The dura mater is a tough (*dur*able), slightly elastic membrane that serves both as a covering for the brain and spinal cord and a lining for the inner surface of the skull. It has two layers. Most of the time the two layers are fused and there is no identifiable boundary between them. The exceptions are the *dural venous sinuses,* in which the two layers separate, forming cavities or channels into which the cerebral veins drain. (*Sinus* means "a cavity or channel," usually for the storage or movement of fluids such as blood.) The venous sinuses are a complex set of cavities and channels within the dura, which forms a collection system for receiving the venous blood flowing down from the brain and for discharging the blood to the internal jugular vein for return to the heart and lungs. Some of the venous sinuses are shown in Figure 1-4.

The dura mater projects inward toward the center of the cranial cavity in several places, forming stiff sheets that divide the cavity into several compartments (Figure 1-4). The dural projections help to support and restrain the brain, brain stem, and cerebellum within the cranial vault. The two major dural projections are called the *falx cerebri* and the *tentorium cerebelli.* The falx cerebri is a long, crescent-shaped band of dura mater that protrudes downward

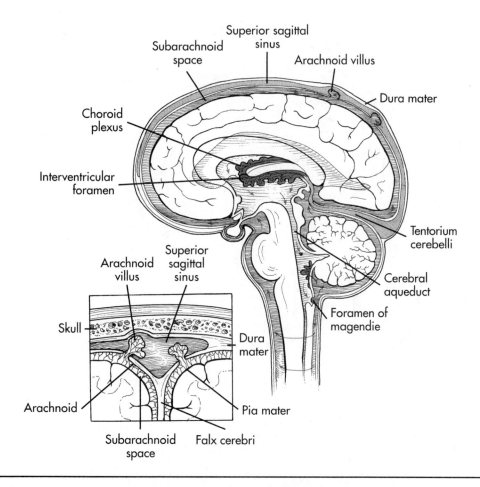

Figure 1-3 ■ **The meninges and related structures. Cerebrospinal fluid circulates throughout the ventricles and subarachnoid space. Its direction of flow is indicated by arrows. Cerebrospinal fluid is passed into the blood via the arachnoid villi, which protrude into the venous sinuses.**

along the midline of the skull, from front to back. The tentorium cerebelli is a dome-shaped sheet of dura mater that protrudes horizontally from the back of the cranial vault, creating two compartments, one above the other. The brain occupies the upper compartment, and the cerebellum occupies the lower compartment.

The outer side of the dura mater adheres to the skull, and the inner side is attached to the arachnoid. Ordinarily there is no space on either side of the dura, but in some pathologic condi-

tions fluid may accumulate between the dura and the skull, or between the dura and the arachnoid. The most frequent source of such accumulation is bleeding from the blood vessels on the surface of the dura mater. When blood vessels on the outer surface of the dura mater bleed, the result is called *extradural* (or *epidural*) *hemorrhage*. (*Hemorrhage* is medical jargon for *bleeding*. *Hematoma* is medical jargon for the resulting accumulation of blood.) When blood vessels on the inner surface of the dura mater

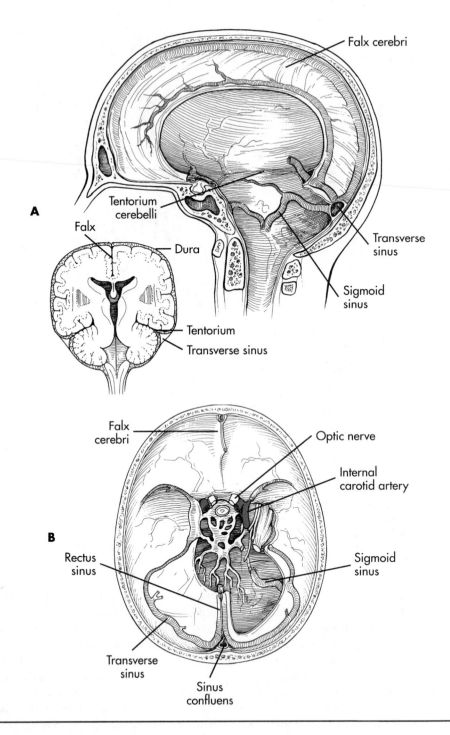

Figure 1-4 ■ **(A) Dural projections and (B) major venous sinuses. The venous sinuses are cavities between sheets of dura into which arterial blood passes on its way back to the heart.**

bleed, the result is called *subdural hemorrhage.* Bleeding from dural blood vessels is most frequently caused by traumatic head injuries, which stretch, shear, tear, or cut the vessels. Such head injuries are often a consequence of motor vehicle accidents, fights, falls, and acts of war.

The arachnoid (from the Greek word *arachne,* which means "spider" or "cobweb") is a web-like sheet of tissue sandwiched between the dura mater and the pia mater. The arachnoid contains no blood vessels and does not conform closely to the contours of the brain. This creates space between the arachnoid and the pia mater, called the *subarachnoid space.* The subarachnoid space is filled with *cerebrospinal fluid* (CSF), a clear, colorless fluid that cushions and protects the brain against trauma, provides a pathway for various metabolic and nutritional compounds to reach the central nervous system, and (perhaps) provides a medium for transport of waste products away from the central nervous system. There are several large spaces at the base of the brain, between the arachnoid and the pia mater. These spaces are filled with cerebrospinal fluid (like the rest of the subarachnoid space), and are called *subarachnoid cisterns.* (*Cistern* is a generic name for cavities or spaces for the storage of fluids.)

The *pia mater* (*pia* is from a Latin word meaning "tender") is a fragile membrane that adheres tightly to the brain's surface. Like the dura mater, it has two layers. The inner layer contains no blood vessels and adheres tightly to the surface of the brain. There are veins and arteries on the outer surface of the pia mater, in the space between the pia and the arachnoid; many blood vessels cross the space. Bleeding into the space between the arachnoid and the pia mater leads to *subarachnoid hemorrhage.* The most frequent cause of subarachnoid hemorrhage is bleeding from weakened and balloon-like outpouchings of an artery, usually at the base of the brain. These weakened outpouchings are called *aneurysms.* The arachnoid protrudes into the venous sinuses at many places. The protrusions

are called *arachnoid villi* (Figure 1-3). The arachnoid villi provide sites at which excess cerebrospinal fluid is transferred into the venous system.

The central nervous system above the spinal cord is shaped somewhat like a mushroom; its stem begins at the top of the spinal cord and broadens gradually into the canopy-like cap formed by the brain hemispheres. As the central nervous system progresses upward from the brain stem to the brain hemispheres, the brain structures progress from more primitive and phylogenetically "older" structures to more advanced and phylogenetically "younger" structures.

For descriptive purposes the part of the central nervous system above the spinal cord is divided into four sections—the *brain stem,* which sits on top of the spinal cord, the *cerebellum,* which sits behind the brain stem and below the brain hemispheres, the *diencephalon,* which is buried deep within the brain hemispheres, and the *cerebrum,* at the top, which contains the brain hemispheres. The cerebrum and diencephalon are often lumped together and called simply *the brain.*

The brain is the largest member of the central nervous system family. It is a gelatinous mass of nerve cells and supportive tissue floating in cerebrospinal fluid within the cranial vault. An average human brain weighs about 3 pounds and is about three-fourths (78%) water. Because of its great water content, the brain has a mushy consistency. If the brain is removed from the skull, its supporting network of membranes, and its flotation system of cerebrospinal fluid, it will slowly sink into a shapeless lump.

The one fourth of the brain that is not water is made up of glial cells, neurons (nerve cells), and connective tissue. Glial cells are the bricks and mortar of the brain. They support and separate the nerve fiber tracts and connective tissue within the brain. Glial cells are five to ten times more numerous than neurons and account for about half of the brain's solid mass. Even so, the brain contains over ten billion neurons, (which means 50 billion to 100 billion glial cells). The brain is a "big spender." It contains only about 2% of total body mass, but receives 20% of cardiac output and consumes 25% of the oxygen used by the body. The brain is not thrifty. It has no metabolic or oxygen reserves and is completely dependent on a constant supply of oxygen and nutrients. Consciousness is lost within 10 seconds after the brain's blood supply is interrupted, and after about 20 seconds the brain's electrical activity stops. If the blood supply to the brain is interrupted for more than two or three minutes, permanent brain damage is almost certain.

The Cerebrum

The cerebrum accounts for about three fourths of the nervous system's mass. The cerebrum is divided into two halves, or *hemispheres,* by a deep fissure, called the *longitudinal cerebral fissure,* which runs from front to back down the center. (Other names for the longitudinal cerebral fissure are the *interhemispheric fissure* or

superior longitudinal fissure.) It seems to be a rule that the more prominent the fissure is, the more names it gets. The falx cerebri projects down into the longitudinal cerebral fissure for most of its length. The hemispheres appear to be identical mirror images. (As we shall see they are not identical functionally.) The surface of the hemispheres is covered by a layer of *cortex* that is rich in nerve cells and tan-gray in color. The cortex is crisscrossed by a network of convolutions, making the brain look something like the surface of a pecan. The convolutions (ridges) are called *gyri* (singular = gyrus, from a Greek word meaning "circle"), and the depressions (valleys) are called *sulci* (singular = sulcus, from a Latin word meaning "furrow" or "ditch"). Very deep sulci often are called *fissures.*

Two prominent fissures serve as landmarks on the brain's lateral surface. One begins at the superior longitudinal fissure (approximately half-way back in each hemisphere) and progresses about halfway down the lateral surface

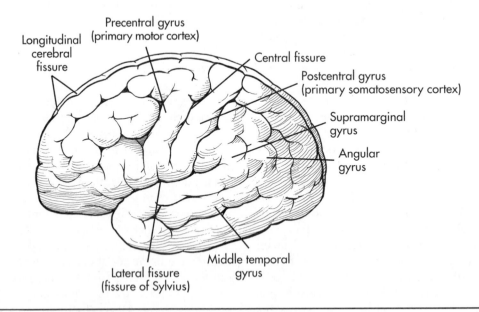

Figure 1-5 ■ **Prominent gyri and sulci on the surface of the human brain. The left brain hemisphere is shown. The gyri and sulci on the surface of the right hemisphere are essentially mirror images of those on the surface of the left hemisphere. There is considerable variability across brains in the location, shape, and prominence of the landmarks, sometimes making them difficult to identify.**

of the hemisphere (Figure 1-5). It is called the *central fissure, fissure of Rolando,* or the *central sulcus.* The other fissure runs from front to back on the lateral surface of each hemisphere. It is called the *lateral cerebral fissure* or *fissure of Sylvius* (Figure 1-5). It is also sometimes called the *frontotemporoparietal fissure,* because it forms one boundary of each of those lobes. The calcarine fissure is a less prominent groove inside the longitudinal fissure at the back of the brain (Figure 1-5). (Note that this short, less prominent fissure gets only one name.)

Each hemisphere historically has been divided into four *lobes,* named after the parts of the skull that cover them (Figure 1-6)—the *frontal lobe,* the *parietal lobe,* the *occipital lobe,* and the *temporal lobe.* The lobes are topographic conventions and do not reflect differences in the structure of the brain.*

---
* Although different brain regions differ in structure, the structural differences do not correspond to the boundaries of the lobes.

The frontal lobes, as their name implies, are the ones in front. The cortex in the frontal lobes accounts for about one third of the surface area of the brain. The lower boundary of each frontal lobe is the *lateral cerebral* (Sylvian) *fissure,* and the posterior boundary is the *central* (Rolandic) *fissure.* The *parietal lobe* forms the upper back part of each hemisphere, behind the central fissure and above the lateral fissure. Its posterior boundary is an imaginary line that lies an inch or two forward from the *occipital pole* (farthest back point in the hemisphere). The *occipital lobes* are at the very back of the brain. They extend from the imaginary line forming the posterior boundary of the parietal lobe to the bottom of the longitudinal fissure in the back of the brain. The *temporal lobe* makes up approximately the bottom third of each hemisphere. The lateral cerebral fissure forms its top boundary, and its bottom boundary is on the underside of the hemisphere, near the midline. Its posterior boundary is the imaginary line marking the anterior border of the occipital lobe.

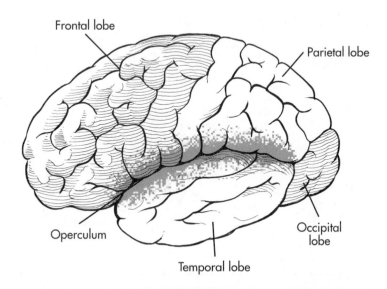

Frontal lobe

Parietal lobe

Operculum

Occipital lobe

Temporal lobe

Figure 1-6 ▪ The lobes of the brain. Much of the occipital lobe is hidden from view within the longitudinal cerebral fissure. The lobes are arbitrary divisions and do not represent either architectural or functional differences.

The *insula* is a patch of cortex that is folded into the lateral cerebral fissure, so it can be seen only if the lateral fissure is spread apart. The insula is sometimes (but not often) called the *island of Reil.* It is hidden from view by folds of the frontal, parietal and temporal lobes, which are called the *operculum.* (*Operculum* comes from a Latin word meaning "cover" or "lid"—in this case the cortex that folds over and covers the insula.)

The Ventricles Deep within the brain dwell four fluid-filled cavities, called *cerebral ventricles*—two *lateral ventricles* (one in each hemisphere), a *third ventricle*, and a *fourth ventricle,* both on the midline of the brain (Figure 1-7). The ventricles are connected by narrow passageways and are filled with *cerebrospinal fluid.* The *lateral ventricles* are the largest and are roughly symmetrical. Each lateral ventricle is connected to the third ventricle by an *interventricular foramen (foramen of Munro).* (As mentioned earlier, a foramen is an aperture or opening in tissue or bone.) The third ventricle is an irregularly-shaped, disk-like cavity that stands on edge on the midline below and between the lateral ventricles. It is connected to the fourth ventricle by the *cerebral aqueduct (aqueduct of Sylvius).* The fourth ventricle is a narrow, tubular cavity extending down through the brain stem, ending at an opening into the subarachnoid space (Figures 1-3, 1-7). The ventricles hold about 15% of the cerebrospinal fluid in the cen-

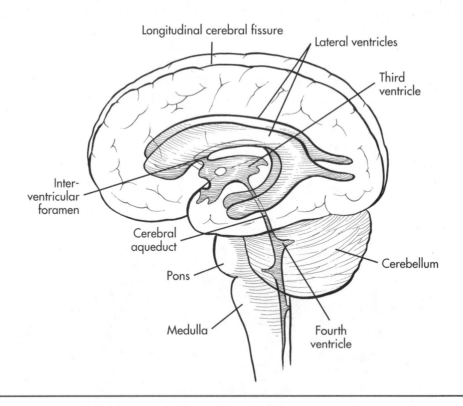

Figure 1-7 ▪ The cerebral ventricles. The ventricles form a fluid-filled space in the center of the brain and brain stem. One lateral ventricle is located deep within each brain hemisphere. The third and fourth ventricles are located on the midline. Most of the fourth ventricle is in the brain stem.

tral nervous system, and the subarachnoid space holds about 85% of the cerebrospinal fluid.

The ventricles contain the *choroid plexus,* which are soft, spongy masses of tissue that are the body's primary producer of cerebrospinal fluid. (Cerebrospinal fluid also is produced by cells on the surface of the brain.) The cerebrospinal fluid circulates throughout the central nervous system. The fluid flows from the lateral ventricles to the third ventricle via the interventricular foramina, and from the third ventricle to the fourth ventricle by way of the cerebral aqueduct (Figure 1-7). It passes from the fourth ventricle into the subarachnoid space through the *median aperture (foramen of Magendi)* and the (two) *lateral apertures (formina of Luschka).*

The Diencephalon The diencephalon (From Greek, meaning "through-brain") is located deep in the substance of the cerebrum, at the top of the brain stem. It contains several structures that play important roles in movement and sensation—the *thalamus* and the *basal ganglia.*

The thalamus is a pair of egg-shaped nuclei, one on each side of the third ventricle (Figure 1-8). (The word *thalamus* comes from a Latin word, meaning "a little nut.") The thalamus serves as a major relay center and way-station for motor information coming down from the motor cortex and for sensory information going up to the sensory cortex. It receives input from many sources (the cerebellum, the basal ganglia, other subcortical regions, and the brain stem) and its fibers project to much of the cortex. Because of its major role as a relay center for information going to the cortex, the thalamus is thought to play a part in regulating the overall electrical activity of the cortex. Many sensory pathways synapse at the thalamus, and perhaps because of this, the thalamus plays an important role in consciousness, alertness, and attention.

The basal ganglia consist of several nuclei adjacent to the thalamus, deep in the substance of the brain (Figure 1-8). Their number varies somewhat, depending on who is writing about them. Most writers include the *caudate nucleus,* the *putamen,* and the *globus pallidus* in the basal ganglia. Some add the *subthalamic nucleus* and the *substantia nigra.* To make things even more complicated, the putamen and the globus pallidus often are lumped together and renamed the *lenticular nucleus.* Topographically, the lenticular nucleus (putamen and globus pallidus) is separated from the thalamus by the posterior limb of the internal capsule, and the lenticular nucleus is separated from the caudate nucleus by the anterior limb.* The subthalamic nucleus, as the name implies, is located just beneath the thalamus, and the substantia nigra is just beneath the subthalamic nucleus. The precise functions of the subthalamic nucleus and the substantia nigra are unknown, although their numerous connections to the other basal ganglia suggest that they collaborate with them in important ways. The substantia nigra, as the name implies, is very darkly colored. Degeneration (and fading) of the substantia nigra is frequently seen in *Parkinson's disease.*

The basal ganglia receive input from multiple sites in the cortex (almost all in the frontal lobe) and send (or relay) information, via the thalamus, to the cortex. The basal ganglia have responsibility for regulation and adjustment of major muscle groups in the trunk and limbs. Their control of these muscle groups produces the postural adjustments necessary for dealing with shifts in body weight and compensate for inertial forces accompanying movement or tilting. Damage in the basal ganglia causes a variety of problems with movement and sensation, depending on the location of the damage. Most damage is characterized by loss of voluntary movements and the appearance of involuntary movements, called *dyskinesia.*

---

* The internal capsule is a dense band of nerve fibers that connects the cerebral cortex to lower center. See Chapter 4 for more on the internal capsule.

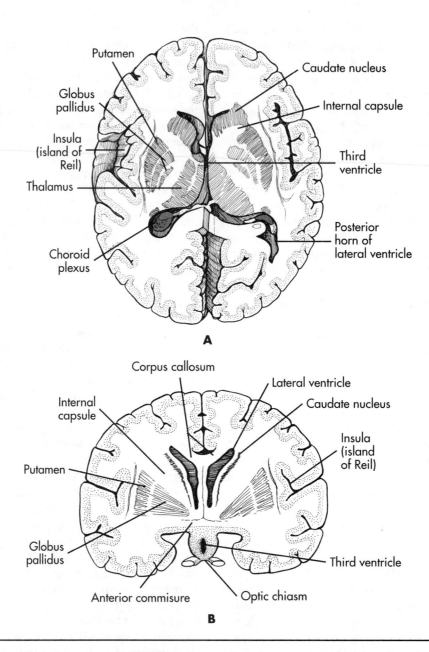

Figure 1-8 ■ The basal ganglia and related structures. (A) The brain has been cut on a horizontal plane at about the middle of the third ventricle. (B) The brain has been cut on a vertical plane just anterior to the thalamus. The corpus callosum is the major interhemispheric nerve fiber tract. It forms the roof of the lateral ventricles. The anterior commissure is a minor interhemispheric fiber tract (*see also* Figure 1-10).

A dense band of motor and sensory nerve fibers called the *internal capsule** passes through the thalamus and basal ganglia. The motor fibers passing through the internal capsule can be divided into three categories depending on where they go after leaving the cortex. *Corticopontine* fibers (sometimes called *corticopontocerebellar fibers*) go from the cortex to the pons, through the anterior part (anterior limb) of the internal capsule, where they connect with fibers going to the cerebellum. *Corticobulbar* fibers go from the cortex to the medulla, where they connect with cranial nerves. (The medulla is sometimes called *the bulb* because of its bulb-like shape.) Corticobulbar fibers pass through the middle of the internal capsule (called the *genu*). *Corticospinal* fibers go from the cortex to the spinal cord, where they connect with the spinal nerves. They pass through the posterior one third of the internal capsule (called the *posterior limb*). Some sensory fibers from the thalamus ascend through the anterior limb of the internal capsule, but most ascend through the posterior limb, from the thalamus to the postcentral gyrus. The sensory fibers in the posterior limb are topographically arranged, with fibers from the face and hand in front of those for the leg. A few fibers pass through the internal capsule on their way to other subcortical sites, especially the basal ganglia. The nerve fibers passing through the internal capsule are responsible for transmission of almost all of the motoric information going from the cortex to lower centers, and for transmission of sensory information go-ing from lower centers to the cortex. Consequently, damage in the internal capsule is almost always followed by muscle paralysis and sensory disruptions.

The Brain Stem The brain stem provides the communicative and structural link between the brain and the spinal cord, although structurally it is simply a continuation of the spinal cord. The *cranial nerves,* which serve the muscles and sensory receptors of the head, originate here. The brain stem also serves as the only pathway by which motor nerve fibers from the brain can reach the spinal cord and as the only pathway by which sensory nerve fibers from lower levels can reach the brain. For this reason, damage in the brain stem often has dire consequences for motor and sensory functions. Brain stem structures regulate some aspects of breathing and heart rate and play a role in integrating complex motor activity. Some brain stem structures participate in regulating the overall level of consciousness, primarily by means of the *reticular formation,* which makes up the brain stem's central core. Because structures in and just above the brain stem control many of the body's vital functions (e.g., breathing, heart rate, and temperature regulation) damage in the brain stem may have disastrous, even fatal, results.

For descriptive purposes, the brain stem is divided into three parts—the *midbrain* (upper), the *pons* (middle), and the *medulla* (lower). The midbrain (mesencephalon) connects the brain stem with the cerebral hemispheres (via the *cerebral peduncles*),* and cranial nerves 3 and 4 (which connect to muscles that move the eyes) originate here. Two midbrain structures, called the *red nucleus* and the *substantia nigra,* are involved in motor control and muscle tension. The midbrain merges into

---

* The term *capsule,* as used in this sense, is misleading. In ordinary use, the word denotes "enclosure" or "case." As used here, it denotes that section of the motor and sensory fibers going from the brain to lower levels that happens to be passing through the thalamus and basal ganglia. The word *capsule* apparently comes from early, gross dissections, where the dense white matter and membrane-like appearance of the nerve fibers, compared with the gray matter of the basal ganglia and thalamus, suggests a capsular structure.

---

* The word *peduncle* comes from a Latin word meaning "foot." *Pedestrian* and *pedal* are more common descendants of that Latin word. In neuroanatomy *peduncle* refers to various stem-like or stalk-like connecting structures in the brain.

the pons at the base of the brain, in front of the cerebellum. The pons can easily be identified because a prominent forward bulge in the brain stem marks its location. The pons contains several nuclei involved in hearing and balance, as well as the nuclei of three cranial nerves. (*Nuclei* are collections of nerve cells dedicated to specific functions. For example the *nucleus ambiguus* sends efferent fibers to the pharynx and larynx and plays an important role in swallowing. Nuclei are differentiated from surrounding tissue by cell type or density.) As noted earlier, the majority of the fourth ventricle is located in the posterior pons, just ahead of the cerebellum (Figure 1-7). Pontine damage typically produces paralysis of muscles responsible for moving the eyes horizontally, but large lesions in the anterior pons may cause *locked-in syndrome,* in which patients are conscious but cannot talk, and are quadriplegic (all limbs are paralyzed). These patients may be able to communicate only by eye blinks or by moving the eyes vertically.

The medulla is a tapered section of the brain stem located between the pons and the spinal cord. It contains the nuclei for five cranial nerves (8 through 12), as well as several nuclei concerned with balance and hearing. The nerve fiber tracts for volitional movement cross from one side of the central nervous system to the other in the medulla. The point at which they cross is called the point of *decussation.* Medullary damage typically causes combinations of vertigo (dizziness), paralysis of muscles in the throat and larynx, and various combinations of sensory loss in the limbs and sometimes the face.

The Cerebellum The cerebellum is just behind the pons and medulla and looks much like a miniature brain (Figure 1-7). The cerebellum has two hemispheres, each with an outer layer of gray matter called the *cerebellar cortex.* The cerebellum does not initiate movements, but coordinates and modulates movements initiated elsewhere (primarily by the motor cortex). The cerebellum plays a major role in regulating the rate, range, direction, and force of movements. Cerebellar damage causes clumsy movements— a condition called *ataxia.*

Nerve Cells and Neural Pathways The activity of the nervous system is produced by nerve cells, or *neurons* (Figure 1-9). Each neuron has a cell body and numerous projections, most of which are short and hair-like. The short, hair-like projections are the receptors for the neuron and are called *dendrites.* One projection is longer, usually thicker, and less hair-like than the others. The longer projection, called the *axon,* sends electrical signals from the neuron's cell body to other neurons. Axons range in length from very short (less than 1 mm) to several feet long. Axons differ in diameter, and as a consequence, they differ in the speed with which they conduct nerve impulses (those with larger diameter conduct impulses faster than those with smaller diameter). Some axons are covered with a thin layer of a white, fatty substance called *myelin.* Myelin provides electrical insulation for nerve axons, much like the plastic coatings on electrical wires.

The point at which the axon of one neuron encounters a dendrite of another is called the *synapse.* The tiny space between an axon and a dendrite is called the *synaptic cleft.* Transmission of nerve impulses across the synaptic cleft is a chemical process. A chemical transmitter substance is released by the axon and drifts across the synaptic cleft, where it excites the dendrite of a second neuron (assuming, of course, that the dendrite is interested in what the axon has to say). The dendrite's excitation causes a change in its electric charge. This change (if it is especially strong or if it is combined with the response of other excited dendrites), causes the second neuron to fire, sending a signal down its axon to excite the dendrites of yet another neuron.

The axons in the nervous system are bundled into *nerve fiber tracts*, which form the white matter within the central nervous system. The white matter is made up of bundles of axons. It

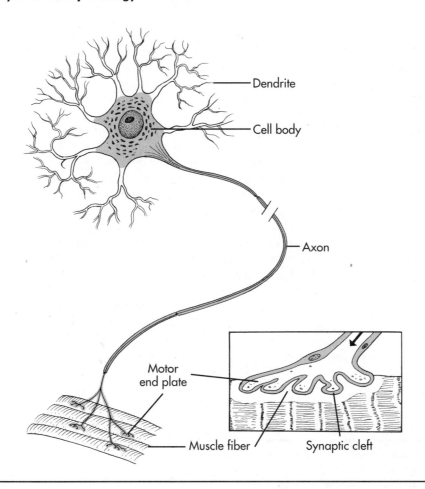

Figure 1-9 ▪ A motor neuron, showing the cell body, axon, and myoneural (muscle-nerve) junction. A motor-end plate (the junction between a neuron and a muscle fiber) is shown on the lower right.

is *white* because the myelin around the axons is white.

Neuoranatomists have divided central nervous system nerve fiber tracts into three major categories—*projection fibers, commissural fibers,* and *association fibers.* Projection fibers are the long-distance carriers of the central nervous system. They carry information from the brain to the brain stem and spinal cord, or from peripheral sensory nerves to the brain via the spinal cord.

Projection fibers that carry command and control signals from the brain to muscles and glands are called *efferent projection fibers.* They originate at neurons in the motor and premotor cortex and progress down through the brain. They converge as they approach the brain stem, through which they pass to enter the spinal cord. From there, connecting nerve fibers are distributed to various muscle groups. As they progress downward, they form a compact, dense fiber band (called, as mentioned earlier, the *internal capsule* where it passes through the thalamus and basal ganglia.)

Projection fibers carrying sensory information from receptors in the periphery to the brain are called *afferent projection fibers.* The sensory process begins in sensory receptor cells scattered throughout the peripheral nervous system. These receptor cells send sensory information to the spinal cord or brain stem via peripheral sensory nerves, which converge and enter the spinal cord and brain stem. As they progress upward through the spinal cord and brain stem, they form a compact dense band of fibers. These fibers synapse with neurons in the thalamus, from where they fan out to destinations in the cortex, primarily in the postcentral gyrus and other parts of the parietal lobe.[*]

Commissural fibers, or *commissures,* are the regional carriers of the central nervous system. They provide communicative links between the brain hemispheres. There are three commis-

---

[*] There is no great mnemonic for remembering *efferent* vs. *afferent.* It may help to remember that in the alphabet *a* precedes *e,* and that sensations (*a*fferent) often lead to responses (*e*fferent).

sures, called the *corpus callosum,* the *anterior commissure,* and the *posterior commissure* (Figure 1-10).

The corpus callosum is by far the largest and most important commissure. It provides the primary pathway for interhemispheric communication and it provides the major structural link between the hemispheres. It is crescent-shaped, with the open side of the crescent facing down. The anterior third is called the *genu,* the central third is called the *rostrum* or *body,* and the posterior third is called the *splenium.* Nerve fibers crossing through the corpus callosum are spatially arranged to minimize their length. Fibers crossing through the genu (the anterior part) connect cortical areas in the anterior frontal lobes; fibers crossing through the rostrum connect cortical areas in the posterior frontal and the anterior parietal lobes; and fibers crossing through the splenium (the back part) connect cortical areas in the posterior parietal and occipital lobes. Damage to the corpus callosum inter-

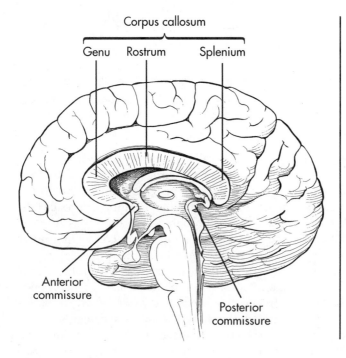

Figure 1-10 ■ The interhemispheric fiber tracts (commissures) of the human brain. The brain hemispheres have been cut apart at the superior longitudinal fissure, and the cut ends of nerve fibers making up the corpus callosum, anterior commissure, and posterior commissure are visible.

rupts communication between the hemispheres and sometimes causes a collection of symptoms called *split-brain syndrome.*

The anterior commissure crosses the midline deep within the brain near the thalamus. The posterior commissure crosses at the posterior base of the brain, just below the posterior end of the corpus callosum. The anterior and posterior commissures are much smaller than the corpus callosum and their importance for interhemispheric communication is debated. However, given that the anterior commissure and the posterior commissure together are about 1/100 the size of the corpus callosum, it seems obvious that the corpus callosum is the major-player in interhemispheric communication.

Association fibers are the local carriers in the central nervous system. They connect cortical areas within a hemisphere. If the cortical areas are close together (in the same lobe) the association fibers connecting them are called simply *association fibers.* If the cortical areas are farther apart (in different lobes) the association fibers between them get a shorter but harder-to-remember name—the name is *fasciculus,* the plural of which is *fasciculi.* (*Fasciculus* comes from a Latin word for "bundle." *Fascist* also

comes from that word.) Fasciculi are long and massive (as fiber tracts go) bundles of nerve fibers connecting widely separated regions within a hemisphere. However, they never cross the midline. (If they did, they would be commissures.) There are three major fasciculi in the human brain. They are the *uncinate fasciculus,* the *arcuate fasciculus,* and the *cingulum* (Figure 1-11). The uncinate fasciculus is a direct pathway connecting the inferior frontal lobe with the anterior temporal lobe in each hemisphere. The cingulum runs along the top of the corpus callosum in each hemisphere and connects deep regions of the frontal and parietal lobes with deep regions of the temporal lobe and midbrain. The uncinate fasciculus and the cingulum apparently play no major part in speech and language. This is not the case for the arcuate fasciculus, sometimes called the *superior longitudinal fasciculus* (Figure 1-10). It is a crescent-shaped fiber tract that connects posterior and central regions of the temporal lobe with posterior and inferior regions of the frontal lobe. From its origin in the temporal lobe, it sweeps up and back around the back of the lateral fissure, about an inch below the cortex. Then it curves forward and downward to the frontal lobe. As we shall see, the ar-

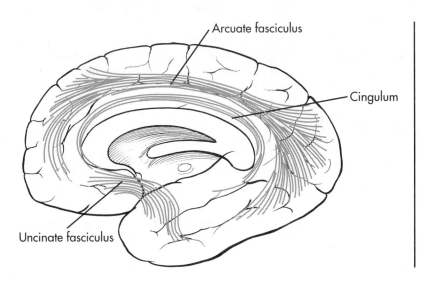

Arcuate fasciculus

Cingulum

Uncinate fasciculus

Figure 1-11 ■ Major fasciculi in the human brain. The arcuate fasciculus is believed to play an important part in many speech and language processes.

cuate fasciculus plays a central role in some models of how the brain deals with language.

The Cerebral Cortex The cerebral cortex covers the outer surfaces of both hemispheres. It varies in thickness, from 1.5 mm in the occipital area to 4 mm (¼ inch) in the precentral area. The cortex is densely packed with neurons and nerve fibers—it contains 7 billion or 8 billion neurons and somewhere in the neighborhood of 100,000 miles of nerve fibers. (If you think about this fact very long, it may give you a headache!) The human cerebral cortex is responsible for planning and executing most volitional motor activity, for conscious processing of sensory information, and for all "higher" mental activity, such as speaking, writing, reasoning and playing the lottery. The convolutions on the brain's surface allow nature to pack considerably more cortex into the skull than it could if the brain were smooth. The average adult human brain has about 2½ square feet of cortex, two thirds of which is hidden in the fissures (Nolte, 1993).

The cortex of the human brain can be divided into two major functional categories—*primary cortex* and *association cortex.* Primary cortex is responsible for specific motor or sensory functions. Association cortex is responsible for combining, refining, interpreting, and elaborating crude sensory information that is transmitted from primary cortical sensory areas. It is also responsible for organizing and planning action sequences to be transmitted to the primary motor cortex. Put simply, association cortex is an interpreter of sensory information and a planner of motor activity.

The first region of primary cortex to be identified according to its functional responsibility was the *primary motor cortex.* It is a strip of cortex just in front of the central fissure, corresponding roughly to the area of the precentral gyrus. The nerve cells in the primary motor cortex are responsible for initiating and controlling voluntary and precise skilled movements of skeletal muscles on the *contralateral* (opposite) side of the body. (The left hemisphere primary

motor cortex controls muscles on the right side of the body, and vice-versa.)

The *primary somatosensory cortex* lies just behind the central fissure and corresponds roughly to the area of the postcentral gyrus. The primary somatosensory cortex is responsible for *somesthetic* (skin, muscle, joint, and tendon) sensation from the contralateral side of the body. (Gross perception of pain, temperature, and light touch are not the exclusive responsibility of this strip of cortex. Lower structures in the brain can mediate these perceptions.)[*]

The *primary auditory cortex* is located on the upper surface of the temporal lobe, at the lateral fissure, in the transverse temporal gyrus (better known as the *gyrus of Heschl*). Each auditory cortex (left and right) receives input from both ears, and together they are responsible for hearing. The *primary visual cortex* is located in the occipital lobe, around the calcarine fissure, and is responsible for vision. Each visual cortex receives half the visual input from each eye. Finally, the *primary olfactory cortex* occupies part of the posterior-inferior frontal lobe and insula and is responsible for our sense of smell. Figure 1-12 shows the location of these functional areas.

The regions of primary cortex are organized so that the surface of the body, the visual fields, or auditory frequencies are projected onto the cortex in topographic arrays, with point-to-point connections between the cortex and tactile receptors in the skin, visual receptors in the eyes, and auditory receptors in the cochlea.[†] Stimulation of primary motor cortex produces gross, un-

---

[*] Some contemporary neurophysiologists (such as Nolte, 1993) combine the motor and somatosensory cortex into a single *sensorimotor cortex,* apparently to illustrate the important role somatosensory information plays in regulation and control of movement. For simplicity's sake the traditional division of precentral and postcentral cortex will be used. However, the reader should keep in mind that the somatosensory cortex plays an important role in regulating and controlling almost all volitional movement.
[†] The olfactory cortex seems not to be arranged topographically.

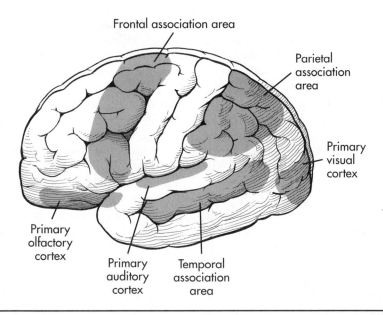

Figure 1-12 ▪ The association areas and primary auditory, visual, and olfactory cortex of the human brain. The association areas, like the lobes, represent arbitrary divisions. No differences in brain architecture mark these divisions, and their size and location vary, depending on who is drawing the picture. The right hemisphere contains mirror-image representations of these cortical areas.

refined movements of major muscle groups, sometimes associated with primitive movement sequences such as licking, chewing, or swallowing. Stimulation of primary somatosensory cortex produces gross, unrefined sensations (such as, numbness, tingling, or electric-shock-like sensations). Stimulating the olfactory cortex typically produces sensations of peculiar odors and tastes. Stimulating the visual cortex typically produces a sense of light flashes. Stimulating the auditory cortex typically produces buzzing or roaring sensations. Damage to primary motor or sensory cortex impairs the motor or sensory functions previously served by the destroyed cortex.

Several association areas in the human brain have been described in the literature. Four are most relevant to neurogenic communication disorders (Figure 1-12). The *frontal association area* is a strip of cortex just in front of the primary motor cortex. It sometimes is called the *premotor cortex.* It plays an important part in planning and initiating complex volitional movements. The *parietal association area* participates in the processing of tactile information and seems to be responsible for body image, position sense, and awareness of extrapersonal space. The *temporal association area* is important for discriminating and processing auditory information and for many language-related processes. The *parieto-occipital association area* seems important for discriminating and processing visual information, including many of the precise visual processes involved in reading.

Stimulation of association cortex usually causes combinations of sensory phenomena (usually unpleasant) and primitive movements of muscle groups (e.g., eye closure or twisting of the body or limbs). Destruction of association cortex usually does not cause specific motor or sensory deficits, but generates deficits related to discrimination, recognition, or comprehension of categories of stimuli, depending on the region of association cortex that has been destroyed.

Hemispheric Specialization The left and right hemispheres of the human brain are structurally similar to one another, but not identical. Right-handed adults' left hemispheres tend to be slightly larger than their right hemispheres, and the lateral fissure in their left hemisphere tends to be slightly longer than the one in their right hemisphere (von Bonin, 1962). However, their parietal lobes go the opposite direction, with the right hemisphere lobe being larger than the lobe in the left hemisphere (Rubens, 1977).* In spite of their structural similarity, it is clear that the two hemispheres are in many respects functionally specialized, with different functions assigned to each hemisphere.

That the two hemispheres of the human brain are functionally different has been known since the late 1800s. In 1861 Paul Broca, a French neurologist, reported that eight patients with language disturbance secondary to brain damage all had lesions in the left hemisphere. Within the next few years the so-called *dominance* of the left hemisphere for language had become widely accepted.† During the next decade most believed that the left hemisphere was dominant for most cognitive functions, with the right hemisphere responsible only for

perceptual and motor functions and perhaps some rudimentary mental processes. Then, in 1874, John Hughlings Jackson asserted that the two hemispheres have different but more or less equal functions. He claimed that the left hemisphere is responsible for language and that the right hemisphere is responsible for visual recognition, discrimination, and recall. In spite of Jackson's assertions, during the next hundred years the right hemisphere's contribution to cognition and intellect was largely neglected, as investigators concentrated on exploring the allocation of responsibilities for language in the left hemisphere. It was not until the middle of the twentieth century that investigators began to explore the organization and function of the right hemisphere in any organized way.

Early theorists who wrote about the different functions of the hemispheres claimed that the left hemisphere is specialized for language and reasoning, while the right hemisphere is specialized for music and visual processes. This concept of hemispheric specialization gradually changed as investigators found that the two hemispheres appeared to operate in fundamentally different ways. Writers began to describe the left hemisphere as "rational and analytic" and the right hemisphere as "intuitive and holistic." Some contemporary models of hemispheric functions depict the left hemisphere as specialized for processing sequential, time-related material, which requires linear (serial) processing, and the right hemisphere as specialized for processing nonlinear arrays, which require holistic, gestalt-like (parallel) processing. Because auditory information often comes in time-ordered sequences (syllables in a word, words in a sentence), for some time investigators thought that the left hemisphere had greater responsibility for auditory events, and because visual information often comes in multidimensional arrays (pictures, scenes, faces), they felt that the right hemisphere had greater responsibility for visual events. However, it subsequently became clear

---

* It is not clear that the converse is true for left-handed adults. One reason for the lack of knowledge about left-handed peoples' brains may be that interhemispheric differences are so small that one must measure and/or weigh a very large number of hemispheres to demonstrate a statistically significant difference between the hemispheres. Left-handed peoples' brains are also much less available for weighing and measuring than those of right-handed peoples' brains.

† Statements about hemispheric specialization, such as this one, may be misleading unless the qualifier "in right-handed adults" is added. Few writers add the qualifier. However, the reader should keep it in mind whenever reading descriptions of the brain hemispheres and what they do.

that these hemispheric differences reflected the nature of the information rather than the modality through which it enters the brain. For example, patients with left-hemisphere damage have difficulty with temporal sequences of visual stimuli and patients with right-hemisphere damage have difficulty with spatial sequences of auditory stimuli (Brookshire and Lommel, 1974; Efron, 1963).

The Frontal Lobes The frontal lobes appear to regulate overall activity levels and to play a role in the precursors to overt behavior (intentions, plans, and patterns for volitional behavior). It is not well understood whether or not the left and right frontal lobes serve different cognitive or behavioral functions, in part because unilateral damage to otherwise normal frontal lobes is relatively rare (Gainotti, 1991). Consequently the two frontal lobes usually are lumped together when frontal lobe syndromes are described.

The Parietal Lobes The parietal lobes have responsibility for perception, integration, and mediation of touch, body awareness, and visuospatial information. The primary sensory cortex, responsible for somesthetic sensation, forms the anterior part of the parietal lobe, and the strip of cortex just behind it appears to be important for interpretation of somesthetic sensory information. Damage in this strip of cortex may lead to *tactile agnosia* (sometimes called *astereognosis*), in which the patient is unable to recognize objects by touch, in spite of intact tactile perception. Damage in either parietal lobe typically causes various visuospatial impairments, in which the patient has difficulty drawing or copying geometric designs, discriminating complex visual stimuli, and appreciating spatial relationships.

The Temporal Lobes The temporal lobes appear to be heavily involved in perception and processing of auditory stimuli. The primary auditory cortices are located in the upper temporal lobes, with auditory and auditory-visual asso-

ciation areas located nearby. The anterior temporal lobes in both hemispheres appear to be important in pitch discrimination and in separating signals from a noise background (as in listening to conversations at a cocktail party). The left temporal lobe appears to have major responsibility for comprehension of verbal material, both spoken and written, and for language processes involving semantics and syntax. The right temporal lobe appears to have important responsibility for interpretation of complex visual stimuli and for recognition and comprehension of nonverbal sounds, including receptive components of music.

The Occipital Lobes The occipital lobes contain the primary visual cortex and visual association areas. Destruction of all or parts of the visual cortex in either hemisphere causes blindness in regions of the contralateral visual fields. Damage in the visual association areas of either hemisphere typically causes *visual agnosia* (inability to recognize visually presented familiar stimuli, even though visual perception is adequate) and distorted visual perceptions. Bilateral destruction of the visual cortex results in a phenomenon called *cortical blindness.* Patients who are cortically blind have extreme difficulty discriminating visual shapes and patterns but remain sensitive to light and dark. In some cases perception of simple visual stimuli may be preserved, although the patient usually has difficulty reporting them or incorporating them into other mental activity.

The Pyramidal System

The pyramidal system begins at pyramidal nerve cells in the cerebral cortex (which are called *pyramidal cells* because they are shaped like pyramids). The pyramidal system is responsible for initiating most, if not all, skilled volitional movement. It is made up of the motor neurons of the primary motor cortex and their axons, which project (through the internal capsule) to synapses with neurons in the brain stem and spinal cord. The pyramidal system is a *direct system. Direct* means that neurons in the primary motor cortex synapse directly with neurons in the brain stem or spinal cord—the only synapse in the circuit is where the cortical neuron meets the neuron in the brain stem or spinal cord. (This means that some of the axons in the pyramidal system are 2 feet to 3 feet long. The longest axons are those that synapse with the lowermost spinal nerves.)

Traditionally, control of skilled movements has been considered the major responsibility of the primary motor cortex, located just in front of the central fissure. The connections between the primary motor cortex and skeletal muscle groups are arranged so that it is possible to create a functional map of the motor cortex, show-

ing which cortical areas are responsible for given parts of the body. Such a map, sometimes called a *homunculus* (little man) is shown in Figure 1-13.* It can be seen from Figure 1-13 that cortical responsibility for muscle groups is arranged in upside-down fashion on the motor cortex. The cortex responsible for the toes and foot is located at the top, and representation for the knee, hip, shoulder, elbow, wrist, hand, and face is located laterally and downward. The representation of the body in Figure 1-13 looks

---

* The word *homunculus* was used in the sixteenth and seventeenth centuries when it referred to an exceedingly minute human body, which was thought to inhabit each sperm cell. Development of the embryo, and subsequent growth from infant to adult, was believed to represent the growth of the homunculus.

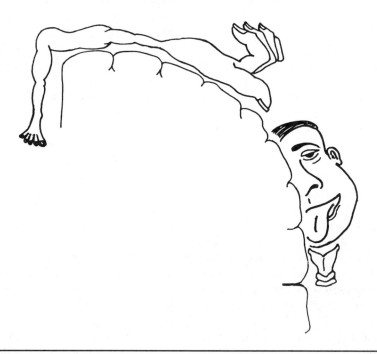

Figure 1-13 ▪ A "homunculus" representing the allocation of motor function in the motor cortex. The size of the body part portrayed in the figure represents the amount of cortex devoted to innervation of the muscles in that body part.

like an extraterrestrial because it is drawn to show the amount of cortical representation assigned to various muscle groups. Differences in cortical representation are related to the precision of movement required from various muscle groups. Movements of the hand, mouth, tongue, larynx, and lips are allocated large amounts of motor cortex relative to the trunk, legs, and upper arms because the former must perform more diverse, intricate, and precise movements.

The *primary somatosensory cortex* is located just behind the central fissure. It is topographically arranged as a mirror image of the motor cortex. Sensation from the face is represented at the lower (lateral) end of the sensory cortex and sensation from the foot is represented at the top, inside the superior longitudinal fissure. The primary somatosensory cortex is not part of the pyramidal system. However, it is described here because of its location near the primary motor cortex, its topographic similarity to the motor cortex, and its importance to skilled movement.

The pyramidal system traditionally is divided into two segments. One segment is made up of *upper motor neurons* (UMNs) and the other is made up of *lower motor neurons* (LMNs). Upper motor neurons are allocated to the central nervous system, but lower motor neurons are consigned to the peripheral nervous system. The cell bodies of the upper motor neurons are located in and near the primary motor cortex. The axons of upper motor neurons pass through the midbrain, brain stem, and spinal cord to synapse with the cell bodies of lower motor neurons in the brain stem and spinal cord. The lower motor neurons synapse with muscles at specialized junctions called *motor endplates*.

The Vestibular-Reticular System

The vestibular-reticular system contains neurons scattered throughout the brain stem and cerebellum. Neurons in the vestibular-reticular system, like pyramidal system neurons, synapse with lower motor neurons. The vestibular-reticular system has responsibility for balance and orientation of the body in space and for maintaining general states of attention and alertness. Some writers combine the vestibular-reticular system with the extrapyramidal system. Although they have structural similarities, they appear to have different functions, so they are kept separate here.

The Extrapyramidal System

The extrapyramidal system arises from many locations in the central nervous system (primarily the basal ganglia) and projects to cranial and spinal nerves. It is an *indirect* system, which means that it is made up of networks of neurons, with chains of neurons and multiple synapses between the origin and destination of any given neural pathway. The extrapyramidal system does not initiate movements, but makes adjustments of muscle tone and posture to maintain a stable base for volitional movements. Because the paths of the pyramidal, vestibular-reticular, and extrapyramidal systems are common throughout much of their course, an injury that affects one usually affects all three. Therefore, combinations of pyramidal, extrapyramidal, and sometimes vestibular signs commonly are seen when any of the divisions is damaged.

Because of its diffuseness, some writers dismiss the concept of the extrapyramidal system as a convenient fiction without neuroarchitectural validity. (The same could be said about many other conventional physiological divisions.) Some neurophysiologists argue that the concept of the extrapyramidal system should be abandoned, and contemporary descriptions of the nervous system sometimes do not mention it. However, the demise of the extrapyramidal system seems likely to be a slow one, because it has a long history and it provides "a convenient shorthand for two broad classes of motor disorders" (Nolte, 1993).

Cranial Nerves and Spinal Nerves

The (somatic) peripheral nervous system serves as a conduit for sensory information from the body's sensory receptors to the central nervous system. It also provides for transmission of motor commands from the central nervous system to the muscles. As mentioned earlier, its major components are the cranial nerves and the spinal nerves.

The *cranial nerves* (at least most of them) synapse with the central nervous system in the midbrain, pons, and medulla.* There are 12 cranial nerves on each side of the body, making 24

---

* Cranial nerves 1 (olfactory) and 2 (optic) are sensory tracts that project directly into the brain above the level of the brain stem. Therefore they should be considered parts of the central nervous system. However, they were called cranial nerves in the nineteenth century, and the custom persists.

in all. Traditionally the pairs are labeled from top to bottom, using the Roman numerals I through XII. This labeling system apparently began with Galen, a Roman physician who died about 200 ad. Contemporary writers (including this one) often substitute Arabic numerals for Roman numerals. Each cranial nerve has a name. Some are descriptive and recognizable (e.g., optic [1], olfactory [2], facial [7], but most are cryptic (e.g., trigeminal [5], vagus [10]). Some serve only motor functions (3, 4, 6, 11, 12), some serve only sensory functions (1, 2, 8), and the rest serve both functions. The cranial nerves, their names, their motor or sensory functions, and where they connect with the central nervous system are summarized in Table 1-1. Several mnemonic devices (some obscene) have been devised by students who must memorize the cranial nerves and their names. The

TABLE 1-1

The cranial nerves

Nerve	Name	Type*	Function	Mnemonic
1	Olfactory	S	Smell, taste	On
2	Optic	S	Vision	old
3	Oculomotor	M	Eye and eyelid movement	Olympus'
4	Trochlear	N	Eye movement	towering
5	Trigeminal	S,M	Sensation from face; motor to masseters, palate, pharynx	tops
6	Abducens	M	Eye movement	A
7	Facial	S,M	Sensation from anterior tongue; motor to facial muscles	Finn
8	Vestibular	S	Balance, hearing	and
9	Glossopharyngeal	S,M	Sensation from posterior tongue, soft palate, pharynx; motor to pharynx	German
10	Vagus	S,M	Motor to larynx, pharynx, viscera; sensation from viscera.	vend
11	Accessory (spinal accessory)	M	Motor to larynx, chest, shoulder	at (some)
12	Hypoglossal	M	Motor to tongue	hops

*M = motor, S = sensory.

following socially acceptable, but not very literary, mnemonic is passed along:

On old Olympus's towering tops
A Finn and German viewed a house

Calling the accessory nerve the *spinal accessory* nerve makes the mnemonic slightly more literary:

On old Olympus's towering tops
A Finn and German vend some hops

Table 1-1 shows how these mnemonic devices work.

The *spinal nerves* are bundles of nerve fibers that leave the spinal cord below the brain stem. There are 31 pairs divided into 5 categories. The categories and the number of pairs in each category are (from top to bottom): *cervical* (8), *thoracic* (12), *lumbar* (5), *sacral* (5), and *coccygeal* (1) (See Figure 1-14). The names of the cranial and spinal nerves often are abbreviated. *C3* stands for the third cervical nerve, *T4* for the fourth thoracic nerve, and so on (Figure 1-14). The spinal nerves conduct motor and sensory impulses to and from the viscera, blood vessels, glands, and muscles. Each spinal nerve has a posterior *dorsal* (sensory) *root* and an anterior *ventral* (motor) *root,* arising from the posterior and anterior columns of the spinal cord, respectively. For this reason, spinal sensory neurons are called *posterior horn cells* and spinal motor neurons are called *anterior horn cells.*

The Spinal Cord

The spinal cord in a normal adult is about 18 inches long. It extends from the first cervical vertebra to the first lumbar vertebra and from there it continues downward as a fine bundle of nerve fibers, which reminded Andreas Laurentius, a seventeenth century German physiologist, of a horse's tail. Accordingly, he named it the *cauda equina* (Latin for "horse's tail"), an appellation that has continued to this day. The spinal cord has an outer layer of *white matter* and a central core of *gray matter* (Figure 1-15). In cross-section, the latter looks somewhat like a butterfly.

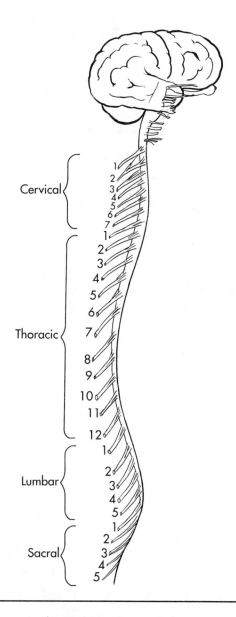

Figure 1-14 ▪ The human central nervous system, showing the vertical location of cranial and spinal nerves, and the division of spinal nerves into cervical, thoracic, lumbar, and sacral nerves.

The white matter contains ascending and descending nerve fibers. The gray matter contains motor and sensory neurons. As mentioned in the previous section, the motor neurons are located primarily in the *anterior horns* of the central gray matter, and the sensory neurons are located in the *posterior horns* of the gray matter (Figure 1-15).

Motor Pathways There are two major motor pathways from the head to the peripheral muscles. The *corticospinal* pathway is the pathway of the *pyramidal system.* The corticospinal pathway begins in the primary motor cortex and ends at synapses with either cranial nerves or spinal cord anterior horn cells. The *spinocerebellar* pathway connects the peripheral nervous system with the cerebellum and brain stem. As noted earlier, the corticospinal pathway is a *crossed* pathway—damage in one brain hemisphere causes impairments on the contralateral side of the body. In contrast, the spinocerebellar pathway is *uncrossed*— damage in a cerebellar hemisphere generates symptoms on the same side of the body.

Sensory Pathways The sensory pathways in the spinal cord are complex. The pathway for *pain and temperature* ascends in the lateral spinal cord to the thalamus and parietal lobe (Figure 1-16). It is a crossed pathway, and the crossing occurs where the peripheral nerve enters the central nervous system. The pathway for *proprioception* (the ability to tell the position of the head and limbs without seeing them) and *stereognosis* (the ability to identify objects by touch) ascends through the dorsal (posterior) spinal cord to the cerebellum and the postcentral gyrus in the parietal lobe. This pathway is also a crossed pathway, but it ascends on the ipsilateral side of the spinal cord and crosses over in the brain stem. The pathway for *light touch* ascends in the ventral (anterior) spinal cord to the brain stem and parietal lobe. This pathway contains both uncrossed fibers and fibers that cross at the brain stem.

The complexity of spinal cord sensory pathways is the bane of students who must learn them, but a blessing for neurologists who must deduce what is wrong with patients who have sensory abnormalities. A neurologist often can identify the location and nature of spinal cord pathology by noting how temperature sensation, proprioception, and stereognosis are affected in various regions of the body.

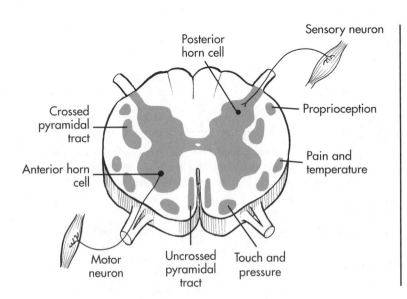

Figure 1-15 ▪ Cross-section of the human spinal cord showing motor and sensory fiber tracts. The posterior columns (which contain the posterior horn cells) primarily serve sensory functions, and the anterior columns (which contain the anterior horn cells) primarily serve motor functions.

Posterior horn cell

Sensory neuron

Crossed pyramidal tract

Proprioception

Anterior horn cell

Pain and temperature

Motor neuron

Uncrossed pyramidal tract

Touch and pressure

The Reflex Arc Some reflexive motor responses are accomplished at the level of the lower motor neuron. This reflexive activity is accomplished by the *reflex arc,* which permits rapid movements without the participation of higher neural systems. The reflex arc has five parts—a sensory receptor, an afferent (sensory) neuron, an interneuron, a motor neuron, and an effector, usually a muscle (Figure 1-16). Stimulation of the sensory receptor causes it to generate an electrical signal, which is transmitted by the afferent neuron to the posterior column of the spinal cord, where the interneuron is located. The interneuron transmits the impulse forward to the motor neuron in the anterior column of the spinal cord. The motor neuron activates a muscle or gland. Because reflexes are executed at the level of the spinal cord, they permit very quick but indiscriminate responses to stimulation. Consequently, many reflexes serve protective functions (e.g., the sneeze, cough, and eye blink reflexes).

How the Nervous System Produces Volitional Movement

The process by which the nervous system produces volitional movement is complex and not completely understood. Several subsystems participate in all but the simplest movements. The *anterior frontal lobes* (it is believed) start the process by producing the intent or motivation for movement. Then the *premotor cortex* sets up a plan for executing the movement and transmits it to the primary motor cortex. The *primary motor cortex* transmits command and control information necessary to execute the plan downward via the *pyramidal tract* to the cranial nerves and spinal nerves. The *vestibular nuclei, midbrain,* and *reticular formation* adjust balance and posture before and during the movement. The *cerebellum* modulates the rate, force, and direction of the movement. The *extrapyramidal system* adjusts muscle tone to make the movement smooth and continuous.*

■ BLOOD SUPPLY TO THE BRAIN

As mentioned previously, the brain is a major consumer of the body's production of oxygen and glucose, both of which get to the brain by way of the blood stream. At any given moment, about

---

* The operations described are not sequential. Systems controlling balance, posture, and limb position no doubt are activated well before movements actually begin, perhaps as early as when the frontal lobes first signal their intent to begin the movement process.

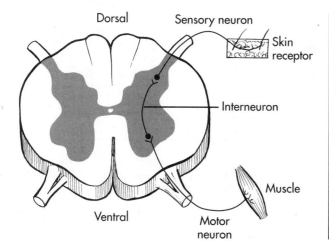

Figure 1-16 ■ The reflex arc. Stimulation of a sensory nerve is transmitted to a motor nerve via an interneuron, making rapid responses to stimuli (usually painful ones) possible without participation of higher centers in the nervous system.

25% of all the blood in the body is in the brain. Because the brain is such a massive consumer of oxygen and glucose and because it has no significant reserves, cutting off the brain's blood supply usually has catastrophic consequences. Consequently, it is not surprising that interrupted blood supply is a common cause of brain injury.

The mechanical process of getting blood to the brain begins at the heart, which provides the pumping pressure to push the blood through the arteries. The heart pumps oxygenated blood into the *aorta,* the major artery from the heart. The blood is distributed from the aorta to two *subclavian arteries* (one on each side). A common carotid artery branches

off from each subclavian artery. The common carotids ascend into the neck where they each divide into an *internal carotid artery* and an *external carotid artery* (This is going to be complicated. Figure 1-17 may help.) The external carotid heads off for the face and can be ignored from here on. The internal carotids proceed upward toward the brain on each side of the neck, near the surface, just behind the angle of the jaw. (If you place your open hand on your neck under the angle of your jaw, you should feel a relatively strong pulse at about your middle or ring finger. That pulse comes from your internal carotid artery.) The carotid arteries eventually connect to opposite sides of the *circle of Willis.*

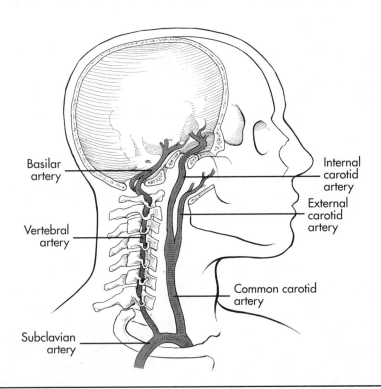

Basilar artery

Vertebral artery

Subclavian artery

Internal carotid artery

External carotid artery

Common carotid artery

Figure 1-17 ■ How the blood gets to the brain. The subclavian arteries branch off from the aorta, which is the major artery from the heart. The common carotid arteries branch off from the subclavian arteries. Each common carotid artery eventually divides into an external and an internal carotid artery. The external carotid arteries supply blood to the face, and the internal carotid arteries supply the central regions of the brain. The vertebral arteries also branch off the subclavian artery; they supply posterior regions of the brain via the basilar artery.

Now let's return to the subclavian arteries and follow them to where each branches into a *vertebral artery* (one on each side). The vertebral arteries follow the anterior surface of the medulla upward until they *anastomose* (join together) at the base of the pons to form the *basilar artery*. The basilar artery continues upward along the midline of the pons and eventually connects into the posterior part of the circle of Willis.

The *circle of Willis* is a circular (or heptagonal) set of arteries at the base of the brain approximately at the midline (Figure 1-18). As mentioned earlier, the internal carotid arteries and the basilar artery connect to the bottom of the circle of Willis. Three pairs of cerebral arteries branch upward from the circle of Willis—two *anterior cerebral arteries,* two *middle cerebral arteries,* and two *posterior cerebral arteries* (one of each in each hemisphere—*see* Figure 1-19). The anterior cerebral artery supplies blood to the upper and anterior regions of the frontal lobes and the corpus callosum. The middle cerebral artery has a fan-shaped distribution and supplies blood to most of the lateral surfaces of the brain hemispheres, plus the thalamus and basal ganglia. The posterior cerebral artery supplies blood to the occipital lobe and the lower parts of the temporal lobe.

The circle of Willis forms a conduit connecting the three major feeder arteries (the two carotid arteries and the basilar artery) to the six cerebral arteries. Because the cerebral arteries all have access, via the circle of Willis, to the blood supplied by any of the feeder arteries, if one feeder artery is blocked, the other two may still provide enough blood to maintain blood supply to the cerebral arteries. However, this "safety valve" function of the circle of Willis is possible only when the blockage is *below* the circle of Willis. Occlusion of a cerebral artery above the circle of Willis inevitably causes brain damage, because the cerebral arteries share no

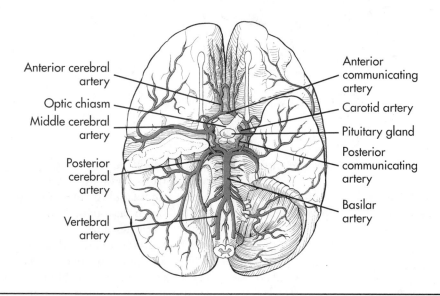

Anterior cerebral artery

Optic chiasm

Middle cerebral artery

Posterior cerebral artery

Vertebral artery

Anterior communicating artery

Carotid artery

Pituitary gland

Posterior communicating artery

Basilar artery

Figure 1-18 ■ How blood is distributed to the brain by the circle of Willis. Occlusions below the circle of Willis usually do not cause as much damage as occlusions above the circle of Willis, because the circle of Willis provides a common pathway for blood coming from the three major feeder arteries (two internal carotid arteries and the basilar artery) to the cerebral arteries that branch off the top of the circle of Willis.

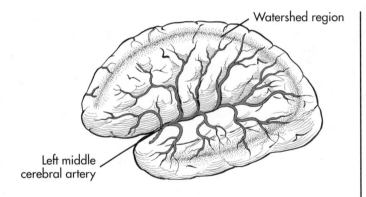

Watershed region

Left middle
cerebral artery

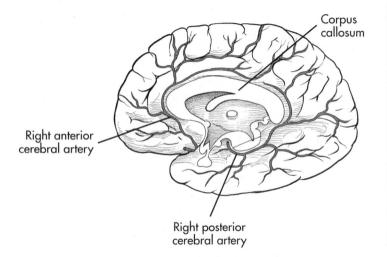

Corpus
callosum

Right anterior
cerebral artery

Right posterior
cerebral artery

Figure 1-19 ■ **The distributions of the cerebral arteries. The watershed region is where the distributions of the cerebral arteries overlap. Occlusions in the watershed region may have relatively small effects on cerebral functions because of collateral circulation from the neighboring artery.**

common source once they leave the circle of Willis.*

The amount of brain tissue affected by occlusion of a cerebral artery depends on where

---

* The compensation provided by the circle of Willis may be less than one might expect, because occlusion of a feeder artery is most common in patients with generalized vascular disease, which compromises blood flow through the arteries. For these patients, collateral flow from the other feeder arteries also is likely to be compromised by the vascular disease. Furthermore, the cerebral arteries and the arteries in the circle of Willis may themselves be narrowed or occluded by the disease.

in the artery the occlusion occurs. Occlusions in the trunk or a main branch of a cerebral artery affect large regions of the brain, whereas occlusions in peripheral branches affect smaller regions. Furthermore, the distributions of the cerebral arteries overlap slightly at their boundaries. Consequently, occlusions at the periphery of an artery's distribution may not cause as much brain damage as one might expect, because of collateral blood supply from an adjacent artery. These areas of overlapping blood supply are called *watershed* areas (Figure 1-19).

■ NEUROLOGIC CAUSES OF ADULT COMMUNICATION DISORDERS

This section describes some major neurologic causes of adult language disorders, primarily aphasia (a disorder that affects comprehension and production of spoken, written, or gestured verbal materials) and the pragmatic communicative impairments exhibited by some adults with right-hemisphere damage. It will not deal with the neurologic causes of dysarthria (speech impairments caused by nervous system damage) or traumatic brain injury (linguistic and cognitive impairments following traumatic injury to the nervous system, caused by car accidents or blows to the head). The neuropathology of dysarthria and traumatic brain injury will be covered in subsequent chapters.

■ STROKE

Stroke is a generic term for the temporary or permanent disturbance of brain function due to vascular disruptions, caused by either loss of blood supply or bleeding. Another more technical term is *cerebrovascular accident* (CVA).[*]

Stroke is the third leading cause of death in the United States. Each year about 500,000 strokes occur, and about 150,000 people die as a consequence of strokes. In any given year there are approximately 2 million survivors of stroke alive in the United States (Caplan, 1988). About 80% of stroke patients survive for at least 1 month after their stroke, but only about one third are alive 10 years later. (This 10-year survival rate may not be as gloomy as it first appears, because most stroke patients are in their 60s or 70s when they have their first stroke. However, there is no doubt that stroke survivors, on the average, have shorter life ex-

pectancy than individuals of comparable age who have not had strokes.) Of those who survive a stroke, about 85% are able to return to their prestroke-living environment, although usually with some level of persisting impairment, while 15% of stroke survivors are so impaired that they require institutional care (Greenberg, Aminoff, & Simon, 1993).

The brain is remarkably intolerant of sudden changes in its oxygen and glucose supply. The onset of communicative disorders following strokes is almost always dramatic, with symptoms developing rapidly and becoming maximally expressed within a few minutes to a few hours. During the first few days after a stroke, parts of the brain that are not actually damaged or destroyed may be functionally impaired, unless the stroke is a very small one. Consequently, major strokes often produce immediate, general disruption of cerebral functions, gradually resolving to more limited *(focal)* disruption of specific processes, depending on what parts of the brain have been permanently damaged.

Strokes can be *ischemic* (a term that means "deprived of blood") or *hemorrhagic* (a term that means "caused by bleeding"), although the occurrence of ischemic stroke is far higher (80% ischemic vs. 20% hemorrhagic). In ischemic stroke (sometimes called *occlusive* stroke), an artery is blocked, with consequent loss of blood supply to the part of the central nervous system served by the artery. If the occlusion lasts more than a few (3 to 5) minutes, death *(necrosis)* of central nervous system tissue is likely. The medical term for death of tissue caused by interruption of its blood supply is *infarct.*

Ischemic Stroke

Ischemic strokes can be either *thrombotic* or *embolic*. In *thrombotic strokes* (cerebral thrombosis), an artery is gradually occluded by a plug of material that accumulates at a given site in the artery. In *embolic strokes,* an artery is suddenly

---

[*] Some professionals dislike the term *cerebrovascular accident* and particularly its acronym *CVA,* because it often leads to misunderstanding. "Confused vascular analysis" has been suggested as an alternate meaning for "CVA."

occluded by material that moves through the vascular system and occludes an artery.

Most cerebral thromboses occur in the large arteries supplying blood to the brain (internal carotids, vertebrals, and the basilar artery). Thromboses are uncommon in smaller arteries. (Arteries become smaller in diameter as they get farther from the heart until they become capillaries, after which the venous system begins.) A thrombosis typically begins in an area of increased turbulence, which means that thromboses favor locations where arteries change direction or divide (at *bends* and *bifurcations*). Debris in the blood stream tends to accumulate at these locations, just as it does in river bends and junctions. In rivers, the debris may include driftwood, cola bottles, and overturned canoes. In arteries the debris consists mainly of fatty substances (lipids) and fibrous material, which accumulate on the lining of the artery. These accumulations are called *atherosclerotic plaque.* (*Atherosclerotic* comes from a combination of Greek words meaning "paste" (athero-) and "hard" (sclero-). *Plaque* comes from a French word meaning "plate" or "slab"). The turbulence and increased velocity of the blood flowing through the narrowed artery abrade and roughen the inner lining of the artery. Plaque forms at these roughened areas and gradually thickens over the course of years, until it may eventually fill the *lumen* (space within the artery). As the size of the lumen diminishes (a condition called *stenosis*), the volume of blood flowing through the narrowed portion decreases (although its velocity increases—the Bernoulli effect). Sometimes the plaque in the arterial wall cracks or ulcerates. Blood platelets and fibrin (a protein found in blood) adhere to the ulceration, accelerating clot development. The clot may eventually occlude the artery, or parts of the clot may break off and become *emboli* traveling through the vascular system. The clots eventually occlude smaller vessels downstream from the original clot.

In *embolic events* (cerebral embolism), an artery is occluded by a fragment of material that travels through the circulatory system until it reaches a blood vessel smaller than its own diameter and lodges, occluding the artery. The material in the embolus may be a blood clot that has broken loose from its site of formation, a fragment of arterial lining, a piece of atherosclerotic plaque, tissue from a tumor, a clump of bacteria, or other solids that may move through the arteries. The most frequent source of emboli are fragments from thromboses in the heart, followed by fragments of atherosclerotic plaque from an artery. Patients with atrial fibrillation ("heart palpitations") are particularly susceptible to cerebral embolism, because the lack of strong atrial contraction promotes pooling and clotting of blood in the left atrium, which then embolizes.

Determining whether the cause of a particular event is thrombotic or embolic is difficult, so the diagnostician may hedge his or her bets by referring to ischemic incidents as *thromboembolic* events. However, thrombotic and embolic events differ in their progression. Because embolic strokes are a consequence of sudden blockage of an artery, their symptoms usually are maximally expressed within a few minutes. Because thrombotic strokes arise from slowly-developing occlusion of an artery, they tend to develop in an irregular stepwise manner, sometimes preceded by transient periods of ischemia.

Many stroke patients have a history of *transient ischemic attacks (TIAs)*, which are by definition temporary (lasting less than 24 hours and usually less than 30 minutes) disruptions of cerebral circulation. TIAs are quickly-developing episodes of sensory disturbance, limb weakness, slurred speech, visual complaints, dizziness, confusion, mild aphasia, or other symptoms that resolve completely. Most transient ischemic attacks are thought to be caused by small emboli that temporarily occlude an artery, then break up or dissolve. Transient ischemic attacks sometimes occur when a stationary thrombus has nearly, but not completely, occluded an artery. When an artery is nearly occluded, otherwise insignificant variations in blood pressure may be sufficient to interrupt blood flow through the artery, causing a transient ischemic attack. Transient ischemic attacks may occasionally (but rarely) be caused by *cerebral vasospasm* of a nearly occluded artery, in which the muscles of the arterial wall contract, further narrowing the lumen and compromising blood flow.

Transient interruptions of blood supply to the brain that last more than 24 hours, but completely resolve within a few days, are sometimes called *reversible ischemic neurologic deficits* (*RINDs*). Interruptions of blood supply to the brain that last more than 24 hours, but leave minor deficits after a few days, are sometimes called *partially reversible ischemic neurologic deficits* (*PRINDs*). The general public, many physicians, and some neurologists forego these categorizations and call any transient episode of sensory disruption, weakness, slurred speech, visual anomalies, dizziness, confusion, or aphasia caused by temporary interruption of blood supply to the brain a *small stroke*.

Transient ischemic attacks and reversible ischemic neurologic deficits are manifestations of cerebrovascular disease. Consequently, their occurrence often presages a completed stroke. According to Greenberg and associates (1993), about one third of patients who have transient ischemic attacks or reversible ischemic neurologic deficits will, within 5 years, have a stroke that leaves them with permanent neurologic deficits.

Hypoperfusion Insufficient blood supply to the brain and brain stem may also be caused by *hypoperfusion,* in which the brain's blood supply is compromised not by occlusion of arteries but by insufficient blood volume. Insufficient blood volume is most commonly caused by massive bleeding elsewhere in the body or by insufficient cardiac pumping capacity (usually from heart disease). The pattern of cerebral damage caused by hypoperfusion is different from that caused by occlusion. Occlusion causes maximal damage to brain tissue in the center of the region supplied by the affected artery or branch. Hypoperfusion causes maximal damage in the

watershed areas (border zones) of the region supplied by the artery or branch. The blood, under low pressure, tends not to penetrate into these border zones, where vessel diameters are small and flow resistance is high. Although hypoperfusion causes cerebral ischemia, it is a not a stroke, and, unlike ischemic strokes, there is usually a gradual onset rather than a sudden one. Because hypoperfusion is a cause of cerebral ischemia (albeit a minor one) it is discussed in this context.

General Effects of Ischemic Stroke Rubens (1977) has described some of the physiologic changes that take place following major ischemic strokes. During the first few days after the stroke, the brain tissue in the area damaged by the stroke swells. If the damaged area is large, the swelling may raise intracranial pressure and cause displacement of brain tissue. Blood flow to both hemispheres decreases and may remain depressed for several months after the stroke. Neurotransmitters are released, not only in the brain substance around the stroke but throughout the brain and into the cerebrospinal fluid. Their presence upsets neuronal metabolism and perhaps contributes to reduced cerebral blood flow. By the end of the first week swelling begins to diminish, and the patient's physical, cognitive, and behavioral conditions begin to improve. The phenomenon of *diaschisis* also seems to play a role in the impairments seen immediately after stroke. In diaschisis there is disruption of brain function in regions away from the site of injury but connected to it by neuronal pathways. For many years, diaschisis was an unproved phenomenon, but studies with positron emission tomography (PET) have confirmed that destruction of brain tissue in one area is followed by reductions in cerebral metabolism in other areas—primarily those that have substantial neuronal connections to the damaged area (Metter and associates, 1983, 1984). Brain swelling, reduction in cerebral blood flow, neurotransmitter release, and diaschisis, either individually or in combination, help to create diffuse impairment of brain functions, behavior, and mental status, which gradually resolves over time.

In the first hours and days after the patient's stroke, the symptoms generated by this diffuse impairment are superimposed on the more focal symptoms caused by death of tissue at the site of the stroke. As time passes, cerebral swelling diminishes, cerebral blood flow to undamaged tissue is restored, and neurotransmitters released by the injury are resorbed. As these physiologic repairs take place, the patient gradually improves, with diffuse impairment of behavior and mental status resolving to a more specific *(focal)* collection of symptoms reflecting the permanent damage caused by the stroke. It is often difficult to predict a patient's eventual neurologic recovery (and their residual level of impairment) during the first few days after a stroke, because the permanent effects of the tissue destruction caused by the stroke are masked by the stroke's temporary effects on brain chemistry and function. Consequently, clinicians often delay making predictions about a patient's eventual level of recovery until these temporary effects have diminished (usually within 2 weeks to a month).

Hemorrhagic Stroke (Cerebral Hemorrhage)

Cerebral hemorrhages are caused by rupture of a cerebral blood vessel. They may be caused by weakness of a vessel wall, by traumatic injury to a vessel, or (rarely) by extreme fluctuations in blood pressure. Hemorrhages from the blood vessels of the meninges or on the surface of the brain are called *extracerebral hemorrhages* because the bleeding is outside the brain proper. Hemorrhages within the brain or brain stem are called *intracerebral hemorrhages* because the bleeding is within the brain substance.

Extracerebral Hemorrhage To complicate matters further, extracerebral hemorrhages can be subclassified as *subarachnoid, subdural,* or *extradural* hemorrhages, depending on where the blood accumulates. If the bleeding is beneath the arachnoid, between the arachnoid and the pia mater, it is called a *subarachnoid hemorrhage.* (Subarachnoid hemorrhages are the most common extracerebral hemorrhages.) If the bleeding is beneath the dura mater, it is called a *subdural hemorrhage,* and if it is above the dura, between the dura mater and the skull, it is called an *extradural (or epidural) hemorrhage.*

Hemorrhages involving the dura mater, whether subdural or extradural, usually are caused by traumatic head injuries, when dural blood vessels are torn or lacerated. *Subarachnoid hemorrhages* usually are caused by leaking or ruptured blood vessels on the surface of the brain, brain stem, or cerebellum. Such leaks often come from *aneurysms.*

Aneurysms are pouches formed in arterial walls. They develop at places where the arterial walls are weak. Blood pressure within the artery causes the weakened section of the arterial wall to stretch, much like an inflating balloon. The resulting malformations are sometimes called *berry aneurysms* because of their berry-like appearance or *saccular aneurysms* because of their sack-like appearance (Figure 1-20). The stretched arterial walls are thin, weak, and susceptible to rupture.

About half of all extracerebral aneurysms occur in the arteries at the base of the brain (in the vertebral arteries, basilar artery, internal carotid arteries, and the circle of Willis). Almost all of the others occur in the anterior and middle cerebral arteries. Very few (2% to 3%) occur in the posterior cerebral artery. If an aneurysm is detected before it ruptures, it may be surgically repaired by clamping or tying off the neck of the aneurysm, by wrapping the aneurysm, or by tying off the artery that supplies blood to it. Sometimes aneurysms that are leaking, but have not ruptured, can be repaired. When an aneurysm ruptures, repair often is impossible. Bleeding into the subarachnoid space follows, and the risk of death or irreversible brain damage escalates.

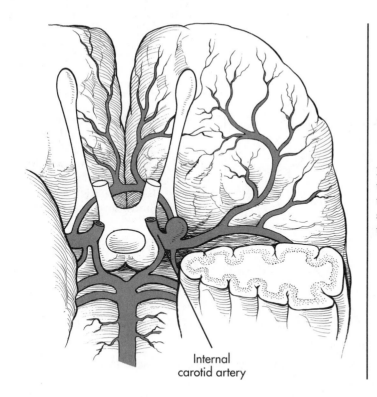

Internal
carotid artery

Figure 1-20 ▪ A "berry" aneurysm on the left anterior communicating artery in the circle of Willis. Aneurysms are most common in the arteries at the base of the brain.

Some subarachnoid hemorrhages come from *arteriovenous malformations* (AVMs). Arteriovenous malformations are collections of dilated, thin-walled veins connected to a tangled mass of equally thin-walled arteries (Figure 1-21). They occur in all parts of the brain, brain stem, and spinal cord, but most large ones develop deep in the cerebral hemispheres. As is true for aneurysms, the vessel walls in arteriovenous malformations usually are weak and sometimes bleed, causing a hemorrhage. Almost all arteriovenous malformations are present at birth and become larger with the passage of time. When arteriovenous malformations become large, they may cause headaches and other central nervous system symptoms. If they are identified before massive bleeding occurs, they may be surgically excised, or the blood vessels that connect to the malformation may be tied off or plugged. According to Adams and Victor (1981)

the risk of bleeding from AVMs is about 1% to 2% per year, which suggests that a patient with an AVM is unlikely to reach her or his 60s or 70s without a hemorrhage.

Intracerebral Hemorrhage Almost all intracerebral hemorrhages (about 90%) occur in patients with high blood pressure. The most obvious reason for this relationship is the pressure on arterial walls caused by hypertension. A less obvious reason is that chronic hypertension leads to degenerative changes in the small penetrating arteries deep in the brain, weakening them and creating *microaneurysms*. These microaneurysms are vulnerable to rupture, with consequent leakage of blood into the brain. This leakage often exerts pressure on adjacent vessels, causing them to rupture, which leads to a *snowball* effect, in which the hemorrhage grows by displacing adjacent brain tissue and stretching and tearing small blood vessels in the

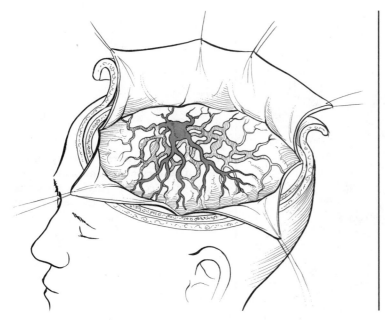

Figure 1-21 ■ An arteriovenous malformation (AVM). AVMs are tangled masses of arteries and veins that gradually increase in size with the passage of time. The greatest risk to patients with AVMs is rupture and subsequent hemorrhage.

vicinity. The most common sites for *intracerebral hemorrhages* are the small penetrating arteries in and around the thalamus and basal ganglia, but they also occur in the brain stem (especially the pons) and the cerebellum.

Intracerebral hemorrhages dissect brain matter along white matter tracts, but tend not to destroy the tracts themselves. An intracerebral hemorrhage may eventually decompress itself by bleeding into the ventricles or subarachnoid space. Because of their location (usually deep in the brain) most intracerebral hemorrhages are not surgically manageable, and surgery usually is attempted only if the bleeding is life-threatening and the hemorrhage is accessible. Medical management usually includes reduction of blood pressure, maintaining adequate respiration, and regulation of fluid intake.

■ OTHER NEUROLOGIC CAUSES OF COMMUNICATION DISORDERS

Most of the other neurologic processes that can cause communicative impairments (excluding, of course, traumatic brain injury) are insidious rather than abrupt in onset. Insidious neurologic processes make their presence known slowly, over a period of time, sometimes with intermittent periods of stabilization or even remission, until the patient receives treatment, becomes incapacitated, or dies.

The major insidious processes that affect the central nervous system are:

- Intracranial tumors
- Hydrocephalus
- Infections and toxins
- Nutritional and metabolic disorders

Any of these processes can cause impaired communication. However, when impaired communication is caused by these processes, dementia or personality disruptions usually accompany the communication impairment. Insidious processes usually do not have a clearly definable time of onset, and patients often do not see their physician when the first symptoms appear because the symptoms are mild and appear innocuous. Consequently, the pathologic process may be advanced when the patient first seeks medical attention. In some cases delay may have no significant consequences, but in other cases (such as intracerebral tumor), delay may have serious and sometimes disastrous results.

Intracranial Tumors

Tumors growing within the cranial vault may be either *primary* (originating there) or *secondary* (originating elsewhere and migrating to intracranial locations). The process by which a tumor appears at a secondary site in the body is called *metastasis,* and such tumors are called *metastatic tumors.*

Primary intracranial tumors are most often found in the cerebrum and the cerebellum. They occur at all ages, but are most common in adults from 25 to 50 years old. The causes of most primary intracranial tumors remain a mystery. Some appear to be related to previous injuries, and there is a tendency for some kinds of intracranial tumors to occur in families.

Intracranial tumors, whether primary or secondary, have similar effects on the central nervous system. The tissue around the tumor swells. This swelling is one of the major causes of observable symptoms in patients with cerebral tumors. If the tumor exerts pressure on circumscribed areas of the brain or brain stem, localized symptoms (motor impairments, sensory loss) may follow. If the tumor causes general swelling of the brain and brain stem, then widespread symptoms of cerebral dysfunction related to pressure and displacement of brain tissue are likely. It is common to see localized symptoms in the early stages of tumor growth, with increasing and more generalized dysfunction as tumor growth and swelling of brain tissue causes intracranial pressure to increase.

When cerebral swelling is severe, *herniation* may occur (Figure 1-22). Large masses in the brain hemispheres (or smaller ones in the brain stem) may force the brain stem downward through the foramen magnum or may squeeze parts of the brain against dural projections (such as the falx cerebri, the tentorium), causing compression, shearing, and bleeding of brain tissues.

According to Pang (1989) the four major types of herniation are:

1. *Subfalcine herniation* is most common and least ominous. It occurs when one brain hemisphere is pushed against the falx cerebri, the rigid sheet of dura that projects downward into the superior longitudinal fissure (Figure 1-22, *B*). Subfalcine herniation does not always generate focal neurologic symptoms, unless the anterior cerebral artery is compressed, in which case the patient may complain of numbness and weakness in the contralateral leg.

2. *Lateral transtentorial herniation* usually occurs as a consequence of masses in the temporal lobe. The mesial surface of the temporal lobe is squeezed against the tentorium, the rigid sheet of dura that separates the space occupied by the brain from that occupied by the cerebellum (Figure 1-22, *C*). The herniation creates pressure on cranial nerve 3, causing ipsilateral pupillary dilation. The pressure also forces the brain substance downward into the foramen magnum, stretching tissues and blood vessels at the base of the brain and in the brain stem. The resulting brain stem ischemia may lead to coma and, if brain stem hemorrhages occur, to irreversible coma or death.

3. *Central transtentorial herniation* is caused by swelling near the apex of the brain or in the frontal lobes. The brain mass is pushed downward into the foramen magnum. As in lateral transtentorial herniation, structures and blood vessels at the base of the brain and in the midbrain are stretched and distorted, with consequent impairment of vital functions. Irreversible coma or death are common consequences.

4. *Tonsillar herniation* is caused by swelling in the cerebellum, pons, or medulla. The cerebellar tonsils (hence the name *tonsillar*) are extruded through the foramen magnum, where they exert pressure on the medulla (Figure 1-22, *D*). The brain stem is displaced

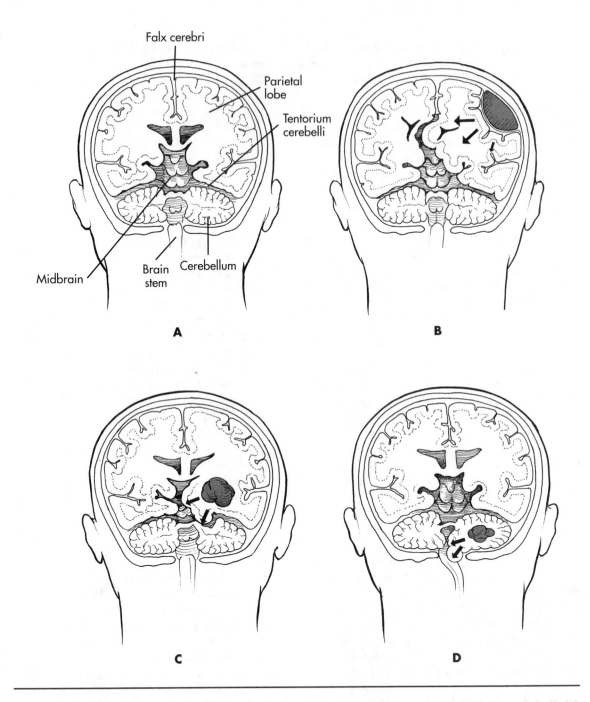

Figure 1-22 ▪ **Examples of herniation syndromes. (A) A cross-section of a normal brain and skull. (B) Displacement of brain tissue caused by a mass above the right parietal lobe, which pushes adjacent regions of the right hemisphere under the falx cerebri (subfalcine herniation). (C) Displacement of the mesial temporal lobe around the tentorium cerebelli by a mass in the temporal lobe (transtentorial herniation). (D) Displacement of the right cerebellar tonsil downward into the foramen magnum by a mass in the right cerebellar hemisphere (tonsillar herniation).**

downward, with consequent shearing and distortion. Respiration is compromised, heart rate decreases, blood pressure rapidly increases, and coma soon follows.

The overall course of patients with intracranial tumors is deterioration. In the early stages, when intracranial pressure is low, the patient may complain of nonspecific alterations in mental function, such as forgetfulness, lack of initiative, drowsiness, blurred or double vision, light-headedness, or vertigo. About one third of patients report headaches early in the course of tumor development. Such headaches can take several forms, but most are not affected by analgesics. Vomiting sometimes occurs in the early stages of tumor growth, and seizures often are seen throughout the course of tumor growth, especially when the tumor is within the brain itself.

Patients with tumors who have elevated intracranial pressure almost always exhibit cognitive impairments, are lethargic, and may be stuporous. In most cases, these patients report unremitting bifrontal and bioccipital headaches that are not affected by analgesics and are present day and night. Vomiting frequently occurs, and the patient may be unsteady and generally clumsy.

The number of symptoms generated by a tumor, and the rate at which symptoms progress are determined by the *size, rate of growth,* and *location* of the tumor. Large tumors generate more extreme symptoms. Faster-growing tumors produce symptoms more quickly than slower-growing ones because the brain adapts to slowly developing processes better than faster developing ones. If the tumor is located in or near areas that serve important functions (sensory and motor cortex, brain stem), a relatively small tumor may quickly generate major symptoms. If the tumor is located in a "silent" area of the brain, it may grow to surprising volume before generating observable symptoms.

Different kinds of intracranial tumors have different rates of growth and differ in malig-

nancy. *Gliomas* are the most common. Gliomas can be divided into several subtypes, but the two most important ones are *astrocytoma* and *glioblastoma multiforme.* Astrocytomas are the most common and the most benign (nonmalignant) of the gliomas. They usually grow slowly, and symptom development may span 5 or 6 years. Postoperative survival of 10 or more years is common. In some cases, astrocytomas may be completely removed, and the patient is considered cured. However, even "benign" astrocytomas can cause substantial neurologic impairments, or even kill the patient if the tumor is strategically located (e.g., in the brain stem).

Glioblastoma multiforme is the next most common glioma. It is also one of the most malignant and rapidly growing of all intracranial tumors. Symptoms typically develop during a 3-month to 1-year period, and the average postsurgical survival is only about 6 to 9 months.

Meningiomas are also relatively common tumors that, as the name implies, arise from the meninges. They are among the most benign of all intracranial tumors because they are slow-growing, well-defined, and usually do not invade the brain substance. For this reason they often can be completely removed. The symptoms of meningiomas are slow to develop because meningiomas are slow-growing. However, when symptoms do appear, meningiomas are among the most localizable of intracranial tumors because they generate pressure at specific places on the cortex and rarely cause general increases in intracranial pressure.

Secondary intracranial tumors (metastatic carcinomas) are tumors that form from cancerous cells that have migrated (usually through the blood stream) from the primary tumor site to the brain, where they settle and grow. The primary sources for metastatic carcinoma of the brain are, in decreasing order of frequency, breast, lungs, and the pharynx and larynx. Metastatic carcinomas of the brain usually are grossly, well-defined, but multiple sites of metastasis within the brain are common. There usually is considerable local swelling around the tumor site. The prognosis for metastatic brain tumor patients usually is poor. The average survival after diagnosis of metastatic brain tumor is 2 months to 6 months.

Hydrocephalus

Hydrocephalus refers to enlargement of the cerebral ventricles, with consequent increase in the volume of the cerebrospinal fluid within them. *Obstructive hydrocephalus* is caused by obstruction of the interventricular passageways through which cerebrospinal fluid circulates. The obstruction blocks the flow of cerebrospinal fluid from the ventricles into the meningeal spaces and spinal column. Sometimes obstructions are caused by material circulating in the cerebrospinal fluid (plugs of bacteria, bits of floating tissue), but more often they are caused by swelling of nearby brain tissue. The most frequent site of obstruction is the *cerebral aqueduct,* connecting the third and fourth ventricles. The cerebral aqueduct is the longest and narrowest of the passageways between the ventricles and consequently is the most susceptible to obstruction (usually because of swelling of adjacent brain tissues or displacement of brain tissue by tumors). Because cerebrospinal fluid is formed in the cerebral ventricles, anything that blocks the exit of cerebrospinal fluid from the ventricles causes the pressure within the ventricles to rise. As the pressure rises the ventricles enlarge, the brain is compressed against the skull, and the patient becomes mentally dulled, lethargic, and hyporesponsive.

The primary medical treatment for obstructive hydrocephalus is *intraventricular shunt.* A cannula (hollow needle) connected to a small flexible tube is passed through the brain into the ventricles. Excess cerebrospinal fluid is then forced (by intraventricular pressure) through the shunt, decreasing the pressure within the ventricles. The tube may be passed into the neck or the abdominal cavity, where the excess fluid is allowed to drip away. The patient's response to shunt placement usually is dramatic, with few long-term residual deficits, unless intracranial pressure has reached exceptionally high levels or has continued for weeks or months.

Nonobstructive hydrocephalus is a generic label for several other conditions that cause ventricular enlargement. One of the most common causes of nonobstructive hydrocephalus is cerebral atrophy. Nonobstructive hydrocephalus is not accompanied by elevated intracranial pressure.

Infections

The central nervous system ordinarily is strongly resistant to bacterial or viral infection, but such infections sometimes occur. The major bacterial infections are *bacterial meningitis* and *brain abscess.* In bacterial meningitis, the pia, arachnoid, and the cerebrospinal fluid become infected, causing inflammation, swelling, and fluid exudate from the meninges. The patient becomes feverish, chilled, and lethargic and complains of headache, drowsiness, and stiff neck. If the infection is severe, the patient may progress into coma. Bacterial meningitis exacerbates quickly and can be fatal if not promptly treated. The standard treatment for the infection is antibiotic medication, which usually cures the infection, although neurologic sequelae may persist.

Brain abscess is caused by introduction of bacteria, fungus, or parasites into brain tissues from a primary infection site elsewhere in the body. Transmission may be through the blood or by migration through tissues. In about 40% of cases, the primary sources of infections are the nasal sinuses, middle ear, or mastoid cells. In about 30% of cases the source is the lungs or cardiovascular tissue. Symptom development in brain abscess is slower than that of bacterial meningitis, and brain abscesses tend to generate localized symptoms such as visual anomalies or sensory loss, rather than the generalized symptoms of meningitis. However, patients with brain abscess, like those with meningitis, often complain of fever, chills, headache, lethargy, and drowsiness. The usual treatment is surgical drainage of the abscess in combination with antibiotic medication. Recovery usually is dramatic, although the patient may be left with chronic deficits related to destruction of brain tissue by the abscess.

Numerous viruses may infect the central nervous system. The two major sources of central nervous system viral infections are: (1) general infections, such as mumps or measles, and (2) viruses transmitted by insect or animal bites, such as equine encephalitis or rabies. The progression of viral infections depends on the virus. Sometimes (as in viral meningitis), symptoms develop quickly, followed by gradual improvement. Sometimes symptoms develop slowly, followed by gradual improvement (e.g., when the body's immune system successfully eliminates the infection). Sometimes (as in acquired immune deficiency syndrome, or AIDS), symptoms develop slowly and continue to worsen, usually ending in death. In some cases, (as in rabies), symptoms develop quickly and dramatically, invariably ending in death. A few antiviral medications that are not toxic to the body have been developed and may be of benefit. Otherwise, treatment of viral infections is palliative, directed toward maintaining the patient's vital functions, providing adequate nutrition, and regulating fluid balance, to help the patient's natural defenses rid the body of the virus.

Toxemia

Toxemia is caused by introduction into the nervous system of substances that inflame or poison nerve tissue. Toxemia may be a result of drug overdoses, drug interactions, bacterial toxins (tetanus, botulism, diphtheria), or heavy metal poisoning (lead, mercury). The course of heavy metal or chemical poisoning (such as may occur in occupational exposure to the compounds) is usually one of decreasing mentation and increasing lethargy, with motor or sensory disruptions generally occurring only in advanced stages of poisoning. Poisoning with bacterial toxins usually follows a more acute course, with symptoms developing quickly, followed by slow recovery, unless the poisoning ends in death. Treatment is usually directed toward removal of the source of the toxin, and, sometimes, purging the system of the toxin.

Metabolic and Nutritional Disorders

Metabolic disorders are common causes of central nervous system dysfunction but, like other insidious processes, rarely cause isolated communication disorders. Severe hypoglycemia may cause deterioration of cerebral function, leading to confusion, stupor, or coma. Thyroid disorders may generate central nervous system symptoms (apathy, confusion, and intellectual deterioration). Treatment of metabolic disorders usually involves correcting or compensating for the metabolic imbalance, and central nervous system symptoms may regress or resolve when the metabolic disturbance is corrected.

Nutritional disorders, though rare in the United States, sometimes cause central nervous system dysfunction and may occasionally generate communicative impairments. One classic nutritional deficiency syndrome is *Wernicke's encephalopathy,* caused by thiamine deficiency, and usually associated with alcoholism. The primary symptoms of Wernicke's encephalopathy are paralysis of some of the muscles that move the eyes, clumsy, staggering gait, and mental confusion. Other vitamin deficiencies, including deficiencies in vitamin B12 and nicotinic acid, may cause variable neurologic symptoms. Neurologic syndromes associated with vitamin or mineral excess may also be seen (e.g., overdose of vitamin A). In the case of nutritional deficiencies, treatment usually involves replenishment of the deficient compound by medication, together with dietary adjustment, and in the case of vitamin or mineral excess, treatment is directed toward reducing the patient's intake of those compounds.

■ KEY CONCEPTS

- The central nervous system (brain, brain stem, cerebellum, spinal cord) is responsible for perceiving and processing sensory input, for formulating, monitoring, and adjusting motoric output, and for maintaining and modulating complex interactions between motor and sensory processes.

- The peripheral nervous system contains sensory receptors and nerve fibers that convey information from the outside world to the central nervous system. It also has sensory receptors and nerve-muscle interfaces that enable the central nervous system to initiate, maintain, and regulate muscle activity.

- The brain receives its blood supply from the *internal carotid* and the *vertebral arteries.* The cerebrum(the brain hemispheres) is supplied by paired *anterior, middle,* and *poste-rior cerebral arteries,* which arise from the *circle of Willis* at the base of the brain.

- Strokes (cerebrovascular accidents) are an important cause of adult communication disorders. *Ischemic strokes* (interruption of blood supply to the brain by blockage of an artery) are more common than *hemorrhagic strokes* (bleeding into the brain or into spaces around the brain). Strokes usually are characterized by rapid onset of neurologic signs and symptoms, followed by slow improvement.

- Most ischemic strokes are related to the presence of *atherosclerosis* (fatty deposits on the inner walls of arteries), and most hemorrhagic strokes are related to the presence of *hypertension* (high blood pressure). Some hemorrhagic strokes are the result of ruptured *aneurysms* (weakened outpouchings of arterial walls).

- Tumors, elevated intraventricular pressure, infections, toxins, metabolic imbalances, and nutritional disorders also can cause neurogenic communication impairments.

Neurologic Assessment

Most patients with neurogenic communication disorders are examined by a physician (usually a neurologist) and sometimes other professionals before they are referred to the speech-language pathologist. The physician's report of the physical and neurologic examination of the patient almost always provides valuable information about the origin, nature, and potential course of the neurologic processes underlying the patient's communication disorders. This chapter provides an overview of how the neurologist uses the patient's *current complaints and medical history,* the *neurologic examination,* and the results of *laboratory tests* to arrive at a diagnosis. The neurologist's evaluation of the patient is an important part of the patient's *medical record,* which is a complete account of the patient's care.

In the typical scenario, the neurologist begins the examination by interviewing the patient and family members to determine what symptoms brought the patient to the neurologist's office, how the symptoms first expressed themselves, and how they changed over time. Following the interview the neurologist carries out a neurologic examination in which the patient's motor, sensory, and mental status are systematically evaluated. During the examination the neurologist pays particular attention to motor, sensory, or mental functions that were discussed in the interview, and if a tentative diagnosis has been made, the neurologist pays particular attention to those parts of the neurologic examination that are likely to support or refute the diagnosis. Finally, the neurologist may order laboratory tests to provide additional information about the nature and severity of the patient's nervous system pathology.

■ THE INTERVIEW AND PHYSICAL EXAMINATION

The *pattern of symptom development* often plays an important part in establishing the cause of the patient's complaints, because many diseases and pathologic processes exhibit characteristic progressions of symptom development. Most degenerative diseases (such as Huntington's chorea) and slowly growing tumors are characterized by gradual and uninterrupted development of symptoms over months or years.

Infections, rapidly-growing tumors, and a few degenerative diseases (e.g., amyotrophic lateral sclerosis) are characterized by rapid and uninterrupted symptom development over days or weeks. Occlusive vascular disease of large arteries typically is characterized by periods of rapid development of symptoms over minutes to hours, followed by intervals of symptom stabilization that can last from days to years. Occlusive vascular disease of small arteries and multiple sclerosis are characterized by gradual development of symptoms over months or years with periods of remission ranging from weeks to months (Figure 2-1).

The *patient's family history* is important because some neurologic diseases are hereditary or familial. *Hereditary* diseases have a definite genetic inheritance pattern; *familial* diseases have a greater than expected occurrence in families but do not exhibit a definite inheritance pattern. Several progressive neurologic diseases are hereditary (e.g., Huntington's disease, myotonic dystrophy, Friedreich's ataxia). Some dementing illnesses and some forms of epilepsy may be familial. When a disease is hereditary and the inheritance pattern is known, the family history alone may permit the neurologist to make a diagnosis. When a disease is known to

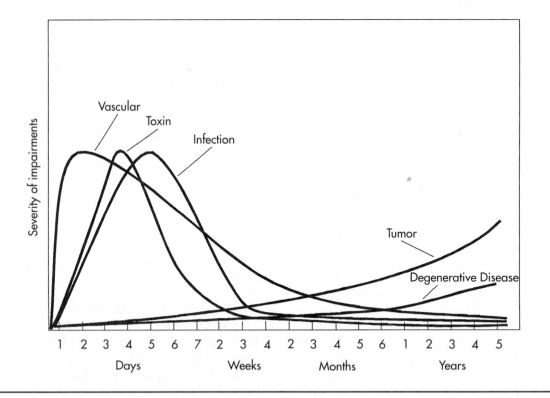

Figure 2-1 ■ The progression of symptoms in major categories of neurologic disease. These curves represent overall trends. Specific diseases within a category may differ somewhat from the trend for the category in which the disease is located. For example, multiple sclerosis is a degenerative disease, with an overall pattern of gradual increasing severity, but there are periods of exacerbation and remission within this overall pattern.

exhibit familial patterns, the history may point to a probable diagnosis, in which case the patient's symptoms and the results of the neurologic examination and laboratory tests serve primarily to confirm or refute the diagnosis.

If someone else has not already done a physical examination before the neurologist sees the patient, the neurologist performs one. The physical examination provides a sense of the patient's general health and physical condition. In the physical examination the neurologist evaluates the patient's *vital signs* (temperature, pulse rate, respiration rate, blood pressure); *general appearance* (evidence of illness, presence of lesions, deformities); *heart, lung, and abdominal sounds* (with a stethoscope); *eyes* (conjunctiva, sclera, pupillary dilation, retinae); *ears* (external auditory canal, tympanic membrane); *mouth* (mucous membranes, teeth, gums, tongue, pharynx); *neck* (muscles, movement, lymph nodes); *thorax and abdomen* (muscles, masses, tenderness, lesions); *genitals* (masses, tenderness, lesions, exudate); and *rectum* (masses, tenderness).

The results of the general physical examination are noted in the patient's medical record. Abnormalities are noted in the record, and a plan for continued assessment of the more important abnormalities may be included at the end of the physician's report of the examination.

■ THE NEUROLOGIC EXAMINATION

In the neurologic examination, the neurologist evaluates the patient's *cranial nerves, motor system, sensory system, equilibrium,* and *consciousness and mentation.* In each part of the examination the neurologist combines information from the patient's *history and current complaints* with information from *examination of the patient* to move toward a diagnosis and formulate a plan of care.

Cranial Nerves

History and Current Complaints Patients with cranial nerve involvement report a variety of symptoms, depending on which cranial

nerves are involved. Patients with optic, olfactory, or auditory nerve involvement complain of diminution or loss of sensation in the affected sensory modality, of distorted perception in the affected modality, or of visual, olfactory, or auditory hallucinations. Patients with involvement of somesthetic sensory branches of cranial nerves complain of diminished sensation or exaggerated sensitivity in the body parts served by the nerve or of hallucinatory tactile phenomena. Patients with involvement of motor branches of cranial nerves complain of diminished strength or paralysis (called *palsy*) of the muscles served by the nerve. When the cranial nerve itself or the cranial nerve nucleus are damaged, motor and sensory deficits are on the same side of the body as the damage. When fibers between a cranial nerve nucleus and the cortex are damaged (the corticobulbar tract), motor and sensory deficits are contralateral to the damage.

Examination of the Patient Neurologic evaluation of the cranial nerves usually follows a top-down format, beginning with CN 1 and ending with CN 12. The neurologist evaluates *CN 1 (olfactory)* by asking the patient to identify odors such as cloves, peppermint, coffee, or tobacco. (Neurologists often forego evaluation of the olfactory nerve in routine neurologic examinations unless there is reason to believe that the olfactory nerve has been injured.)

To evaluate *CN 2 (optic),* the neurologist tests the patient's visual acuity, color vision (sometimes), and visual fields. The neurologist also estimates the size of the patient's pupils, notes whether they are equal or unequal in size, and tests their responsiveness to light (do the pupils constrict when a bright light is shone into the eye?) and accommodation (do the pupils constrict when the eyes converge to focus on nearby objects?). Abnormalities in pupillary responses to light and accommodation can be caused by various conditions, some of which involve the optic nerve. While examining the patient's eyes the neurologist also evaluates the condition of the optic disk (a yellowish, oval region of the retina located at the posterior pole of the eye) using an ophthalmoscope. This part of the examination provides information about a variety of conditions, most of which do not involve the optic nerve. Optic disk swelling (*papilledema*) may suggest increased intracranial pressure, local inflammation, or an ischemic condition. Fading (pallor) of the optic disk, together with impaired visual acuity or visual field blindness, may suggest inflammation, nutritional deficiency, or degenerative disease.

The neurologist evaluates the cranial nerves serving the eye muscles *(CN 3 [oculomotor] CN4 [trochlear],* and *CN 6 [abducens])* by observing the position of the patient's eyes and eyelids at rest and their activity during volitional movements. Injury to the oculomotor nerve produces drooping of the eyelid *(ptosis)* on the affected side (caused by paralysis of the muscles that raise the eyelid), and downward and outward rotation of the affected eye (caused by paralysis of the muscles that rotate the eye upward and inward, leaving nothing to oppose the action of the muscles that rotate the eye downward and outward). Patients with oculomotor nerve dysfunction often report *diplopia* (double vision) in the affected eye (because the affected eye is not looking in the same direction as the unaffected eye), except when the patient looks downward and outward (so that both the affected and unaffected eye are looking in the same direction). Injury to the trochlear nerve causes upward deflection of the affected eye during forward gaze. The patient may experience diplopia when looking downward because the affected eye does not move downward as the unaffected eye does. Injury to the abducens nerve causes adduction (inward deflection) of the affected eye at rest and inability to rotate the eye outward (laterally). The patient usually reports diplopia when looking toward the side of the affected eye. The presence of *nystagmus* (rhythmic oscillation of the eyes) may suggest weakness in some of the muscles that move the

eyeball. The neurologist observes the patient's eyes as the patient looks straight ahead, up, down, laterally, and medially. Nystagmus that occurs when the patient looks in specific directions *(gaze-evoked nystagmus)* may suggest weakness in the muscles that move the eyeball in the direction of the nystagmus.

The neurologist evaluates the function of *CN 5 (trigeminal)* by testing the corneal reflex (blinking when the eyeball is touched with a wisp of cotton) and the jaw-jerk reflex (elicited by tapping the patient's open jaw). Exaggeration of these reflexes implicates corticobulbar tracts above the CN 5 nucleus, and abolition implicates CN 5 on that side. The motor branch of the trigeminal nerve innervates the muscles of mastication (chewing), so the neurologist tests its function by asking the patient to open and close the jaw against resistance. Injury compromises the patient's ability to close the mouth or to chew. The patient's jaw may deviate to the side of the injured nerve on opening (because of loss of muscle tone on that side), and the patient's resistance is weak when the examiner pushes the patient's jaw away from the side of the injured nerve (because the weak muscle on that side cannot oppose the movement). The neurologist assesses the sensory function of the trigeminal nerve by testing the patient's sensitivity to touch, pain, and temperature in the face and anterior scalp. The sensory branch of the trigeminal nerve has three divisions— ophthalmic, maxillary, and mandibular. The ophthalmic division provides sensation to the eye, upper eyelid, bridge of the nose, and anterior scalp. The maxillary division provides sensation to the cheeks, nose, upper teeth and lip, hard palate, and nasopharynx. The mandibular division provides sensation to the skin of the lower jaw, outer ear, lower teeth and gums, floor of mouth, and inside surfaces of the cheek. Injury in any of the three divisions causes loss of tactile sensation in the regions served by the division. Irritation of the trigeminal nerve causes severe paroxysmal facial pain *(trigeminal neu-*

ralgia or *tic douloureux)* and sometimes causes excessive contraction of the muscles of mastication *(trismus).*

The neurologist tests the function of *CN 7 (facial)* by testing the patient's ability to move the muscles involved in facial expression. Injury to the facial nerve causes weakness or paralysis of those muscles. Patients with facial nerve damage cannot close the eyelid tightly, wrinkle the forehead, or pucker the lips and they may lose taste in the anterior two thirds of the tongue. At rest, the patient's eyebrow and eyelid on the side of the injured nerve droop, the nasolabial fold on that side is flattened. The patient's mouth droops on the affected side and may be drawn upward on the unaffected side. Paralysis of all the facial muscles on one side is caused by damage in the cranial nerve nucleus or the cranial nerve proper (a condition called *peripheral 7th nerve palsy).* Paralysis only in the lower facial muscles is caused by damage in the corticobulbar tracts above the facial nerve nucleus (a condition called *central 7th nerve palsy).* Central 7th nerve palsies are caused by damage in the *contralateral* corticobulbar tracts, and peripheral 7th nerve palsies are caused by damage in the *ipsilateral* cranial nerve nucleus or cranial nerve.

The neurologist tests the function of the acoustic branch of *CN 8 (acoustic-vestibular)* by testing the patient's hearing acuity for whispered speech, ticking clocks or watches, and tuning forks (which are used to test both air-conduction and bone-conduction hearing). The function of the vestibular branch of CN 8 is (sometimes, but not routinely) evaluated by *caloric testing,* in which cold or warm water is injected into the ear canal and the appearance of nystagmus is monitored. Normally, nystagmus appears within about 20 seconds after the water is placed in the ear canal. If the vestibular branch of CN 8 is affected, the nystagmus may fail to appear, appear later than usual, and/or disappear earlier than usual.

The neurologist tests the sensory functions of *CN 9 (glossopharyngeal) and CN 10 (vagus)*

by evaluating the patient's sensitivity to touch on the posterior wall of the pharynx and tests the presence of a gag or swallowing reflex on stimulation of the posterior tongue and pharynx. Diminished or abolished sensation and gag and swallow reflexes implicate the sensory divisions of CN 9 and CN 10. Loss of taste sensation in the posterior third of the tongue implicates CN 9. The neurologist evaluates the motor function of CN 9 and CN 10 by asking the patient to swallow and by observing the position of the velum (soft palate). Injury to CN 9 causes the midline of the velum to be displaced toward the side away from the injured nerve both at rest and when the patient phonates (because of the unopposed action of the contralateral muscles).

The neurologist evaluates the function of *CN 11 (accessory/spinal accessory)* by testing the patient's ability to turn the head, to resist the neurologist's attempts to rotate the patient's head, to shrug the shoulders, and to elevate the shoulders against resistance. Injury to CN 11 causes the patient's shoulder on the affected side to droop, interferes with arm movements above the shoulders on the affected side, and interferes with head turning toward the side opposite that of the injured nerve (the head is rotated to the *right* with the *left* sternomastoid muscle).

The neurologist evaluates the function of *CN 12 (hypoglossal)* by testing the patient's ability to protrude the tongue and move it from side to side, both freely and against resistance. Injury to CN 12 causes the patient's tongue to deviate toward the side of the injured cranial nerve on protrusion (because the muscle that pulls the tongue forward on that side is weak or paralyzed). Injury also prevents the patient from volitionally moving the tongue to the corner of the mouth on the side of the injured nerve and prevents the patient from pushing the tongue into the cheek against resistance on that side (because the muscle that pulls the tongue toward that side is weak or paralyzed).

The neurologist's active testing of muscle strength and movement during evaluation of cranial nerve functions is accompanied by observation of muscles at rest to look for signs of involuntary movements *(fasciculations, fibrillations)* and *atrophy* (wasting away), both of which are signs of compromised innervation. These phenomena are discussed later in this chapter.

Assessment of Visual Fields As noted above, the neurologist's examination of CN 2 (the optic nerve) usually includes assessment of the patient's visual fields. The presence of visual field blindness suggests damage in an optic nerve or the optic tract that connects the optic nerve with the visual cortex.* The nature of the patient's visual field blindness provides the neurologist with important clues about the location of the neurologic damage causing the blindness. This is true because of how the human visual system is arranged (Figure 2-2). Optic nerve fibers from the right half of each retina project to the visual cortex in the right hemisphere, and fibers from the left half of each retina project to the visual cortex in the left hemisphere. The left half of each retina receives visual input from the right side of visual space, and the right half of each retina receives input from the left side of visual space. This means that visual information from the right side of visual space goes to the left hemisphere and visual information from the left side of visual space goes to the right hemisphere (Figure 2-2).

The neurologist tests the patient's visual fields by covering one of the patient's eyes and asking the patient to look straight ahead while the neurologist introduces visual stimuli (usually the neurologist's wiggling index finger) into various sectors of the patient's visual fields. Patients with blindness in parts of the visual field do not report stimuli that are presented in the affected regions of the visual field. The kinds of visual field deficits observed may suggest (or confirm) the location of the lesion (or lesions) responsible for the patient's deficits. If a lesion destroys the visual fibers posterior to the optic chiasm the patient is blind in the contralateral visual half field (Figure 2-3, *C*). Such blindness is called *homonymous hemianopsia* (or *hemianopia*) and occurs following deep lesions in the temporal lobe or lower parietal lobe. (*Homonymous* means that the same part of the visual field is affected in each eye.) Destruction of the visual cortex in one hemisphere also causes contralateral homonymous hemianopsia (Figure 2-3, *D*).

If a lesion destroys one optic nerve, the patient is blind in that eye (Figure 2-3, *A*). If a lesion destroys the crossing fibers at the optic chiasm, the patient exhibits *bitemporal hemianopsia* (blindness in the lateral visual fields for both eyes), because the fibers that transmit visual information from lateral visual space in both eye fields are destroyed (Figure 2-3, *B*).

Sometimes visual field blindness affects less than one half of the visual field. This blindness is called *quadrantanopsia* (quadrantic hemianopsia). Technically, quadrantanopsia means that vision in one fourth of the visual field is lost, but in practice this appellation is applied to blindness affecting anywhere from about one third of the visual field to patches comprising one eighth of the visual field or less. Quadrantanopsia typically is caused by damage in the upper or lower optic radiations on their way to the visual cortex. Lesions in the inferior parietal lobe that destroy the uppermost optic radiations typically cause blindness in the lower quadrant of the contralateral visual field. Lesions in the temporal lobe that destroy the lowermost optic radiations typically cause blindness in the upper quadrant of the contralateral visual field. (Inferiorly placed lesions that are posterior to the optic chiasm produce contralateral superior quadrant blindness, and vice versa.)

---

* The nerve fibers serving vision are called the *optic nerve* between the eye and the optic chiasm, and the *optic tract* from the optic chiasm to the visual cortex. The optic nerve is outside the brain proper and the optic tract is mostly within the brain substance.

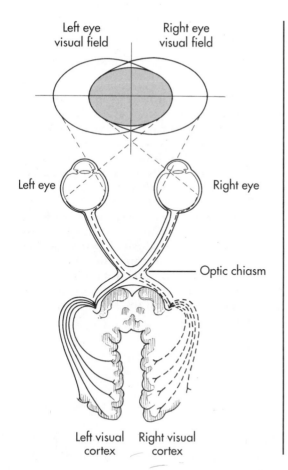

Figure 2-2 ■ The human visual system. Each hemisphere receives visual input from contralateral visual space. Visual fibers from the nasal (inner) half of the retina in each eye cross at the optic chiasm and project to visual cortex in the contralateral hemisphere. Visual fibers from the temporal (outer) half of each retina do not cross and project to visual cortex in the ipsilateral hemisphere.

If the neurologist is uncertain about the presence or extent of a patient's visual field blindness, he or she may refer the patient for a specialized test called *perimetry,* in which the patient's visual fields are tested with a specialized instrument called a *perimeter.* In perimetry, small visual stimuli (dots, points of light) are moved through the patient's visual fields in semicircular paths. The patient's report of the presence of stimuli and the coordinates at which the stimuli are seen or not seen are recorded. These records are used to produce a graphic depiction of the patient's intact and deficient visual fields. Some examples of perimetry plots are provided in Figure 2-4.

A phenomenon called *macular sparing* often is seen in visual-field blindness. The macula

of the retina is a small, circular area near its center. It is the area of greatest visual acuity. In macular sparing, vision in the center of the visual field for the affected eye (that part served by the macula) is spared so that the hemianopsia or quadrantanopsia is incomplete. Macular sparing is common in hemianopsias caused by posterior cerebral artery occlusions that destroy the visual cortex in the occipital lobe. Macular sparing occurs for two reasons—(1) a large area of visual cortex is devoted to the macula, relative to the peripheral retina and (2) the distributions of the posterior cerebral artery and the middle cerebral artery overlap near the cortical area assigned to the macula, making collateral blood supply available to this section of cortex.

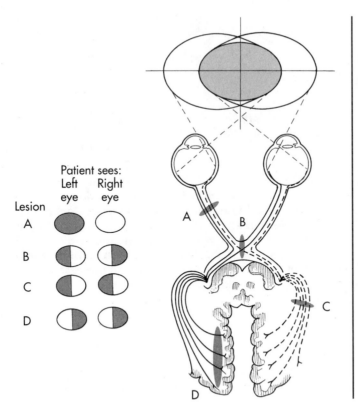

Patient sees:
Left   Right
eye   eye
Lesion
A
B
C
D

Figure 2-3 ▪ How damage in the human visual system affects vision. (A) Lesions in the optic nerve cause blindness in the eye served by the nerve. (B) Lesions that destroy the optic chiasm cause loss of vision in both lateral eye fields because they destroy the crossing fibers from the nasal half of the retina in each eye. Lesions posterior to the optic chiasm (C and D) cause contralateral visual field blindness because they interrupt the fibers from the nasal half of the retina in the contralateral eye and the fibers from the temporal half of the retina in the ipsilateral eye.

If the optic tract or the visual cortex are completely destroyed, macular sparing does not follow.

Bilateral destruction of the visual cortex results in a phenomenon called *cortical blindness*. Patients who are cortically blind cannot discriminate shapes and patterns but may be sensitive to light and dark. Sometimes perception of simple visual stimuli may be preserved, although the patient usually has difficulty reporting them or incorporating them into mental activity. Occasionally, patients with cortical blindness may claim that they can see and produce elaborate confabulations when asked to describe their surroundings. This condition is called *Anton's syndrome*, or *visual anosagnosia.**

---
* *Anosagnosia* means "denial of illness."

When one 45-year-old cortically blind patient was confronted with evidence that he could not see, he responded:

> "Well, it's no wonder that I can't see what color your shirt is in such poor light. Take me outside into the sunshine and I'll be able to tell you what color it is."

The Motor System

History and Current Complaints Patients with motor deficits usually complain of weakness, clumsiness, stiffness, or heaviness in the affected body parts. The patient's description of problems with movement and control help the neurologist to determine the potential involvement of the motor cortex, neural pathways, the cerebellum, the extrapyramidal system, or nerve-muscle junctions. This information can

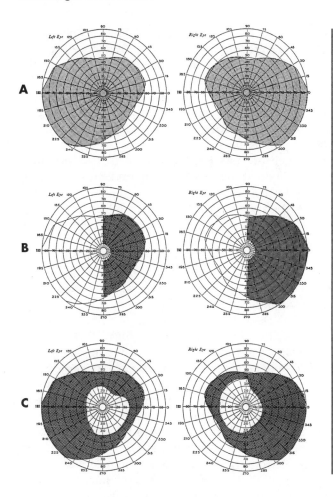

Figure 2-4 ■ Examples of three perimetry plots. (A) Normal visual fields. The lightly shaded areas show the area of vision for each eye. (B) Right homonymous hemianopsia (blindness in the right visual field of both eyes). The dark areas show the area of blindness for each eye. (C) Bitemporal hemianopsia (blindness in the lateral visual fields of both eyes).

subsequently be embellished in the neurologic examination. Patients with damage in upper motor neurons or the motor cortex usually complain of generalized weakness on one side of the body or weakness of the arm, hand, finger, or leg. Patients with leg weakness often report episodes of falling. Patients with cerebellar damage complain more of clumsiness than of weakness (slurred speech and clumsiness involving the arm, hand, and fingers, and/or the leg and foot on both sides of the body). Patients with basal ganglia damage complain of stiffness, difficulty initiating movement, and tremor of the hands and fingers. Patients with disturbances of nerve-muscle transmission usually

complain of excessive fatigue, double vision, and slurred speech.

Examination At the beginning of the examination, the neurologist observes the patient as she or he enters the room and sits down. The neurologist observes the patient's general appearance, posture, walking gait, and behavior and notes characteristics that may suggest abnormalities in the patient's motor system (stooped or slumping posture, slow, effortful or clumsy movements, diminished, spontaneous movement or its converse, hyperactivity, evidence of muscle atrophy [wasting away], and the presence of abnormal and/or unintentional movements). Muscle atrophy suggests lower motor neuron pathology. The presence of unintentional movements suggests extrapyramidal system pathology. Following this period of observation (which usually takes only a few minutes and may be completed during the interview), the neurologist evaluates the functional state of the patient's motor system during movement. During this part of the examination, the neurologist systematically evaluates the patient's *muscle tone, muscle strength,* and the range over which the patient's muscles can be stretched or flexed *(range of movement).*

Muscle Tone and Range of Movement The neurologist evaluates *muscle tone* (the tension remaining in a muscle or muscle group when it is voluntarily relaxed), by palpating (squeezing) individual muscles, moving the patient's limbs while the patient neither assists nor resists the movement *(passive movement),* and sometimes by shaking one or more limbs. The neurologist evaluates *range of movement* by moving each limb through its full range while the patient keeps the muscles relaxed and notes any resistance to movement or the patient's complaints of pain during movement.

Increased resistance to passive movement is called *hypertonia.* There are two major categories of hypertonia, *spasticity* and *rigidity.* In *spasticity* the muscles of the limb are tense and hard and resist stretching. Spastic muscles respond more vigorously to fast stretch than to slow stretch. If the examiner begins to move a limb slowly and then increases the rate at which the limb is moved, the limb's resistance to movement increases suddenly. This phenomenon is called the *spastic catch.* Spastic muscles are most resistant to movement at the beginning of passive movement and their resistance diminishes as the limb is moved at a constant rate through its range. This is called the *clasp-knife phenomenon* (which only readers who have used clasp-knives may appreciate). Spasticity is almost always caused by an upper motor neuron lesion either in the motor cortex or in corticospinal tracts.

In *rigidity* the relaxed limb evenly resists movement in any direction. Rigidity is a prominent characteristic of many extrapyramidal diseases, including Parkinson's disease. The source of the rigidity is increased resting tone of the muscles. The rigid muscles are hard and resist both active and passive movement. Rigidity is more prominent in flexor muscles than in extensor muscles, which gives the patient a stooped posture. Tendon reflexes (e.g., the knee-jerk) are not accentuated by rigidity and their amplitude may be diminished by the patient's increased muscle tone. If rigidity affects the facial muscles, the patient exhibits an unchanging, expressionless, mask-like countenance (called *masked facies*), which is a prominent feature of advanced stages of Parkinson's disease.

Decreased resistance to passive movement is called *hypotonia* or *flaccidity.* When flaccid limbs are shaken, they are unusually floppy and bounce to and fro (the *rag doll* phenomenon). Flaccid muscles usually are weak or paralyzed and provide little or no resistance to passive movement. Hypotonic limbs often can be hyperextended. Pronounced weakness or paralysis usually accompanies the hypotonia. Diminished muscle tone arises from many diseases affecting the nervous system or muscles. Consequently, hypotonia by itself usually is of little diagnostic significance.

Muscle Strength The neurologist assesses the strength of muscles by asking the patient to move them, either freely or against resistance, and asking the patient to maintain his or her contraction against pressure exerted by the neurologist. The strength of muscle groups usually is quantified on a 6-point (0-5) scale (Table 2-1).

Muscle weakness can be caused by damage in the brain, brain stem, spinal cord, the extrapyramidal system, the neuromuscular junction, or in the muscles themselves. Damage in the brain, brain stem, or spinal cord (above the level at which corticospinal fibers decussate) causes motor impairments on the contralateral side of the

Standards suggested by the Medical Research Council for rating muscle strength

Rating	Description
5	Normal strength
4	Active movement against resistance and gravity
3	Active movement against gravity but not resistance
2	Active movement only when gravity is eliminated
1	Flicker or trace of contraction
0	No contraction

Scale for rating reflexes

Rating	Description
0	Absent
1+	Diminished
2+	Normal
3+	Brisk (faster, greater amplitude)
4+	Clonus (rhythmic contraction and relaxation)

body. Usually, numerous muscle groups or all the muscles on one side of the body are affected. (As noted earlier, the affected muscles are spastic.) Damage in cranial nerves or spinal nerves typically produces weakness in the muscle groups served by the affected nerves on the same side as the affected nerves. For example, damage restricted to CN 7 (facial) causes flaccid paralysis in the muscles of the lower face on the same side as the nerve damage, but the muscles of the tongue, palate, and upper face retain strength and motility, and the muscles of the lower face on the other side are unaffected. (As noted earlier, the affected muscles are flaccid.) When pathology involves the muscles themselves (myopathy) or the neuromuscular junction, one typically does not see a right-side-left-side division between affected and unaffected muscles. Instead, a generalized weakness or weakness of large muscle groups in which the weakness is not related to the midline of the body is seen. (That is, the muscles in the shoulders and thighs may be weaker than those in the arms and legs or muscles in the hands and feet may be affected more than proximal muscles, and so forth.)

Paralysis or severe weakness of one limb is called *monoplegia.* Paralysis of both limbs on the same side is called *hemiplegia.* Paralysis of both legs is called *paraplegia* and paralysis of all four limbs is called *quadriplegia.* The suffix denoting weakness is *"paresis."* Substituting *"paresis"* for *"plegia"* provides equivalent terminology denoting limb weakness (monoparesis, hemiparesis, paraparesis, and quadriparesis).

Reflexes The neurologist usually evaluates the patient's reflexes concurrently with muscle strength. Reflexes are evaluated because nervous system damage may abolish, diminish, or exaggerate reflexes that normally are present and may cause the appearance of abnormal (pathologic) reflexes, which should not be present in adults. The neurologist evaluates both *superficial* and *deep* reflexes, comparing the presence and magnitude of reflexes on one side of the body to those on the other side. Like muscle strength, the presence and magnitude of reflexes usually is quantified with a rating scale. Table 2-2 gives an example of such a rating scale.

Superficial reflexes are elicited by stroking, touching, or brushing the surface of body parts. Normal superficial reflexes include the *gag reflex* (gagging or retching when the back of the tongue or the oropharynx is stimulated), the *swallow reflex* (initiation of swallowing when the back of the tongue and pharyngeal walls are stimulated), the *corneal reflex* (blinking when something lightly touches the cornea), and the *plantar flexor reflex* (bending downward of the toes when the sole of the foot is stroked). Pathologic, superficial reflexes include the *plantar extensor (Babinski) reflex,* the *palmar (grasp) reflex,* and the *sucking reflex.* The plantar extensor reflex is elicited by forcefully stroking the sole of the foot, at which time the toes bend upward and fan out, in contrast with the (normal) plantar flexor reflex, in which the toes bend downward and do not fan. The palmar (grasp) reflex is characterized by involuntary grasping of objects touching or stroking the hand. If the grasp reflex is strong, the patient may be unable to voluntarily release objects held in the affected hand (such as the neurologist's necktie). The sucking reflex consists of reflexive sucking movements elicited by touching or stroking the patient's lips. Pathologic superficial reflexes are sometimes called *primitive reflexes* in part because many of the reflexes are present in infants and disappear as the infant matures.

Deep reflexes (sometimes called *tendon reflexes*) are elicited by tapping or suddenly stretching muscles or tendons, which causes brief contraction of the muscle whose tendon is tapped or stretched. Perhaps the best known deep reflex is the *patellar reflex* or knee-jerk reflex, which is elicited by tapping the patellar tendon just below the kneecap. Deep reflexes may be *exaggerated, diminished,* or *absent* (a condition called *areflexia*).

Exaggerated reflexes, either alone or in combination with the appearance of pathologic reflexes, suggest damage in the upper motor neurons (corticobulbar and corticospinal tracts), which releases the reflexes from the inhibitory control ordinarily maintained by the cortex and midbrain structures. Diminished or absent reflexes suggest damage in the peripheral nervous system (lower motor neurons, sensory fibers, or the reflex arc itself).

Volitional Movements The neurologist also evaluates the *speed, accuracy,* and *coordination* of volitional movements (those carried out by the patient without assistance). *Slowness of volitional movements* can come from many sources. Common nervous system sources include lower motor neuron disease (weakness), upper motor neuron disease (spasticity), extrapyramidal disease (rigidity), and peripheral myopathy (weakness). Diminished *accuracy* of volitional movements (in the absence of deficits in strength or sensation that compromise movement accuracy) usually suggests damage in the extrapyramidal system or the cerebellum. Extrapyramidal damage, in addition to producing overall slowing of volitional movements, frequently produces involuntary movements called *dyskinesia.* These involuntary movements are superimposed on (and sometimes replace) volitional movements. The form of the involuntary movements often provides helpful clues regarding the part of the nervous system that has been damaged.

Tremor is a pattern of cyclic, small-amplitude involuntary movements primarily affecting the arms, legs, and head. Distal muscles (those farthest from the trunk) are more likely to exhibit tremor than proximal muscles (those nearest the trunk). Some tremor is present in normal muscles (called *benign* or *physiological* tremor) but is so slight that it is not usually noticeable. Pathologic tremor may appear in relaxed muscles *(resting tremor),* during certain postures *(postural tremor),* or only during movement *(intention tremor). Resting tremor* is a characteristic sign of Parkinson's disease. The tremor often begins in the hand or foot and over the years it gradually spreads to involve other muscle groups, which causes rhythmic flexion and extension of the fingers, hand, and/or foot. When the tremor affects the fingers, the thumb and fingers characteristically are flexed and the thumbtips rub against the fingertips, giving the tremor its characteristic *pill-rolling* quality.

Chorea (from the Greek word for "dance") refers to involuntary and unpredictable movements that are quick, sometimes forceful, and abrupt *(choreiform movements).* In mild cases, patients may appear persistently restless and their choreiform movements may resemble clumsy voluntary movements. (Some patients attempt to disguise the choreiform movements by incorporating them into voluntary movements. However, the strategy usually fails; the combination of voluntary and involuntary movements usually appears grotesque and exaggerated.) When the muscles of patients with chorea are at rest, they tend to be hypotonic, but muscle strength usually is normal. (However, sustained muscle contraction may be interrupted by involuntary movements, leading to a phenomenon called *milkmaid's grasp.*) *Ballism* (or *hemiballism* if it affects only one side of the body) is an extreme form of chorea. In ballism, the involuntary limb movements are violent, and the limbs are flung wildly about, sometimes creating danger for the patient's limbs and for anyone who may be standing or sitting nearby. Like other varieties of pathologic movements, choreiform movements disappear during sleep. Chorea often is a manifestation of hereditary neurologic disease but sometimes appears as a consequence of anoxia, brain hemorrhage, central nervous system intoxication, cerebrovascular disorders, or damage in the extrapyramidal system.

Athetosis (from a Greek word meaning "without position or place") refers to a condition in which resting muscle groups are disturbed by slow, writhing, sinuous movements. Athetosis is especially prominent in the proximal limb muscles and neck. The movements are involuntary and purposeless and often appear to flow from one muscle group to another. Athetoid movements are often associated with chorea, in which case the disorder may be called *choreoathetosis.* Athetosis may be caused by birth trauma or anoxia that produces pathology in the basal ganglia or extrapyramidal system.

Dystonia is a condition in which muscle groups (especially those in the limbs and neck) maintain abnormal, involuntary contractions or postures over long durations. Because the contractions persist and because they cause gross deformation, dystonia is sometimes called *torsion spasm.* In its less severe forms, dystonia may resemble athetosis, and the terms are sometimes used interchangeably. Dystonia often is inherited but also may occur in conjunction with acquired neurologic diseases. Dystonia sometimes occurs as a consequence of prolonged medication (or overmedication) with various psychoactive drugs (such as tranquilizers) or drugs for the control of Parkinson's disease (e.g., Levadopa).

In *myoclonus,* individual muscle groups contract sporadically and irregularly and in short bursts, causing abrupt, brief, twitching movements of the muscle. The contractions may range from nearly imperceptible movements of a single muscle group to overt movements involving multiple groups of muscles. Myoclonic movements typically are irregular in duration and rate and are most easily observed when the affected muscles are at rest. Myoclonus may be seen in epilepsy, dementia, and some cerebellar disorders and occasionally it occurs as the only symptom of nervous system disease.

Fasciculations are fine, rapid, irregular, twitching movements caused by contractions of groups of muscle fibers. The contractions are not large enough to cause overt limb, head, or facial movements but are observable as dimpling or rippling of the skin over the affected muscles. The presence of fasciculations, in combination with weakness and/or muscle atrophy, suggests damage in lower motor neurons (anterior horn cells in the spinal cord and cranial nerve nuclei in the brain stem). Isolated fasciculations may occur in normal persons and when they are not accompanied by muscle weakness or atrophy, they should not be regarded as a sign of nervous system pathology.

Fibrillations are contractions of a single muscle fiber or a small group of fibers. They are too small to be seen but are measurable with sensitive instruments. Fibrillations, like fasciculations, are signs of damage in lower motor neurons.

Tics (sometimes called *habit spasms*) are stereotypic, repetitive movements such as blinking, coughing, clearing the throat, or sniffing that appear when the individual is nervous or under stress. Tics can be volitionally inhibited, but when the individual's attention is no longer focused on the tic, they reappear. Tics have no known relationship to nervous system pathology.

Central nervous system pathology sometimes causes clumsiness or incoordination of volitional movements not caused by muscle weakness. These disruptions are called *ataxia* (from Greek words meaning "out of order"). Several forms of ataxia have been described in the neurology literature, but by far the most frequently occurring one is *cerebellar ataxia* (which is caused, not surprisingly, by cerebellar damage). Although the average speed and velocity of movements may be normal, acceleration at the beginning of movements is slowed, and braking at the end of movements lags, causing overshoot of the target. If the patient is asked to hold a limb in position against resistance provided by the neurologist, who abruptly removes the resistance, the ataxic patient characteristically is unable to relax the muscles quickly, and the limb swings uncontrollably in the direction of the previous resistance (the *rebound* phenomenon). Complex volitional movements or movements that require rapid changes in direction are the most obviously affected in ataxia, and complex movements may be broken down into a succession of small, individual movements with a jerky, segmented quality (called *decomposition of movement*). Rapid, alternating movements, such as alternately turning the hands palm up, then palm down, are slow and awkward and their range and force are distorted *(dysmetria)*. Volitional movements may be accompanied by a characteristic tremor, which appears as a rhythmic oscillation at a right angle to the direction of the movement.

Gait For patients who can stand and walk, observation of the patient's standing and walk-ing often provides screening information that may help the neurologist determine the nature and location of nervous system pathology. The patient is asked to stand, walk a short distance at a comfortable rate, turn and retrace his or her steps, then sit down. If the patient accomplishes this without appreciable difficulty, she or he may be asked to run, walk on the heels or the balls of the feet, or walk heel-to-toe along a straight path (a test that should be familiar to motor vehicle drivers stopped by law enforcement officers on suspicion of driving under the influence of alcohol or drugs). During these activities, the neurologist evaluates the patient's sitting, standing, and walking posture; the ease with which the patient moves between sitting and standing positions; the ease with which the patient starts and stops walking; stride length; walking rhythm; the rhythm and amplitude of arm and leg movements; the presence of involuntary movements; and the distance between the feet.

Patients with *unilateral corticospinal damage* (hemiplegia, severe hemiparesis) walk with what is called a *circumducted gait*—the patient tilts toward the nonaffected side and swings the paralyzed leg out and forward from the hip without flexing the knee (this movement is called *circumduction* of the leg). The patient's spastic arm is flexed and held close to the body. Patients with mild hemiparesis may swing the affected leg normally but drag the foot because of weakness in the muscles that lift the leg. (These patients often become regular customers at a shoe repair shop because the shoe on the affected side wears excessively.)

Patients with *lower motor neuron disease* or *peripheral myopathy* may have difficulty standing and maintaining erect posture if their leg and hip muscles are involved. If the muscles in the front of the lower leg are affected, the patient may exhibit *foot drop,* in which the toes and ball of the foot hang down as the foot is lifted, which leads the patient to lift his or her leg abnormally high to allow their toes to clear the ground *(steppage gait)*. (Patients with impaired position sense of the legs also may exhibit steppage gait. They lift their feet higher than necessary because they can't tell how far the foot is lifted. However, their toes don't dangle as they step.) The patient may exhibit *waddling gait,* if the trunk and hip muscles are involved, which is caused by tipping of the pelvis toward the non–weight-bearing side.

Patients with *extrapyramidal damage* may exhibit disruptions in sitting and standing posture and in walking because of the presence of dyskinesia. Patients with *chorea,* if they can walk at all, do so in irregular fashion; their progress is interrupted by sudden dipping and lurching produced by irregular and involuntary muscle contractions in their legs and trunk (sometimes called *dancing gait*). Patients with *athetosis* and some patients with *dystonia* may have difficulty maintaining erect posture because of slow, sinuous, and writhing movements of the arms and legs. (Patients with severe athetosis or dystonia usually cannot stand or walk unaided.) Patients with *Parkinson's disease* assume a stooped, forward-leaning posture on standing and when asked to walk they may experience difficulty starting and stopping. The patient typically shuffles for a few steps, before making more normal, but still shortened strides. Occasionally the patient's steps become very short and rapid, until he or she is nearly running in tiny shuffling steps (called *festinating gait*).

Patients who have *cerebellar disease* and can walk typically do so with a broad-based stance while keeping their feet wide apart. Their steps are clumsy and irregular in both length and rhythm, they lurch from side-to-side, they turn with difficulty, and they have a tendency to fall to one side. Walking heel-to-toe is extremely difficult and usually impossible for these patients. (Because the clumsy, staggering gait of patients with cerebellar disease resembles that of intoxicated people, they are sometimes mistakenly thought to be intoxicated by those they meet in public.)

Somesthetic Sensation

History and Current Complaints Patients with pathology in the system serving somesthetic (bodily) sensation may complain of *pain, numbness,* or *abnormal sensations.* Of the three complaints, pain usually poses the most difficult diagnostic problem. Pain is one of the body's responses to tissue damage. It is an important symptom in many diseases (not only those involving the nervous system). However, not all pain is a sign of disease and not all pain is a consequence of tissue damage (e.g., the pain associated with muscle cramps, intestinal "gas" pains, and most headaches). The patient's history usually provides the neurologist with clues to the cause of the pain, and the neurologic examination defines the extent to which the pain is caused by nervous system involvement. Knowing what relieves or exacerbates the pain may help the neurologist determine its source. When pain is exacerbated with movement or effort or if pain changes with changes in posture, its source may be mechanical (compression of nerves, inflammation of joints). If the pain is unaffected by movement, effort, or posture, its source may be inflammation of peripheral nerves or lesions affecting sensory pathways in the central nervous system.

Other kinds of unusual sensations also give the neurologist clues to the location and nature of nervous system pathology. Numbness or loss of sensitivity usually point to damage in cranial nerves, spinal nerves, or sensory nerve fiber tracts. Abnormal sensitivity to stimulation (called *hyperesthesia*) or abnormal sensations in the absence of stimulation (e.g., tingling or burning, called *paresthesia*) suggest a disturbance in the peripheral nerves or central sensory pathways. Sensory loss in an entire limb or on one side of the body suggests damage in ascending spinal cord tracts or the sensory cortex (complete loss is called *anesthesia,* partial loss is called *hypesthesia*). Patterns of sensory loss that are inconsistent with what the neurologist knows about the sensory system may suggest a functional rather than an organic cause.

Examination Armed with information from the history, the neurologist proceeds to objective examination of the patient's somatic (body) sensation. Sensory abnormalities may affect *deep sensation* (from the muscles, tendons, and joints), *superficial sensation* (from the skin), or both. *Deep sensation* includes (1) *joint sense* (the ability to tell the position of the limbs without seeing them), (2) *deep pain sensation* from muscles, tendons, and joints, and (3) *sensitivity to vibration*. *Superficial sensation* includes the perception of *light touch, superficial pain* (pinprick), and *temperature*. Evaluation of these three categories of sensation is useful in diagnosing pathology affecting the spinal cord. The categories of sensations affected by spinal cord pathology and the parts of the body exhibiting sensory disruption permit the neurologist to predict the level within the spinal cord at which the pathology exists (spinal cord lesions typically produce sensory deficits below the level of the lesion). They also allow the neurologist to predict if the lesion affects the front, back, middle or sides of the spinal cord.

Diminished *deep sensation* (for position and vibration) implicates the posterior sensory tracts in the spinal cord or large sensory fibers in peripheral nerves on the same side as the diminished sensitivity. However, some deep pain sensation (but not joint sense or vibratory sense) is carried by fibers in the anterior spinal cord. Consequently, impaired sensitivity to deep pain with preserved joint sense and vibration sensitivity suggests damage in the anterior spinal cord.

Superficial sensation (light touch, pinprick, and temperature) is carried by sensory tracts in the anterolateral spinal cord. Consequently, impairment of all superficial sensation suggests damage in the lateral spinal cord. However, some fibers conveying light touch sensation to the sensory cortex also ascend in posterior sensory tracts on the same side as the peripheral sensory receptors, and in anterior tracts contralateral to the sensory receptors. Consequently, diminished sensitivity to light touch and preservation of sensitivity to pinprick and temperature suggest involvement of either the posterior tract on the side of the lesion or the anterior tract, contralateral to the lesion.

Regional loss of superficial sensation, rather than loss on one side of the body or loss below a given level of the spinal cord, suggests damage either in cranial or spinal nerves. Knowing the usual distribution of sensory regions for the cranial and spinal nerves (the regions are called *dermatomes*) helps the neurologist decide which cranial or spinal nerves are affected (Figure 2-5). When the area of sensory impairment matches the dermatome for a cranial nerve or spinal nerve, the neurologist can, with considerable confidence, conclude that the patient's neuropathology involves that cranial nerve or spinal nerve.

Double simultaneous stimulation sometimes is used to detect slight impairments in sensory function. In double simultaneous stimulation, two symmetrical points on the body are simultaneously touched. If the patient's sensory function is diminished on one side, the patient reports only the stimulation on the less impaired side. Inability to detect the stimulus on the impaired side during double simultaneous stimulation is called *extinction* and is associated with cortical lesions.

Some patients lose the ability to identify objects by touch and palpation even though their ability to report superficial sensation is unimpaired. They report light touch and pinprick without error yet cannot identify common objects (such as a comb or a key) when the objects are placed, out of sight, in either hand. Problems in *recognition* of objects by touch is called *astereognosis*. Patients with damage in the sensory cortex of the parietal lobe or adjacent regions often exhibit astereognosis.

Equilibrium

History and Current Complaints Patients with impairments of *equilibrium* usually complain of feeling dizzy or light-headed or report

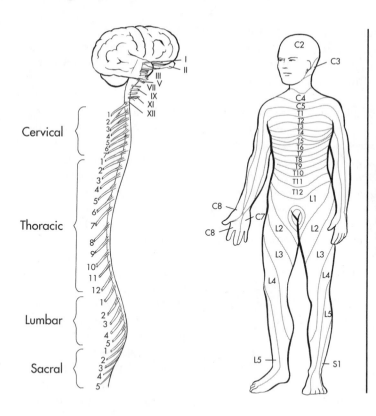

Figure 2-5 ■ **The pattern of skin sensation on the human body as it relates to cranial nerves and spinal nerves. Each cranial nerve and spinal nerve serves a specific region (these regions are called *dermatomes*).**

subjective illusions of movement or changes in position. When a patient complains of *dizziness,* the neurologist is likely to ask questions to find out what, exactly, the patient means by "dizziness." Some patients may be referring to *vertigo*—the sensation that the body or the environment are moving (usually rotating) when in fact they are not. Vertigo usually is caused by problems in the inner ear, the vestibular branch of the acoustic nerve (CN 8), or the brain stem. The presence of persisting or recurring vertigo may suggest involvement of the vestibular system or, less frequently, the brain stem and/or cerebellum. Severe vertigo with sudden onset often is a result of vascular problems in the brain stem or cerebellum. Episodic vertigo may be a result of transient insufficiency of cerebral blood flow or Meniere's disease (increased pressure in inner ear structures that play a role in equilibrium). Progressive vertigo may be a result of toxi-

city, some vitamin deficiencies, or degenerative neurologic disease. Attacks of true vertigo are most often accompanied by nausea, vomiting, pallor, and sweating, and any head movement increases the severity of the attack. Some patients may complain of light-headedness, faintness, or giddiness. Such sensations sometimes are experienced by normal, healthy individuals, in which case they may be related to anxiety, hyperventilation, sudden changes in head position, or other transitory conditions. Most patients with true vertigo quickly learn that they must remain immobile during an attack.

Examination The neurologist is likely to pay particular attention to the parts of the neurologic examination in which the patient's *stance, gait,* and *nystagmus* are evaluated. Examination of motor function may also contribute information concerning the source of the patient's problems with equilibrium.

Patients with disequilibrium typically stand with their feet wide apart. When these patients are asked to stand with their feet together, they customarily are reluctant to do so and may be unwilling or unable to bring their feet completely together. Patients whose disequilibrium is caused by loss of proprioceptive feedback from the legs and feet usually can compensate for the loss by relying on visual input to maintain balance. When these patients close their eyes, they become increasingly unsteady and may fall *(Romberg's sign)*. Patients whose disequilibrium is caused by cerebellar pathology are unsteady with eyes open or closed, although the unsteadiness is worse with eyes closed.

Patients with disequilibrium typically walk with a wide-based gait. When a patient's disequilibrium is caused by loss of proprioceptive feedback, he or she is likely to walk with *steppage gait* (see pp. 56-57). Patients with vestibular disease and loss of proprioceptive feedback usually walk better when provided support (a cane or the examiner's arm), and patients with either disease do much worse when walking in the dark or with eyes closed. Asking patients with disequilibrium to walk with feet close together or heel-to-toe along a straight line always exaggerates their symptoms.

Nystagmus (abnormal and involuntary oscillation of the eyes, either at rest or when tracking a visual target) is commonly seen in patients with vestibular disorders and is sometimes seen in patients with cerebellar pathology. *Caloric testing,* in which cold and/or warm water is introduced into the ear canal, often produces characteristic patterns of nystagmus in patients with vestibular pathology. The relationships between the nature of a patient's nystagmus and the nervous system pathology that causes it are too complex to be dealt with here, but these relationships often point directly to the site of the patient's nervous system pathology. The reader who wishes to know about these relationships can find them described in any contemporary neurology textbook.

Consciousness and Mentation

History and Current Complaints Changes in consciousness or mentation may be caused by a great variety of diseases and pathologic states. In general, changes in mentation or consciousness are attributed to the brain hemispheres and, to a somewhat lesser extent, the brain stem. Such changes may be experienced by patients with cerebrovascular disease, head injury, alcohol or drug ingestion, central nervous system infections, brain tumors, brain abscesses, metabolic disturbances, nutritional deficiencies, dementing illness, and several other diseases and conditions. When a patient experiences changes in mentation or consciousness, the neurologist is likely to be concerned with determining if the changes represent one of the following categories.

- *Confusion* (often called *acute confusional state*). Confused patients usually exhibit normal or slightly lowered overall levels of consciousness but are grossly impaired in their orientation to the environment (where they are, what day it is, and so on), have diminished attention span and memory, and cannot think clearly. Acute confusional states usually are transitory, but sometimes (e.g., following stroke), an initial period of confusion may evolve to a more circumscribed, but longer-lasting syndrome (e.g., aphasia).

- *Lethargy* or *somnolence.* Lethargic or somnolent patients are drowsy, fall asleep at inappropriate times, sleep longer than usual, and are difficult to awaken. These states sometimes are transitory and separated by periods of normal alertness and attention or they may be progressive, ending in coma and death.

- *Amnesia.* Amnesia is complete loss of memory for a limited interval. Amnesic patients usually are aware of and distressed by the missing memories. Amnesic states are often present in psychiatric illness and are a frequent consequence of traumatic brain injury.

Confusional states, lethargy, and amnesia come from a variety of causes, including drug and alcohol intoxication or withdrawal, endocrine disturbances, nutritional disorders, infections, cerebrovascular disorders, head trauma, and psychiatric illness.

- *Syncope.* Syncope (fainting spells) denotes transitory loss of consciousness caused by briefly reduced blood supply to the brain. Syncopal episodes usually are accompanied by autonomic irregularities—rapid respiration, rapid and feeble pulse, pallor, perspiration, and cold, clammy skin. Syncope may be caused by diminished cardiac output, abnormally low blood pressure, dehydration, drugs, or stress and anxiety.
- *Fugue state.* Fugue state is a temporary disturbance of consciousness, lasting from a few minutes to several days. During this time, the patient engages in normal activities of daily life. However, the patient does not later remember the events or activities that took place during the fugue state. Fugue states are seen in combination with psychiatric illness and (rarely) as a consequence of epilepsy.

Although *epileptic seizures* include loss of consciousness, they are more dramatic and somewhat better understood and their diagnosis is somewhat more straightforward than the changes in consciousness and mentation described previously. Seizures are caused by abnormal patterns of neuronal discharge in the brain. These discharges interfere with normal brain activity and may cause periods of depressed mental function, confusion, uncontrollable muscle contraction and relaxation, and usually, loss of consciousness.

If a patient reports a history of seizures, the neurologist will be interested in how frequently they occur, how long they typically last, what kinds of events precipitate them, whether disturbances of sensation or mentation *(aura)* precede them, and what the patient's mental and physical state was following the seizures.

Seizures usually suggest damage in the brain hemispheres. Seizures may also be caused by alcohol or drug withdrawal, central nervous system infections, hypoglycemia (abnormally low blood sugar), and several other diseases. Seizure-like phenomena sometimes occur as a consequence of psychiatric conditions *(pseudoseizures).*

Seizures have been divided into two major categories, reflecting differences in what happens to the patient during the seizure:

- *Generalized seizures* are seizures in which the patient loses consciousness. In *gran mal* seizures, sometimes called *convulsions,* there is massive discharge of neurons in the brain, causing contraction of almost all the muscles of the body, followed by a series of intermittent *clonic* jerks. Gran mal seizures last from 1 minute to 3 minutes on the average and are never remembered by the patient (perhaps because they lose consciousness). In *absence* seizures (formerly called *petit mal* seizures), the loss of consciousness lasts only a few seconds, and the patient usually does not fall. The patient may stare, stop moving and talking, drop things, and/or move the head and limbs aimlessly and involuntarily.
- *Partial seizures* (sometimes called *focal seizures*) are seizures in which there is localized discharge of neurons in the brain, with the pattern of discharge varying widely across patients. The patient who experiences a partial seizure usually experiences clonic movements of individual muscle groups but does not lose consciousness, although typically there is some clouding of consciousness and disruption of mental activity. Partial seizures may last from a few seconds to several minutes or even (rarely) hours. The magnitude of the seizure activity is related to how much of the brain is involved in the abnormal patterns of neuronal discharge. Partial seizures suggest localized areas of discharge, and generalized seizures suggest that major portions of both brain hemispheres are involved.

Examination The breadth and amount of detail in the neurologist's mental status examination is likely to vary, depending on the neurologist's interests and orientation as well as on the degree to which the patient's mental functioning appears compromised. Standard neurologic examinations usually provide for rudimentary (screening) assessment of the patient's level of consciousness, attention and concentration, orientation and memory, mood and behavior, thought content, and language and speech.

In a screening examination of mental status the patients' *level of consciousness* typically is described in terms of their general level of arousal (awake and alert, lethargic, somnolent, stuporous, or comatose) and their responsiveness to stimulation (whether they are responsive and appropriate, responsive and inappropriate, or unresponsive). The patients' level of *attention and concentration* typically is described in terms of their ability to complete tasks requiring low levels of sustained and focused mental effort, such as counting backward or reciting the alphabet backward. The patients' *orientation* typically is described in terms of their ability to answer questions about themselves *(person),* where they are *(place),* and what day, date, and time it is *(time).* (If the patient is considered oriented to person, place, and time, the neurologist's report may describe him or her as "oriented X3".) The patients' *mood and behavior* typically are described in terms of their nature (e.g., apathetic, elated, depressed) and stability (stable vs. variable). The *patient's thought content* is described in terms of its appropriateness and rationality and whether hallucinations or delusions are present. The patient's *memory* typically is assessed by asking the patient to remember and recall short lists of numbers or words. The patient's *language and speech* typically are assessed by asking the patient to carry out simple spoken commands, to repeat words and phrases, to name pictures or objects, to read words and sentences, and to write words and short sentences.

Several more or less standardized screening tests of mental status have been published. One of the most widely used by neurologists is the *Mini Mental State Examination* (MMSE; Folstein, Folstein, & McHugh; 1975). The MMSE takes from 5 minutes to 10 minutes to administer and contains 11 items to screen orientation, attention, naming, repetition, comprehension, writing, and copying (Table 2-3). Normal adults typically score from 25 to 30 points (of a possible 30 points). Scores below 25 usually are considered an indication of compromised mental status.

■ LABORATORY TESTS

Laboratory tests provide information about the patient that cannot be obtained from the interview and physical examination. In addition to standard laboratory tests, such as analysis of blood and urine, the neurologist may order special tests to aid in the diagnosis of the patient's neurologic disorder.

Radiologic Studies

In *radiologic studies,* x-rays are passed through body tissues onto a sheet of photographic film to create a negative image of internal structures. The x-rays easily pass through low-density tissues but are blocked by dense tissues such as bone. Consequently, low-density tissues appear as dark areas on the x-ray plate, and higher-density tissues appear as lighter images. Sometimes fluid containing a substance that blocks x-rays *(radio-opaque* fluid called *contrast medium)* may be injected into structures that ordinarily would not appear on an x-ray, such as veins or arteries. The images obtained from such tests are said to be *contrast enhanced.*

Standard x-rays of the skull, spine, or both may provide useful information regarding the probable causes of a patient's symptoms. X-rays of the skull (skull films) may show fractures, abnormal deposits, or abnormal calcification of structures within the skull (Figure 2-6). X-rays of the spine (spine films) may provide evidence of

The Mini Mental State Examination

Item	Points
Orientation	
What is today's date?	1 point
What is the year?	1 point
What is the month?	1 point
What day is today?	1 point
What season is it right now?	1 point
What is the name of this hospital (clinic)?	1 point
What floor are we on?	1 point
What city (town) are we in?	1 point
What county are we in?	1 point
What state are we in?	1 point

Immediate Recall

I'm going to say three words. Say them after me and try to remember them. (Repeat if necessary until patient can say them. Record number of trials: _____)   *1 point for each word correct*

Baby	Daughter	Village	Ball	Apple
Garden	River	Heaven	Flag	Penny
Leader	Table	Finger	Tree	Table

Attention and Calculation (give one of the following two)

Count backwards from 100 by 7s.
100 93 86 79 72 65   *1 point for each number correct (up to 5)*

Or: I'm going to say a word, and I want you to spell it backwards. Spell **world** backward.
D L R O W   *1 point for each correct letter until first wrong letter*

Recall

What were the three words that I asked you to remember?   *1 point for each correct item*

Language

Name pencil, watch.   *1 point for each correct name*

Repeat after me: "No ifs, ands, or buts."   *1 point for completely correct repetition*

Comprehension. Give the patient a sheet of paper: [Take the paper in your right hand], [fold it in half], and [put it on your lap].   *1 point for each bracketed segment*

Read and do the following: Close your eyes (printed).   *1 point*

Write a sentence.   *1 point for any grammatical sentence*

Copy: *1 point for correct copy*

Modified From Folstein, Folstein and McHugh, 1975.
Total Score: (maximum = 30 points)

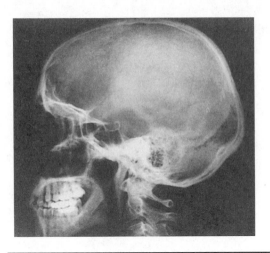

Figure 2-6 ▪ An x-ray image of a normal adult skull. (From Ballinger PW: *Merrill's atlas of radiographic positions and radiologic procedures,* ed 8, vol 2, St. Louis, 1991, Mosby.)

congenital deformities, fractures, displacement of intervertebral discs, degenerative changes, or tumors involving the verterbrae and spinal cord.

Cerebral angiography (or *cerebral arteriography*) is a method by which the veins and arteries of the brain and brain stem can be visualized (Figure 2–7). In this procedure, a contrast medium is injected into one of the arteries that supply blood to the brain (usually a carotid artery, but occasionally a vertebral artery), and a sequence of x-rays of the head is taken. The contrast medium fills the injected artery and its branches and eventually makes its way into the cerebral veins so that when the sequential x-ray plates are developed one can visualize the circulation through the larger cerebral vessels. (Angiograms do not show the smallest vessels.)

Angiograms are useful in detecting occlusions of arteries or their branches, because occluded vessels do not fill with contrast medium and are not visible on angiography. Blood vessels that are narrowed but not occluded (a condition called *stenosis*) fill slowly. Slow filling of vessels is detected by evaluating the progress of the contrast medium through the blood vessels from the beginning to the end of the x-ray plates. Angiography may show the presence of space-occupying lesions, such as tumors or abscesses, if the lesion displaces cerebral blood vessels from their customary locations. A recently developed procedure, called *digital-subtraction* angiography, provides improved image quality while lessening the amount of contrast medium that must be injected into the vascular system. This is accomplished by a computer-averaging technique, in which the signals from nonvascular structures are deleted from the image, yielding an enhanced image of vascular structures.

Myelograms, like arteriograms, involve injection of radio-opaque fluid into the central nervous system, but in myelography the fluid is injected into the subarachnoid space around the spinal cord. After the fluid is injected, one or more x-rays of the spine are taken. Myelograms permit visualization of the subarachnoid space surrounding the spinal cord and permit indirect visualization of the spinal cord and spinal nerves, which are silhouetted against the contrast medium. Myelograms are useful in diagnosing spinal cord or spinal nerve compression, structural abnormalities of the spine, and tumors or deformities of the spinal cord or spinal nerve roots. However, CT or MRI scanning of the spine often provides a simpler and less invasive procedure for obtaining the information provided by myelography.

Computed tomography (also called *CT scanning* or *CAT scanning,* for *computed axial tomography*), makes use of a computer to process and analyze information. In CT scanning the patient is placed in the center of a circular arrangement of x-ray generators and detectors, which rotate axially around the patient. X-rays pass through the parts of the patient's body being scanned and are picked up by detectors on the other side of the circle. The signals from the detectors are passed on to a computer that analyzes them and generates photograph-like

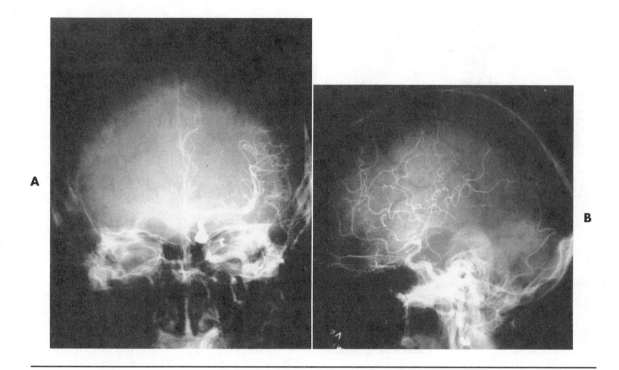

Figure 2-7 ▪ A normal cerebral angiogram. (A) The image is taken from the front. The anterior cerebral artery proceeds upward on the midline, and the middle cerebral artery proceeds laterally and upward on the right side of the image. (B) The image is taken from the side. The middle cerebral artery and portions of the posterior cerebral artery can be seen. The carotid artery is visible in both illustrations.

images that represent cross-sections of the body (Figure 2-8). The scanner moves up or down the body in regular steps so that a series of images representing consecutive layers or "slices" of the body are obtained.

The combination of a narrow beam of x-rays, sensitive detectors, and computer enhancement of signals permit visualization of soft tissues not visible on standard x-rays. In many instances CT scanning has replaced other tests because it provides better visualization of internal structures with less risk to the patient. The primary drawback of CT scanning is that it exposes the patient to radiation. Consequently, CT scans are not a routine part of the neurologic examination. Within the past decade several

imaging procedures that do not require that the patient be exposed to radiation have been developed.

Nonradiologic Imaging Studies *B-mode carotid imaging* (sometimes called *echo arteriography*) is a noninvasive technique for visualizing superficial (extracranial) blood vessels with ultrasound. It is frequently used to study the carotid arteries in the neck. A transducer that emits high-frequency sound waves is placed against the neck over the carotid artery. The sound waves are transmitted into the neck, where some are reflected back, depending on the acoustic absorption characteristics of the tissues beneath the transmitter. A detector picks up the reflected sound waves and a computer

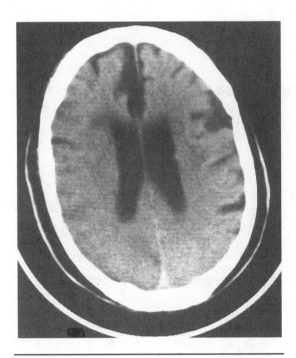

Figure 2-8 ■ A CT scan of a patient with a long history of neurologic problems. The lateral ventricles (butterfly shaped dark areas in center) are enlarged and the sulci are widened, suggesting atrophy of brain tissues. Dark areas in the anterior left hemisphere near the midline and in the lateral aspect of the right frontal lobe suggest regions of tissue destruction, probably by strokes.

analyzes the variations in the waves and generates an image of the tissues scanned. Echo arteriograms are most useful for detecting stenosis or ulceration in the carotid arteries, although they cannot reliably differentiate between severe stenosis and complete occlusion.

Transcranial Doppler ultrasound is an experimental, noninvasive technique for measuring blood pressure and flow in the cerebral arteries. High-frequency sound waves are transmitted into the head by a probe attached to a computer. The computer manipulates the characteristics of the sound waves in order to target

a particular blood vessel. If the blood within the vessel is moving, the frequency of the reflected sound waves is altered in a predictable way (the *Doppler effect*).* A detector picks up the reflected sound waves and passes them to the computer. The computer analyzes changes in the frequency of the reflected waves (the Doppler effect) and generates a graphic image representing blood pressure and flow within the artery.

Magnetic Resonance Imaging (MRI) is a recently developed technique that generates photograph-like images that look somewhat like the images generated by CT scans. However, MRI scanning has two important advantages over CT scanning; it does not expose the patient to radiation and it usually provides images with greater detail than those from CT scanning. Magnetic resonance imaging operates on the principle that the nuclei of hydrogen atoms behave somewhat like small bar magnets; if they are placed in a strong magnetic field, they orient themselves in the same direction and in line with the magnetic field. In MRI the body part to be imaged is placed within such a magnetic field. Then, when the hydrogen nuclei in the body tissues have all aligned themselves with the magnetic field, a short pulse of electromagnetic energy is introduced into the field, causing the hydrogen nuclei to be momentarily deflected from alignment. As the nuclei swing back into alignment with the magnetic field, they emit tiny electromagnetic signals. A set of detectors measures these signals and sends them to a computer, which constructs a photograph-like image from the signals (Figure 2-9). In MRI scanning, as in CT scanning, the detec-

---

* The Doppler effect is experienced in everyday life when a rapidly-moving vehicle with horn or siren blaring passes a bystander. As the vehicle passes by, the pitch of the sound made by the horn or siren drops. This happens because the movement of the vehicle away from the listener adds to the distance between the cycles of the sound wave, lowering its frequency.

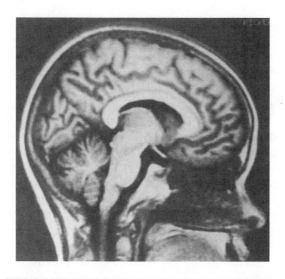

Figure 2-9 ▪ A magnetic resonance image (MRI) of the head. This image shows a vertical "slice" at the midline of the brain. The brain hemisphere, cerebellum, corpus callosum, and brain stem are clearly visible. (From Oldendorf W, Oldendorf W, Jr: *MRI primer,* Philadelphia, 1991, Lippencott-Raven Publishers.)

tors are moved in steps along the axis of the body to yield images representing consecutive layers or "slices" of the body parts scanned. MRI is sensitive to differences in the chemical composition of tissues, whereas CT scanning is sensitive to differences in the density of tissues. For this reason, MRI can show differences between tissues that have similar density but different chemical composition, such as gray matter and white matter in the brain (differences that cannot be seen in CT scans). MRI scanning is superior to CT scanning for imaging the temporal lobes, brain stem, cerebellum, and spinal cord, and for detecting arteriovenous malformations and aneurysms. As mentioned previously, MRI requires no radiation, and so far there is no evidence that the magnetic fields used in MRI are a risk to patients. However, MRI cannot be used when patients have metal (pins, plates, pacemakers) in their body because of the magnetic

field. MRI scans take a long time, and the patient must remain motionless in a noisy, confining space, sometimes leading to claustrophobia and blurring of the MRI image because of patient movement *(movement artifacts).*

Regional cerebral blood flow measurement (rCBF) is a procedure for estimating blood flow in various brain regions. Because cerebral blood flow and cerebral metabolism usually are related, rCBF provides indirect estimates of regional cerebral metabolism rather than static images of structures. rCBF can be measured in several ways, most of which require introduction of compounds that emit small amounts of radioactivity into the blood, either directly by injection of a liquid or indirectly by having the patient breathe air containing small amounts of a slightly radioactive gas, which is eventually absorbed into the blood. When the radioactive element reaches the brain, specialized scanners detect the subatomic particles (photons, posi-trons) emitted by the radioactive element, convert these events into electrical signals, and send the signals to a computer, which analyzes them and generates an image representing the blood flow in various brain regions. rCBF studies are useful in detecting vasospasm following hemorrhages and can provide information about compensatory blood flow in patients with documented cerebrovascular lesions.

Positron Emission Tomography (PET) also measures the metabolic activity of regions of the brain. The patient is given a solution of metabolically active material (usually glucose) tagged with a positron-emitting isotope (oxygen, fluorine, carbon, or nitrogen). The glucose eventually makes its way to the brain, where it is metabolized. The glucose and the isotope concentrate at areas of high metabolism (which are the areas of greatest neural activity and greatest blood flow). The positrons emitted by the isotope are picked up by a set of detectors and the signals are amplified and sent to a computer, which processes them to generate an image representing the regional metabolic activity of the brain (Figure 2-10). PET scanning is at this time primarily a research tool. PET scans are expensive (the scanning facility needs a cyclotron together with physicists and chemists to prepare the isotope) and are currently found only in large institutions—usually those with large medical research operations. PET scans can provide estimates of regional cerebral blood flow and may also permit visualization of hypofunction in brain regions in which blood flow is not compromised and in which no structural damage is visible on standard CT scans (Metter and associates 1984; Metter and associates 1983).

Electrophysiologic Studies Several diagnostic procedures yield recordings of the electrical activity in various parts of the nervous system. In these procedures, arrays of electrodes

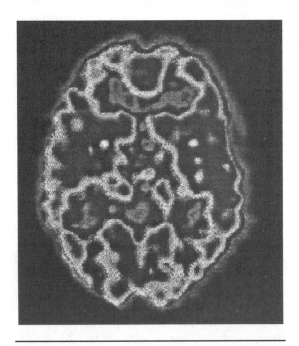

Figure 2-10 ■ A positron-emission tomography (PET) scan of a normal adult's brain in a resting state. Variations in shading represent different levels of metabolic activity. The images generated by PET scanners are in color, and different colors represent different levels of metabolic activity.

are placed at strategic locations to monitor the electrical activity in adjacent tissue. This low-voltage activity is amplified and sent to a recording device (usually a pen on a moving strip of graph paper), which generates a visual representation of the activity.

The *electroencephalogram* (EEG) yields a graphic record of the electrical activity of the cerebral cortex. It is obtained by placing an array of recording electrodes on the scalp. The electrodes detect the tiny electrical signals generated by the brain cortex. These signals are amplified until they are capable of operating pens that write the signals out on a moving strip of paper. The activity from a number of electrodes is traced on the paper, so that tracings of the electrical activity at several cortical locations (usually 16) are obtained. The amplitude and pattern of the waveforms in the tracings, together with the location of anomalous patterns of activity, permit the neurologist to make inferences about what is happening physiologically in the patient's brain. Localized brain lesions often cause *focal disturbances* in the EEG record in the vicinity of the lesion. The disturbance usually takes the form of aberrations in rhythm and amplitude (Figure 2-11). General disturbances of brain function usually cause general abnormalities in the EEG record across all recording sites (Figure 2-11). EEG recording is particularly useful for detecting and localizing seizure activity. In some cases, the EEG may help to distinguish between cortical and subcortical lesions in patients with overt neurologic signs of stroke. (If the EEG record from a stroke patient is normal, the stroke is likely to be subcortical; if the EEG is abnormal the stroke is likely to be cortical.) When a patient is in deep coma, EEG recordings may be used to estimate the severity of brain injury and predict whether or not the patient will return to consciousness.

An adaptation of EEG recording is *measurement of evoked cortical potentials* (also called *evoked response testing*). When evoked cortical potentials are measured the patient is placed in a quiet, dark room with recording electrodes on her or his scalp. When the patient's EEG has stabilized, tactile, auditory, or visual stimuli are presented, and the electrical activity of the cortex is measured from the electrodes. The signals from the electrodes are averaged by a computer across several stimulations. The computer calculates the cortical activity occurring at each of many time intervals following each stimulus. Changes in activity that regularly follow each stimulus are added together, and irregular (random) changes are ignored. A graphic printout of the averaged waveform attributable to stimulation is then generated. Alterations of computed waveforms for the *visual evoked response* (generated by visual stimulation), *brainstem evoked response* (generated by auditory stimulation), and *somatosensory evoked response* (generated by weak electrical stimulation of peripheral sensory nerves) suggest damage to the central nervous system conduction pathways serving those sensory modalities—damage that may not be detectable by clinical neurologic examination.

In *electromyography* fine needle electrodes are inserted into muscles to record their electrical activity. Relaxed muscles normally produce no spontaneous electrical activity, but when the muscles contract they produce bursts of electrical activity that are fairly predictable in terms of their amplitude, frequency, duration, and pattern. Spontaneous discharges in resting muscles (fibrillations, fasciculations) may indicate peripheral nerve disease. Other variations in amplitude, frequency, duration, or pattern may indicate disease in anterior horn cells, neuromuscular junctions, or the muscles themselves.

Nerve conduction studies are performed when peripheral neuropathy is suspected. In nerve conduction studies a nerve fiber (either

| R = right | F = frontal | P = parietal | AT = anterior temporal | T = temporal |
| L = left | O = occipital | Pc = precentral | Pf = posterior frontal | E = ear |

Calibration: 50 microvolts (vertical) and 1 second (horizontal).

Normal Adult

Petit Mal Epilepsy. This 6-year-old boy had one of his "blank spells," in which he was transiently unaware of surroundings and blinked his eyelids, during the recording.

Figure 2-11 ▪ Examples of normal and abnormal EEGs. On the left is a recording from an adult with no EEG abnormalities. On the right is a recording from a patient with petit mal epilepsy, showing general disruption of cortical activity. (From Waxman S: *Correlative neuroanatomy, ed 23,* Stanford, Conn., 1996, Appleton & Lange.)

motor or sensory) is stimulated at one point and the response is measured at another point along the fiber. The time between the stimulation and the response is called the *nerve conduction velocity.* Variations in nerve conduction velocities sometimes are helpful in diagnosing the nature and extent of peripheral nerve damage.

Tests Involving Analysis of Body Tissue or Fluids In some cases, an adequate diagnosis cannot be made on the basis of the history, neurologic examination, and laboratory tests alone, and more invasive (and potentially dangerous) tests must be carried out. These tests involve removal of a sample of tissue or fluids and laboratory analysis of the sample.

A *lumbar puncture* (sometimes called *spinal tap*) may be performed if the neurologist suspects infection or hemorrhage in the patient's central nervous system. In a spinal tap, a hypodermic needle is inserted between the vertebrae in the lower spine, below the level of the spinal cord, and a sample of cerebrospinal fluid is taken for analysis. When the needle is inserted, the pressure with which the fluid flows into the syringe is measured. (Increased pressure may suggest blockage in the circulation of CSF, the presence of space-occupying pathology such as a tumor or abscess, or swelling of brain tissue.) The CSF is analyzed for the presence of cells, bacteria, parasites, or viruses and its chemical composition is determined, including the amount of glucose and protein in the fluid. The presence of red blood cells or a yellowish color *(xanthochromia)* are signs of bleeding into the ventricles, meningeal spaces, or spinal cord. The presence of bacteria, parasites, or viruses proves infection with those agents. Increased protein content may suggest meningeal inflammation, a tumor, or obstructions within the spinal canal. CSF glucose levels often are lowered by infections.

Biopsies (removal of a sample of tissue for laboratory analysis) may be performed when less invasive procedures do not yield a definite diagnosis. Most biopsies of nervous system tissue are *needle biopsies* (sometimes called *aspiration biopsies*), in which a hollow needle is inserted into the tissue of interest and a small amount of tissue is removed by applying suction to the needle. Sometimes *open biopsies,* in which samples of tissue are surgically excised, may be performed when the tissue is readily accessible to the surgeon's scalpel. *Biopsy of brain tissue* sometimes is ordered to determine the nature of brain tumors, to identify the nature of infectious agents (as in brain abscess), or to permit diagnosis of certain degenerative diseases. *Muscle biopsy* may be ordered to determine if muscle weakness is caused by neuropathy or by disease of the muscle itself. *Biopsy of nerve tissue* may occasionally be ordered to determine the underlying nature of peripheral neurologic disease. Biopsy of an artery may be ordered to identify inflammatory or degenerative diseases involving the arterial system. Biopsies are among the least requested laboratory tests ordered by neurologists and are ordered only when less invasive procedures have failed to yield a diagnosis.

■ RECORDING THE RESULTS OF THE NEUROLOGIC EXAMINATION

The neurologist records the results of the neurologic examination in the patient's medical record, where it usually is the first entry in the daily record of the patient's care. The neurologist's report of the examination usually ends with a *problem list,* in which the patient's current significant medical problems are recorded. The neurologist's report of the neurologic examination almost always provides important information for others involved in the patient's care.

■ KEY CONCEPTS

- The neurologist establishes a diagnosis, arrives at a prognosis, and decides on a plan of treatment based on information obtained from an interview with the patient, a physical and neurologic examination, and the results of laboratory tests.

- During her or his examination of the patient, the neurologist explores the patient's family history, medical history, and current complaints. The neurologist also tests the patient's sensory and motor functions and assesses the patient's basic cognitive and mental status.

- The neurologist supplements the information obtained during her or his examination of the patient with information from laboratory tests. The results of imaging studies, such as CT scans, MRI scans, or angiography often play an important part in determining the causes of the patient's symptoms and signs.

- The neurologist summarizes the results of the interview, physical examination, and neurologic examination, together with diagnoses and a plan of care, in the patient's medical record.

Assessing Adults Who Have Neurogenic Communication Impairments

Novice clinicians can be intimidated by the complexity of neurogenic communication disorders and the seeming impossibility of making sense of a sometimes bewildering array of signs and symptoms.* Watching a skilled speech-language pathologist evaluate a patient who has a neurogenic communication disorder can be a mystifying experience for the novice. They watch the speech-language pathologist take the patient through an array of tests, which share no discernable common purpose, terminate some tests before completion, modify others without apparent reason, improvise new tests on the spot, and eventually arrive at a diagnosis of the patient's communication disorder, offer a prognosis, and decide about the advisability and nature of treatment.

The skilled clinician's idiosyncratic approach to assessment reflects their experience and clinical knowledge. The skilled clinician is familiar with the signs, symptoms, and usual course of many syndromes, which makes him or her adept

---

* *Symptom:* "Any morbid phenomenon or departure from normal in function, appearance, or sensation, *experienced by the patient* and indicative of disease" (*Stedmans Medical Dictionary,* p. 1376). *Sign:* Any abnormality discoverable by the physician at his examination of the patient" (*Stedmans Medical Dictionary,* p. 1283; italics added). Symptoms are subjective data reported by the patient; signs are objective data observed by the physician.

at interpreting the significance of individual bits of information as they are received. When skilled clinicians recognize that an emerging pattern of test results is consistent with a known syndrome, they deviate from their usual testing routine to focus on tests whose results will support or argue against the presence of the syndrome. Each new bit of information that fits with the developing pattern increases the clinician's confidence that the patient's signs and symptoms represent the syndrome, while conflicting information moves the clinician toward an alternative diagnosis.

Skilled clinicians use their clinical knowledge without consciously thinking about it, and it seems likely that much of what they know they cannot verbalize. Add to that the likelihood that much of what they do is based as much on intuition as on rules or principles, and it should not be surprising that clinical methods are learned more by observation, practice, and imitation than by direct instruction.

Although there really is no substitute for experience, there are some general principles that govern the collection and analysis of clinical data. These principles relate, in a general way, to the well-known *scientific method,* formalized by John Dewey in the 1930s and taught to nearly every secondary school and college student since that time.

- Identify the problem.
- Propose a solution (formulate a hypothesis).
- Develop procedures to test the hypothesis.
- Collect data relevant to the hypothesis.
- Analyze the data.
- Modify the hypothesis, formulate a new one, or reach a conclusion based on the analysis.

The principles of the scientific method have been repackaged by numerous authors for clinical purposes. The new package usually is called the *clinical method.*

The solution of any clinical problem is reached by a series of inferences and deductions—each an attempt to explain an item in the history of an illness or a physical finding. Diagnosis is the mental act of integrating all the interpretations and selecting the *one* explanation most compatible with all the facts of clinical observation (Adams & Victor, 1981, p. 3).

The general steps in the clinical method are:

- Gather information about the patient's impairments from the referral, the history, and examination of the patient.
- Evaluate the patient's subjective reports (symptoms) and the objective test results (signs) to determine which are relevant.
- Determine if a distinctive cluster of symptoms and signs representing a *syndrome* exists.
- Look for correlations among symptoms and signs to identify the parts of the body or the underlying physical or mental processes responsible for the observed symptoms and signs.
- If the patient's symptoms and signs represent a syndrome for which information about the course and eventual outcome of the patient's condition are available, offer a *prognosis* regarding the patient's eventual recovery.
- Use information from the patient's history, the examination of the patient, and knowledge of the patient's life situation to formulate a conclusion about the *functional effects* of the patient's condition—the degree to which the patient's condition affects his or her competence and independence in daily life.

Distinguishing between *facts* and *information* is an important part of assessing neurogenic communication disorders. Facts may relate to different categories of information (e.g., the patient is male, 55 years old, is missing his left index finger, complains of shortness of breath and pain in the left arm, has a rash on his chest, and has an abnormal electrocardiogram). However, these facts are of little clinical use until someone evaluates their relationship to each other and looks for similarities between the patient's history, symptoms, and signs and those of patients previously examined by the clinician or reported by other practitioners. In this way the clinician separates the important facts from the trivial or irrelevant ones—a process that imparts diagnostic meaning to the facts. (The *facts* have acquired *meaning* and have become *information.*) A physician, given the foregoing facts about a patient, might select the patient's complaint of shortness of breath, arm pain, and the abnormal electrocardiogram as significant facts suggestive of cardiac problems and focus the interview, examination, and laboratory tests on that possibility.

As each piece of information about the patient is received, the clinician evaluates it for its meaning (information content) and relates it to other information about the patient. This process continues until the clinician is satisfied that he or she understands the nature of the patient's problems (at which time the clinician might apply a diagnostic label and shift his or her attention to arriving at a prognosis and making decisions about management).

In summary, the clinician gathers facts from the history, the medical record, the interview with the patient, and the results of testing. With each new fact, the clinician looks for relationships that might suggest a diagnosis. As additional facts become known, the clinician evaluates the consistency of the new facts with the working diagnosis. When new facts suggest that the working diagnosis is no longer valid, the clinician considers alternative diagnoses and may change tests or examination procedures to gather facts that are relevant to the new diagnosis. When alternative explanations for the pattern of facts have been eliminated, the clinician settles on the diagnosis most compatible with the facts of the history, the interview, and the examination.

Harvey and associates (1988, p. 2) have summarized the principles that govern the clinical method:

1. The collection and analysis of clinical information are essentially the application of the scientific method to the solution of a clinical problem.
2. These methods can be taught and learned; it is not an art in which one is either gifted or not. Proficiency can be improved by consciously considering the meaning of each piece of information as it is received.
3. The process is rapidly iterative. The cycle is repeated within the time interval of asking a few questions or making physical observations. This explains the mystery of why the novice fails to ask the key question or seek the key physical finding.
4. The process is an ongoing one. There are no irrefutable hypotheses, only unrefuted hypotheses. In clinical terms, the physician should not arrive at a diagnosis and abandon any further consideration of alternative explanations. He must remain alert for information that does not fit with his current hypothesis and for sources of new information that might make him alter his considerations. When uncertain, he should continue to seek ways of testing the tentative diagnosis.
5. Consideration of a diagnosis that can neither be confirmed nor excluded fails to advance the decision-making process. Such a diagnosis is directly parallel to a scientific hypothesis that cannot be tested.
6. Finally, clinical problem-solving is as sensitive to flawed or missing information as are scientific experiments. A major difference lies in the fact that clinical decisions must often be made on what is acknowledged to be incomplete evidence.

The foregoing material deals primarily with *how* the assessment takes place. Some *when, where, what,* and *why* questions that are asked before, during, and after the assessment are: When does the clinician first learn about the patient? When does the clinician first meet the patient? When does testing begin? Where does the clinician find information about the patient's personal history? Where does the clinician find out about the patient's medical problems? What does brain damage do to the patient's ability to take tests? How does the clinician review a medical chart? How does the clinician conduct a patient interview? These and other questions related to assessment of adults with neurogenic communication disorders are addressed in the following sections.

When a patient with a communication disorder is referred, the speech-language pathologist typically begins by gathering background information about the patient. This information provides a context from which the clinician can make predictions about the nature and severity of the patient's impairments and decide which tests are likely to be most appropriate. The information providing this context comes from three sources—*the referral, the patient's medical record,* and *the interview.*

■ THE REFERRAL

Most patients with neurogenic communication disorders are referred to a speech-language pathologist by a physician. The physician recruits specialists (including speech-language pathologists) into the patient's program of care by means of *consultation requests* (sometimes called *referrals*). The information included in the consultation request provides the speech-language pathologist with a general sense both of the patient and what the referring physician would like the speech-language pathologist to do. Most consultation requests include:

- Personal information about the patient (name, birthdate, social security number, and such).
- Information about the patient's location (hospital ward, service, unit).
- A brief description of what the physician would like from the consultant.
- The physician's name (and sometimes their phone and/or pager numbers).
- A space for the consultant's response.

Consultation requests do, however, span a wide range of completeness, accuracy, and legibility.

The good requests are legibly written,* include a short description of the patient's major current problems, provide a diagnosis (sometimes provisional), and include a brief statement of the services requested. Most requests contain numerous abbreviations, both standard and nonstandard, and many are telegraphic. Figure 3-1 gives an example of a consultation request form as it might be received by a speech-language pathologist.

The consultation request in Figure 3-1 was sent from Dr. Ericcson, a fictional neurologist on a neurology ward, and concerns a fictional patient named Arthur Shaw. The provisional diagnosis suggests that Mr. Shaw has had a stroke (cerebrovascular accident) involving the left middle cerebral artery and that he exhibits severe aphasia. The physician has left it to the speech-language pathologist to decide where to see the patient. The "reason for request" section, when decoded, yields the following information about Mr. Shaw:

> Mr. Shaw is a 55-year-old right-handed male, who has had (is one day status post) a recent left middle cerebral artery cerebrovascular accident. He has right upper extremity (arm) and right lower extremity (leg) weakness and appears globally aphasic. He has a history of diabetes mellitus and hypertension (high blood pressure).[†]

Consultation requests such as this provide the speech-language pathologist with an important first look at the patient, the patient's history,

---

* The advent of computerized consultation and referral procedures has had a major positive side effect, in that consultation requests are typed into a central computer and printed out on a consultation request form. Consequently, those receiving the request no longer are burdened with deciphering the scrawl in which handwritten requests often are produced. Unfortunately, computerized referrals have had little effect on the arcane and nonstandard abbreviations and terms used by some physicians, nor have they had any measurable salutary effects on their spelling, clarity of style, and literary merit.

† See Appendix A for a list of common medical abbreviations and their definitions.

Medical record	Consultation request/referral	
To: Speech pathology	**From:** Ward 2N neurology	**Date:** 08/12/96 14:30

Provisional diagnosis: L MCA CVA, global asphia

Requested by: Ericcson, G. 4498	Place: Consultant's choice	Urgency: Routine

Reason for request:
55 y/o R-H M 1 day s/p recent L MCA CVA. RUE RLE weakn. Globally aphas. Hx DM, HTN. Pls eval pt.'s spch & lang & make recs.

Consultation report

Signature and title:			Date:	
Id#:	Organization/service:	Reg#:		Ward:

Patient Id:
  Shaw, Arthur 5/17/41
  503-42-9680   SF 522 3/94
  2K435-32 NEU   **Consultation request**

Figure 3-1 ■ A consultation request as it might be received by a speech-language pathologist. The shaded areas contain information provided by the physician.

the nature and severity of the patient's neurologic impairments, and (sometimes) the probable future course of the patient's condition. By
making inferences from the information in the
consultation request, the speech-language
pathologist may develop an impression of the
patient that goes well beyond the sketchy information provided.

The information provided in the consultation
request suggests several hypotheses about Mr.
Shaw, his communication impairments, and his
life situation:

- Mr. Shaw is right-handed and has damage
  in the distribution of the left middle cerebral artery. Therefore he is very likely to be
  aphasic—a hypothesis supported by the
  neurologist's description.
- Mr. Shaw is weak but not paralyzed on his
  right side. This suggests that the stroke has
  not compromised the entire central region
  of the left hemisphere. Consequently, he
  may not be globally aphasic, as the neurologist's description indicates.*
- Mr. Shaw's stroke is very recent. Therefore he is likely to be in a period of relatively rapid spontaneous recovery. The
  severity of his communication (and physical) impairments is likely to diminish over
  the next few weeks.
- Mr. Shaw is 55 years old. This means that
  he probably was employed when he had
  his stroke. Consequently, his stroke may

have important financial consequences for
Mr. Shaw and his family.
- Mr. Shaw is diabetic and hypertensive.
  These medical problems could complicate
  his physical recovery.
- Mr. Shaw is currently on a neurology ward.
  The average length of stay on neurology
  wards (and other acute-care wards) is only
  a few days. This may affect how much testing, family education, and counseling the
  speech-language pathologist can accomplish before discharge.
- Mr. Shaw and his family are likely to be in
  the initial stages of coming to grips with
  what has happened and they may need education, support, and reassurance to deal
  with what has happened and to plan for
  the future.

This example shows how information contained in a consultation request permits the
speech-language pathologist to make inferences
about the patient that go well beyond what
is explicitly provided in the request. Such
inference-making is in many ways an idiosyncratic process that depends on the speech-
language pathologist's experience, knowledge,
and talent for making inferences. Although it is
impossible to describe the process by which
such inferences are made, it is possible to describe some of the sources of information that
may lead to the inferences.

Sources of Information in Referrals

The Referring Service or Ward. Where
the consultation comes from usually has implications for the patient's probable length of stay,
her or his physical and medical condition, and
the speech-language pathologist's role in the patient's care.

Patients in *intensive care units (ICUs)* are
likely to be weak, seriously ill, or comatose.
Some patients may have tracheostomies (openings into the trachea to provide an alternative
airway or to facilitate treatment of respiratory
impairments). Intensive care unit patients are

---

* Sometimes patients with severe Broca's or Wernickes'
aphasia are reported by physicians to be globally aphasic because they appear to comprehend little or nothing and produce little if any intelligible speech. Physicians sometimes
call patients with severe Broca's aphasia "globally aphasic"
because their inability to talk makes testing of comprehension (which usually is relatively good) difficult. Physicians
sometimes call patients with severe Wernicke's aphasia
"globally aphasic" because their severe comprehension impairments and vague, empty, and circumlocutory speech
give an impression of globally impaired language. Globally
aphasic patients usually are paralyzed on one side. The fact
that Mr. Shaw is weak but not paralyzed on his right side
suggests that he may not be globally aphasic.

confined to bed, usually with feeding, medication, or drainage tubes or monitoring equipment attached. Patients in intensive care units usually remain there only until their medical condition stabilizes and they no longer need intensive around-the-clock monitoring and care (although a few seriously ill ones may remain there for several weeks). When they leave the ICU, most patients are transferred to a medical/surgical ward. Patients in intensive care units usually are referred to a speech-language pathologist because they cannot communicate basic needs or because they have known or suspected swallowing impairments. The speech-language pathologist's typical role with these patients is to establish a system by which the patient can communicate basic needs to unit personnel, to evaluate the patient's swallowing, or both.

Most patients on *medical/surgical wards* (including neurology wards, which are a subcategory of medical wards) are discharged within 3 to 5 days, although some patients with serious illnesses or those recovering from major surgery may stay longer. (One of the most dramatic consequences of managed care and health care reform is a striking shortening of the length of time patients spend in hospitals.) Patients on medical/surgical wards usually have acute or evolving medical problems (e.g., recent stroke, pneumonia, or recent surgery). Most patients can get out of bed and many are ambulatory,* although some may require a cane, crutches, a walker, or a wheelchair to get around. Consultation requests to speech-language pathologists from medical/surgical wards are made for many reasons. Some may seek an opinion regarding the presence and severity of a communication or swallowing impairment. Some may request assessment of a patient's speech, language, and cognitive status.

Some may request assessment and recommendations for treatment. Some may seek the speech-language pathologist's help in resolving a diagnostic dilemma. The emphasis in referrals from medical/surgical wards tends to be toward assessment and diagnosis—patients usually are discharged before treatment of their communication impairments becomes an important part of their overall plan of care.

Patients on *rehabilitation wards* usually stay for several weeks. Few are acutely ill and almost all are ambulatory, although most get around with the help of canes, crutches, a walker, or a wheelchair. Most patients receive occupational, physical, and/or recreational therapy, and sometimes other therapies while they are on the ward. Consequently, the speech-language pathologist is likely to serve on a treatment team with the patient's physician and rehabilitation therapists. Patients on rehabilitation wards usually get there by transfer from other wards. For this reason, referrals from rehabilitation wards may be for patients whom the speech-language pathologist has already seen following referral from another ward or from intensive care units, in which case part or all of the assessment and perhaps some treatment may have been done by the time the patient is referred from the rehabilitation ward. Because of their relatively long stays, patients on rehabilitation wards usually can get a good start on treatment of their communication impairments before they leave the hospital.

Patients in *extended care centers* usually stay for weeks or months. Almost all are ambulatory. Few are acutely ill, but most, if not all, have chronic medical problems (e.g., stroke-related impairments or pulmonary disease) and some may be receiving continuing treatment for chronic disease (for example, kidney dialysis, radiation therapy, or chemotherapy). The speech-language pathologist's focus for these patients is likely to be treatment, although an occasional patient may require only an assessment and diagnostic workup.

---

* The primary meaning of *ambulatory* is "capable of walking about." Its secondary meaning is "not confined to bed," which is the meaning used in the text.

Outpatients sometimes make up a significant part of a speech-language pathology clinic's caseload. Most outpatients are individuals who have been discharged from the hospital but need continuing treatment for communication impairments and are ambulatory. Not many are acutely ill but many have chronic low-level medical problems such as diabetes, cardiovascular disease, or pulmonary disease. Some may have degenerative disease such as multiple sclerosis or cerebellar degeneration and some may be recovering from strokes, other neurologic incidents, or surgery. Physicians refer outpatients to speech-language pathology for many reasons but most frequently they wish either to know the cause and nature of a patient's communication impairments or to know if treatment of a patient's communication impairments is appropriate.

Demographic Information. Demographic information about the patient contained in the referral provides information about his or her communication history and potential communicative needs. The patient's *age* may indicate whether the patient is working or retired and whether dependent children live at home. Incapacitation of younger patients who are below retirement age is likely to have important financial consequences for the patient and family. As a patient's age increases, so does the probability that the patient's spouse will be medically or physically impaired, which compromises his or her ability to care for the patient. As a patient's age increases, the greater the probability that she or he does not have a living spouse, that the burden of care will fall upon children or other relatives, and that the patient will be placed in an extended care facility on discharge from the medical center. Finally, as age increases, physical resilience diminishes and the likelihood of complicating medical conditions increases, with consequent negative effects on the prognosis for recovery.

A patient's *handedness* may influence the speech-language pathologist's guesses about the patient's probable communication impairments. If the patient is right-handed and has left-hemisphere brain damage, he or she is very likely to be aphasic. If a patient is right-handed and has right-hemisphere brain damage, the probability that he or she will exhibit symptoms of nondominant hemisphere pathology increases.

The *medical diagnosis* provides another indicator of a patient's potential communication impairments. Because stroke, traumatic brain injury, and degenerative disease have different prognoses, a patient's neurologic diagnosis has important implications for the patient's recovery. The location of a patient's nervous system pathology has implications for the nature of the patient's symptoms. For example, damage in the brain hemispheres is likely to affect higher mental processes (language and cognition), whereas damage in the brain stem is likely to have important effects on motor and sensory functions, while sparing higher mental processes. The extent of a patient's nervous system pathology usually is directly related to the number and severity of the patient's symptoms and, in a less direct way, to the eventual outcome of treatment.

The Request The *nature of the services requested* directly communicates the likely role of the speech-language pathologist in the patient's care. Some consultation requests are specific about what the referring physician would like from the speech-language pathologist. A physician may refer a patient with progressive neurologic disease and ask the speech-language pathologist to establish baseline measures of speech and language against which the progression of the patient's disease can be measured. A physician may refer a patient with a questionable neurologic diagnosis and ask the speech-language pathologist to administer tests to help clarify the diagnosis. A physician may refer an aphasic patient whose competence to make financial and legal decisions is questionable and ask the speech-language pathologist to evaluate the degree to which the patient's comprehension impairments affect her or his financial and legal competence. However, most consultation requests are generic (e.g., for assessment or treatment of the patient's communication impairments) and leave the specifics to the speech-language pathologist.

Occasionally, a consultation request will focus on one aspect of a patient's care but neglect other aspects to which the speech-language pathologist can contribute. For example, a patient with a brain-stem stroke may be referred for evaluation of her or his swallowing with no mention of coexisting dysarthria. The sagacious speech-language pathologist, recognizing that dysarthria is a common consequence of brain stem injuries, might suggest to the referring physician that the evaluation be extended to include speech as well as swallowing. However, the physician retains primary responsibility for the patient's overall plan of care. Changes or additions to the plan of care prescribed by the physician can be made only with the physician's knowledge and consent.

■ REVIEWING THE MEDICAL RECORD

With referral in hand and a general sense of what to expect in mind, the speech-language pathologist proceeds to the patient's ward to tap the second major source of information about the patient—the patient's medical record. The medical record is a legal document that provides a complete record of the patient's medical care. Medical records are divided into sections, with different kinds of information in each section. How medical records are divided depends to some extent on the medical facility in which the record is located but most resemble the arrangement described below. The speech-language pathologist reviews the medical record and extracts information relating to the patient's potential communication impairments. This information is summarized, either freehand or, more often, on a form for that purpose.

Patient Identification The patient identification section usually is at the bottom of each page in the record and includes the patient's name, date of birth, social security number, and ward. It may also contain other information about the patient, such as home telephone number and diagnostic or other codes.

Personal History The patient's personal history contains demographic information about the patient (occupation, marital status, children, where the patient lives and with whom, vocation, and work history). Information about the patient's emotional and social history may also appear here (e.g., the presence of previous or current emotional or personal problems, the nature of the patient's relationships with others, and whether the patient has a history of alcoholism or other substance abuse). In Figure 3-2 the neurologist has summarized Mr. Shaw's personal history at the beginning of the neurologic examination.

Medical History As described in Chapter 2, the medical history usually comes from a physician who interviews the patient, with the information from the interview sometimes supplemented by information from previous medical records. The medical history describes the patient's previous illnesses, injuries, or medical conditions and current disabilities and complaints. Past cerebrovascular disorders, disorientation, confusion, slurred speech, loss of consciousness, or seizures are noted, as are chronic medical conditions such as diabetes, vascular disease, heart disease, pulmonary disease, hearing loss, or visual problems.

Figure 3-2 shows the neurologist's summary of Mr. Shaw's medical history, which is a characteristic one for stroke patients. Diabetes and hypertension each increase the risk of stroke and when they appear in combination, the risk is greater than when either appears separately. Mrs. Shaw's description of the March, 1995 incident, when combined with his diabetes and hypertension, suggests the occurrence of a transient ischemic

Medical record	**Neurologic examination**

Personal history: Mr. Shaw is a 55-y/o accountant (college grad). Married, with two children; son 28, daughter 24, neither living at home. Wife (Florence) is a secondary-school teacher. Nonsmoker × 10 yrs. Occasional social ETOH—nonabuser. Both parents deceased (mid-80s), apparently of natural causes. Employed at time of apparent neurologic incident.

Medical history: Past medical history includes adult-onset diabetes mellitus diagnosed in 1991, hypertension diagnosed 1993, and a possible TIA in March of last year. The patient's wife reports that at the time of the apparent TIA they were watching television when the patient became confused, did not answer questions, and seemed not to understand. The patient's symptoms apparently cleared in an hour or two, and they did not seek medical advice or assistance. Medications on admission include tolbutamide 500 mg twice a day, chlorothiazide 500 mg twice a day, which apparently control the patient's hypertension and diabetes, and occasionally aspirin.

Background: The patient was accompanied to this medical center by his wife, who provided this information. The patient apparently was in good health until this apparent neurologic event, which occurred at approximately 0815 hrs this day. The patient was getting dressed for work when he experienced a sudden onset of speech difficulties and leg weakness. The patient did not vomit, lose consciousness, or report double vision, nausea or vertigo. He arrived at the emergency room at this medical center at 0905 hrs. The neurologic examination began at approximately 0920 hrs.

Habits: The patient is an exsmoker (0.5 ppd × 10 years) and has not smoked for approximately the past 10 years. The patient apparently drinks three or four glasses of wine per week and other alcoholic drinks occasionally, but his wife reports that he has never been a heavy drinker.

Physical examination: The patient looks his stated age and is in no apparent distress. He appears alert and is oriented × 3. **Vital signs:** Blood pressure 162/89, pulse 72, temperature 98.6, respiration 18. **HEENT exam:** No signs of trauma or deformation. Moist mucous membranes. Neck negative for lymphadenopathy or thyromegaly. No carotid bruit. **Cardiovascular exam:** Normal S1, S2, without gallop or murmurs. **Lungs:** Clear to auscultation. **Abdomen:** Soft and nontender. No organomegaly or palpable masses. **Lower extremities:** No pedal edema. **Neurologic examination:** The patient is globally aphasic. Listening comprehension evaluation showed that he is able to follow very simple commands like "close your eyes" or "open your mouth." He is unable to give yes-no answers to questions. He is a little bit confused as to right/left commands. He is unable to do complex commands. Reading evaluation showed the patient unable to identify a letter. He had paraphasic errors in single-word identification (e.g., "wrisp" for "wrist"). The patient was unable to follow commands on reading because of inability to comprehend. Expression evaluation showed that the patient was unable to read a narrative. He was unable to repeat "no ifs, ands, or buts." He was also unable to name objects like watch or pin.

Cranial nerve examination: It was difficult to examine the patient's visual acuity because of his aphasia. Acuity appears within normal limits, but the patient exhibits a questionable right-sided field cut. Funduscopic examination showed no evidence of papilledema. His pupils are 3mm to 4 mm bilaterally, round, equal, and reactive to light and accommodation. He had intact extraocular movements. His corneal reflexes are present bilaterally. His jaw jerk was +1. He had symmetrical nasolabial folds and wrinkles. His tongue is midline and so is his uvula. He has symmetrical gag reflex bilaterally. He has symmetrical strength in his shoulders bilaterally. **Motor examination:** The patient has no pronator drift and no involuntary movements. His muscle tone is normal bilaterally. His strength appears 5/5 on the left and 4/5 in the right upper extremity and 3/5 in the right lower extremity. Grasp reflex on right. He had external rotation in his right lower extremity. His coordination exam was unremarkable for dysmetria. Deep tendon reflexes are +2 on the left and +3 on the right, except +1 in both ankles. Plantar reflex on right. **Sensory examination:** Impossible to establish accurately because of patient's aphasia. However, the patient withdraws both lower and upper extremities to pinprick stimuli. **Gait:** The patient walks slowly, but with symmetrical arm swings bilaterally. Mild dragging of right foot.

Problem list:

    1. Probable LH stroke
    2. Aphasia
    3. Hypertension
    4. Adult-onset diabetes mellitus

                  (Signed)

                          G. Ericsson

Date: 8/11/96   G. Ericsson, MD

Patient Id:
      Shaw, Arthur 5/17/41
      503-42-9680   **Medical record**
      2K435-32 NEU   **Neurologic examination**

Figure 3-2 ■ **A neurologic examination report.**

attack.* The events that brought Mr. Shaw to the hospital (see "background" in Figure 3-2) also are characteristic of stroke and their nature and progression suggest an occlusive, rather than a hemorrhagic, stroke. The symptoms developed early in the day and their onset was abrupt, with gradual exacerbation over the next few hours. Occlusive strokes tend to occur early in the day and are not strongly related to physical exertion. The symptoms of an occlusive stroke gradually increase, often in a stepwise manner, following onset. Hemorrhagic strokes tend to occur during physical exertion, and symptom development usually is rapid, often accompanied by headache, nausea, and sometimes vomiting. Mr. Shaw's past history of smoking and his moderate alcohol consumption are unlikely to have much to do with the cause of his current symptoms.

Physical and Neurologic Examination
The results of the physician's examination of the patient (including the neurologic examination) are reported here. (See Chapter 2 for a description of the neurologic examination.) The physician's report of the examination usually ends with a *problem list,* in which relevant preexisting and current symptoms and complaints are summarized.

The neurologist's report of Mr. Shaw's physical and neurologic examination follows the standard format (Figure 3-2). The report begins with the neurologist's observations of Mr. Shaw's appearance, mood and orientation (*oriented ×3* means oriented to *person (who are you?), place (where are you?),* and *time (what day, month, year is it?)*. The report continues with a summary of Mr. Shaw's physical examination. Mr. Shaw's *vital signs* are within normal limits,

except for slightly elevated blood pressure. The remainder of the physical examination is generally unremarkable. (*Lymphadenopathy* means "enlarged lymph glands," *thyromegaly* means "enlarged thyroid gland." *Bruit* is the rushing sound blood makes in a constricted or roughened artery—in this case the carotid artery in the neck. *S1, S2, gallop, murmur* are heart sounds. *Auscultation* means "listened to," usually by means of a stethoscope. *Organomegaly* means "enlarged organs." *Palpable* means "detectable by touch." *Pedal edema* means "swelling of feet or ankles.")

The neurologist's description of Mr. Shaw's speech and comprehension suggests that Mr. Shaw is aphasic, with severely impaired comprehension. Because little information about Mr. Shaw's speech is provided, it is not clear from the neurologist's report whether Mr. Shaw is globally aphasic or has severe Wernicke's aphasia.

The neurologist's examination of Mr. Shaw's cranial nerve functions follows the standard top-down format, beginning with visual acuity (CN 2)* and moving on to eye movements and pupillary responses (CN 3, 4, 6), face (5, 7), tongue, larynx, pharynx (CN 9, 10, 11, 12), and shoulders (CN 11). (CN 7 [balance and hearing] often is tested indirectly by observing the patient's response to spoken questions and instructions during the examination and by observing the patient's balance during tests involving standing and walking.) The results of testing Mr. Shaw's cranial nerves do not suggest cranial nerve damage but indicate damage in the posterior left hemisphere. (Symmetric nasolabial folds and wrinkles suggest no significant upper motor neuron damage in corticobulbar tracts serving the lower face, which in turn suggests no major frontal lobe involvement and slightly diminishes

---

* Normal, healthy adults may occasionally experience similar transitory alterations of consciousness and mentation, which are not symptoms of cerebrovascular disease and are not warning signs for future strokes. Benign reasons for such incidents include constriction of cerebral arteries, hyperventilation, and transitory hypotension (low-blood pressure).

---

* The neurologist's omission of CN 1 testing (smell, taste) is typical. CN 1 is rarely tested in routine neurologic examinations unless the neurologist has reason to suspect pathology in the olfactory nerve or olfactory cortex.

the probability that Mr. Shaw is globally aphasic.) The neurologist reports a slightly diminished jaw-jerk reflex, which is of minor significance, given the negative results of other cranial nerve functions.

The neurologist's examination of Mr. Shaw's motor functions reveals slight weakness on Mr. Shaw's right side (with his leg somewhat weaker than his arm), brisk reflexes on his right side (but diminished in both ankles), a grasp reflex in his right hand, and a probable plantar (Babinski) reflex in his right foot. These findings are consistent with damage affecting the upper motor neurons on Mr. Shaw's left side. That his weakness is slight is consistent with posterior brain damage, which spares the majority of corticospinal tracts. A *grasp reflex* is an involuntary closing of the hand when the patient's palm is stroked. It is a sign of upper motor neuron damage in the contralateral corticospinal tract. *Pronator drift* is a sign of muscle weakness, and it is seen when the patient is asked to hold his arms out straight in front, with palms up and eyes closed. Weakness in the arm muscles causes the weak arm to rotate toward a more natural palms-down position, and sometimes the weak arm sags in response to the pull of gravity. Mild weakness in leg muscles sometimes causes the leg to rotate outward, especially when the patient is lying down.

The neurologist's examination of Mr. Shaw's somesthetic sensory functions and gait are generally unremarkable except for a slight right foot-drag, which is consistent with the motor examination. Overall, the neurologic examination suggests that Mr. Shaw has had a stroke involving the posterior left hemisphere, with possible mild involvement extending into the frontal lobe. The most probable communication diagnosis appears to be one of Wernicke's aphasia and not global aphasia.

Doctor's Orders Doctor's orders are written by the patient's primary physician (and sometimes by other physicians) to stipulate how the patient is to be cared for. The orders may include medications, special precautions, tests and consultations, diet, monitoring of fluid or caloric intake, rehabilitation services, and other important aspects of the patient's in-hospital care. Each order is signed by the physician writing the order and when the order is carried out, the person who carries it out initials the order and writes the time at which it was carried out. Information from this section of the medical record adds to the speech-language pathologist's sense of the plan of care. The speech-language pathologist will wish to find out what laboratory tests have been ordered, what medications have been prescribed, whether diet modifications or restrictions have been ordered, whether other therapies such as physical therapy or occupational therapy have been ordered, and what other specialists have been consulted. This information alerts the speech-language pathologist to the need for collaboration with others involved in the patient's care and, in the case of other therapies, will alert the speech-language pathologist to the need for coordinating the patient's speech clinic appointments with others.

Figure 3-3 shows the neurologist's orders for the period immediately following Mr. Shaw's admission to the neurology ward. The first order is for a CT scan of Mr. Shaw's head to rule out cerebral hemorrhage as the cause of his neurologic deficits. Head CT scans are one of the first laboratory tests ordered for patients with probable strokes, because the medical treatment of hemorrhagic strokes is markedly different from that of occlusive strokes. Treatment of occlusive strokes often entails administration of blood thinners (anticoagulants), which make hemorrhagic strokes worse. Consequently, ruling out cerebral hemorrhage is a critical concern in the early phase of treatment. The next order in the medical record is for an electrocardiogram, perhaps to rule out coronary artery disease or atrial fibrillations as a

Medical record		Doctor's orders	
Date and time	**Prob no**	**Orders**	**Nurse's initials**
8/11/96 1035	1	**Lab:** Head CT with contrast. R/O hemorrhage vs occlusion. _Ericsson_	_JAN_ 1045
8/11/96 1035	1	**LAB:** EKG. 55-y/o male with probable CVA, aphasia. _Ericsson_	_JAN_ 1045
8/11/96 1035	1	Activity: Up in chair as tolerated. _Ericsson_	_JAN_ 1045
8/11/96 1035	3, 4	Meds: Chlorothiazide 0.5g. b.i.d. Tolbutamide 0.5g. b.i.d. _Ericsson_	_JAN_ 1055
8/11/96 1035	1,3	Diet: Low fat, no added salt. _Ericsson_	_JAN_ 1055
8/11/96 1035	1	**Lab:** Coag time, sed rate. _Ericsson_	_JAN_ 1100
8/12/96 0905	1	**Lab:** Carotid u/s. R/O stenosis. _Ericsson_	_JAN_ 0930
8/12/96 1420	2	Speech pathology consult: 55 y/o R-H M 1 day s/p L MCA CVA. RUE, RLE weakn. Globally aphas. Hx DM, HTN. Pls eval pt.'s spch & lang & make recs. _Ericsson_	_MRB_ 1435
8/12/96 1420	1, 2	Social work consult: 55 y/o M 1 day s/p L MCA CVA. Globally aphasic. Pls assist with d/c planning. _Ericsson_	_MRB_ 1440
8/12/96 1420	1	Rehab consult: 55 y/o M 1 day s/p L MCA CVA. Globally aphasic. RUE, RLE weakness. Pls assess and make rec's. _Ericsson_	_JAN_ 1440
8/12/96 1600	1	Activity: No restrictions on ward. Pt. not to leave ward w/o supervision. _Ericsson_	_JAN_ 1620
8/12/96 1600	1	**Lab:** Serum triglycerides, cholesterol, _Ericsson_	_MRB_ 1620

Patient Id:
   Shaw, Arthur 5/17/41
   503-42-9680   **Medical record**
   2K435-32 NEU   **Doctor's orders**

Figure 3-3 ▪ **Excerpts from doctor's orders in a hypothetical medical record.**

source of emboli.* The next order gives permission for Mr. Shaw to be out of bed and sitting in a chair but not to walk unassisted—a routine precaution for patients in the first day or two post-stroke. The next order prescribes continuation of the medications Mr. Shaw has been taking for his hypertension and diabetes (to be given twice a day). The neurologist prescribes a standard low-fat, low-salt diet. In most medical facilities, a dietician sees all newly admitted patients and recommends diets to meet their nutritional and hydration needs. The last order on Day 1 is for laboratory tests of coagulation time and sedimentation rate, which reflect the time it takes Mr. Shaw's blood to clot. Shorter-than-normal coagulation time and faster-than-normal sedimentation rate suggest a greater likelihood of blood clots in the vascular system and may be an indication that anticoagulant therapy is needed.

On Day 2 the neurologist orders a carotid ultrasound to determine if Mr. Shaw has stenosis of his carotid arteries. The order suggests that the neurologist is moving toward a diagnosis of occlusive stroke rather than hemorrhagic stroke. Neurologists often order carotid ultrasound tests early in the care of patients with suspected occlusive strokes. If the results show stenosis, the probability that the patient's stroke is occlusive rises. If the stenosis is severe, the neurologist may order a follow-up cerebral angiogram to get a more precise indication of the location, severity, and nature of the stenosis than can be gotten from the somewhat fuzzy image provided by the carotid ultrasound. The neurologist also orders referrals to speech pathology, social work, and rehabilitation medicine and amends his previous day's order to permit Mr. Shaw to move

---

* *Atrial fibrillations* are irregularities in the heartbeat in which the normal rhythmic contractions of heart muscles are replaced by rapid and irregular contractions. The rapid and irregular contractions can cause blood clots or fragments of tissue to break loose and travel through the blood stream.

about the ward without assistance (probably in response to his observations and those of ward personnel that walking poses no risk to Mr. Shaw). Finally, the neurologist orders laboratory analysis of a sample of Mr. Shaw's blood to determine if the level of fatty compounds that play a part in atherosclerosis is elevated.

Progress Notes Progress notes are written by physicians, nurses, and other patient-care personnel to provide a chronologic record of the patient's physical, behavioral, and mental status during his or her hospitalization. Day-to-day changes in the patient's behavior or condition are routinely described in progress notes, and the results of assessments (including the speech-language pathologist's assessment of communication) are found there. Entries in the progress notes by physicians, nurses, ward personnel, and other specialists provide information about the patient's alertness, orientation, and mood, his or her responses to caregivers and to other patients on the ward, and may indicate whether the patient can walk, dress, bathe, and accomplish other activities of daily living. Reports from other specialists such as psychologists, social workers, and physical therapists provide the speech-language pathologist with insights into aspects of the patient's condition not covered by the physical and neurologic examination, and perusal of the specialists' goals and objectives helps the speech-language pathologist get a sense of their plans for the patient's care. If the patient is evaluated or treated by other services such as occupational therapy, physical therapy, psychology, vocational counseling, or social work, their reports and comments will be found in the progress notes. The physician's interpretations of laboratory tests also may be found there. The first progress note usually is written by the admitting physician and consists of a brief description of the patient, a summary of the patient's history, and a concise summary of the significant aspects of the physical and neurologic examination. The physician's initial progress note usually ends with the physician's conclusions about diagnostic issues and her or his plan for the immediate future care of the patient.

Figure 3-4 is a page of progress notes from Mr. Shaw's medical record. It begins with the neurologist's admitting note, which follows the format described above, and it summarizes the findings of the neurologic examination presented in Figure 3-2. The A/P (assessment/plan) section describes the neurologist's diagnostic hunches and plans for the patient's care. From reading the neurologist's plans for carotid ultrasound and MRI angiogram, it appears that he suspects an occlusive stroke but has decided not to give Mr. Shaw anticoagulant medications (probably because he wants to see the results of the CT scan first). If the CT shows no hemorrhage, the neurologist plans to administer anticoagulant medications. Finally, the neurologist plans to involve rehabilitation medicine, speech pathology, social work, and ophthalmology in Mr. Shaw's care, no doubt to deal with his weakness, aphasia, post-hospital placement, and potential visual field blindness, respectively.

The progress notes continue with several entries by nursing personnel, which give a picture of Mr. Shaw as ambulatory, alert, and oriented but with significant communication impairments. Several comments suggest that Mr. Shaw's aphasia is Wernicke's-like ("understanding seems to be a major problem," "tends to ramble," "doesn't appear frustrated or even acknowledge the communication block," "doesn't always get what you say"). However, he appears to be pleasant, cooperative, and helpful, suggesting that control of behavioral abnormalities is unlikely to be a major management issue. The last entry is by the speech-language pathologist, who acknowledges receipt of the consultation request, gives her initial impressions, and directs the reader to a language screening assessment elsewhere in the progress notes.

Laboratory Test Reports Most medical records have a separate section for laboratory test reports. Results of tests such as blood tests, CT scans, EEGs, and reports of surgical procedures are found here. The speech-language pathologist reviews this section of the medical record to discover what laboratory tests have been ordered and notes the results of the completed tests, paying particular attention to the results of CT and MRI scans, angiograms, cerebrospinal fluid cultures, and any other tests that have implications for the patient's communication impairments.

Figure 3-5 and Figure 3-6 contain examples of two reports like those that can be found in the laboratory test reports section of a medical record. Figure 3-5 shows the neuroradiologist's report of a head CT scan performed on Mr. Shaw. It suggests that Mr. Shaw has had an occlusive stroke in the white matter of the brain beneath the left temporoparietal cortex, which extends into the cortex. The stroke was caused by occlusion in the posterior distribution of the middle cerebral artery. Importantly, there is no evidence of a hemorrhagic stroke.

Figure 3-6 shows the radiologist's report of Mr. Shaw's carotid ultrasound test. It indicates that Mr. Shaw has thickening of the arterial walls and atherosclerotic plaque distributed throughout both carotid arteries. Neither Mr. Shaw's left nor his right common carotid artery is significantly narrowed, but both internal carotid arteries show significant stenosis, with the right artery more so than the left. Mr. Shaw's left external carotid artery also may be narrowed, as indicated by increased blood velocities during the systolic phase of Mr. Shaw's heartbeat.

Figure 3-7 shows how a speech-language pathologist transfers information from Mr. Shaw's medical record to a form used in a speech-language pathology clinic. The form includes personal information about Mr. Shaw, labels his communication disorder, and summarizes the information from Mr. Shaw's medical

Medical record	Progress notes
Date, time	**Note**
8/11/96 1015	Neurology admit note: 55-y/o man s/p L MCA stroke 8/11/96 approx. 8:15 a.m. Pt. apparently in good health previously. Sudden onset RUE, RLE weakness, slurred speech. Brought to MC by wife. No apparent preceding symptoms or headache. **PMH:** AODM, × 5 yrs. HTN × 3 yrs. Poss. TIA 3/95. **PE:** BP 162/89, P 72. T 98.6 R 18. Lungs clear. Neck supple, mental status: Pt. awake & responsive, though inappropriate. Responds "I'm fine." Cannot give name or repeat. Follows midline commands—close eyes, open mouth. Cannot follow complex commands. CN: EOM full, no nystagmus. Pupils equal, reactive. Face symmetric. Tongue midline. Palate midline, elevates symmetrically. Motor. Unable to follow specific commands. Appears to give normal resistance in arms and legs. Can walk with support. R leg externally rotated when lying. Inc. grasp, plantar on R. Coordination: able to follow and locate moving target. **A/P:** Pt presents with acute alteration in language and comprehension. Also subtle signs of motor deficit on R. Obtain CT or MRI to r/o bleed. Stroke vs TIA most likely diagnosis. Obtain carotid ultrasound for risk factors. Consider MRI angiogram for vascular abnormalities. No clear indication for anticoagulation. Consider ASA or ticlopidine if CT shows no bleed. Will consult rehab, spch, sw, opth. *G. Ericsson*
8/11/96 1105	**Nursing admission note:** Pt. alert, oriented in no apparent distress. Wife present, participated in orientation to ward. Pt. is responsive to stimulation, but unable to respond with appropriate answers. Can transfer from bed to chair w/o assistance. Sits upright w/o tipping. Walks with assistance, but seems to have no problems with strength, balance, judgment. No signs of confusion. Continent × 2. May need assistance with ADLs for a few days. Not an apparent fall risk. Patient can talk, but doesn't always make sense. Can say name, "I'm fine," "o.k.," etc. Understanding seems to be a major problem. *J Nelson*
8/11/96 1245	**Nursing note:** Pt. alert, oriented. Pleasant & cooperative. Tends to ramble. Needs to be kept on one subject as much as possible. Wife came in with pt. Very concerned. Needs reassurance, support. *J Nelson*
8/11/96 1500	**Nursing note:** Pt. ambulating w/o assistance. Had late lunch. Appetite good. Pleasant and helpful. Offers no complaints. *M Benson*
8/11/96 1805	**Nursing note:** Patient seems to have severe receptive and expressive communication probs. Doesn't appear frustrated or even acknowledge the communication block. Needs seem to be met. No problems with ADLs. *M Benson*
8/11/96 2200	**Nursing note:** Pt. sleeping calmly. No apparent prob's. *G. Taylor*
8/12/96 0610	**Nursing note:** Slept all night. No complaints. Awake and alert. Carried out ADLs w/o assistance. Doesn't always get what you say. Sometimes helps to repeat, remind pt. of topic. *L. Smith*
8/12/96 1000	**Speech-language pathology note:** Consultation request received. Pt. seen briefly @ bedside. Impression: moderate-severe Wernicke's aphasia. Full report to follow. *G. Becker, PhD, CCC, SLP*

Patient Id:
    Shaw, Arthur 5/17/41
    503-42-9680
    2K435-32 NEU   **Medical record**
                                 Progress notes

Figure 3-4 ▪ A series of progress notes from a hypothetical medical record. The notes are not necessarily continuous. Ordinarily, there would be several more notes entered on the patient's first day on the ward.

**Medical record
Radiographic report**

Name: Shaw, Arthur	**Ward:** 2N, Neuro
Id#: 503 42 9680	**Req. MD:** Ericsson
Age: 55	**Case #:** 3937

Date of examination: August 12,1996: 1433
Examination: CT head with contrast

Clinical history:
55-year-old male with suspected LH stroke 8/11/96. Rule out hemorrhage.

Comparisons: There are no previous studies available for comparison.

Findings: Enhanced CT scan of the head. A new area of decreased attenuation in the left temporoparietal white matter and extending into the overlying cortex consistent with a new occlusive infarct. No evidence of hemorrhage. The ventricles are in a midline position without evidence of mass effect.

Impressions: New area of infarction in the left temporo-parietal region consistent with occlusion of posterior branch of left middle cerebral artery. See above findings.

Films were read by: *Mary C. Richman*

       Mary C. Richman, MD, Neuroradiologist

Figure 3-5 ▪ An example of a CT scan report from a hypothetical medical record.

record. The information in this form provides a quick reference for speech pathology clinic personnel who may be involved in Mr. Shaw's care and serves as a record of Mr. Shaw's medical history and current problems, should that information be needed in the future when his medical records are not readily available.

The speech-language pathologist's review of a patient's medical record provides her or him with a general sense of the patient's medical and neurologic problems and potential communication impairments, a general impression of the patient's behavioral and emotional state, and a preliminary plan for the patient's care. These impressions are firmed up by an interview with the patient and testing sufficient to solidify the impressions. Then the speech-language pathologist writes a response to the consultation request. The speech-language pathologist's re-

sponse to the neurologist's consultation request for Mr. Shaw is shown in Figure 3-8.

The speech-language pathologist's response to the consultation request follows a common format. It begins with the consultant's subjective observations, proceeds to a description of objective test results, follows with the consultant's interpretation of test results and conclusions regarding the nature of the patient's problems and their probable time-course, and ends with recommendations for dealing with the problems that led to the referral. The response to the consultation request is brief and to the point (physicians and other health-care personnel rarely have, or take, the time to read long and complex reports). Tests are described in everyday language, and examples of test items are provided. (The names of most tests of communication ability and scores on them have little meaning to most non–speech-language-

Medical record
Radiographic report

Name: Shaw, Arthur	**Ward:** 2N, Neuro
Id#: 503 42 9680	**Req, MD:** Ericsson
Age: 55	**Case #:** 2302

Date of examination: August 13, 1996: 0803
Examination: Noninvasive carotid w imaging

Clinical history:
55-year-old male with suspected LH stroke 8/11/96. Rule out carotid stenosis.

Comparisons: There are no previous studies available for comparison.

Findings: Intimal thickening and focal areas of soft plaque are identified throughout both carotid systems.

The right common carotid artery has no associated hemodynamically significant stenosis. The right internal carotid artery has increased peak systolic velocities of 160 cm per second. This is consistent with a severe stenosis (60% to 79%) of the right internal carotid artery. The right external carotid artery demonstrates no hemodynamically significant stenosis.

The left common carotid demonstrates no associated hemodynamically significant stenosis. The left internal carotid artery has slightly increased peak systolic velocities of 130 cm to 140 cm per second with a diastolic velocity of 40 cm per second. This is consistent with a mild to moderate stenosis (20% to 59%) of the left internal carotid artery. There are increased peak systolic velocities in the left external carotid artery consistent with an underlying stenosis.

Impressions:
1. Severe stenosis (60% to 79%) of the right internal carotid artery.
2. Mild to moderate stenosis (20% to 59%) of the left internal carotid artery.
3. Increased peak systolic velocities of left external carotid artery consistent with underlying stenosis.
4. Right vertebral artery not visualized on this examination.

Films were read by: *Warren E Davies*

Warren E. Davies, MD, Radiologist

Figure 3-6 ■ **An example of a carotid ultrasound report from a hypothetical medical record.**

pathologists). The format of the speech-language pathologist's report makes it easy for the person making the consultation request to get the information from the report quickly and without appreciable effort. This helps to ensure the report will be read by the requestor (and others) and that those who read it will get the information they need to appreciate the effects of the patient's communication impairments on the plan of care.

The impressions generated by the speech-language pathologist's review of the patient's medical record are subsequently put to the test when the speech-language pathologist interviews the patient and family members. The speech-language pathologist may also be put to the test in the interview and subsequent test sessions by behavioral, cognitive, and emotional perturbations exhibited by brain-damaged pa-

Speech pathology service

Patient information		
Patient name: Shaw, Arthur	**Soc sec number:** 503 42 9680	**Referral date;** 8/12/96
Home address: 6877 Lakeview Court Riverview, MN 55444-1212	**Occupation:** Accountant **Marital status:** M (Florence) **Education:** College (BA)	**Physician:** Ericsson 4498 **Med diagnoses:** LMCA CVA. aphasia
Birthdate: 7/26/41	**Home phone:** 612-555-9888	
Referring ward: 2N (Neuro)	**Referring service:** Neurology	**SPS** file #:6888

Communication, swallowing disorders	
Problem #1: Aphasia	**Date of onset:** 8/11/96
Problem #2:	**Date of onset:**
Problem #3:	**Date of onset:**

Medical information

Previous medical history: Adult onset diabetes mellitus diagnosed 1991. Controlled by oral medications. Hypertension diagnosed November, 1993. Pt.'s wife mentioned brief episode of numbness in pt.'s RUE, March, '95. MD: "poss. TIA."

History of present illness: The patient apparently was in good health until the morning of August 11. He was dressing for work when he experienced sudden onset of right-sided weakness and slurred speech. He alerted his wife who called an ambulance that brought him to the emergency room at this medical center. On arrival he exhibited extreme weakness and exaggerated reflexes on his right side. His speech apparently was fluent with verbal paraphasias and some jargon and his comprehension was grossly impaired. Since that time he apparently has been improving slowly, although he seems still to have a substantial aphasia. Nursing notes suggest that he is oriented and alert.

Laboratory results: CT scan: "New area of decreased attenuation in the left temporo-parietal white matter, extending into cortex, c/w new occlusive infarct. No evidence of hemorrhage. Carotid u/s: Severe stenosis R TCA (60%-79%), mild-moderate stenosis LTCA (20%-50%).

BP: 162/89.

Medications: Tolbutamide, chlorothiazide

Other: Low-fat, low-salt diet. Consult to SW: "Pls assist with d/c planning." Consult to Rehab: "RUE, RLE weakness, pls assess and make rec's."

Clinician: G. Becker **Signature:** G. Becker, PhD, CCC-SLP **Date:** 8/12/96

Figure 3-7 ■ An example of a standard form used to record information from a patient's medical record.

Medical record	Consultation request/referral	
To: Speech pathology	**From:** Ward 2N neurology	**Date:** 08/12/96 14:30

Provisional diagnosis: L MCA CVA, global aphasia

Requested by: Ericcson, G. 4498	Place: Consultant's choice	Urgency: Routine

Reason for request: 55 y/o R-H M 1 day s/p recent L MCA CVA. RUE RLE weakn. Globally aphas. Hx DM, HTN. Pls eval pt.'s spch & lang & make recs.

Consultation report

Mr. Shaw's speech and language was evaluated in the Speech pathology clinic on 8/14/96.

Subjective observations: Mr. Shaw is a 55-year-old man who experienced a left middle cerebral artery CVA on August 11, 1996. Mr Shaw was brought to the speech pathology clinic in a wheelchair although he later claimed that he can walk: "I guess I'm a little unsteady on my feet." During the evaluation he was cooperative, attentive, alert, and task-oriented, although the presence of a severe auditory comprehension impairment markedly compromised his conversational and test-taking abilities.

Objective measures: Several speech and language tests were administered. Mr. Shaw's performance suggested:
- Severe impairment of listening comprehension. Mr. Shaw can correctly identify drawings of common objects named by the examiner on about 50% of trials. He can follow one-step commands ("Pick up the spoon") with about 50% accuracy, but cannot follow 2-step commands ("Point to the pencil and give me the key.")
- Severe impairment of speech production. Mr. Shaw's speech, both in conversation and during testing, is vague, devoid of meaning, and littered with verbal paraphasias ("chair" for "table") and literal paraphasias ("spomb" for "comb"). Occasional neologisms (nonwords) are also observed. However, the mechanics of Mr. Shaw's speech production are relatively unaffected—he speaks smoothly and effortlessly, with essentially normal rate, intonation, and stress patterns.
- Severely compromised reading ability. Mr. Shaw can read a few simple concrete words ("man," "dog") but cannot read multisyllabic words or longer units. Failed attempts are characterized by paraphasias and neologisms.
- Severely compromised writing ability. Mr. Shaw could copy his name, with effort, but could write nothing intelligible either spontaneously or to dictation.

Impressions and conclusions: Mr. Shaw currently exhibits symptoms consistent with severe Wernicke's (receptive) aphasia. Because of the recent onset of Mr. Shaw's aphasia, the severity of his language impairments should diminish during the next several weeks, although he is likely to remain moderately aphasic even when full neurologic recovery has taken place. His return to employability appears, at this time, unlikely.

Recommendations:
1. Additional assessment of Mr. Shaw's listening comprehension to determine the extent and nature of his comprehension impairments.
2. A period of trial treatment to improve auditory comprehension and self-monitoring to determine Mr. Shaw's potential to benefit from treatment.
3. Speech-language pathologist to meet with Mr. Shaw's wife and other concerned family members to answer questions and discuss Mr. Shaw's potential return home.

The patient was examined: [x] yes [ ] no
The patient's medical record was reviewed: [x] yes [ ] no

Signature and title: *G. Becker*	G. Becker, PhD CCC-SLP	Date: 08/14/96	
Id#: 133591	**Organization/service:** Speech pathology	**Reg#:** —	**Ward:** —

Patient Id:
  Shaw, Arthur 5/17/41
  503-42-9680   **SF 522 3/94**
  2K435-32 NEU   **Consultation request**

Figure 3-8 ■ The speech-language pathologist's response to the consultation request for Mr. Shaw.

tients. These behavioral perturbations can have serious effects on how brain-damaged patients respond to unusual, unexpected, or challenging situations, such as interviews with strangers in white coats or tests with unusual or difficult materials.

■ BEHAVIORAL, COGNITIVE, AND EMOTIONAL CONSEQUENCES OF BRAIN DAMAGE

Brain damage creates impairments in reading, writing, speaking, and listening and affects the way patients approach tasks, solve problems, respond to stimuli, monitor their performance, interact with others, and view themselves. The presence of these consequences of brain injury depends on several factors, including the patient's previous personality and intellect, the location and severity of the patient's brain damage, and how those around the patient respond to him or her. These behavioral, cognitive, and emotional consequences of brain damage may complicate the interview, interfere with assessment, get in the way of treatment, and compromise the patient's daily-life independence and self-sufficiency.

Responsiveness

Many brain-damaged patients have difficulty getting purposeful behavior started and sustaining behavior once they get it going. Patients with mild initiation problems are passive but compliant. They tend not to initiate purposeful behavior but respond appropriately when requested to (especially in highly-structured contexts). Many of these patients readily talk about plans and projects but fail to put their talk into action. Because these patients are capable of doing much more than they spontaneously do, family members and associates may consider them lazy, unmotivated, uncooperative, or stubborn. The most seriously affected patients produce almost no self-initiated behavior beyond routine self-care and household activities. They seem apathetic and uninterested in what goes on around them. When pushed to respond they do, but their responses are slow and terse, though they may be normal in structure and content.

Some brain-damaged patients are *hyperresponsive* and *impulsive*. Their responses to people, events, and situations are quick, indiscriminate, and sometimes inappropriate. Mentally they seem to be caught up by their first impressions. They fail to appreciate subtle or abstract aspects of events or situations, which leads them to misinterpret the events or situations. These patients' impulsiveness and their failure to appreciate nonliteral meaning and intent often creates havoc in social, personal, and financial matters.

Other brain-damaged patients are the antithesis of impulsive. These patients behave as if they do not trust their perception and interpretation of what goes on around them and doubt their capacity for responding appropriately to challenging events and situations. These self-doubts make them indecisive, hesitant, and slow to respond when they feel challenged or threatened, and when they do respond, their self-doubts can cause them to revise, qualify, or elaborate on responses that were adequate and appropriate in the first place. The excessive cautiousness of these patients affects their test-taking behavior and their performance in treatment activities, wherein they tend to perform below their capabilities. Their cautiousness often compromises their social well-being by leading them to withdraw from all but the most comfortable and predictable daily-life relationships.

Horner and LaPointe (1979) characterized brain-damaged adults' tendency toward impulsiveness or cautiousness as variations in *cognitive style*. According to Horner and LaPointe, patients with *reflective style* proceed through tasks slowly, take a long time to respond, and (usually) make few errors. Patients with *impulsive style* proceed through tasks quickly, respond quickly, and (usually) make many errors. Horner and LaPointe recommended that clinicians structure assessment procedures to identify patients' characteristic cognitive style and that clinicians modify assessment and treatment procedures to help patients compensate for exaggerated impulsiveness or reflectiveness. According to Horner and LaPointe, patients who go slowly but make many errors need training in the task or revision of the task to make it easier. Patients who proceed through a task slowly and make no errors may be speeded up, as long as speeding them up does not generate errors. Patients who respond quickly and make many errors may be helped by slowing them down. Patients who respond quickly but make no errors in a task probably need a more difficult task (see Box below).

Perseveration Perseveration refers to repetition of responses when they are no longer appropriate, (as when a patient who has correctly named a pencil calls the next several objects pencils or when a patient who has correctly given his name in response to the examiner's request for it continues to give his name in response to the examiner's questions about his address and vocation). The frequency and persistence of perseverative responses seem to be related to the severity of brain damage, although the relationship is not perfect. Perseverative behaviors may be seen following unilateral damage in either brain hemisphere, following generalized damage caused by traumatic injuries, and in the middle to late stages of dementia. Perseveration often appears in the first days and weeks following brain injury and usually diminishes (and sometimes disappears) as the patient recovers.

Diminished Response Flexibility Most brain-damaged patients have difficulty changing their responses when tasks or response requirements change. Some may perseverate. Others exhibit temporary disruptions of performance when tasks or response requirements change. Porch (1994), writing about aphasic adults, described this latter phenomenon as a "tuning in" problem, and Brookshire (1992), also writing about aphasic adults, described it as "slow rise time." Both labels describe patients who are slow at refocusing or reallocating attention when situational requirements change. Some patients with diffuse brain damage exhibit transitory disruptions of performance as new tasks are introduced, not because of slowness at allocating attentional resources, but because they are slow at developing a strategy for dealing with the new task requirements.

Cognitive Changes

Concreteness and Difficulty with Abstract Concepts Concreteness, or what Goldstein (1948) referred to as "loss of the abstract attitude," is a common consequence of brain injury (especially diffuse damage or damage in the right brain hemisphere). Goldstein was referring to brain-damaged patients' tendency to be caught up by the obvious literal meaning of abstract material. These patients frequently have difficulty appreciating the figurative meaning of idioms and metaphor (*She had a heavy heart. He paid the piper*) and may have difficulty with humor, sarcasm, proverbs, and other materials in which intended meaning cannot be represented by literal interpretations. Concreteness may contribute to some brain-injured patients' tendencies toward *egocentrism* (inability to appreciate another person's point of view). Concreteness often has major effects on brain-damaged patients' problem-solving, because they see only the simplest and most obvious so-

	Low Error Rate	High Error Rate
Responds quickly	Increase task difficulty	Slow patient down
Responds slowly	Speed patient up	Make task easier

lutions and cannot appreciate less obvious but more satisfactory solutions. Sometimes apparent concreteness can be a result of impulsiveness but more often it reflects an underlying cognitive impairment that prevents the patient from appreciating the implied meaning of abstract material.

Impaired Self-Monitoring Many brain-damaged adults do poorly at monitoring their performance, both in structured assessment and treatment activities and in unstructured social situations. Impaired self-monitoring can have wide-ranging effects, including obliviousness to errors during testing and treatment and inappropriate behavior in social situations. It is a common consequence of both focal and diffuse brain injuries. There is no strong relationship between impaired self-monitoring and damage to specific brain regions, although it tends to be more frequent following frontal lobe or temporal lobe damage than damage in other brain regions. In general, patients with diffuse brain damage are more likely to be impaired in self-monitoring than those with focal lesions.

Impaired Anticipation of Errors Some brain-damaged adults are good at recognizing their errors but cannot anticipate or prevent them. Their errors typically appear "out of the blue" without delay, hesitation, editing, or foreknowledge of the impending errors. Their reactions to errors can range from bemusement to chagrin. Patients with posterior brain damage are more likely to be bemused; those with anterior brain damage are more likely to be chagrined. When brain-damaged adults attempt to self-correct their errors, their attempts sometimes lead them away from the intended response, rather than toward it.

Difficulty Focusing and Sustaining Attention Many brain-damaged adults are slow at focusing attention and cannot maintain optimum levels of attention over time. Those who are slow at focusing attention have difficulty when tasks or response requirements change. When these patients are tested, they may miss the first items in a test or subtest but respond adequately to later items. Patients who have difficulty sustaining attention typically get worse as testing progresses, even when the difficulty of test items does not change. Some patients' attentional processes seem to fluctuate over time, so that intervals of poor performance alternate with intervals of adequate performance, with the changes in performance seemingly unrelated to changes in tasks, stimuli, or response requirements. The intervals of poor performance may last from a few seconds to (rarely) minutes, after which performance recovers. It is not clear what causes these fluctuations in performance, and there is no strong relationship between the presence of attentional impairments and the location of patients' brain injuries, although traumatic brain injuries are well-known precursors to attentional impairments.

Sequential Ordering Impairments Some brain-injured patients have difficulty perceiving, retaining, reporting, and reproducing sequential information. This phenomenon was first described by Efron (1963) and subsequently elaborated on by Brookshire (1974, 1975). These patients have difficulty in test or treatment activities in which temporally ordered sequences of responses are required (e.g., pointing, in order, to a series of objects or pictures named by the clinician). Sometimes these patients do better if the clinician provides cues to the proper sequence of responses by means of the spatial arrangement of stimuli (such as from left to right, in the order in which the responses to them are to be made). Damage in the frontal lobe of the language-dominant hemisphere is a frequent cause of sequential ordering impairments, although impairments occasionally are seen following damage in other brain regions.

Disturbances of Personality and Emotion

Emotional Lability Brain damage sometimes contributes to exaggerated swings in emotional expression (a condition called *emotional* *lability*).* Emotionally labile patients' expression of emotion is appropriate (they express sadness and happiness in appropriate contexts), but the magnitude of their emotional response is disproportionate to the eliciting stimulus. Emotional lability associated with brain damage frequently is expressed as uncontrollable crying in response to neutral or mildly emotional stimuli (e.g., a patient bursts into tears when asked if she or he has children). Neurologists and others sometimes call this phenomenon *pseudobulbar affect,* because it can occur as a consequence of bilateral damage to corticospinal and corticobulbar tracts above the pons. (As mentioned earlier, the pons is sometimes called the *bulb;* hence the term *pseudobulbar.*) For these patients, lability may represent loss of cortical inhibition of emotional responses originating in lower, phylogenetically more primitive structures. Emotional lability sometimes takes the form of inappropriate laughter in situations that are not humorous or takes the form of excessive laughter in response to mildly amusing stimuli (especially when the patient feels stressed, challenged, or threatened).

Irritability and Low Frustration Tolerance Some brain-damaged patients are prone to emotional outbursts, usually as a consequence of lowered frustration tolerance. These patients explode emotionally when they are stressed or pushed to their limits or beyond. This is a response that Schuell, Jenkins, & Jimenez-Pabon (1965) call *catastrophic reaction.* There are several differences between emotionally labile patients and patients with low frustration tolerance. Emotionally labile patients can be pushed into emotional breakdown

---

* Emotional lability can occur in association with or as a consequence of conditions that have nothing to do with brain injury; for example in some psychiatric states and intoxication, or as a reaction to stress, confusion, or embarrassment. The discussion in this section excludes lability from those other causes.

by innocuous or mildly stressful events, but patients with low frustration tolerance typically lose control only when pushed too far. The outbreaks of emotionally labile patients appear suddenly and without warning, but patients with low frustration tolerance often give visible signs of an impending explosion and become progressively agitated and show other signs of autonomic arousal as they approach the threshold for an outburst. Those who live and work around patients with low frustration tolerance soon learn to recognize the precursors to emotional outbursts and they may prevent them by changing the situation or otherwise lowering the patient's level of arousal.

The foregoing effects of brain damage on cognitive, perceptual, and behavioral functions can influence brain-injured patients' responses to the interview and affect their test performance. The clinician who knows that brain damage can create cognitive, perceptual, and behavioral disturbances can plan for them. Planning for them minimizes their effects on the interview, on testing, and on treatment.

■ INTERVIEWING THE PATIENT

The interview provides the speech-language pathologist's first direct look at the patient's communication abilities, physical condition, orientation and attention, visual and hearing acuity, behavioral inclinations, and other characteristics that might affect how (or if) the subsequent assessment is carried out. Getting the interpersonal relationship off to a good start usually is as important as the information gathering function of the interview. There is no one best way to do this, and different clinicians may approach a given patient in different ways with equivalent results. The most successful clinicians, however, share two common attributes— they care about the patient and let it show and they treat the patient with respect. In addition to caring about and respecting the patient, good interviewers comply with the following general principles that govern how the interview takes place.

Conduct the Interview in a Quiet Place, Free From Distractions Many first interviews are held at bedside in the patient's room. This is fine if the room is quiet without much other activity, because the patient is likely to be more relaxed and comfortable in the familiar surroundings of her or his own room. However, the advantage of familiar surroundings is easily overwhelmed by noise or distracting activity elsewhere in the room. If the patient's room is not quiet and free of distractions, find another place nearby (a day room, conference room, an empty patient room, or, if nothing is available on the patient's ward, move the interview to a quiet room off the ward).

Include Family Members or Significant Others in the Interview Family members and significant others should be invited to participate in the interview. If the patient's communication impairments are mild or moderate, family members and significant others can corroborate what the patient reports and can help the patient remember, produce, or clarify information. If the patient's communication impairments are severe, family members and significant others may be the primary (or only) source of information and the patient's role may be that of confirmation and corroboration. If a patient is able to communicate only rudimentary information with great difficulty, the speech-language pathologist may schedule some time with family members and significant others to get the information that the patient cannot provide. The following suggestions relate to the patient interview but they also apply to interviews with family members and significant others.

Tell the Patient Who You Are In teaching hospitals, patients are seen by a confusing mix of physicians, residents, medical students, trainees, and others, many of whom pop in and out of the patient's room without introduction

or explanation. Helping the patient sort out this mix of people usually makes for a more relaxed and less-stressed patient. Regrettably, physicians sometimes neglect to tell patients that they are referring them to other specialists. Therefore it is important that you make certain that the patient knows right away who you are and what your role is in her or his care. Introduce yourself and tell the patient what your responsibilities are:

> I'm Dr./Ms./Mr. Smith. I'm from the speech clinic. I'll be working with you to find out what kinds of problems you might be having with talking, writing, and understanding, and what we might be able to do about them.

Tell the patient how you fit into the treatment team:

> Your doctor will take care of your medical problems. The physical therapist will work on your walking and help you regain strength in your arm. I'll be working with you on talking, writing, and understanding.

Boll (1994) recommends that the interviewer begin by asking the patient why he or she has been referred. According to Boll, the patient's response gives the interviewer a sense of the patient's comprehension of the circumstances, his or her level of interest and motivation, his or her comfort with the arrangements, and the adequacy with which the referral has been handled by the referring parties. According to Boll, it also gives the interviewer a sense of whether the patient has been informed about the nature of the interview and whether the information has been understood, ignored, or forgotten.

Make the Patient Comfortable Spend a few minutes in conversation to allow the patient to relax and talk about familiar topics. Ask the patient some general questions about themselves (*"Where are you from? What kind of work do you/did you do? Are you married? Do you have children/grandchildren?"*). This usually helps put the patient at ease, especially if the interviewer can discover common ground (knowledge of the patient's home town, street address, mutual interests, and so forth).* Sit down during the interview. A standing interviewer conversing with a seated patient can be intimidating, and, regardless of the length of the interview, standing during the interview may give the patient a feeling that you won't be staying long or that the interview will be a brief and perhaps unwelcome addition to your busy schedule. Try to give patients the sense that getting to know them and their concerns is important to you.

Get the Patient's Story Begin with a general question (*"How are you feeling today?"*) and follow up with whatever additional questions or commentary seem appropriate. Then move on to the patient's communication problems. (*"Are you having difficulty talking? Tell me about it."*) Find out how the patient feels about the problems. Some patients may be traumatized about communication abnormalities that most people would consider minor annoyances (while others are unconcerned about impairments that seriously interfere with their communication). Make mental notes of what the patient says and pursue any interesting leads.[†] Note other significant aspects of the patient's condition and behavior, such as whether the patient is ambulatory and able to sit up and attend for the length of time needed for testing, the patient's mood, orientation and mental sta-

tus, the patient's visual and auditory acuity, and whether the patient wears eyeglasses or a hearing aid.

Be a Patient, Concerned, and Understanding Listener Give the patient time to tell her or his story. Don't interrupt and don't lead unless the patient gets bogged down in trivial details or goes off on tangents that clearly are unrelated to the purpose of the interview. Ask questions to follow up on potentially meaningful information, but do not steer the patient to provide the answers that you expect based on your preconceptions of what ought to be. Don't be oversolicitous and overly sympathetic. Adult patients don't need and often resent overdone expressions of concern and sympathy. Receive what the patient says objectively and matter-of-factly, and treat the interview as a problem-solving enterprise between the patient and the interviewer.

Talk to the Patient at Her or His Level Use everyday language and avoid the use of jargon and technical terminology that may confuse or intimidate the patient. Monitor the patient's alertness and understanding and repeat and paraphrase if necessary. Pay careful attention to the patient's eye contact, facial expression, and body language as indicators of their frustration, anxiety, or miscomprehension. Don't talk *at* the patient but talk *with* the patient. Engage him or her as a partner in the interview. Accommodate to the patient's interaction style but avoid excessive familiarity. Be friendly but objective. Use humor sparingly and judiciously but don't avoid it. Judiciously used and properly timed humor can help to humanize the interview, dissipate tension, and reassure the patient without minimizing the seriousness of the patient's situation.

Do Your Homework Before the Interview Before the interview get a general sense of the patient's major problems and concerns from the medical record and from conversations with physicians and others involved in the patient's care. This knowledge will enable you to

---

* Some patients react emotionally to questions about family and occupation, because the questions make them despondent about compromised family and work relationships and responsibilities. The interviewer must be sensitive to the potential effect of such topics and should be prepared to change the subject if the patient shows signs of emotional upset.

† Rarely do patients provide background information that is so detailed and complex that the speech-language pathologist cannot remember it without the aid of written notes. More importantly, the speech-language pathologist's note-taking may be intimidating to the patient and get in the way of establishing a relationship with the patient, which is one of the objectives of the early part of the interview.

ask the appropriate questions and make appropriate comments at the right times and will enable you to elicit relevant information and pursue a line of inquiry that is directed toward testing diagnostic questions. It may also help you avoid material that may elicit emotional responses from the patient or make him or her feel apprehensive or threatened.

Treat the Patient as an Adult Who Merits Respect Never ask questions or convey an attitude that makes the patient feel inadequate, juvenile, or incompetent. Sometimes it helps to point out to the patient that her or his neurologic injury may have made it difficult or impossible to do some of the things that she or he used to do easily and that many other abilities remain unaffected. If a topic or line of questioning appears to embarrass the patient or make him or her anxious, it may be best to move on to a different topic. If the abandoned line of questioning appears important, you can come back to it later and lead into it more carefully. An important but subtle indicator of respect is the way in which the clinician addresses the patient. It is never appropriate to address the patient by her or his first name during the clinician's early contacts with the patient, although it may become appropriate later when the clinician and the patient have gotten better acquainted. However, the clinician should ask the patient how she or he would prefer to be addressed. Some older patients resent the use of their first names by those involved in their care, especially when the person providing care is appreciably younger than the patient.

Prepare the Patient for What Comes Next If you plan additional testing, prepare the patient for it. Give the patient a general idea of the kinds of tests you plan to administer and why you are going to administer them. Tell the patient the day and time of testing if you know them. Answer the patient's questions and deal with any concerns he or she express.

By the end of the interview the patient and the clinician should be comfortable with each other, and the patient should be comfortable with the idea of being tested. The clinician should have accumulated a large amount of information about the patient from the medical record and the interview, and should have a good idea of what tests to begin with and the approximate level of difficulty of the first few tests. Information from the referral, the patient's medical records, and the interview helps to determine which tests are selected. The clinician's experiences with the patient during the interview largely determine the level of difficulty at which testing begins.

■ TESTING THE PATIENT

The bulk of testing usually is done in the speech-language pathology clinic, although screening tests may be administered in the patient's room. Before the testing begins the clinician takes a few minutes to explain the purpose of the tests, answer the patient's questions, and obtain the patient's consent for testing. Lezak (1995) provides guidelines regarding what the patient should be told before any test is administered.

Explain the Purpose of Testing Tell the patient why he or she has been referred to the speech-language pathologist, why testing is necessary, and how the information from the tests will be used (e.g., to determine if the patient has a communication impairment, to understand the patient's communication problems, to decide about the need for treatment, to decide how to treat the patient's communication problems, or to measure the patient's progress).

Describe the Nature of the Tests Likely to Be Given The patient might be told that the tests will be concerned with identifying and measuring impairments in speaking, listening, reading, and writing.

Tell the Patient What Will Be Done to Protect His or Her Privacy and the Confidentiality of Test Results The patient might be told that only persons in the medical center who are involved in the patient's care will have access to the results of testing and that access will be given to others only with the written permission of the patient and/or her or his legal representative.

Tell the Patient Who Will Report Test Results to the Patient and Family and When They Will Be Reported The speech-language pathologist usually reports the test results, but the physician or another professional may also do so.

Give the Patient a Brief Explanation of Test Procedures The patient usually is told that he or she will be asked to do a variety of tasks involving speaking, listening, reading, and writing, and that some of them will be easy and others may be difficult. They also may be told how long test sessions usually last and that testing can be terminated if the patient becomes tired or wishes to end the test.

Find Out How the Patient Feels About Taking the Tests Some patients may be uneasy or apprehensive about testing because they feel that being tested is a sign of weakness, lack of intelligence, or childishness on their part. When this happens, reiterating the purposes of testing may be sufficient to dispel the patient's concerns. However, the patient (or the patient's legal representative) always has the right to refuse any or all testing.

If audiotape or videotape recordings of the patient's performance are made, the speech-language pathologist must explain:

> *The purposes of the recording*—for example, to allow the patient and the speech-language pathologist to evaluate the patient's progress.
> *Who will have access to the recordings*—for example, the speech-language pathologist, the patient's physician, and student trainees.
> *What will be done with the recordings when the patient is no longer receiving speech-language pathology services*—for example, given to the patient, or erased.

When audiotape or videotape recordings are made, many facilities require that the patient and/or her or his legal representative read and sign a printed consent form giving permission for the recordings. Patients with severe communication impairments may not understand all of the material on the consent form, but the speech-language pathologist should convey as much of it as the patient's comprehension permits and should give the patient an opportunity to communicate his or her feelings and to ask questions. When a patient seems not to comprehend the information, it should be conveyed to the patient's spouse, significant other, caregiver, or legal representative who may then give consent for testing.

Some General Principles for Testing Adults with Brain Injuries

Testing adults who have brain injuries poses special challenges. Because brain injured adults may exhibit a bewildering array of behavioral, cognitive/linguistic, and psychological abnormalities, those who test them often are called upon to exhibit unusual levels of patience, empathy, and understanding, in addition to being expert in test administration and interpretation of patients' responses to test items. There is no substitute for experience in testing brain injured adults just as there is no substitute for experience in other complex activities such as making a souffle or driving a taxicab in New York City. However, observation of the following set of general principles can help beginning clinicians compensate for lack of experience.

Do Your Homework The conscientious clinician comes to the first test session with a plan for assessing the patient's communication based largely on information from the patient's medical record and the interview. From reading the medical record the clinician has learned something about the patient's background, life situation, and current problems, and from the interview the clinician has gotten a sense of the patient's cognitive abilities, personality, social behavior, and communication impairments. The clinician may have formulated a tentative diagnosis and usually will have in mind a plan for testing (where to begin and how to proceed). This knowledge about the patient, together with the resulting plan, help to make testing systematic and efficient so that each test builds on the one before, and ensures that all necessary tests, but no unnecessary ones are given.

Choose an Appropriate Place for Testing The test environment should be quiet, well-lit, and free from distractions. Furnishings should be comfortable but functional—a good-sized table and two comfortable chairs are a minimum requirement. The test materials should be accessible to the examiner but out of sight until they are needed. If audio or video recordings are to be made, microphones and cameras should be in unobtrusive locations.

Schedule Testing to Maximize the Patient's Performance Most hospitalized patients with neurogenic communication disorders have surprisingly busy schedules. Laboratory tests, appointments with counselors and social workers, physical and occupational therapy appointments, and other activities fill the patient's day. To compound the problem, most brain-damaged patients no longer have the stamina they had before their injury and by late morning or early afternoon they are exhausted and need nothing so much as a nap. Consequently, the shrewd speech-language pathologist schedules testing sessions early in the day while the patient is still fresh, and if testing sessions must be scheduled later in the day, the clinician ensures that the patient has had a chance to rest before the test session.

Marshall & King (1972) confirmed the negative effects of fatigue on the communication performance of aphasic adults. They tested aphasic adults' communication ability following either a period of exertion or following a rest period. They reported that most subjects' communication performance was negatively affected by previous exertion and recommended that testing be accomplished early in the morning and before strenuous activities such as phys-

ical or corrective therapy appointments. However, some of Marshall and King's subjects' communicative performance was unaffected by the exercise and a few even improved slightly on some subtests when they were tested after an exercise session. Consequently, clinicians may find that some brain-injured patients tolerate strenuous activity better than others.

Make Testing a Collaborative Effort The examiner must never forget that the patient is an adult who may be anxious, apprehensive, bewildered, and frightened by his or her neurologic and behavioral symptoms. The clinician should point out that because the purpose of testing is to get a sense of the nature and severity of the patient's impairments, together with an accurate picture of what the patient can still do, both difficult and easy tests are necessary. Testing should be approached matter-of-factly but in an atmosphere of support and understanding. Pointing out to the patient that the assessment process is a collaborative effort by the patient and the clinician may help give the patient a sense that she or he is an active participant in the process. Schuell, Jenkins, and Jimenez-Pabon (1965) claim therapeutic benefits for testing when it is approached as a joint effort by the clinician and the patient:

> . . . searching exploration of aphasic disabilities can be a therapeutic rather than a traumatic procedure. This is true because the process of testing establishes communication on a level that is highly meaningful to the patient. As a result, he feels less isolated and less anxious. By means of the tests, the examiner leads the patient toward objectivity by helping him understand the nature of his problems and their limits. The patient discovers things he is able to do, which tends to restore confidence and alleviate depression. Patients become less and less defensive as confidence in the clinician increases (p. 168).

Select Tests That are Appropriate for the Patient Skilled clinicians usually have a general sense of the nature of the patient's probable impairments and the patient's likely level of impairment in areas of deficiency before testing begins. This knowledge helps the clinician focus testing on the patient's probable impairments and ensures that testing begins at a level appropriate to the patient.

The assessment process often begins with administration of a generic test battery (e.g., a standardized aphasia test battery). Generic test batteries provide a general description of a patients' performance in a variety of tasks and at various levels of difficulty within tasks. The tests are useful for identifying communication disabilities, estimating their severity, and describing their nature. Some tests can be used to assign patients to diagnostic categories and some can be used to predict the eventual level of a patient's recovery of communicative ability. Generic test batteries provide broad coverage of a domain of linguistic, cognitive, or behavioral attributes in a reasonable amount of time (1 to 3 hours). Generic test batteries provide clinicians with a look at many aspects of a patient's communication performance (speaking, listening, writing, and reading) but the look does not always have great depth. In some respects generic test batteries function as screening devices because they are good at detecting communication impairments but not so good at specifying their exact nature or severity.

Weisenberg and McBride (1935), Schuell (1965), and Porch (1967) have each discussed characteristics that generic test batteries for aphasic adults should have. Most of these characteristics also apply to test batteries for assessing communicative impairments other than aphasia. The following list is a blend of recommendations made by Weisenberg & McBride, Schuell, and Porch:

- The test battery should sample a large number of performances at different levels of difficulty in several related tasks so that all potentially disturbed performances are evaluated.
- The test battery should allow the user to determine the level at which performance is error-free, the level at which performance

completely breaks down, and several intervening levels within each test or subtest.
- The test battery should sample, in a consistent way, the input modalities through which test instructions are delivered, the processes used while tasks are performed, and the output modalities necessary for carrying out the tasks.
- The test battery should be standardized so that results are reliable from test to test and examiner to examiner. It should provide for control of relevant variables such as method of stimulus presentation, instructions to the patient, and response scoring.
- The test battery should record patient performance in such a way that the quality of responses as well as their correctness is recorded.
- Subtests in the test battery should include a sufficient number of items to permit the user to reliably determine a patient's average performance on each subtest and to minimize variability generated by sporadic fluctuations in the patient's performance.
- The test battery should suggest the reasons for a patient's deficient performance on test items.
- The test battery should permit predictions regarding a patient's eventual recovery of communication.

Because no two brain-injured patients are likely to exhibit exactly the same pattern of deficits, clinicians rarely rely exclusively on a generic test battery for evaluating every patient within a diagnostic category. Most clinicians begin with a generic test battery to get a general impression of the patient's level of performance under well-controlled test conditions and to establish the general pattern and overall severity of the patient's deficits. Then they branch off with standardized or nonstandardized tests appropriate for the patient's pattern of impairments. The generic test battery permits them to get a look at the patient's performance under standardized test conditions, to compare the patient's performance with that of norm groups, and to establish reliable baseline levels of performance. The follow-up testing permits them to describe the patient's own unique pattern of impairments and preserved abilities.

Let the Patient's Performance Guide What and How You Test Skilled clinicians are alert to signals suggesting that they should branch off from their usual test routine. These signals come from many places, such as the patient's history, the diagnosis, the clinician's previous experience with similar patients, the patient's current test performance, and sometimes from a clinical hunch. When skilled clinicians receive such signals they diverge from their test routine to follow up on leads provided by the patient's performance. They do this by modifying standard tests or improvising new tests to specify the variables that affect the patient's performance. This sometimes requires that the focus of testing change repeatedly throughout the examination until the nature and severity of the patient's impairments become clear.

An important part of this process is what Lezak (1995) calls *testing the limits.* Clinicians test the limits by going beyond the standard procedures for administering a given test to explore the reasons for a patient's compromised performance. For example, a clinician might allow a patient who fails a standard test of written spelling to spell the same words orally. Normal oral spelling performance would prove that the deficient performance on the standard test was not because the patient could not spell, but perhaps because she or he could not write. If the patient were to fail the oral spelling test, the clinician might have the patient choose correctly spelled words from sets of printed words in which the correctly spelled word is shown with incorrectly spelled foils. According to Lezak (1995):

> "The limits should be tested whenever there is suspicion that an impairment of some function other than the one under consideration is interfering with an adequate demonstration of that function" (p. 129).

An important benefit of personalizing tests and procedures to the patient is a substantial gain in efficiency. Patients and clinicians do not spend large amounts of time on tests in which the patient's performance is normal or on tests that are too difficult (in which the patient experiences repeated failure). The results of tests in which the patient either makes no errors or makes only errors are of little diagnostic or therapeutic use, and administering them may be a waste of precious clinic time. Furthermore, administering tests that are outside the patient's range may have negative affects on the patient. Tests that are too easy may bore or insult the patient and too-difficult tests may frustrate and anger him or her, interfering with performance on other tests that normally might be within the patient's capabilities.

Use Standardized Tests and Test Procedures Whenever You Wish to Generalize to Other Patients or Other Test Occasions Standardized tests and test batteries usually are not sufficient by themselves to describe a particular patient's pattern of performance. This does not mean that skilled clinicians should avoid them. There is no substitute for standardized tests when the clinician wishes to compare a patient's test performance with that of other patients or with non–brain-damaged adults, compare a patient's performance across several test occasions, or communicate about the patient with other professionals. For any of these purposes, uniform test procedures are necessary, and standardized tests are more likely than nonstandardized tests to have uniform test procedures. Standardized tests also can contribute to efficiency in testing. Most are structured to minimize redundancy, maximize precision, and minimize the complexities of test administration, scoring, and interpretation. However, standardized test batteries can contribute to inefficiency by forcing the patient to undergo more testing than necessary. Skilled clinicians often minimize this inefficiency by administering only selected subtests from standardized test batteries. The subtests are selected to target aspects of performance that the clinician finds most important for a particular patient.*

Most standardized tests come with information about their *validity,* or the degree to which they actually measure what they purport to measure. Various kinds of validity have been described in the literature, but the most frequently described kinds are *content validity* and *construct validity.* In general, *content validity* relates to how well the content of a test (items, tasks, or questions) represents the domain of concern (e.g., intelligence), and *construct validity* relates to how well the content of a test relates to an underlying theory, model, or concept of a process or structure. Consider, for example, a test for measuring comprehension of spoken discourse. To evaluate the test's *content validity* one would ask if the items in the test actually require comprehension of spoken discourse. To evaluate the test's *construct validity,* one would ask if the content of the test and the test procedures are compatible with one or more theories, models, or concepts of discourse comprehension. Clinicians tend to be concerned more with *content validity* than with *construct validity.* They want to know that a test of auditory comprehension actually tests comprehension, that a test of memory actually tests memory, and that a test of sustained attention actually tests a patient's ability to maintain attentiveness over time.

The scores on a test are of little value unless there is a way of relating a given patient's performance to that of normal adults or to the performance of other adults in the same diagnostic category. For example, knowing that a traumatically brain-injured patient responded correctly

to 15 of 25 items in a reading test is, in itself, of little clinical value. However, if one knows that non–brain-damaged adults, on the average, correctly answer 23 of 25 items, one can say that the patient's performance is well below the normal average. If one knows that only 10% of non–brain-damaged adults get 10 or more items wrong, one can say that the patient's reading performance would place him at the tenth percentile of a typical group of non–brain-damaged adults. If one knows that the average fourth-grade student correctly answers 15 of 25 items, one can say that the patient's performance is equivalent to that of average fourth-graders. And if one knows that only 10% of traumatically brain-injured adults correctly answer 15 or more of the 25, one can say that the patient's performance places him at the percentile for traumatically brain-injured adults. Such comparisons of a patients performance with that of normal adults or with the performance of other patients having similar diagnoses are made by means of *norms.* Unfortunately, not all published tests provide norms and some that do provide insufficient or inappropriate ones. It is not always easy to tell if the norms in a test manual are adequate and appropriate. However, the following general indicators should help weed out the very deficient ones.

The *size of the norm group* must be large enough to ensure that the sample is representative of the population to which the norms apply and to ensure that statistics calculated on performance of the norm group are reliable and replicable. There is no simple answer to the question of how large a normative sample must be. It depends partly on how much variability in performance there is in the norm group and partly on how much error users are willing to tolerate in comparing individuals to the norm group. When there is little variability in performance among individuals in the norm group, a relatively small sample may suffice. This sometimes happens when a group of non–brain-damaged adults is tested with a test designed for

---

* This is most practical when norms are available for each subtest in the battery. The availability of such norms permits the clinician to compare the patient's performance with that of groups of individuals—usually a group of "normal" adults and one or more groups of adults representing various diagnostic categories (e.g., adults with aphasia) subtest by subtest.

assessing adults with brain injuries (few of the non–brain-damaged adults make any errors on the test and those that do make very few). Because the performance of the non–brain-damaged adults is extremely homogeneous, increasing the size of the norm group beyond that necessary to establish that non–brain-damaged adults rarely make errors adds little if anything to the accuracy of the norms. In such cases, 20 to 30 individuals in the norm group may be sufficient.

In fact, normative samples as small as 10 may be sufficient in such situations. However, most statisticians and many others concerned with making inferences from a sample to a population often are uneasy about the validity of statistics calculated on samples smaller than 20. Consequently, one rarely sees norm groups smaller than 20, even when the performance of the group is extremely homogeneous. The issue of sample size in such situations may in fact be moot, because statistics that assume normal distributions of scores cannot be calculated on extremely homogeneous data because such data are not distributed normally. Nevertheless, a sample size of 20 seems to represent the lower level of the "comfort zone" for most test designers and publishers. The situation changes when there is appreciable variability in performance across members of the norm group. Then the principle becomes *bigger is better.*

Brain-injured adults are a heterogeneous group, and their performance on any test sensitive to the effects of brain injury is likely to show substantial interindividual variability. Because of this, tests designed for brain-injured adults cannot get by with norm groups of 20 or 30. The chances are good that norms based on brain-damaged groups of fewer than 50 or 60 will be unreliable and norms based on brain-damaged groups of less than 100 should be interpreted cautiously.

Evaluate the Representativeness of the Normative Sample The degree to which the characteristics of the individuals in the normative sample are representative of the population from which the sample is drawn is important. Which characteristics are important depends to some extent on the nature of the test and the population represented by the sample, but characteristics that may affect test performance are the most likely candidates. When the norm group represents an impaired population, the severity and nature of the impairments of those in the norm group should resemble the severity and nature of the impairments present in the population. When the norm group represents a "normal" population, the norm group should resemble the population on any variables that are likely to affect test performance (for tests of language and cognition, these variables almost always include age, education, and intellect).

Evaluate the Appropriateness of Normative Statistics The performance of individuals is compared with that of the norm group by means of *statistics.* The simplest statistics are the *mean* (the average score for the group) and the *range* of scores. With the mean, the user of a test can tell if a particular patient falls at, above, or below the average of the norm group. With the range, the user can tell if anyone in the norm group scored higher or lower than the patient. However, neither of these statistics gives much precision in comparing a patient's performance with the norm group. More precise comparative statements can be made when the test manual provides *standard deviations* or *percentiles* in addition to the mean for the norm group. Standard deviations are statistical abstractions based on the concept of the "normal curve." Percentiles are calculated from means and standard deviations and permit test users to say exactly where in the norm group a given patient would fall—that is, what percentage of the norm group would fall above or below the patient's score. Most statistics books provide tables showing the percent of observations that lie within various segments of the normal distribution. It is reasonably easy to use these tables to calculate percentiles from means and standard deviations.

Obtain a Large Enough Sample of the Patient's Behavior to Ensure Test-Retest Stability When brain-injured adults are tested with materials that challenge but do not overwhelm them, their performance usually fluctuates from item to item within tests. For example, a patient asked to name a set of 10 line drawings on 3 successive presentations of the set may miss 3 items on the first presentation, 5 items on the second, and 2 items on the third. In general, increasing the number of items diminishes such test-to-test variability, at least up to a point, after which further increasing the number of items has little effect on the stability of performance. There is no answer to the question, "How many items are enough?" Most test designers and clinicians seem to agree that 10 items in a subtest usually are adequate for testing most brain-damaged adults. Most test designers and clinicians also would likely agree that tests containing five or fewer items are too short to ensure adequate test-retest stability.

■ PURPOSES OF TESTING

The speech-language pathologist may test patients with neurogenic communication disorders for several reasons. The most common are:

- To diagnose a patient's communication disorder
- To arrive at a prognosis for a patient's recovery of communication abilities
- To determine the nature and severity of a patient's communication disorder
- To make decisions about the appropriateness and potential focus of treatment
- To measure a patient's recovery of communication abilities, the efficacy of treatment, or both

The initial evaluation of a patient's communication abilities typically is directed toward some combination of the first four reasons and, in fact, it may be impossible to separate them. Determining the severity and nature of a patient's communication disorder usually has implications for the diagnosis, the prognosis, and decisions about treatment. A diagnosis may have prognostic implications and may affect decisions regarding treatment (as when the patient's communication disorder suggests a degenerative neurologic disease). Nevertheless, the speech-language pathologist may now and then have a more limited objective in testing a patient (e.g., when a patient with a mild communication disorder is referred by a physician who needs help in determining if the patient has an underlying neurologic disease). In such a case the emphasis is on diagnosis, and the prognosis and treatment are secondary or perhaps not considered at all.

Deciding on a Diagnosis

To diagnose a patient's communication disorder means to attach a label to it. Diagnostic labels are "shorthand for characterizing the constellation of symptoms" (Albert and associates, 1981, p. 19) and are an efficient way of communicating large amounts of descriptive information about a patient in a few words. (Provided, of course, that those reading the diagnostic labels understand their implications.)

Diagnosis by speech-language pathologists takes several forms. Sometimes a speech-language pathologist wishes to differentiate a patient's communication disorder from other communication disorders that might resemble it (a process called *differential diagnosis*). For example, the speech-language pathologist may wish to determine if a patient's communication disorder represents aphasia, dysarthria, apraxia of speech, or some form of dementing illness. Sometimes a speech-language pathologist knows, based on a patient's history and medical record, that the patient's communication disorder represents a general class of communication disorders but wishes to arrive at a more specific diagnosis. For example, she or he may conclude that a patient is dysarthric, based on information about the location of the patient's brain damage and the neurologist's description of the patient's speech, but may wish to determine which of several dysarthria syndromes best fit the patient's speech characteristics.

Labeling a patient's communication disorder often suggests the location of the nervous system pathology responsible for the patient's symptoms. For example, the label *Wernicke's aphasia* suggests damage in the temporal lobe in the language-dominant hemisphere, and the label *hypokinetic dysarthria* suggests damage in the basal ganglia and the extrapyramidal system. However, applying a diagnostic label to a patient's communication disorder often plays a minor part in specifying the location of the patient's neurologic damage, because many times the neurologic examination and the results of imaging studies (CT, MRI) have localized the patient's nervous system pathology before the patient gets to the speech-language pathologist. Those involved in the patient's care (including the speech-language pathologist) often know the location and (less often) the nature of the patient's nervous system pathology before the first test of communication abilities is administered.

Speech-language pathologists sometimes make a provisional diagnosis of a patient's communication disorder before they actually see the patient based on information in the patient's medical record. For example, if a patient's medical record shows that she or he has had a brain stem stroke, it is very likely that the patient will be dysarthric but not aphasic and not demented (unless there is also a history of previous stroke or other neurologic disease affecting the brain). Davis (1983), was discussing aphasia when he wrote:

> In clinical practice, a test is seldom used to diagnose aphasia, in the sense that a clinician has no idea what the disorder is until the test is analyzed. . . . Having read a patient's chart, an experienced clinical aphasiologist need only talk to a patient before reaching an initial conclusion about not only the presence of aphasia but also the type of aphasia (p. 211).

Davis's assertion is true not only for patients with aphasia but also for patients with other communication disorders. By the time they have finished reviewing a patient's medical record and completed the interview, experienced speech-language pathologists usually have a diagnosis in mind. Testing the patient may serve only to confirm (and perhaps to elaborate on) the speech-language pathologist's preliminary diagnosis.

Attaching a diagnostic label to a neurologically impaired patient's communication disorder usually is not the primary concern of most speech-language pathologists. Their primary concern usually is to determine the nature and severity of the patient's communication impairments and to make decisions about the appropriateness and content of treatment. However, this does not mean that diagnostic labeling has no place in the speech-language pathologist's business day. Those referring a patient to the speech-language pathologist may expect a diagnostic label, and using a diagnostic label in a report may substitute for lengthy description. For example, reporting that a patient exhibits behaviors consistent with *conduction aphasia* communicates extensive information about the nature of the patient's speech, her or his comprehension of language, and the probable location of the brain damage responsible for the patient's aphasia, all in two words. Likewise, reporting that a patient exhibits *flaccid dysarthria* says a lot about the probable nature of the patient's articulatory impairments as well as the likely location of the central nervous system damage responsible for the impairments.

Making a Prognosis

A prognosis is a prediction about the course (sometimes) and the eventual outcome (usually) of a disease or condition. Prognoses typically are based on actuarial information from studies of large groups of individuals with the disease or condition. These studies can be either *prospective* or *retrospective*. In *prospective studies,* patients in the early stages of a disease or condition are identified and various characteristics of the patients (the prognostic variables) are assessed at the beginning of the study. The patients are then followed to determine outcome. At some predetermined future time, the outcomes are tallied and the relationships between the prognostic variables and the outcomes are evaluated to identify the prognostic variables that are most strongly related to outcome. In *retrospective studies* the records of a group of patients who have already experienced outcomes are reviewed to evaluate the relationships between various prognostic variables and outcome (both determined from the records). Retrospective studies almost always are scientifically weaker than prospective studies because the prognostic variables are not defined in advance of the study, the data are not collected using standardized procedures, and the definitions of outcome measures tend to be less precise than those in prospective studies.

Most studies of prognostic variables related to recovery of communication following nervous system pathology are retrospective. The records of groups of patients who have recovered various levels of communication ability are reviewed, and the relationships between patients' recovery (usually defined as scores on standardized tests of communication ability) and various prognostic variables are evaluated. Numerous studies and opinion pieces have been published in the search for prognostic variables that might predict brain-damaged adults' recovery of communication. These variables fall into three categories: *neurologic findings, associated conditions,* and *patient variables.*

Neurologic Findings In addition to their function as a shorthand for communicating a lot of information about the patient in a few words, many neurologic diagnoses have prognostic significance. Longstreth and associates (1992) link diagnosis, prognosis, and treatment when they assert:

A diagnosis that has no prognostic implications does little more than describe a constellation of patient characteristics. Prognosis links diagnosis to outcomes and identifies the diseases that warrant treatment. Treatment becomes an intervention intended to modify prognosis. Thus, in clinical neurology, the concepts of diagnosis, prognosis, and treatment are inseparable, with prognosis as the keystone (p. 29).

This opinion might be regarded by some speech-language pathologists as extreme, because the prognostic implications of many diagnostic labels for communication disorders are fuzzy at best. For example, diagnosing a patient's communication disorder as *Wernicke's aphasia* provides little in the way of prognosis, except that as a group, patients with Wernicke's aphasia recover slightly less well than those with Broca's aphasia (Kertesz, 1979). In contrast, many neurologic diagnoses carry considerably more prognostic weight, because the time-course and outcome of many neurologic conditions are well understood.

The speech-language pathologist who wishes to predict a patient's recovery of communication pays close attention to the neurologic diagnosis, because changes in a patient's communication abilities usually parallel changes in his or her physical and medical condition. Consequently, knowing the usual course of recovery (or deterioration) for common neurologic diagnoses can contribute in important ways to the speech-language pathologist's predictions regarding patients' recovery of communication abilities. When the usual course of a patient's neurologic disease is well known and highly predictable, the speech-language pathologist's prognosis for recovery of communication also is likely to be quite accurate (although perhaps redundant once the neurologic diagnosis has been made).

Notes or comments in a patient's medical record relating to the location and extent of a patient's nervous system pathology can affect the speech-language pathologist's prognosis. The location of the pathology is important because pathology affecting nervous system structures and systems that are directly involved in language and related processes carry greater negative implications than pathology affecting more peripherally related structures and systems. For example, damage in the central zone of the language-dominant hemisphere typically creates more severe and persistent aphasia than damage in more peripheral areas. Likewise, damage in the brain stem affecting the cranial nerves responsible for muscle and sensory systems involved in speech typically causes severe and persistent dysarthria, whereas damage in fiber tracts above the brain stem usually produces milder and less persistent disruption of speech.

The extent of nervous system pathology also affects prognosis. Large lesions, multiple lesions, and damage disseminated throughout the nervous system or throughout parts of the nervous system important for communication are negative prognostic indicators. The speech-language pathologist might revise downward his estimate of communicative recovery for a patient with a confirmed recent left-hemisphere stroke on learning that the patient's CT scan showed a previous stroke in the right hemisphere. Sometimes indicators of the extent of nervous system pathology are indirect. For example, the presence and duration of coma are considered important prognostic indicators for patients with traumatic brain injuries (Jennett and associates, 1979) and, to a lesser extent, for patients with aphasia caused by stroke (Caronna & Levy, 1983). In most cases the presence and duration of coma are strongly related to the extent of brain injury, with longer duration of coma suggesting greater destruction of brain tissue.

The time post onset of a patient's neurogenic communication disorder is an important prognostic variable for patients with communication impairments secondary to strokes or traumatic brain injuries, because most neurologic recovery takes place early post onset, with gradual lessening of recovery as time post onset increases. However, ischemic and hemorrhagic strokes have different courses of recovery. The *pattern* of recovery depends largely on whether the stroke was ischemic or hemorrhagic, and the *eventual level* of recovery depends largely on the amount of brain tissue destroyed and the location of the destruction.

Neurologic recovery from *ischemic strokes* is greatest in the first week or two, with gradually decelerating recovery until the patient's condition stabilizes (Figure 3-9). Recovery is greatest for patients in the middle severity ranges. Patients who remain severely impaired when the acute effects of the stroke have dissipated (2 to 4 weeks post-stroke) usually have large areas of tissue destruction in the brain. Because of this, such patients are likely to remain severely impaired. Patients with extremely mild impairments in the first days and weeks post-stroke also may show little neurologic recovery because they have little room to recover—small amounts of improvement bring them back to (or near) their premorbid levels.

How long it takes for recovery from ischemic strokes to be completed has not been specified. Most recovery of language takes place within the first 3 months post onset (Culton, 1969; Sarno and Levita, 1971), and most neurologic recovery takes place in the first 6 months post onset (Basso, Capitani, and Vignolo, 1979), although some slow neurologic recovery may continue for additional months or years (Caplan, 1993).

Neurologic recovery from *hemorrhagic strokes* usually follows a different course from that for occlusive strokes. Patients with hemorrhagic strokes often show little improvement for the first 4 to 8 weeks post onset followed by a period of rapid recovery (Figure 3-9). Recovery then slows and stabilizes, usually at a level above that for occlusive stroke patients with equivalent deficits at onset. Most patients with hemorrhagic strokes, like those with ischemic strokes, have essentially completed their neurologic recovery by 6 months post onset.

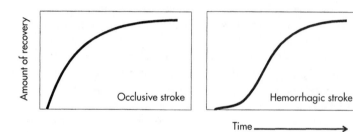
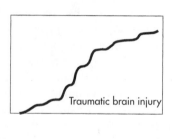

Time ⟶

Figure 3-9 ■ **The general course of neurologic recovery according to the etiology of the neurologic disorder. The graphs represent the average course of recovery for groups of patients. The recovery of individual patients often differs from the group average. These curves are based primarily on clinical experience and anecdotal evidence. There is little empirical evidence documenting differences in the course of neurologic recovery between groups of patients with occlusive or hemorrhagic strokes or traumatic brain injuries.**

The neurologic diagnosis, the location and extent of the nervous system pathology responsible for a patient's communication impairments, and the time post onset of the patient's impairments provide the speech-language pathologist with some of the most dependable prognostic indicators. However, several other prognostic indicators, though less dependable, frequently play a part in determining a patient's prognosis. These indicators can conveniently be divided into *associated conditions* and *patient variables.*

Associated Conditions Associated conditions are medical conditions or physical findings that do not directly affect communication but have indirect affects on the magnitude of the patient's communication impairments and may compromise the patient's recovery and her or his response to treatment. Several associated conditions have been shown to affect recovery from neurogenic communication disorders. A patient's *general health* can have important effects on recovery of communication abilities following neurologic events. The presence of illnesses such as diabetes, heart disease, pulmonary disease and other such chronic diseases are thought to impede physiologic and behavioral recovery from nervous system

pathology (Marshall & Phillips, 1983; Eisenson, 1964; Candelise and associates, 1985). *Associated sensory and motor impairments* also have some prognostic significance. The presence of hemiplegia, perceptual disturbances, seizures, and motor impairments have all been mentioned as indicators of a poor prognosis (Keenan & Brassell, 1975; Van Buskirk, 1955), although some investigators have reported no relationship between the presence of hemiplegia or seizures and recovery from aphasia (Glonig and associates, 1976; Smith, 1972).

Patient Variables Patient variables are patient characteristics such as age, gender, education, occupation, premorbid intelligence, handedness, personality, and emotional state. Many of these variables have been studied as potential predictor variables. Overall, the relationships between patient demographic variables and recovery of communication abilities tend to be weak and most have been the subject of contradictory findings (See Darley, 1982; Davis, 1983; and Rosenbek, LaPointe, & Wertz, 1989 for reviews of these findings.) The most that can be said of patient demographic variables is that they appear to have some weak effects on recovery, but the effects of any single demographic variable are easily overshadowed by the more potent effects of variables such as the location and severity of nervous system pathology.

The Nature and Severity of Communication Impairments The nature of a patient's communication impairment sometimes has prognostic significance. For example, there is evidence that patients with Broca's aphasia recover somewhat better than those with Wernicke's aphasia when aphasia severity is equivalent, and that patients with traumatic brain injuries recover better than those with brain injuries caused by strokes.* The overall severity of a patient's communication impairment at the time of testing is a reasonably dependable indicator of future recovery from neurogenic communication impairments. In general, patients with severe communication impairments do not recover as well as those with milder impairments, although there may be striking exceptions. However, making a prognosis based on the overall severity of a patient's communication impairment is in many respects a subjective process, because the predictive validity of the standardized tests for measuring the severity of a patient's communication impairment has not been established (Tompkins, 1995).

A few tests provide systematic procedures for making prognostic statements based on patients' test performance. Some tests make use of a *patient profile approach,* in which a patient is given a series of tests and a profile of the patient's performance is developed. The clinician then matches the patient's profile with the profiles of previously studied groups of patients whose recovery is known, with the expectation that the patient's recovery should match that of previously studied patients with the same profile. The *Minnesota Test for Differential Diagnosis of Aphasia* (MTDDA; Schuell, 1965) is a good example of the patient profile approach to prediction. The MTDDA permits clinicians to assign aphasic patients to one of five major groups and two minor groups based on their test performance. The MTDDA test manual gives a prognosis for each group, based on the recovery of previously-studied patients. For example MTDDA Group 1 usually has "excellent recovery of all language skills" (Schuell, 1965, p. 9), while for MTDDA Group 5 "language does not become functional or voluntary in any modality" (Schuell, 1965, p. 14).

Other tests permit the use of a more sophisticated *statistical prediction approach* (Porch, Collins, Wertz, & Friden; 1980). The *statistical prediction approach,* like the other approaches, makes predictions based on the characteristics of previously studied patients. Unlike the other approaches, the statistical prediction approach uses sophisticated statistical analyses to determine the relative contributions of several variables, alone and in combination, to observed recovery. These procedures provide quantitative information about which variables are most strongly related to recovery and which combinations of variables provide the most accurate predictions. They also permit quite precise predictions regarding the actual level of recovery to be expected. However, the predictions are not perfect; there is always some error in prediction associated with even the strongest prognostic variables.

A good example of the *statistical prediction approach* is Porch's (1981) *HOAP (high-overall prediction)* procedure for predicting recovery from aphasia. In the HOAP procedure, the patient is tested at one month post onset with the *Porch Index of Communicative Ability* (PICA; Porch, 1981), which has 18 subtests. The clinician then calculates an average score for the nine subtests with the highest scores. This average is then used to enter a table in the PICA manual, from which the patient's 6-month overall PICA performance can be predicted.

For patients tested at more than 1 month post onset but less than 6 months post onset, a

---

* Because patients with traumatic brain injuries usually are younger than stroke patients no doubt makes an important contribution to this relationship.

variant on the HOAP method, called the *HOAP slope* method, can be used to predict recovery at 6 months. The patient is tested with the PICA and an average score for the nine subtests with the highest scores is calculated. This score is used to place the patient on one of several recovery slopes, which permit the clinician to predict the patient's overall PICA performance at 6 months post onset (Figure 3-10).

Even at its best, predicting brain-injured adults' recovery of communication is subject to substantial error. No prognostic variables have been strongly and unequivocally tied to recovery of communication, and many prognostic variables have been the subject of conflicting claims in the literature. Even the sophisticated *patient profile* and *statistical prediction* ap-

proaches (which are quite accurate when predicting the average recovery of groups of patients) often yield inaccurate predictions for individual patients (Aten & Lyon, 1978; Porch & Callaghan, 1981; Wertz, Dronkers, & Hume, 1993). For this reason, many clinicians opt for a short period of *prognostic treatment* (Rosenbek, LaPointe, & Wertz; 1989) to increase the precision of their predictions. In prognostic treatment the clinician and patient spend several sessions (usually 5 to 10) in treatment procedures designed to determine if the patient can perform treatment tasks and can generalize from clinic sessions to daily life. Prognostic treatment usually is the most dependable way to predict whether a patient will benefit from treatment. It also seems to be a good way to pre-

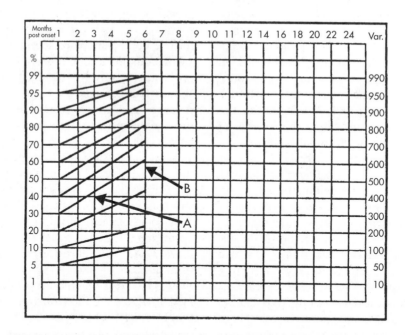

Figure 3-10 ▪ High-Overall Prediction (HOAP) slopes (Porch, 1981). An aphasic patient's 6-month-post-onset Porch Index of Communicative Ability (PICA; Porch 1981) overall percentile score is predicted by finding the patient's current PICA overall percentile score in the family of HOAP slopes and projecting the 6-month overall score based on the angle of the closest slope in the family. A patient who scored at the 40th percentile at 3 months post onset *(A)* should improve to approximately the 58th percentile *(B)* at 6 months post onset.

dict a brain-injured patient's recovery of communication with or without treatment.

Regardless of how it is done, predicting newly referred patients' recovery (or loss) of communication abilities often is an important concern of speech-language pathologists. Patients and their families concerned about the potential effects of the patient's communication disabilities on familial, social, and financial circumstances may press the speech-language pathologist for a prognostic opinion. Physicians and other health-care workers may need the speech-language pathologist's prognosis to help them plan the patient's discharge and arrange for follow-up care. Social workers may need a prognostic opinion to make appropriate social and vocational arrangements for the patient and family. Attorneys may request a prognostic opinion to establish the patient's legal competence or lack thereof. Funding agencies may require that the speech-language pathologist provide evidence for a favorable prognosis before they will approve payment for the patient's treatment. Finally, the speech-language pathologist must decide on the patient's chances of recovery, with or without treatment, before deciding whether to treat the patient's communication impairments.

Measuring Recovery and Response to Treatment

Measuring patient performance across time is an important part of the clinical management of patients with neurogenic communication impairments. Such measurement is integral to establishing baselines against which the effects of treatment can be measured and for describing changes in patients' performance during treatment. Well-defined baselines are the principal element in studies of the evolution of neurologic diseases or pathologic processes and they often are the key to understanding the progression of a particular patient's impairments and predicting outcome for that patient. Defining a baseline for a patient with a neurogenic communication disorder requires administration of a test or set of tests at regular intervals to measure the patient's performance in the domain of interest. A patient with progressive dementia might be evaluated with a story retelling test at 1-month intervals to evaluate the degree to which organization, recall, and production of story elements are affected by the patient's dementia. A semicomatose patient might be evaluated with successive tests of alertness and attention to determine when the patient might be a candidate for a more comprehensive evaluation. A patient with progressive muscle weakness might be evaluated with successive tests of articulatory proficiency to monitor the course of the disease and to determine the advisability of treating the patient's dysarthria.

Figure 3-11 shows how baseline measurements were used to help a neurologist decide on a diagnosis for a 63-year-old woman who was brought to the neurology clinic with vague complaints about difficulty concentrating and memory lapses. The patient's neurologic examination was unremarkable and she scored within normal limits on a screening test of memory and cognition. The neurologist referred the patient to speech-language pathology with a request for help in determining if the patient had a progressive condition, and if so, whether the patient was in the early stages of progressive dementia or some other neurologic disease. The speech-language pathologist chose three tests as baseline measures: a test of *proverb interpretation,* a *story retelling* test, and a *picture naming* test. The speech-language pathologist reasoned that performance on the *proverb interpretation* and *story retelling* tests should be sensitive to dementing illness because they make heavy demands on abstract reasoning and memory (both of which should be affected early in the course of dementia). The *picture naming* test was included because the speech-language pathologist knew that picture naming rarely is affected in the early stages of dementia. If the patient's performance on the *proverb interpretation* and

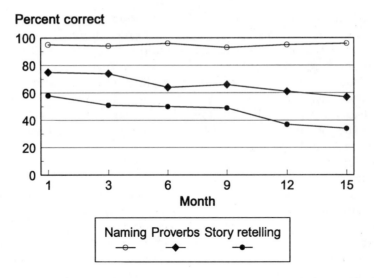

Figure 3-11 ▪ Baseline measurements for a patient who was eventually diagnosed as having dementia. Naming performance remained stable throughout the period of baseline measurement, while performance on tests of proverb interpretation and story retelling gradually worsened.

story retelling tests declined while her performance on the *picture naming* test remained stable, a diagnosis of early dementia would become more plausible. The speech-language pathologist tested the patient at 3-month intervals, concurrent with her appointments in the neurology clinic. The baselines in Figure 3-11 show the patient's performance across five test sessions. The patient's naming performance remained stable and within the normal range across all five tests, but her proverb interpretation and story retelling performance gradually declined. The patient's neurologic examination remained unremarkable across the five test sessions, except for a questionable decline in performance on screening tests of cognition in the sixth session. The patient's baseline pattern of performance led the neurologist to conclude that the patient was in the early stages of progressive dementia, a diagnosis which was confirmed by subsequent evaluations during the following year.

Figure 3-12 shows how a baseline was used to establish the stability of an aphasic patient's performance prior to initiation of a treatment program and then to measure the effects of the treatment program. The patient was referred to the speech-language pathology clinic 3 months after a left-hemisphere stroke, which left her with moderate aphasia. Before beginning treatment the speech-language pathologist established baseline performance levels for listening comprehension, reading comprehension, and naming (Figure 3-12). The patient's performance on all three tests was stable across three weekly baseline tests, so in week 4 the speech-language pathologist began a treatment program focused on listening comprehension. The beginning of treatment was followed by an upturn in the baselines for listening and reading comprehension but not the naming baseline, suggesting that the treatment had a positive effect on the patient's language comprehension (both listening and reading) but not on the patient's naming.

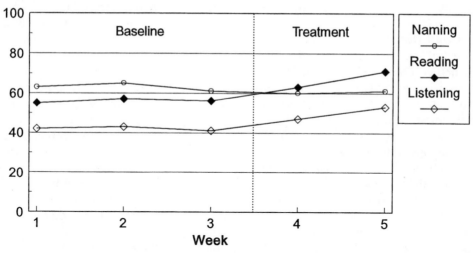

Figure 3-12 ▪ **Baseline measurements used to evaluate the effects of a treatment program. No treatment was given during weeks 1 to 3, but the patient's performance on tests of listening comprehension, reading, and confrontation naming was tested each week. Treatment of listening comprehension began in week 4, and the patient's performance on the listening and reading comprehension tests improved, while performance on the naming test did not change.**

These examples show how baseline measurements can serve important clinical functions. Because speech and language are sensitive indicators of neurologic status, baselines representing a patient's speech and language performance can help to resolve uncertain neurologic diagnoses. For patient's receiving treatment for neurogenic communication impairments, baseline measures can speak to the appropriateness and effectiveness of the treatment.

Measuring Efficacy, Outcome, and Functional Communication

Single-subject experimental designs are excellent vehicles for establishing baseline performance, for measuring patients' response to treatment, and for alerting the clinician to the need for changes in treatment proce-

dures.* They also have potential for contributing to our knowledge about the efficacy of treatment for neurogenic communication disorders and for evaluating the extent to which changes in performance obtained in treatment generalize in a meaningful way to patients' daily life communication performance. These aspects of assessment will become more important as health-care providers become increasingly preoccupied with balancing the costs of rehabilitation against its positive effects on patients' daily

---

* Single-subject experimental designs typically make use of baselines to show the effects of treatment. See Barlow & Herson (1984) Kratchowill (1978), McReynolds & Kearns (1983), or any of several other books on single-subject research for detailed discussion of single-subject experimental designs. See Connell & Thompson (1986), Kearns (1986), and McReynolds & Kearns (1986) for a tutorial on the use of single-subject designs in speech-language pathology.

life independence. The concepts of *efficacy, outcome,* and *functional communication* are central to these considerations.

Efficacy and Outcome When the word *efficacy* is used in the rehabilitation literature, it refers to whether a treatment has a positive effect on a disease or condition. When the word *outcome* is used, it refers to whether treatment provided meaningful benefit to the patient in her or his daily life environment. In speech-language pathology, efficacy usually is defined as a positive change on a standardized test of communication ability. That a treatment is *efficacious* does not necessarily mean that it had a *meaningful positive outcome.* Consider, for example a treatment program that generates a significant increase in an aphasic patient's performance on *The Boston Naming Test* (Kaplan, Goodglass, & Weintraub, 1983). The *Boston Naming Test* requires the test-taker to provide the names of line drawings of common and uncommon objects. If one's measure of efficacy were improvement on the *Boston Naming Test,* the treatment could be called *efficacious.* However, it might not have had a *meaningful positive outcome,* because improved ability to name pictured objects may not provide meaningful benefit to the patient in her or his daily life environment.* To decide if a treatment is efficacious, one asks, "What happened to the patient's test performance?" To decide if a treatment has a positive outcome, one asks, "What happened to the patient's daily life performance?"

---

* A treatment could conceivably have a meaningful positive outcome even though it had not been shown to be efficacious. This unusual situation could occur if, for example, one chose performance on *the Boston Naming Test* as the measure of efficacy for a treatment program that provided broad-based language stimulation, and no naming training. One might then see no significant change in patients' *Boston Naming Test* scores (the measure of efficacy) but find a meaningful positive change in ratings of the patient's communicative success in daily-life activities (a measure of outcome).

The issues of efficacy and outcome are exemplified by a study of the efficacy of aphasia therapy by Wertz and associates (1986). In this study, a *clinic* group received 12 weeks of treatment by a speech-language pathologist followed by 12 weeks of no treatment. A *deferred* group received 12 weeks of no treatment followed by 12 weeks of treatment by a speech-language pathologist.* At the end of the first 12 weeks, the clinic group's overall percentile score on the *Porch Index of Communicative Ability* (PICA; Porch, 1981) was 5.93 points higher than that of the deferred group—a statistically significant difference. This result led Wertz and associates to conclude that their treatment was efficacious—it yielded a statistically significant change in their measure of treatment effect (PICA overall percentile). Whether the treatment had a meaningful positive outcome is not clear, because no one knows if an improvement of 5.93 overall percentile points on the PICA signifies a meaningful change in patients' daily life communicative functioning.

Most studies of treatment benefits for patients with neurogenic communication disorders are efficacy studies. The indicators of efficacy are positive changes in performance on standardized tests of communication, perhaps because these tests are sensitive, reliable, and valid indicators of the communication performance of adults under carefully controlled test conditions. Few treatment studies of adults with neurogenic communication disorders have incorporated measures of outcome as indicators of daily life benefit, perhaps because few standardized outcome measures with proven sensitivity, reliability, and validity were available when the studies were carried out.

In contrast, many medical studies of treatment effects have incorporated measures that speak to both efficacy and outcome. Consider,

---

* The design was more complex than this. These aspects of the study are chosen to illustrate the concepts of efficacy and outcome.

for example, a study of the effects of treatment of hypertension (Veterans Administration, 1972). This study compared the effects of a combination of antihypertensive medications with the effects of a placebo administered to large groups of adults with hypertension. The measure of treatment effects was the frequency of occurrence of five adverse events: *sudden death, heart attack, congestive heart failure, increased hypertension,* and *ruptured aneurysm,* all known to be consequences of hypertension. At the end of the study 8.5% of the group given the antihypertensive medications had experienced adverse events, whereas 22.2% of the group given the placebo had experienced adverse events. Because the occurrence of these adverse events is likely to have profound negative effects on patients and their families, it is reasonable to conclude that the treatment regimen was both efficacious (the difference in the rate of adverse events between the groups was statistically significant) and that it *had a positive outcome* (the treatment improved patients' daily life well-being).

The word *functional* is strongly associated with the concept of *outcome* (so much so that the combination *functional outcome* has become commonplace in the rehabilitation literature). When used in this context, functional means *affecting the patient's daily life competence or well-being,* making the combination *functional outcome* something of a redundancy. Hundreds of articles and dozens of measuring instruments with functional somewhere in their title have appeared in the literature in the past 15 or 20 years, and it is now true that in speech-language pathology an emphasis on functionality in writing clinical goals and outcomes is almost mandatory.

> It has become almost impossible to write a treatment plan or submit a claim to a third-party payor without using the word "functional." A speech-language pathologist must identify "functional" goals, using "functional" tasks, and show "functional" gains, or reimbursement for treatment is likely to be denied (Elman & Bernstein-Ellis, 1995, p. 1).

In spite of the frequency of the word *functional* in contemporary clinical writings and practice, no standard definition of functional exists and its meaning varies depending on who is using it and what their purposes are.

The label *functional communication* is commonly used by speech-language pathologists to describe an approach to assessment and treatment that focuses on patients' daily-life communicative success or lack thereof. It emphasizes the means by which patients get the message across and it represents a movement away from a traditional emphasis on *language* to an emphasis on *communication* (the successful transfer of information from speaker or writer to listener or reader). This movement has been especially evident with regard to aphasia, but the emphasis on communication has spilled over to the other neurogenic communication disorders as well. The general idea is that successful communication does not depend on the linguistic accuracy of messages, but that speakers (and writers) can communicate successfully in spite of errors in word choice, syntax, or the phonologic-graphemic form of messages. It is this sense of the term that underlies several approaches to treatment, such as *Promoting Aphasics' Communicative Effectiveness* (Davis & Wilcox, 1985). Functional treatment approaches typically rely on activities that are structured to resemble the patient's daily-life communication environment and tend to focus on socially relevant aspects of communication, such as social conventions (greetings, farewells, and the like) and adherence to conversational rules.

When the word functional is used by organizations that manage and pay for health care services, it often means *able to communicate basic needs and wants.* Because these organizations may be unwilling to pay for treatment to move patients beyond this level, defining the term in this way may save them money by eliminating their obligation to pay for treatment of patients with mild or moderate communication impairments (because they can already communicate basic wants and needs), and by ending payment for patients with more severe impairments as soon as they reach the minimal level of communication competence represented by the provider's definition of *functional*.

Impairment, Disability, and Handicap Much of current thinking about efficacy, outcome, and functional communication has been influenced by the concepts of *impairment, disability,* and *handicap* (World Health Organization, 1980). Impairment, according the World Health Organization, represents a structural or functional abnormality within a person. *Brain damage* and *hemiplegia* are examples of a structural and a functional abnormality that would be called impairments. *Disability* represents the effects of an impairment or collection of impairments on a specific skill or ability. *Aphasia* and *poor ambulation* are examples of disabilities that might be caused by brain damage and hemiplegia (their respective underlying impairments). *Handicap* represents the effects of one or more disabilities on the individual's ability to carry out daily life roles. *Diminished ability to function as a spouse or parent* is an example of a handicap that might be caused by aphasia.

The concepts of impairment, disability, and handicap have had strong effects on contemporary thinking about the nature of health care services and how health care services should be paid for. The past decade has seen the development of numerous measuring instruments for assessing the level of handicap created by diseases or conditions and the degree to which treatment serves to alleviate handicaps. Most of these measuring instruments are *rating scales* by which patients' level of handicap in a given domain can be subjectively estimated. A few are standardized tests by which patients' performance in a given domain can be objectively scored. The rating scales and standardized tests share a common attribute: that of focusing on what is called functional outcome.

Functional Outcome How functional outcome is measured greatly depends on the purpose of those doing the measuring. The two major reasons for functional outcome measures are *program evaluation* and *patient evaluation.* In program evaluation the primary objective is to identify the most efficient providers of health care service—"those who provide the greatest amount of functional improvement over the shortest period of time for the least cost" (Warren, 1992, p. 63). The concept underlying program evaluation is that in a competitive marketplace health care providers who reduce costs but maintain the quality of services and produce good outcomes will survive and prosper, while those who do not, will not. The emphasis in program evaluation is on the financial health of the program rather than on treatment outcomes for individual patients.

The measures typically used for program evaluation are *rating scales.* Patients' functional abilities in the domain(s) of interest are rated when they enter the program and again when they leave the program. Judgments about the quality of the program are based on the amount of improvement in ratings of functionality between entry and exit and the level of functionality of patients completing the program. The rating scales used in program evaluation are not specific to a given disease or condition (e.g., stroke) and they are not specific to a given discipline (e.g., speech-language pathology). They usually provide for global ratings of broadly defined categories of abilities likely to be important in daily life (e.g., *self-care*). Consequently, they are insensitive to small changes in a patient's level of performance on the categories rated in the scale and they are not sensitive to changes in component abilities that may contribute to performance in one or more of the broadly defined categories.

The best known and most widely used measure of functional outcome in rehabilitation is a rating scale called *The Functional Independence Measure* (FIM; State University of New

York at Buffalo Research Foundation, 1993). The FIM was developed to measure outcome in rehabilitation medicine programs. It provides a 7-point scale to assess *self-care, sphincter control, mobility, locomotion, communication,* and *social cognition* in 18 activities of daily life (Figure 3-13). The 7-point scale is divided into

Functional independence measure

FIM

Copyright 1987 Research Foundation - State University of New York

COPY FREELY–BUT DO NOT CHANGE

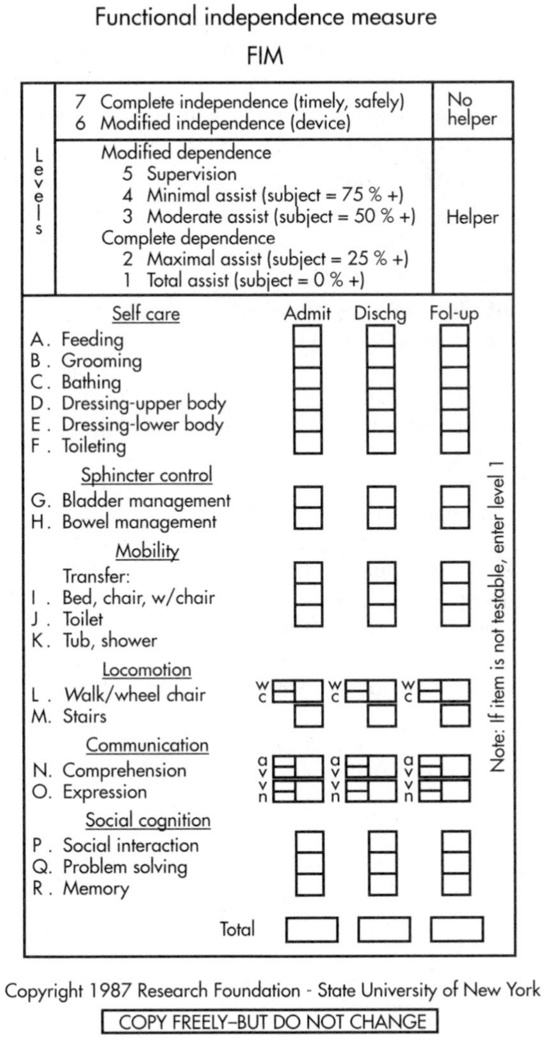

Figure 3-13 ▪ The functional independence measure (FIM).

three levels. At the *independent* (no helper) level, patients do not require assistance to carry out the activities addressed by the FIM. Patients at the *dependent* (helper) level require assistance from someone else to carry out the activities and the rating declines as the amount of assistance required by the patient increases. The dependent level is subdivided into two levels *(modified dependence, complete dependence)* based on the frequency with which assistance is needed by a patient. The FIM has been criticized for lack of reliability in rating levels of independence (Adamovich, 1990), and its use for rating functional independence in communication has been criticized because of its insensitivity to changes in communication abilities (Warren, 1992). Nevertheless, it remains the preeminent outcome measure for program evaluation in rehabilitation medicine.

The combination of increased emphasis on functional outcome by health-care providers and dissatisfaction with the FIM as a measure of communicative adequacy led the American Speech-Language-Hearing Association (ASHA) to develop a measure of functional communication called *ASHA FACS* (for *ASHA Functional Assessment of Communication Skills for Adults;* American Speech-Language-Hearing Association, 1994). ASHA FACS permits users to rate a patient's communicative adequacy in four domains: *social communication, communication of basic needs, daily planning,* and *reading/writing/number concepts* (Table 3-1). The communicative adequacy of each behavior shown in Table 3-1 is estimated with a *7-point Scale of Communicative Independence* which, like the FIM, rates behaviors in terms of how much assistance is needed to perform them:

- Does with no assistance (7)
- Does with minimal assistance (6)
- Does with minimal to moderate assistance (5)
- Does with moderate assistance (4)
- Does with moderate to maximal assistance (3)

- Does with maximal assistance (2)
- Does not do, even with maximal assistance (1)
- No basis for rating

In addition to ratings of the individual communication behaviors, the patient's overall performance in each of the four ASHA FACS domains is rated in terms of its *adequacy, appropriateness, promptness,* and *communicative sharing.*

The FIM and ASHA FACS, like most instruments designed for program evaluation, yield general estimates of a patient's functional ability in a small number of domains chosen because they are likely to be important in determining the patient's independence in daily life. These instruments may provide reasonably accurate estimates of a patient's daily life independence and self-sufficiency in the domains addressed but do not have sufficient sensitivity and do not provide enough detail to be very useful in planning treatment or in tracking a patient's response to treatment. Detail and sensitivity come from instruments designed for *patient evaluation* rather than for *program evaluation.*

The first measure of functional communication to be widely used for patient evaluation in speech-language pathology was the *Functional Communication Profile* (FCP; Sarno, 1969). According to Sarno, the FCP was designed to

---

TABLE 3-1

Assessment domains for ASHA Functional Assessment of Communication Skills for Adults (ASHA FACS)

Social communication	Communications of basic needs	Daily planning	Reading/writing/ number concepts
Uses names of familiar people	Recognizes familiar faces/voices	Tells time	Understands environmental signs
Expresses agreement/disagreement	Makes strong likes/ dislikes known	Dials telephone numbers	Uses reference materials
Explains how to do something	Expresses feelings	Keeps scheduled appointments	Follows written directions
Requests information	Requests help	Uses a calendar	Understands printed material
Participates in telephone conversations	Makes needs/wants known	Follows a map	Prints/writes/types name
Answers yes/no questions	Responds in an emergency		Completes forms
Follows directions			Makes short lists
Understands facial expression/tone of voice			Writes messages
Understands nonliteral meaning and intent			Understands signs with numbers
Understands conversation in noisy surroundings			Makes money transactions
Understands TV/radio			Understands units of measurement
Participates in conversations			
Recognizes/corrects errors			

Data From American Speech-Language-Hearing Association, 1994.

quantify the communication behaviors a patient actually uses when interacting with others, regardless of the severity of the patient's impairment. The clinician who wishes to rate a patient's functional communication with the FCP interviews the patient and then rates the patient on five categories of communication behavior considered common in everyday life (Table 3-2). The behaviors are rated on a 9-point scale in which the patient's current ability is rated as a proportion of her or his premorbid ability.

The Communicative Effectiveness Index (CETI; Lomas and associates; 1989) is a more recent rating scale for estimating aphasic adults' ability to communicate in several daily life situations. The situations were selected by Lomas and associates, based on interviews with stroke survivors and spouses. In the interviews the stroke survivors and spouses were asked to identify situations in which a stroke survivor has to "get his meaning across and to understand what someone else means" (p. 115). The situations given by the stroke survivors and spouses were then partitioned into four categories representing:

- *Basic needs* (such as toileting, eating, grooming, positioning)
- *Life skills* (such as shopping, home maintenance, use of telephone, understanding traffic signals)
- *Social needs* (such as dinner conversation, playing cards, writing to a friend)
- *Health threat* (such as calling for help, giving or receiving information about one's medical condition)

The list of situations generated by the stroke survivors and spouses was then refined to yield a list of 16 items.* (Table 3-3). Results reported

by Lomas and associates suggest that the CETI has acceptable internal reliability (CETI items test the same domain), adequate test-retest reliability (CETI results do not change unpredictably from test to test), and acceptable interrater reliability (different examiners rating the same patient agree). The procedures used to select items for the CETI support its face validity (it appears to measure what it was intended to measure), although strong evidence for its validity as a measure of daily life communication performance (such as correlations between ratings and actual daily life performance) is not provided in the published report.*

Communicative Abilities in Daily Living (CADL; Holland, 1980) differs from the other measures of functional communication in that it scores a patient's actual performance in an interview and in various simulated daily life communication activities rather than subjectively rating the patient's presumed ability.

> "The fact that the CADL is scored relative to getting a message across rather than to correctness or incorrectness *per se* is one of its major departures from traditional tests of language and communication. The CADL's other major departure is in its conceptualization of test items. Rather than being a series of acontextual attempts addressed to isolating a number of language modalities (speaking, reading, writing, comprehension, etc.), most CADL items are molecular communicative interactions not easily described by language modality. Additionally, many items are richly supplied with context and often require understanding of the context for appropriate communicating. Finally, a number of nonverbal communicative events are sampled" (Holland, 1980; p. 29).

---

* Lomas and associates do not identify which items in the CETI represent each of these categories, and it is clear that the 16 items in the CETI are not distributed equally across the four categories. Four or 5 "basic need" items, 10 "social need" items, 1 "health threat" item, and 0 or 1 "life skill" items were counted, using intuitions about which behaviors represented each category.

---

* Lomas and associates reported strong and significant correlations between spouses' CETI ratings and their ratings of their spouses overall communicative ability and considered those correlations evidence of CETI's construct validity. However, it seems that strong correlations would be expected, because the same people did both ratings, apparently in the same rating session.

Abilities rated with the Functional Communication Profile

Category	Behavior
Movement	Ability to imitate oral movements
	Attempt to communicate
	Ability to indicate "yes" and "no"
	Indicating floor to elevator operator
	Use of gestures
Speaking	Saying greetings
	Saying own name
	Saying nouns
	Saying verbs
	Saying noun-verb combinations
	Saying phrases (nonautomatic)
	Giving directions
	Speaking on the telephone
	Saying short, complete sentences (nonautomatic)
	Saying long sentences (nonautomatic)
Understanding	Awareness of gross environmental sounds
	Awareness of emotional voice tone
	Understanding of own name
	Awareness of speech
	Recognition of family names
	Recognition of names of familiar objects
	Understanding action verbs
	Understanding gestured directions
	Understanding verbal directions
	Understanding simple conversation with one person
	Understanding television
	Understanding conversation with more than two people
	Understanding movies
	Understanding complicated verbal directions
	Understanding rapid, complex conversation
Reading	Reading single words
	Reading rehabilitation program card
	Reading street signs
	Reading newspaper headlines
	Reading letters
	Reading newspaper articles
	Reading magazines
	Reading books
Other	Writing name
	Time orientation
	Copying ability
	Writing from dictation
	Handling money
	Using writing in lieu of speech
	Calculation ability

Data From Sarno, 1969.

Situations rated by the Communicative Effectiveness Index (CETI)

Item	Situation
1	Getting someone's attention
2	Getting involved in group conversations about him/her
3	Giving "yes" and "no" answers appropriately
4	Communicating his/her emotions
5	Indicating that he/she understands what is being said to him/her
6	Having coffee, time visits and conversations with friends and neighbors
7	Having a one-to-one conversation with you
8	Saying the name of someone whose face is in front of him/her
9	Communicating physical needs such as aches and pains
10	Having a spontaneous conversation
11	Responding to or communicating anything (including "yes" or "no") without words
12	Starting a conversation with people who are not close family
13	Understanding writing
14	Being a part of a conversation when it is fast and there are a number of people involved
15	Participating in a conversation with strangers
16	Describing or discussing something at length

Data from Lomas and associates, 1989.

CADL testing begins with an interview, which begins with the examiner saying, *("Hello, Mr./Mrs.* _____,*")* and waiting for a response from the patient. The interviewer then elicits personal information from the patient, occasionally making mistakes (e.g., saying, *("Your first name is* _____ *(wrong name) isn't it?")* and noting if the patient corrects the examiner. Following the interview, the examiner gives the patient an appointment card for a pretend visit to a doctor's office. The patient's understanding of the appointment card and ability to carry out the appointment are assessed by means of questions and pictorial props. For example, the patient is shown a picture of the control panel of an elevator while the examiner says, *("You are on the elevator. Remember, Dr. Clark's office is on the third floor. What must you do?")* (Pointing to the "3" button in the picture or an appropriate verbal response are acceptable.) Subsequently, the examiner puts out a sign that says "Receptionist" and says, *("Now I'm the receptionist. May I help you?")* There follow several items in which the patient and examiner role-play the patient-receptionist interaction. Then the examiner takes away the sign, puts on a white coat and stethoscope, and says, *("Now you're inside the doctor's office and I'm the doctor. Well Mr./Mrs.* _____, **what has been bothering you lately?")** Several more role-played interactions between the patient and "doctor" follow. A series of questions follows supported by pictorial, tape-recorded, or object props. (Examples: A picture of a car fuel gauge with the needle pointing to empty is shown as the examiner asks, *("What's wrong here?")* A tape-recorded sound of dishes breaking is played as the examiner asks the patient to point to a picture to show what the sound is.) Patients' responses to CADL items are scored on a 3-point scale. Failed communications are scored

0, "in the ballpark" attempts are scored *1,* and fully successful attempts are scored *2.* The CADL manual provides a means for assigning individual CADL test items to one or more of 10 categories (Table 3-4). Twenty-two of the 68 CADL items each represent a single category, and the remainder represent more than one. A table in the CADL manual gives an item-by-item breakdown of which CADL items represent each category.

The CADL is normed on institutionalized and noninstitutionalized normal and aphasic adults, and the CADL manual provides mean scores, standard deviations, and ranges for the groups partitioned according to several variables such as gender, age, and institutionalization. As part of the standardization of the CADL measure, Holland and her associates compared aphasic adults' CADL performance with their actual communication behaviors in daily life, as measured by observers in the aphasic adults' daily life environments. Correlations between CADL scores and observed communication behaviors

were in the .60 to .70 range, suggesting that CADL scores have a moderately strong relationship to observed daily life communicative performance.* The correlations between CADL and the *Functional Communication Profile* (Sarno, 1969) was .87, suggesting that the two instruments measure much the same things. Intriguingly, the correlation between CADL and the *Porch Index of Communicative Ability* (PICA; Porch, 1981) was 6 points higher, at .93, leaving us to wonder if PICA scores also are moderately strong predictors of daily life communication performance.

---

* These correlations explain about half of the total variance in scores. The correlation between observed communicative performance and the *Porch Index of Communicative Ability* (Porch, 1981) was .55, and the correlation between observed performance and the *Boston Diagnostic Aphasia Examination* (Goodglass & Kaplan, 1983) was .49, suggesting that these two measures do a mediocre to fair job of predicting daily-life communicative performance. Their correlations with observed communicative performance explains 25% to 30% of the total variance in scores.

T A B L E   3 - 4

Categories to which items were assigned in Communicative Abilities in Daily Living and the number of items assigned to each category

Category	Number of items
Reading, writing, and using numbers to estimate, calculate, and judge time	21
Speech acts (using speech, gesture, or writing to communicate information and intent)	21
Using verbal and nonverbal context supplied by the examiner	17
Role playing	10
Sequencing and relationship-dependent communicative behavior (performing sequences of behavior, appreciating cause-effect relationships)	9
Social conventions (greeting, accepting apologies, leave-taking, etc.)	8
Divergences (generation of logical alternatives from given information)	7
Nonverbal symbolic communication (recognizing nonverbal symbols, facial expressions)	7
Deixis (movement-related or movement-dependent communicative behavior; e.g., come-go, bring-take)	6
Appreciating and understanding humor, absurdity, and metaphor	4

Data from Holland, 1980.

Measures of functional communication such as the foregoing are likely to become increasingly important in the future as changes in the way health care is provided and paid for accentuate the need for reliable, sensitive, and valid indicators of daily life communication performance. Those who wish to be paid for services provided to patients with neurogenic communication disorders will be required to show that the services provide meaningful benefits to the patients served. Health care providers will require that treatment planning and treatment procedures explicitly address daily life communication performance. Consequently, development of efficient, sensitive, reliable, and valid measures that are indicators of daily life communication performance will be an important responsibility of those concerned with clinical management of neurogenic communication disorders during the next decade.

■ KEY CONCEPTS

- Assessment of adults with neurogenic communication impairments is an iterative, problem-solving process in which the clinician integrates information from the referral, the patient's medical record, observation of the patient, conversations with family members and patient-care personnel, and test results to make a diagnosis, establish a prognosis, and plan treatment goals and procedures.

- Brain damage affects the way in which patients approach and solve problems, respond to stimulation, monitor their performance, interact with others, and view themselves. These characteristics affect the way in which clinicians interview brain-damaged patients, carry out assessment, plan treatment, and establish goals and prognoses.

- Interviewing the patient allows the clinician to get a sense of the patient as a person, permits the patient to become comfortable with the clinician, and provides the clinician with a sense of the patient's mood, perceptual abilities, cognitive status, and communication abilities and impairments. The clinician uses information gained in the interview to select the initial tests to be administered and to modify standard testing procedures to accommodate the patient's emotional, cognitive, perceptual, and communicative condition.

- Administering standardized and nonstandardized tests provides the clinician with the information needed to plan the content and methods of treatment, modify treatment based on patient performance, and predict treatment outcome.

- Standardized tests form the core of the clinician's information-gathering system and nonstandardized or informal tests permit the clinician to explore and document unique performance patterns that may not be captured by standardized tests.

Assessing Aphasia and Related Disorders

■ NEUROANATOMIC EXPLANATIONS OF APHASIA AND RELATED DISORDERS

Neuroanatomic explanations of aphasia are based on connectionist models of brain processes developed during the nineteenth century and elaborated during the first half of the twentieth century. The first versions of these models were conceived in the early 1800s by European neurologists and anatomists who, in addition to arguing fiercely among themselves about who was right, began the sometimes haphazard process of finding out which parts of the brain did what. The primary subjects for their investigations were patients whose brains had been damaged by stroke, trauma, or, less frequently, other causes. Information about brain-behavior relationships was laboriously accumulated by a small group of investigators who recorded their patients' symptoms, and when the patients eventually died, the investigators obtained their brains and determined which parts had been damaged. When damage to a given part of the brain regularly produced a certain pattern of impairment, it seemed reasonable to assign the impaired functions to the damaged part of the brain *(localization of function)*.

The localizationist effort received its first major impetus from Franz Gall, a German anatomist who, in the early 1800s, published elaborate maps of the brain in which various human "faculties" (such as bravery, honesty, and love) were assigned to specific brain regions (Figure 4-1). Gall believed that brain regions responsible for unusually well-developed faculties were themselves unusually well developed. He reasoned that hyperdeveloped brain regions pressed outward on the skull, creating bumps and bulges that a skilled practitioner could analyze, thereby determining the individual's unique pattern of talents and weaknesses. Gall's methods were naturalistic and naive by today's standards. He obtained the evidence for his conclusions from observation of friends, family members, associates, and his patients. (Gall assigned responsibility for language to the frontal lobes because several of his acquaintances with well-developed verbal skills had protruding foreheads and bulging eyes.) Today Gall's maps are used primarily as illustrations in treatises on the history of neurology and in advertisements for neurological books and journals.

Localizationist models of aphasia got their first major boost from the work of Paul Broca, a

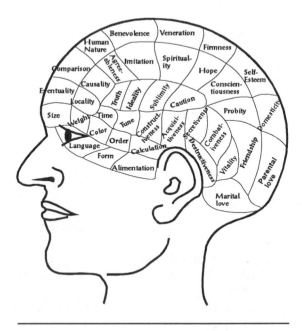

Figure 4-1 ■ A phrenological diagram, showing the sites of various human "faculties" in the brain.

French neurologist, who in the 1860s published a series of papers in which he asserted that loss of "articulate speech" was caused by damage in the posterior-inferior frontal lobe of the left hemisphere. Localizationalist models got another boost in 1874 when Karl Wernicke, a young German neuropsychiatrist, published a description of what he called "sensory aphasia" caused by lesions in the posterior temporal lobe. In subsequent publications Wernicke went on to construct an elaborate account (for the time) of the relationships between language functions and brain regions (an account which has survived, with minor modifications and some elaboration, until contemporary times).

The localizationists did not have the stage all to themselves. A vociferous group of antilocalizationists also was active both in the clinics and in the medical literature of the time. This group maintained that the brain operates as an integrated whole and they considered absurd the localizationists' propensity for fractionating mental activity and assigning it to various brain regions. The published work of Marie Jean-Pierre Flourens, a contemporary of Gall's, is considered by many to represent the beginning of the antilocalizationist movement. Flourens' beliefs were subsequently built upon by others, notably John Hughlings Jackson, a British neurologist in the 1860s; Pierre Marie, a French neurologist in the early 1900s; and Henry Head, another British neurologist in the 1920s. The antilocalizationists had a point but had relatively little effect on the neurologic establishment, partly because the new localizationists were right as often as they were wrong and partly because localization provided neurologists with a reasonably reliable way of telling what part of a patient's brain had been damaged without having to take it out and look at it.

Language and Cerebral Dominance

One of the earliest assertions of the localizationalists was that the left hemisphere of right-handed adults is responsible for language. This assertion had its beginnings in Broca's case reports and was reinforced by repeated observations of language disturbances following left-hemisphere damage in right-handed people. Based on a scattering of case reports (and, no doubt, on logic and a desire for symmetry) it became generally accepted that left-handed peoples' brains were mirror images of right-handed peoples' brains; namely that the right hemisphere of left-handed peoples' brains carried the language load. This belief began to fall apart in the 1950s when published reports (Goodglass & Quadfasel, 1954; Penfield & Roberts, 1959) began suggesting that left-handed people who became aphasic seemed not to have heard of the localizationists' assertions (at least half of them had damage only in the left hemisphere). Russell and Espir (1961) subsequently studied a group of 58 left-handed adults who had sustained traumatic brain injuries. Thirty-six percent of those with left-hemisphere damage but only 13% of those with right-hemisphere damage had significant language impairments.

The population of left-handed people with right-hemisphere dominance for language declined still further with the results of a study reported by Milner (1975). Milner injected sodium amytal into the carotid arteries of a group of left-handed adults. Sodium amytal is an anesthetic, and injection of sodium amytal into a carotid artery anesthetizes the brain hemisphere on that side. The person undergoing amytal testing loses the ability to speak when the language-competent hemisphere is anesthetized. Only 18% of Milner's left-handed subjects stopped talking when their right hemispheres were anesthetized, while 69% stopped talking when their left hemispheres were given the drug. Thirteen percent lost speech when either hemisphere was anesthetized, suggesting that their brain hemispheres shared language responsibilities. The results of a retrospective study by Naeser and Borod (1986) support Milner's findings. They reviewed the medical records of 31 left-handed aphasic adults. Only 4 adults (13%) had right-hemisphere brain damage.

It seems clear that most adults, regardless of handedness, depend on the left hemisphere for language. However, left-handed peoples' brains may be more flexible than right-handed peoples' brains regarding whose hemisphere gets the language responsibilities. Left-handed people who become aphasic seem to have less severe aphasia and recover language better than their right-handed counterparts, regardless of which hemisphere is affected (Glonig and associates, 1969; Goodglass, 1993; Luria, 1970). Milner's (1975) finding that 13% of left-handed adults became aphasic when either hemisphere was anesthetized provides additional support for the notion that left-handed peoples' brains are less constrained than those of right-handed people when it comes to which hemisphere takes care of language.

The question of whether we are born with one hemisphere specialized for language has not been answered, although opinions from researchers seem to favor the idea that we are not born that way. Studies of children and adolescents who sustain brain damage suggest that left hemisphere specialization for language develops as we mature and is not complete before adulthood. A child born with a nonfunctional left hemisphere usually develops normal language unless the right hemisphere is also damaged. A child or adolescent who becomes aphasic almost always recovers far more language than an adult with comparable damage.* The brain's ability to relocate and reassign functions served by damaged tissue diminishes with age. The older the patient is at the time of brain injury, the more severe the persisting conse-

---

* *Cerebral plasticity* is the term used to describe the brain's ability to reassign functions once served by damaged or destroyed tissue to other brain regions. Children's brains are said to be more "plastic" than those of adults, because functions taken care of by damaged or excised regions apparently can be delegated to other regions, often with little permanent impairment.

quences of the injury are likely to be. A 30-year-old aphasic stroke patient usually recovers more language than a 50-year-old or 60-year-old aphasic stroke patient with equivalent brain damage (Lenneberg, 1967; Osgood & Miron, 1963).

The PeriSylvian Region and Language

Connectionist explanations of language impairment following brain damage emphasize the importance of the region surrounding the Sylvian fissure (the *periSylvian* region) in the left hemisphere. Permanent damage anywhere in the periSylvian region in adult brains almost always causes language impairment. The periSylvian region in the left frontal lobe (sometimes called *the anterior language zone*) plays an important part in planning and executing language behavior (speech, writing, and perhaps gesture). The periSylvian region in the left temporal and parietal lobes (sometimes called the *posterior language zone*) is important for comprehending and recalling linguistic material and for formulating linguistic messages with appropriate syntactic structure and semantic content.

The hub of the anterior language zone is the posterior-inferior frontal lobe, which is just in front of the primary motor cortex. This patch of cortex is called *Broca's area* (Figure 4-2). It is named after Paul Broca, the French neurologist who first described its role in speech. Broca's area is next to the primary motor cortex for the speech muscles. Sometimes it is called the *motor speech area* because apparently it is responsible for planning and organizing speech movements for the primary motor cortex. *Broca's aphasia* is said to be the major consequence of damage in Broca's area.

The hub of the posterior language zone is *Wernicke's area*, which is in the posterior superior left temporal lobe (Figure 4-2). Wernicke's area is named after the German neuropsychiatrist (mentioned earlier) who first described an aphasia syndrome caused by temporal lobe damage. Sometimes Wernicke's area is called the *auditory association cortex*. It is thought to be important for

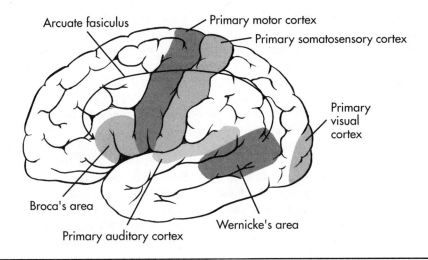

Figure 4-2 ▪ **Important cortical regions and connecting pathways in connectionist explanations of how the brain produces language.**

storage and retrieval of the mental representations of words, for storage and retrieval of word meanings, and for knowledge and use of grammatical and linguistic rules. Damage in Wernicke's area causes *Wernicke's aphasia.*

Wernicke's area receives a large part of its input from the *primary auditory cortex (Gyrus of Heschl),* which is on the top surface of the temporal lobe within the Sylvian fissure of each hemisphere (Figure 4-2). The primary auditory cortex has major responsibility for perception and discrimination of auditory stimuli. Each auditory cortex receives information from both ears, although the contralateral ear has a slight advantage.*

* Destruction of the primary auditory cortex in one hemisphere does not cause lasting deafness, but only mild hearing loss (usually in the contralateral ear) and occasionally some difficulty localizing sounds. Destruction of the primary auditory cortex in both hemispheres causes *cortical deafness,* in which the patient initially loses all auditory sensitivity. For some patients with bilateral destruction of auditory cortex, some hearing sensitivity slowly returns and the patient's pure-tone audiogram may even reach normal. However, perception of speech and other complex auditory stimuli almost always remains profoundly impaired (Jerger and associates, 1969).

Wernicke's area communicates with Broca's area and other frontal regions of the brain by way of the *arcuate fasciculus,* which is a band of nerve fibers that runs between the mid temporal lobe and the lower portions of the frontal lobe via the parietal lobe (Figure 4-2). The arcuate fasciculus is the primary route by which linguistic messages formulated in Wernicke's area are transmitted forward to Broca's area.

The region in and around the *angular gyrus,* at the junction of the temporal, parietal, and occipital lobes, is important for processes involved in reading and writing. Damage to this region usually produces severe impairments in reading (called *alexia*) and severe writing impairments (called *agraphia*).

How the Brain Performs Language

The connectionist model provides a metaphor for describing how the left hemisphere makes sense of incoming verbal messages and how it formulates, plans, and executes verbal and gestural responses. The connectionist model portrays the brain's processing of language as a telephone system of sorts in which various centers send messages back and forth over a system of connecting circuits. The brain does not work like a telephone system, and the connectionist model is simplistic, fuzzy, and in many respects inaccurate. Nevertheless it is a convenient metaphor for what actually happens and it provides a practical way for students to get a general sense of how damage in the brain yields fairly predictable impairments of language and behavior.

Comprehension of Speech According to the connectionist model, when a normal adult comprehends spoken messages (let's call our normal adult *"Fred"* and to keep things simple let's make him right handed), the message goes from Fred's ears via ascending fibers to the primary auditory cortices in each of Fred's temporal lobes. The auditory cortices encode the acoustic information and send the encoded message off to Wernicke's area in the left hemisphere.* When Wernicke's area realizes that the message is speech, it sorts through its store of semantic representations to find meanings for the words in the message, consults its book of syntactic rules to determine the relationships among the words, and constructs a representation of the message's overall meaning. Fred's brain also evaluates the situation to determine if the literal meaning of the sentence actually represents the speaker's intent. (Some sentences, such as *"Can you open the window?"* are implied requests, not meant to be interpreted literally. A *"yes"* or *"no"* response ordinarily wouldn't be appropriate.) When Wernicke's area has figured out the sentence's meaning and knows whether the message should be interpreted literally or figuratively, it sends instructions to other parts of Fred's brain regarding how he should respond (e.g., talk, write, gesture, or open the window).†

---

* The information from the auditory cortex in the right hemisphere gets to Wernicke's area via fibers passing through the corpus callosum just behind its center.
† Fred's right brain hemisphere apparently plays an important part in making nonliteral interpretations.

Comprehension of Printed Materials (Reading) When Fred's brain has to deal with printed messages, the process resembles that for comprehension of speech, except that Fred's visual cortex is the message's first stop in the brain. Fred's visual cortex encodes the information coming from the eyes in a form that his Wernicke's area can understand and sends it to Wernicke's area.* From there the process resembles that for auditory comprehension. Wernicke's area constructs a representation of the message's meaning and sends the relevant information to the other parts of Fred's brain that are to be involved in the response.

Spontaneous Speech When Fred speaks a sentence spontaneously, Wernicke's area searches the lexicon for the words needed to express the message and constructs a sentence that complies with phonologic, syntactic, and semantic rules. Wernicke's area then sends the neurally coded sentence forward via the arcuate fasciculus to Broca's area. Broca's area translates the code into an action plan and sends the plan to Fred's primary motor cortex. The primary motor cortex puts the finishing touches on the message and sends it down, via the pyramidal system, to the cranial nerves, which set the speech muscles into motion. As the speech muscles produce the message, Wernicke's area monitors it to ensure that what it sent is what is said. If it is not correct, Wernicke's area shifts the system into repair mode.

Repetition According to the connectionist model, repetition of words, phrases, and sentences tests the entire circuit for reception and production of verbal messages from the primary auditory cortex through the motor cortex for speech. Suppose Fred is asked to repeat a phrase such as *"Nelson Rockefeller drives a Lincoln Continental."* The first stop in the brain is Fred's primary auditory cortex, where the in-

---

* The information from the visual cortex in the right hemisphere gets to Wernicke's area via fibers passing through the posterior corpus callosum.

coming message is perceived and translated into a neural code that Wernicke's area will understand. Then the coded message is sent off to Wernicke's area, where the meaning of the message (that Fred should say *"Nelson Rockefeller drives a Lincoln Continental."*) is extracted. Wernicke's area then codes the sentence in a form that Broca's area can work with and sends it off via the arcuate fasciculus. When the message arrives at Broca's area, Broca's area recodes the phrase into an articulatory plan for the speech muscles and sends it to the primary motor cortex. The primary motor cortex sends the message down pyramidal fibers to the cranial nerves, which move the speech muscles. Wernicke's area monitors the output and initiates corrective routines if necessary.

Oral Reading If Fred is asked to read printed material aloud, processes similar to those involved in speech repetition take place once the message has reached Wernicke's area. However, Wernicke's area gets the message from the visual cortex rather than the auditory cortex.

Writing When Fred writes a message, his Wernicke's area formulates a message containing the appropriate words in syntactically acceptable order, gets the spelling right, and sends it via the arcuate fasciculus to the premotor cortex for Fred's hand and arm, which sets up the appropriate movement plans and sends them to his motor cortex. Fred's eyes and Wernicke's area collaborate to monitor what he writes. If Wernicke's area is not satisfied, Fred may erase, revise, correct spelling errors, or make other repairs to his written message.

Gestural Responses to Spoken Commands In this task, the neural processes are similar to those for speech, except that the information from Wernicke's area is sent to the premotor area for Fred's hand and arm just above Broca's area rather than to the premotor cortex for the speech muscles (Broca's area). If the gestural response is to be carried out by Fred's right hand and arm (contralateral to his

language-dominant hemisphere), the message goes from Wernicke's area to the premotor cortex in the dominant hemisphere and then to the motor cortex in the same hemisphere, which sends the message to his right hand. If the response is to be carried out by Fred's left hand and arm (on the same side as his language-dominant hemisphere), the message goes from Wernicke's area to the premotor cortex in the left hemisphere, from there it is sent via the corpus callosum to the motor cortex in the right hemisphere and then down the corticospinal tract to Fred's left hand. (The premotor cortex in Fred's left hemisphere plans volitional movements for both sides of Fred's body.)

Damage in the centers and pathways postulated by the connectionist model causes distinctive patterns of speech, language, and motor-planning disorders. Some of these patterns are caused by destruction of important centers (such as Broca's area and Wernicke's area), and other patterns are caused by damage in the pathways connecting the centers (such as the arcuate fasciculus). Classification of aphasic patients into classic connectionist syndromes relies heavily on relationships among *speech fluency, paraphasia, repetition,* and *language comprehension.*

Speech fluency is an important concept for understanding the connectionist model because connectionist aphasia syndromes often are divided into *fluent* and *nonfluent* types. In general, the speech of aphasic patients with damage anterior to the central sulcus (fissure of Rolando) is *nonfluent* and that of aphasic patients with lesions posterior to the central sulcus is *fluent.*

Speech fluency refers to the prosodic or melodic characteristics of speech. The speech of patients with fluent aphasia flows smoothly and effortlessly, and fluent aphasic speakers manipulate speech rate, intonation, and emphatic stress in much the same way as normal speakers do. The speech of patients with nonfluent aphasia is halting and produced with great effort.

Their speech rate is markedly slowed, their intonational patterns are constricted, and changes in loudness related to emphatic stress are markedly diminished or disappear.

Over the years, the terms *fluent* and *nonfluent* have acquired meaning that goes beyond the mechanics of speech to its syntactic, grammatical, and semantic content:

> Fluent (aphasic patients) have normal or near normal speech rates and use a variety of different grammatical constructions; function words and grammatical inflections are present, and usually syntactically appropriate. Intonation patterns are present and usually appropriate. Nonfluent (aphasic patients) have slow and labored speech. The variety of grammatical constructions is often restricted and intonation may be reduced or absent; function words and grammatical affixes may be omitted, and patients may rely a lot on nouns (Howard & Hatfield, 1987, p. 147).

Paraphasia is another important concept in connectionistic models of aphasia. Paraphasia can be loosely defined as *errors in speaking produced by a person with aphasia.* (The circularity of this definition has not affected its durability in the literature.) Two kinds of paraphasias have been described, although there is some confusion about which speech errors qualify as paraphasias. *Literal paraphasias* (sometimes called *phonemic paraphasias*) are phonologic errors. They are caused by substitution of incorrect sounds for correct ones (e.g., *shooshbruss* for *toothbrush*) or by transpositions of sounds within words (e.g., *tevilision* for *television*). *Verbal paraphasias* (sometimes called *semantic paraphasias*) are errors in which an incorrect word (usually semantically related to the target) is substituted for the target word (e.g., *door* for *window,* or *knife* for *fork*).

According to Canter (1973), the term *literal paraphasia* denotes a *pattern* of articulatory errors, which means that the label should not be attached to individual articulatory errors, especially those made by patients who are dysarthric rather than aphasic. Consequently, the clinician must consider not only the nature of the speech errors but also the context in which they occur to tell if they are truly literal paraphasias. When an aphasic patient makes speech-sound errors in a context of fluent, effortless speech they are likely to be literal paraphasias. When they occur in a context of nonfluent, effortful articulatory posturing they are likely to represent the phonetic dissolution usually associated with motor-planning disorders (apraxia of speech).

As noted earlier, *speech repetition* tests the entire connectionist circuit from the auditory cortex through the motor cortex for speech. For this reason, repetition tasks get a major place in the testing routine of clinicians intent on assigning aphasic patients to connectionist syndromes. As we will see, dissociations between speech repetition and language comprehension are important signs in discriminating among fluent aphasic syndromes.

Aphasia Caused by Destruction of Cortical Centers for Language

Three of the most common aphasia syndromes (*Broca's aphasia, Wernicke's aphasia,* and *global aphasia*) are caused by damage in cortical regions considered important for comprehension, formulation, and production of language. These regions are located in the central part of the language dominant hemisphere, in the area served by the middle cerebral artery. Broca's aphasia prototypically is caused by occlusion of the anterior branch of the middle cerebral artery, and Wernicke's aphasia is caused by occlusion of the posterior branch. Global aphasia usually is caused by occlusion of the artery's main trunk.

Broca's Aphasia Broca's aphasia may be called *expressive aphasia, motor aphasia,* or *anterior aphasia.* Because Broca's area is close to the primary motor cortex for the face, hand, and arm, and because descending pyramidal tract fibers run alongside Broca's area, patients with Broca's aphasia usually have right-sided hemiplegia or hemiparesis.

Broca's area makes up the lower part of the *premotor cortex,* which is a strip of cortex just in front of the primary motor cortex. The premotor cortex seems to be responsible for planning skilled volitional movements for the primary motor cortices in both hemispheres. Because Broca's area is adjacent to the primary motor cortex for the speech muscles, it gets the responsibility for planning speech movements.

Patients with Broca's aphasia talk as if the motor plans for speech have gone awry. Their words come slowly, laboriously, and haltingly. They put unusually long pauses between words and sometimes within words. Their intonation and stress patterns are markedly diminished, giving their speech a monotonous quality. Misarticulations are prominent, with occasional distortions of consonants and vowels (a phenomenon sometimes called *phonetic dissolution*). Patients with Broca's aphasia are laconic—their utterances are short and consist mostly of content words (nouns, verbs, and sometimes adjectives, but rarely adverbs). Most function words (conjunctions, articles, and prepositions) are missing from their speech, leading some writers to describe their speech as *agrammatic* or *telegraphic.* What follows is a transcript of a patient with Broca's aphasia describing the "cookie theft" picture from the *Boston Diagnostic Aphasia Examination* (BDAE; Goodglass & Kaplan, 1983, Figure 4-25).

> *Uh. . .mother and dad . . . no . . . mother . . . dishes . . . uh . . . runnin over . . . water . . . and floor . . . and they . . . uh . . . wipin disses . . . and . . . uh . . . two kids . . . uh . . . stool . . . and cookie . . . cookie jar . . . uh . . . cabinet and stool . . . uh . . . tippin over . . . and . . . uh . . . that . . . bad . . . and somebody . . . gonna get hurt.*

Patients with Broca's aphasia write as they talk: slowly and laboriously. Their written language typically consists of strings of content words sprinkled with misspellings and distortions or omissions of letters. Letters are clumsily formed (perhaps in part because the presence of hemiplegia forces the patient to write with the nonpreferred hand) and their effortfully printed sentences often slant downward across the page. They rarely write in cursive form. Figure 4-3 shows a sample of writing from a patient with Broca's aphasia who is describing in writing what one does with the 10 test objects (*cigarette, comb, fork, key, knife, match, pen, pencil, quarter, toothbrush*) from the *Porch Index of Communicative Ability* (PICA; Porch, 1981a).

Patients with Broca's aphasia comprehend spoken and written language better than they speak or write although they are slow readers (careful testing will almost always reveal impair-

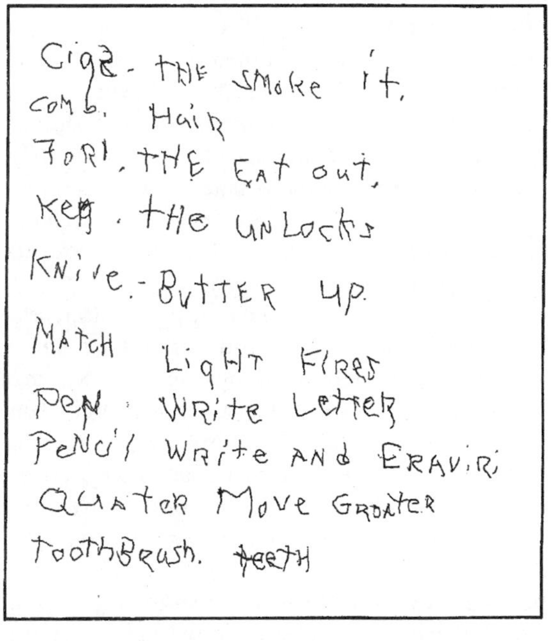

Figure 4-3 ■ A sample of writing produced by a patient with Broca's aphasia.

ment of both reading and listening comprehension). Their self-monitoring usually is well preserved. When they make errors in speech or writing or are unsuccessful in communicating they typically repeat or attempt repairs. Patients with Broca's aphasia usually are aware of their physical and communicative impairments, sometimes excruciatingly so, which may be why some (especially those with severe impairments) are easily upset by failed communication attempts, sometimes to the point of emotional outbursts. Patients with Broca's aphasia usually are cooperative and task-oriented in testing and treatment activities. They are good at remembering treatment procedures and goals from day to day and may spontaneously generalize responses acquired in treatment sessions to their daily life environment.

Wernicke's Aphasia Like Broca's aphasia, Wernicke's aphasia sometimes is called by other names. *Sensory aphasia, receptive aphasia,* and *posterior aphasia* are the most common names. One of the most striking language characteristics of patients with Wernicke's aphasia is their impaired comprehension of spoken and printed verbal materials. Patients with severe Wernicke's aphasia fail to comprehend even simple spoken or written materials although some may get a smattering of what is said in conversations. Patients with mild or moderate Wernicke's aphasia usually get the overall point of conversations but miss many specifics.

Patients with Wernicke's aphasia often exhibit dissociations between the sound (or sight) of words and their meanings and in extreme cases may be unable to discriminate between phonologically valid nonwords *(spome)* and real words *(spoon)*. Their language comprehension may be additionally compromised by blurring of semantic distinctions among words, rendering them unable to appreciate differences between words with related meanings *(good* vs. *wonderful)* and causing some patients with Wernicke's aphasia to lose their sense of semantic typicality (e.g., whether *carrot* is a more typical vegetable than *artichoke).*

The semantic impairments of patients with Wernicke's aphasia are exacerbated by impaired short-term retention and recall of verbal materials. They perform poorly on tests of short-term memory such as repeating strings of numbers or recalling word lists. When they are asked to perform sequences of manipulative or gestural responses to spoken or printed commands (such as *"Put the pencil beside the spoon and the quarter beside the box."),* their performance quickly deteriorates as the commands become longer.

In contrast with the slow, laborious, and halting speech of patients with Broca's aphasia, patients with Wernicke's aphasia talk smoothly, effortlessly, and usually copiously. Patients with Wernicke's aphasia can produce long, syntactically well-formed sentences with normal intonation and stress patterns although they may pause and muddle about when experiencing word retrieval difficulties, which are common. Because the mechanics of speech are preserved in Wernicke's aphasia does not mean, however, that patients with Wernicke's aphasia have no difficulty communicating by talking. Their connected speech may be littered with verbal paraphasias (substitution of one word for another), occasional literal paraphasias (substitution or transposition of sounds within words), and *neologisms* (nonwords such as *carabis).* Patients with severe Wernicke's aphasia may produce *jargon* (strings of neologisms with a sprinkling of connecting words).

When asked to tell the examiner what he had for breakfast, a patient with severe Wernicke's aphasia responded with, *That's frinking the ambuvali binai the frigilator.**

---

* Interestingly, these patients often produce strings of words in which the major content words are replaced by neologisms, but in which the connectives (articles, conjunctions, prepositions) are real words. The strings also seem syntactically well formed (Goodglass, 1993).

Wernicke's aphasic patients with severe word-retrieval impairments may produce what is called *empty speech* by substituting general words such as *thing* or *stuff* or pronouns without referents for more specific words.

> A patient with moderate Wernicke's aphasia was attempting to explain what he had done on a shopping trip the previous day. He concluded with, *I went down to the thing to do the other one and she was only the last one that ever did it.*

Some Wernicke's aphasic patients talk around missing words—a behavior called *circumlocution.*

> A patient with moderate Wernicke's aphasia was attempting to tell the examiner what she had had for breakfast that morning. She was unable to come up with the needed words so she circumlocuted to get her intended meaning across.
>
> *This morning for—that meal—the first thing this morning—what I ate—I dined on—chickens, but little—and pig—pork—hen fruit and some bacon, I guess.*

The ease with which Wernicke's aphasic patients produce speech, their circumlocution, and their deficient self-monitoring may contribute to their well-known inclination to talk at great length unless forcibly interrupted. This phenomenon is called *press of speech* or *logorrhea.*

> **Clinician (To a patient with mild Wernicke's aphasia):** *Tell me what you do with a comb.*
>
> **Patient:** *What do I do with a comb? Well a comb is a utensil or some such thing that can be used for arranging and rearranging the hair on the head both by men and by women. One could also make music with it by putting a piece of paper behind it and blowing through it. Sometimes it could be used in art—in sculpture, for example, to make a series of lines in soft clay. It's usually made of plastic and usually black although it comes in other colors. It is carried in the pocket until its needed, when it is taken out and used, then put back in the pocket. Is that what you had in mind?*

The handwriting of patients with Wernicke's aphasia usually resembles their speech. They write effortlessly and their letters are well formed and legible. Most write in cursive form rather than in printed form. Although their handwriting may be mechanically normal, like their speech, it is often deficient in content. Patients who produce verbal paraphasias in speech also produce them in writing. Patients who speak neologistically write neologistically. (Interestingly, the letters in neologistic words usually are grouped in clusters that are consistent with letter groupings for real words.) Patients with press of speech when they talk exhibit press of writing when they write.

Figure 4-4 shows a writing sample generated by a Wernicke's aphasic patient with mild aphasia describing what one does with the 10 test items from the PICA.

Most patients with Wernicke's aphasia are alert, attentive and task oriented. Those with

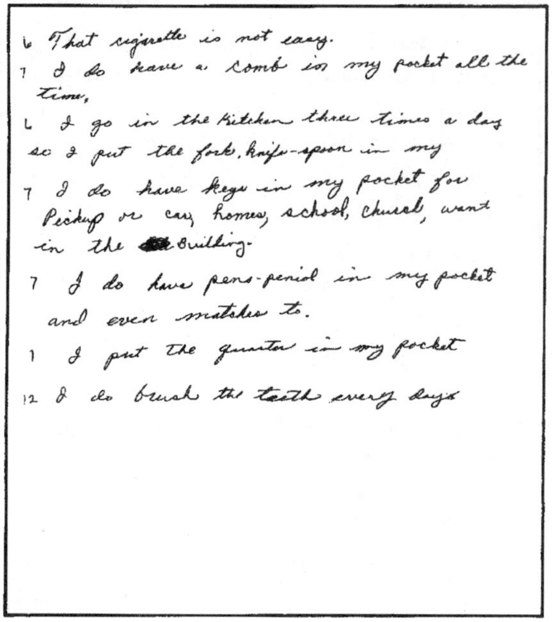

6 That cigarette is not easy.

7 I do have a comb in my pocket all the time,

6 I go in the kitchen three times a day so I put the fork, knife-spoon in my

7 I do have keys in my pocket for Pickup or car homes, school, church, want in the ████ building.

7 I do have pens-pencil in my pocket and even matches to.

1 I put the quarter in my pocket

12 I do brush the teeth every days

Figure 4-4 ▪ A sample of writing produced by a patient with Wernicke's aphasia.

mild Wernicke's aphasia are aware of their errors (at least most of them), the content of their speech is semantically appropriate, and they generally follow conversational rules such as those governing turn taking. Patients with moderate Wernicke's aphasia rarely notice errors or attempt repairs. They are attentive and cooperative in testing and treatment, but many cannot stay on task in testing and treatment activities without regular intervention by the clinician. In conversations, patients with Wernicke's aphasia tend to go off on tangents and talk at length about unrelated or trivial topics.

Most patients with severe Wernicke's aphasia are attentive but their profound comprehension impairments greatly interfere with their performance of all but the simplest verbal tasks. These patients are uniformly oblivious to errors and communication failure but appear sensitive at least to the basic rules governing conversational interactions; they acknowledge and attend to their conversational partner and respect turn-taking rules although once they get the conversational floor they tend to run on.

Patients with Wernicke's aphasia usually show less outward concern about their communication impairments than patients with Broca's aphasia. Part of Wernicke's aphasia patients' unconcern may relate to their lack of awareness, but many who do recognize errors and understand that they have communication impairments are remarkably complacent and unconcerned.

Because Wernicke's area is not close to the motor cortex, most patients with Wernicke's aphasia are not hemiparetic or hemiplegic unless the lesion extends into the frontal lobe or descending pyramidal tracts (in which case the aphasia might be more appropriately labeled *global aphasia).* However, fibers in the optic tract pass under Wernicke's area on their way to the visual cortex. Lesions extending deep into the temporal lobe often destroy these fibers, causing contralateral visual field blindness (described in Chapter 2).

Global Aphasia As mentioned earlier, global aphasia most often follows occlusion of the trunk of the middle cerebral artery, which causes massive damage extending throughout the periSylvian region.* The effects on the patient are comparably massive. Globally aphasic patients invariably exhibit severe impairments in all language functions. Most cannot perform even the simplest tests of listening comprehension and most cannot reliably answer simple yes-no questions, although some may respond to conversations in a way that suggests that they

---

* However, cases of global aphasia have been reported in which either Wernicke's area or Broca's area is spared (Basso and associates, 1985; Vignolo and associates, 1986) and following subcortical damage in the thalamus and basal ganglia (Naeser and associates, 1982).

get at least a rudimentary sense of what is said.* Few globally aphasic patients can read even simple words and their reading of sentences or texts is invariably nonfunctional. The speech of globally aphasic patients is severely limited, usually consisting of a few single words, stereotypical utterances (such as *"one-one-one, kakie-kakie-kakie"*), overlearned phrases (such as *"how-dee-do"*), or expletives. Over time, some globally aphasic patients become proficient at communicating in a limited way with a combination of intoned stereotypic utterances, gesture, and facial expression, but verbal communication remains largely nonfunctional.

Most globally aphasic patients are attentive, alert, task-oriented, and socially appropriate, which helps to differentiate the globally aphasic patient from the confused or demented patient. They usually can perform nonverbal tasks (matching objects or pictures, matching pictures to objects) satisfactorily, and some may perform normally or nearly so on nonverbal (performance) tests of intellect.

Aphasia Caused by Damage to Association Fiber Tracts Important to Language

Several aphasia syndromes are caused by damage in association fiber tracts that connect Wernicke's area with Broca's area or by damage to tracts that connect Wernicke's area and Broca's area to the rest of the brain. In *conduction aphasia* the pathway connecting (language-competent) Wernicke's area to (speech-competent) Broca's area is affected. In the *transcortical aphasias,* pathways connecting the periSylvian region with other regions of the brain are affected. The brain damage producing

these aphasia syndromes may involve the cortex but always extends beneath the cortex to affect association fiber tracts.

Conduction Aphasia Conduction aphasia typically is caused by lesions affecting the arcuate fasciculus, but sparing Wernicke's area and Broca's area. The defining behavioral characteristics of conduction aphasia are *grossly impaired repetition* and *relatively preserved language comprehension.** Language comprehension is preserved in conduction aphasia because the primary auditory cortex and Wernicke's area are spared. Conduction aphasic patients have extraordinary difficulty repeating what they hear because of poor transmission of information between Wernicke's area and Broca's area. Conduction aphasic patients speak fluently (speech rate, intonation, and stress patterns are normal) but they are prone to literal paraphasias and produce occasional verbal paraphasias. Their spontaneous speech is better than their repetition, although literal paraphasias and pauses generated by word-retrieval difficulties are common. Patients with conduction aphasia have difficulty reading aloud because oral reading, like repetition, depends on the connections between Wernicke's area and Broca's area. Conduction aphasic patients' problems with oral reading do not extend to their reading comprehension, which, like their auditory comprehension, is relatively good.

Conduction aphasic patients' handwriting typically is well formed and legible, but self-formulated writing and writing to dictation usually contain spelling errors and transpositions of syllables and words. They are better at saying what they think than repeating what they hear and they can write self-formulated material bet-

---

* Some globally aphasic patients who do not respond appropriately to any other spoken materials may respond appropriately to "whole body commands" such as *"stand up, turn around, lie down"* and so forth. The reason for this phenomenon is not clear, but Albert and associates (1981) suggest that it may be attributable to right-hemisphere participation in responding to such commands.

---

* This is not to say that conduction aphasic patients' comprehension is intact. They typically exhibit mild to moderate comprehension impairments. The point is that their ability to repeat phrases and sentences is strikingly worse than their ability to comprehend the same phrases and sentences.

ter than they can write what is said to them.

Conduction aphasic patients are alert, attentive, and task oriented. They are aware of errors in speech and writing and attempt repairs. When conduction aphasic patients produce paraphasias, many seem surprised by what they say, and comments to that effect are not unusual. Patients with conduction aphasia typically produce conversational asides (*"Why can't I say that?" "What's going on here?"*) normally and without conscious effort. Their first attempts at self-correcting a response often are unsuccessful, and long strings of unsuccessful repair attempts are common, with the patient often getting farther and farther from the target, until she or he throws in the towel or the examiner supplies the target word or words.

A patient with conduction aphasia was trying to produce the word *circus: It's a kriskus. . . . No, that's not right, but it's near. . . . Sirsis. . . . No. . . . This is very strange that I can't say this word. . . . How about kirsis? . . . No. . . . I'll have to by that. Kriskus? For some reason I can't say it right now.*

Transcortical aphasias (sometimes called *isolation syndromes*) are caused by dominant-hemisphere brain damage that spares the central region (Wernicke's area, Broca's area, and the arcuate fasciculus) but disconnects (*isolates*) all or parts of the central region from the rest of the brain. Because association fibers are compromised in the transcortical aphasias, Lichtheim, in 1885, called what we now know as transcortical aphasia *commissural dysphasia* or *white matter dysphasia*.

The disconnection causing transcortical aphasias is a result of damage in the border zone (watershed region) surrounding the territory of the middle cerebral artery. Damage in this wa-

tershed region most often comes from severe narrowing of the middle cerebral artery, which produces hypoperfusion in the watershed region. Less frequently, watershed damage is caused by embolic strokes.

Preserved repetition is a defining characteristic of the transcortical aphasias. Because Wernicke's area, Broca's area, and the arcuate fasciculus are spared, repetition of spoken words, phrases, and sentences is preserved, although other language functions may be substantially compromised. Three kinds of transcortical aphasia have been described in the literature: *transcortical motor aphasia, transcortical sensory aphasia,* and *mixed transcortical aphasia.*

Transcortical Motor Aphasia The classic cause of transcortical motor aphasia is damage in the anterior superior frontal lobe. The defining characteristics of transcortical motor aphasia are *marked reduction in speech output, good repetition* and *good auditory comprehension.* The reduced speech output of transcortical motor aphasic patients seems to be a consequence of their anterior frontal lobe involvement. The anterior frontal lobes are important for initiation and maintenance of purposeful activity. It follows, then, that patients with damage in the anterior frontal lobe of the language-dominant hemisphere should have problems initiating and maintaining speech output. (Luria (1966) called this syndrome *dynamic aphasia* and its behavioral manifestation *pathologic inertia.*) Large anterior frontal lobe lesions extending into the posterior frontal lobe may cause transcortical motor aphasia accompanied by right hemiparesis (or, less frequently, right hemiplegia). Wernicke's area is not affected in transcortical motor aphasia, so these patients' auditory comprehension is preserved. The arcuate fasciculus is spared, so patients with transcortical motor aphasia are good at repeating what they hear and are good at oral reading.

Although they are attentive, task-oriented, and cooperative, patients with transcortical motor aphasia are terrible conversationalists; they are content to sit silently while the conversational partner carries the entire communicative burden. When, after considerable urging, a patient with transcortical motor aphasia eventually speaks, she or he usually produces a perfunctory word or two and lapses into silence. However, if the interaction is highly structured and only a few highly predictable words are called for, these patients respond fluently and without delay. The surprising thing about transcortical aphasic patients is how well they talk when asked to repeat phrases or sentences, once they get started. Once these patients begin talking they can repeat long and complex phrases and sentences fluently and without error.

A patient with transcortical motor aphasia was asked, *What did you do for a living?* After a long delay he responded, *bakery,* and lapsed into silence. Repeated requests by the examiner to *tell me more* elicited only the word *bakery.* When the examiner subsequently tested the patient's repetition, the patient repeated fluently and without delay, *Before I had my stroke I worked as a baker in a large wholesale bakery in Minneapolis, Minnesota.*

Transcortical Sensory Aphasia (Posterior Isolation Syndrome) Like transcortical motor aphasia, transcortical sensory aphasia is caused by brain damage that spares Wernicke's area, the arcuate fasciculus, and Broca's area. However, in this case the damage is in the high parietal lobe. Like patients with transcortical motor aphasia, those with transcortical sensory aphasia do well when asked to repeat phrases or sentences after the examiner. Unlike patients with transcortical motor aphasia, those with transcortical sensory aphasia speak without having to be cajoled by their conversational part-

ner. In fact, some patients with transcortical sensory aphasia seem compelled to repeat what is said to them even when instructed not to do so. In a test situation they often repeat what the examiner asks them to do before responding, and in conversations they may incorporate what is said to them into their responses (Goodglass, 1993).

A test of sentence comprehension was administered to a patient with transcortical sensory aphasia. He was asked, *Does the sun rise in the west?* He responded, *Does the sun rise in the west?—The sun rises in the west—in the west—the sun rises—Yes—I should think the sun does rise in the west—yes the sun rises in the west.*

Because the brain damage that produces transcortical sensory aphasia isolates Wernicke's area from much of the parietal lobe and from the visual cortex, patients with transcortical sensory aphasia always have major impairments in listening and reading comprehension. In some ways patients with transcortical sensory aphasia resemble patients with Wernicke's aphasia; they speak fluently and their speech is empty, with numerous verbal paraphasias. Most are unaware of their errors and do not attempt to self-correct. However, they usually do not exhibit *press of speech,* as many Wernicke's aphasic patients do, and their excellent repetition clearly differentiates them from patients with Wernicke's aphasia. A striking characteristic of patients with transcortical sensory aphasia is their ability to repeat or read aloud long and complex sentences that they are unable to comprehend. They may be at a loss when asked to perform even simple manipulations in response to spoken directions but they flawlessly repeat much longer ones.

A patient with transcortical sensory aphasia was befuddled by simple commands such as *Pick up the pencil,* but without hesitation repeated after the examiner *Put the comb beside the matches, point to the quarter, and give me the spoon.*

Because the brain damage that produces transcortical sensory aphasia involves the parieto-occipital-temporal junction, transcortical sensory aphasic patients invariably have severely impaired reading comprehension (although oral reading is preserved), and they may have right-sided visual field blindness (usually inferior quadrantanopsia).

Mixed Transcortical Aphasia This rare syndrome is sometimes called *isolation of the speech area* (Geschwind, Quadfasel, & Segarra, 1968). These patients retain their ability to repeat what is said to them in the presence of profound impairment of all other communicative functions. The prototypical patient with isolation of the speech area "is nonfluent (in fact does not speak at all unless spoken to), does not comprehend spoken language, cannot name, cannot read or write, but can repeat what is said by the examiner (Benson, 1979, p. 46)." These patients often have a striking tendency to repeat, in parrot-like fashion, what is said to them, and if the examiner says the first few words of familiar songs or rhymes, these patients often complete the phrase and may go on to provide one or more following lines.

Mixed transcortical aphasia is caused by damage that spares Broca's area, Wernicke's area, and the arcuate fasciculus but isolates those areas from the rest of the brain. Its most frequent cause is stenosis of the internal carotid artery, which compromises blood flow throughout the watershed area of the language-dominant hemisphere. Mixed transcortical aphasia also has been reported following cerebral hypoxia, severe cerebral swelling, and multiple embolic strokes affecting the peripheral branches of the middle cerebral artery.

An Aphasia Syndrome Without a Clear Localization

Whether *anomic aphasia* exists as a separate syndrome is not clear (Albert and associates, 1981). Goodglass (1993) comments, "Of all the aphasia subtypes, anomic aphasia is the one that appears as a result of diverse causes and as a result of lesion sites that are remote from each other (p. 214)." The label usually is applied to patients whose major symptom is word retrieval difficulties in spontaneous speech and naming tasks. Anomic aphasic patients' spontaneous speech is fluent and grammatically correct but marked by word retrieval failures. The word-retrieval failures generate unusual pauses, circumlocution (talking around missing words), and substitution of nonspecific words such as *thing* for missing words. These patients usually have subtle comprehension impairments and may have other mild language impairments.

Goodglass (1993) described four varieties of anomic aphasia. According to Goodglass, patients with *frontal anomia* represent mild versions of transcortical motor aphasia. The major characteristic of these patients is the remarkable degree to which their word retrieval improves if the examiner provides the first sound of the target word. Patients with *anomia of the angular gyrus region* speak fluently but with frequent word-retrieval failures. The phenomena that set this syndrome apart from the other anomic syndromes are intermittent occasions in which the patient, upon failing to retrieve a word, fails to recognize it when it is supplied by the examiner. These patients often exhibit alienation of word meaning; they may repeat a word over and over without recognition. According to Goodglass, this syndrome may be a mild form of transcortical sensory aphasia.

Patients with *anomia of the inferior temporal gyrus* have severe word-retrieval problems but speak fluently and grammatically and have near-normal reading, writing, and presumably (although Goodglass does not mention it) near-normal auditory comprehension. Patients with *anomia as an expression of residual aphasia* may represent the most frequently occurring anomic aphasia syndrome. These are patients who have passed through a more severe form of any of the other aphasia syndromes and have recovered nearly normal language function but continue to exhibit mild to moderate impairments of word retrieval.

It is not clear if Goodglass's anomic aphasia syndromes are unique syndromes or if they simply represent milder versions of other aphasia syndromes, which seems likely. Anomia certainly is not a localizing phenomenon. As Goodglass notes, it can occur with damage in many different regions of the brain and in combination with a variety of other aphasic symptoms.

Table 4-1 summarizes the important characteristics of the connectionist aphasia syndromes.

■ RELATED DISORDERS

Nonlinguistic disorders sometimes occur in combination with the linguistic disorders characterizing the aphasia syndromes. *Disconnection syndromes* happen when the language-competent brain hemisphere is isolated from its nonlinguistic counterpart. *Visual field blindness* may accompany aphasia caused by temporal lobe or parietal lobe damage. *Apraxia* often occurs in combination with aphasia caused by frontal lobe damage. A variety of perceptual impairments called *agnosias* may follow cortical damage.

Disconnection Syndromes

Disconnection syndromes are created when the nerve fibers crossing between the hemispheres in the corpus callosum are damaged or destroyed. *Complete disconnection syndromes* usually are created by neurosurgeons who cut

the connections between the hemispheres (a procedure called *commissurotomy*) to keep epileptic seizures originating in one hemisphere from spreading across the corpus callosum to the other hemisphere. *Partial disconnection syndromes* sometimes are caused by strokes, tumors, or (rarely) traumatic injuries. The most frequent causes of partial disconnection syndromes are strokes involving the anterior or posterior cerebral arteries, which provide most of the blood supply to the corpus callosum. Occlusion of the anterior cerebral artery can produce *anterior disconnection syndrome,* and occlusion of the posterior cerebral artery can produce *posterior disconnection syndrome.*

Patients with *anterior disconnection syndrome* cannot carry out verbal commands requiring responses by their left hand and are unable to talk about or name objects held in the left hand. However, they can draw the objects, demonstrate their function, or choose an unseen but palpated object from a group with their left hand but not their right.* These phenomena occur because the sensory areas for the left hand (in the right hemisphere) are disconnected from the language-competent left hemisphere by destruction of the anterior corpus callosum. If the lesion extends laterally into the left frontal lobe, patients with anterior disconnection syndrome may exhibit symptoms of transcortical motor aphasia.

The most common impairments of patients with *posterior disconnection syndrome* are reading impairments attributable to isolation of the visual cortex from Wernicke's area, caused by interruption of visual fibers crossing in the posterior corpus callosum. These patients' reading impairments are measurable only by special testing in which printed words or pictures are flashed into the eyes in such a way that the image goes only to the right hemisphere. When this is done, these patients behave like those with complete disconnection syndrome.

---

* Assuming that the patients are right-handed.

T A B L E 4 - 1

Characteristics of connectionist aphasia syndromes

Aphasia syndrome	Lesion location	Fluency	Speech	Word retrieval	Repetition	Comprehension
Broca	Posterior, inferior frontal lobe	Nonfluent, telegraphic	Phonetic dissolution*	Fair, but misarticulated	Labored, misarticulated, telegraphic	Fair to good
Wernicke	Posterior, superior temporal lobe	Fluent, empty	Verbal (semantic) paraphasia	Poor, with verbal paraphasias	Fluent, verbal paraphasias, grossly restricted retention span	Poor
Conduction	Parietal lobe	Fluent, sensical	Literal (phonemic) paraphasia	Fair, with literal paraphasias	Fluent, literal paraphasias, some restriction of retention span	Fair to good
Anomic	Temporal, parietal lobe	Fluent, sensical	Verbal (semantic) paraphasia	Fair, with verbal paraphasias	Good	Fair to good
Transcortical motor (anterior isolation syndrome)	Anterior, superior frontal lobe	Fluent, sparse†	Variable	Variable, with delays in initiation	Good, but delays in initiation	Good
Transcortical sensory (posterior isolation syndrome)	Posterior, parietal superior lobe	Fluent, empty	Variable	Poor	Good	Poor
Global	Large, perisylvian	Nonfluent	Literal, verbal paraphasia, verbal stereotypies	Poor	Poor. Literal, verbal paraphasias, grossly restricted retention span	Poor

*Phonetic dissolution: *Distortion* of consonants (and sometimes vowels) a result of disrupted articulatory programming (apraxia of speech). In contrast, literal paraphasia involve *substitution* of a correctly articulated, but inappropriate, sound for another.
†With unusual delays in initiation. Utterances tend to be one or two words long.

Patients with posterior disconnection syndrome sometimes have an unusual reading impairment called *alexia without agraphia*. Patients with alexia without agraphia have severely impaired reading comprehension but retain their ability to write spontaneously and to copy printed materials although they cannot subsequently read aloud what they have written. Alexia without agraphia is caused by a complex lesion (or combination of lesions) that destroys the left visual cortex and the connections between the right visual cortex and the left hemisphere (Figure 4-5). As a consequence, visual information from the language-incompetent right hemisphere cannot reach the language-competent left hemisphere, and the patient does not appreciate the meaning of printed materials. The patient still can write because the connections between Wernicke's area (which formulates the messages) and the anterior motor planning and execution regions (which do the writing) are intact. Patients with posterior disconnection syndrome do not exhibit the tactile disconnection symptoms seen in anterior disconnection syndrome. They can name, describe, and otherwise talk (or write) about unseen objects palpated with either hand.

Another syndrome, *alexia with agraphia*, is caused by lesions in the region of the angular gyrus at the posterior end of the Sylvian fissure. These lesions disconnect the visual cortex from Wernicke's area and disconnect Wernicke's area from anterior motor planning and execution areas. Consequently, visual information from printed materials cannot be communicated either to Wernicke's area or from Wernicke's area to the anterior motor planning and execution areas, leaving the patient unable either to read or to write.

Patients with *complete disconnection syndrome* exhibit a symptom complex that is a combination of anterior and posterior disconnection syndromes. These patients are unable to name common objects held out of sight in the left hand because the sensory input from the hand goes into the mute right hemisphere, which has no way of transferring the information to the verbal left hemisphere. These same patients name objects held in the right hand with alacrity. If printed words or pictures of ob-

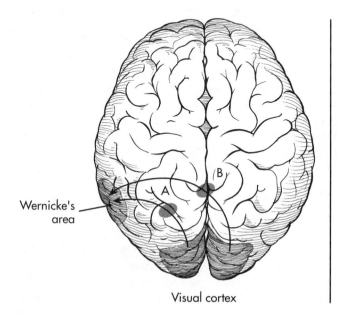

Wernicke's
area

Visual cortex

Figure 4-5 ■ How brain damage produces alexia without agraphia. The visual cortex in the left and right hemispheres is isolated from Wernicke's area by a lesion that destroys the left visual cortex or disconnects the left visual cortex from Wernicke's area *(A),* and another lesion that interrupts the visual fibers crossing through the corpus callosum from the right visual cortex *(B).*

jects are flashed into the eyes in such a way that the image goes only to the right hemisphere, the patient can report seeing them but cannot name them or otherwise talk about them. However, if the patient is allowed to choose from several words or pictures that are flashed into the right hemisphere, the patient can choose the correct one with the left hand but not the right hand. If printed commands calling for arm or hand movements are flashed into the right hemisphere, the patient cannot respond. If the commands are flashed into the left hemisphere the patient responds correctly with the right hand but not the left hand.

If a patient with complete disconnection syndrome is blindfolded and given objects to palpate in one hand or the other, then allowed to choose the palpated object from a group of objects, they choose correctly when the palpated object and the choice objects are palpated with the same hand but not when the test object is palpated with one hand and the choice objects are palpated with the other. (The brain cannot get the sensory information from the hand that palpated the object across the corpus callosum to tell the other hand what to search for.)

Right-handed people with complete disconnection syndromes can name objects held in the right hand. If they are allowed to name the objects, they can then choose the correct match with either hand because both hemispheres have heard the spoken name. Likewise if they can sneak a peek at the test object from under the blindfold, they can choose the correct match with either hand because the visual information goes to both hemispheres. Commisurotomized patients do not ordinarily encounter situations that restrict stimulus input to one hemisphere outside the clinic or laboratory. Consequently, they usually get along normally in daily life.

Visual Field Blindness

Aphasic patients with temporal or low parietal lobe damage often exhibit contralateral visual field blindness. (See Chapter 2 for more on how lesions in the visual system cause perceptual problems.) Because the visual fibers reach the visual cortex through the lower parietal and temporal lobes, visual field blindness commonly accompanies the posterior aphasias (primarily Wernicke's and conduction aphasia). It is unusual to see anterior aphasia or hemiplegia in combination with visual field blindness unless the aphasia is severe and global. It is also unusual to see visual field blindness in combination with transcortical sensory aphasia, because lesions in the watershed region of the language-dominant hemisphere rarely impinge on visual fibers.

Apraxia

Apraxia is a label for several different syndromes characterized by difficulty carrying out volitional movement sequences in the absence of sensory loss or paralysis sufficient to explain the difficulty. Apraxia often accompanies aphasia, especially aphasia caused by damage in the frontal lobe or anterior parietal lobe.

Liepmann (1900) described two kinds of apraxia, which he called *ideational apraxia* and *ideomotor apraxia*. Liepmann characterized *ideational apraxia* as a disruption of the *ideas* needed to *understand* the use of objects. Individuals with ideational apraxia are unable to carry out movement sequences that lead to a given result (such as filling a pipe and lighting it). According to Liepmann, ideational apraxia is caused by damage in the left parietal lobe and always affects both sides of the body. Patients with ideational apraxia are unable to carry out the movement sequences even if they are given real objects to use in the movements.

Ideomotor apraxia represents disruption of the *plans* needed to *demonstrate* actions. Ideomotor apraxia is caused by frontal lobe damage and may be either unilateral or bilateral. Patients with ideomotor apraxia usually can carry out movement sequences if they are given real objects to use in the movements. The patient with ideomotor apraxia may be unable to show the examiner how one would use a hammer when asked to pretend that he is using it but usually performs the movements when given a hammer, some nails, and a board. Several varieties of ideomotor apraxia have been identified, including *buccofacial apraxia, limb apraxia,* and *apraxia of speech.* (A fourth variety so-called *dressing apraxia* is sometimes seen in right hemisphere pathology but is not a true apraxia.)*

In *buccofacial apraxia* (oral nonverbal apraxia) the patient is unable to execute volitional sequences of movements with the tongue, jaw, lips, and other oral structures. The presence of buccofacial apraxia is revealed by asking the patient to demonstrate movements such as whistling, blowing dust off a shelf, sucking up through a straw, and sniffing a flower. In *limb apraxia* the patient is unable to carry out sequences of volitional movements with the arm, wrist, and hand. Limb apraxia usually is bilateral, but the presence of hemiplegia usually masks the limb apraxia on one side. Limb apraxia is more severe *distally* (away from the torso) than *proximally* (near the torso) so that patients with limb apraxia perform shoulder and elbow movements better than they perform wrist and finger movements. The presence of limb apraxias is revealed by asking the patient to demonstrate movement sequences such as flipping a coin, winding a watch, thumbing a ride, using a hammer, and waving goodbye.

For many years, the presence of apraxia was taken as evidence for damage in the premotor cortex, regarded as the center for motor planning. In recent years this view of the etiology of apraxia has been somewhat modified. Bucking-

ham (1979), for example, has postulated two kinds of apraxia: *center* apraxia and *disconnection* apraxia.* According to Buckingham, *center* apraxia is caused by damage to a cortical center for praxis. *Disconnection* apraxia is caused by disconnection of regions of the left hemisphere that can comprehend spoken commands from regions that can plan and carry out responses to the commands.

According to Buckingham, the key difference between these syndromes is in patients' responses to nonverbal requests for movements of apractic body parts. Patients with center apraxia are unable to execute movements in response to the examiner's requests, whether the movements are requested verbally by asking the patient to perform them or nonverbally by showing a picture depicting the requested movement. This is because the center for planning the movements is damaged. Conversely, patients with disconnection apraxia are unable to perform movements in response to verbal requests but can do them if the requests are made nonverbally because making the request nonverbally bypasses the pathways involved in comprehension of the request.[†]

Both sides of the body are routinely tested for limb apraxias unless one side is paralyzed. The nondominant limb is tested first because limb apraxia can be unilateral, and if it is, the nondominant limb is the unilaterally apraxic limb. If a patient is unilaterally apraxic and the examiner tests the (unaffected) dominant limb first, the patient may be able to perform the movement sequence with the apractic nondominant limb by watching the performance of the dominant limb and mimicking it with the nondominant limb.

The relationship between dominance and unilateral apraxia is interpretable by a connec-

---

* Patients with dressing apraxia have difficulty getting into articles of clothing. They may put articles of clothing on backward or inside-out and may attempt to put arms through trousers legs or legs through shirt or blouse sleeves. Dressing apraxia apparently represents a combination of disrupted body image and disturbed appreciation of the body's relationship to surrounding space.

---

* *Center apraxia* and *disconnection apraxia* are my labels, not Buckingham's.

† Patients with disconnection apraxia are likely to exhibit conduction aphasia because of the location of the brain damage

tionistic model. According to the model, the left hemisphere pathways from the primary auditory cortex to Wernicke's area to the premotor and motor cortex via the arcuate fasciculus are crucial for performing movements in response to spoken commands. (In order to keep things simple, the patient is assumed to be right-handed.)

According to the model, the spoken request for the movement is first perceived at the primary auditory cortex (Figure 4-6). The message then is sent to Wernicke's area where its meaning is deduced. A neurally-coded response to the message then is sent via the arcuate fasciculus to the premotor cortex where the plan for the movement sequence is drawn up. If the patient is to carry out the movement sequence with the right (dominant) hand and arm, the plan is sent from the premotor cortex to the pri-

mary motor cortex in the left hemisphere. If the patient is to carry out the movement sequence with his or her left (nondominant) hand and arm, the plan is sent from the left hemisphere premotor cortex across the corpus callosum to the motor cortex in the right hemisphere. (The left premotor area for the hand and arm plans movement sequences for both sides of the body, just as Broca's area plans all speech movements.)

Destruction of Wernicke's area prevents the patient from comprehending the meaning of spoken requests for limb movements. The patient fails to execute the movement with either limb but not because he or she is apraxic. Damage in the arcuate fasciculus prevents the sense of the command from getting to the premotor cortex. The patient fails to execute the movement with either limb but exhibits disconnec-

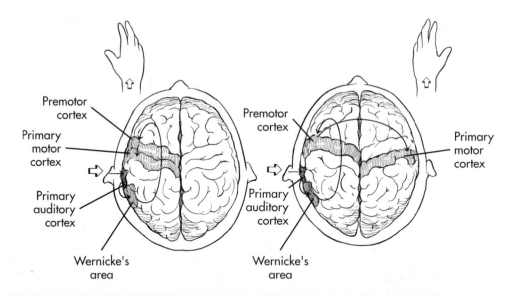

Figure 4-6 ▪ A connectionist explanation for limb apraxia. The spoken command requesting a limb movement is perceived by the primary auditory cortex, comprehended by Wernicke's areas, and sent via the arcuate fasciculus to the premotor cortex for the hand where a plan for the movement is formulated. The premotor cortex sends the plan to the motor cortex for execution. If the movement is to be carried out by the right hand, the plan is sent to the motor cortex in the left hemisphere. If the movement is to be carried out by the left hand, the plan is sent across the corpus callosum to the motor cortex in the right hemisphere.

tion apraxia. Destruction of the motor planning regions in the premotor cortex causes center apraxia. If the pathways from the left primary auditory cortex through the left premotor cortex are spared, but the crossing fibers that connect the premotor cortex in the left hemisphere with the right hemisphere motor cortex are interrupted, the patient exhibits unilateral apraxia of the left hand because the patient's left hand is isolated from the motor plans for the response.

Diagnosis of Apraxia

In diagnosing apraxia, the examiner must be careful to exclude alternative explanations for the movement disabilities observed. Alternative explanations include the following.

Paralysis or Weakness Apraxic individuals usually can perform movements that are a spontaneous response to natural occurrences in the environment, as well as movements that are part of automatic movement sequences. The presence of automatic and unplanned movements rules out weakness and paralysis as explanations for presumed apraxia.

Sensory Loss Sensory loss in apparently apraxic body parts should make the examiner cautious about diagnosing apraxia, especially if the apparently apraxic movements do not appear in unplanned, automatic movements. Sensory loss, by itself, is not a likely explanation for movement disorders, including apraxia. However, its presence requires that the examiner exclude it as a potential cause for what seems to be an apraxia.

Comprehension Deficit The examiner must be certain that inability to comprehend the instructions used in testing for apraxia is not misinterpreted as apraxia. One can estimate a patient's comprehension and at the same time test his or her knowledge of movement patterns by demonstrating a series of different movement sequences, while asking the patient with each sequence, *"Am I (for example) using a hammer?"* If the patient responds appropriately, one can assume that auditory comprehension and knowledge of the movements requested are good enough to eliminate them as explanations for the movement disabilities observed.

Incoordination Patients with incoordination generally perform movement sequences in response to the examiner's requests but with clumsiness and distortion. These patients can be distinguished from patients with apraxia by the consistent presence of clumsiness and incoordination in unplanned, automatic movements.

Apraxia of Speech

Apraxia of speech first appeared in the literature in the late 1800s and early 1900s lumped together with oral nonverbal apraxia into a syndrome called *oral apraxia.* During the first half of the twentieth century, writers began separating apraxic speech movements from apraxic nonspeech movements, and labels such as *apraxic dysarthria, peripheral motor aphasia, articulatory dysarthria,* and *apraxia of vocal expression* appeared in the literature. Darley (1969) settled on the label *apraxia of speech,* and since then most speech-language pathologists (and many others) have used this label for a collection of articulatory impairments, described by Darley, Aronson, and Brown (1975) as follows:

> Apraxia of speech is a distinct motor speech disorder distinguishable from the dysarthrias (speech disorders due to impaired innervation of speech musculature) and aphasia (a language disorder due to impairment of the brain mechanism for decoding and encoding the symbol system used in spoken and written communication). Apraxia of speech is a disorder of motor speech programming manifested primarily by errors in articulation and secondarily by compensatory alterations of prosody. The speaker shows reduced efficiency in accomplishing the oral postures necessary for phoneme production and the sequences of those postures for production of words. The disorder is frequently associated with aphasia but may also occur in isolation. Oral (nonspeech) apraxia may co-occur.

Apraxia of speech is characterized by highly variable articulation errors embedded in a pattern of speech made slow and effortful by trial-and-error gropings for the desired articulatory postures. The off-target productions are usually complications of articulatory performance, that is, substitutions (many of them unrelated to the target phoneme), additions, repetitions, and prolongations. Less frequently the errors are simplifications, that is, distortions and omissions. Errors are most often on consonants occurring initially in words, predominantly on those phonemes and clusters of phonemes requiring more complex muscular adjustment. Errors are exacerbated by increase in length of words and the linguistic and psychologic "weight" of a word in a sentence. They are not significantly influenced by auditory, visual, or instructional set variables. Islands of fluent, error-free speech highlight the marked discrepancy between efficient automatic-reactive productions and inefficient volitional-purposive productions (p 267).

Apraxia of speech (sometimes called *verbal apraxia*) resembles other forms of ideomotor apraxia in several ways. It is not caused by weakness, paralysis, or sensory loss in the speech muscles. Unplanned, automatic speech is much less clumsy and effortful than speech requested by the examiner. Speech elicited by natural contexts is less effortful and sounds more nearly normal than speech elicited in artificial contexts (such as a typical speech evaluation).

Several characteristics of apraxia of speech differentiate it from other neurogenic communication impairments that otherwise resemble it (particularly dysarthria and aphasia). Two important identifying characteristics are *articulatory error patterns* and *consistency of errors.*

Articulatory Error Patterns Darley, Aronson, & Brown (1975) and Wertz, LaPointe, & Rosenbek (1984), among others, have described characteristic articulatory error patterns of patients with apraxia of speech. These error patterns define relationships between articulatory or linguistic characteristics and error probabilities.

Wertz and associates (1984) describe the following error patterns:

- Substitution errors are more frequent than distortion, omission, or addition errors. Many substitution errors involve substituting a more difficult sound for an easier one. However, recent physiologic and acoustic studies of voice onset, phoneme duration, and movement patterns suggest that what listeners perceive as substitutions may actually be extreme phonetic distortion errors (Kearns & Simmons, 1988).
- Errors are more likely to be errors in placement of the articulators than errors of voicing, manner, or resonance.
- Most errors resemble the target sound.
- Consonant clusters are more likely to be in error than single consonants.
- Front-of-the-mouth sounds are more likely to be correct than sounds produced farther back in the mouth.

Wertz and associates (1984) suggest that the following characteristics are true for apraxic speakers as a group but may not always be true for a given apraxic speaker:

- Voiceless sounds are more frequently substituted for voiced sounds than vice-versa.
- Anticipatory errors (producing a sound before it occurs in a word or phrase, as in *thoothbrush* for *toothbrush*) are more frequent than either perseverative errors (saying a sound again, later in a word or phrase, when it is not appropriate, as in *manina* for *manila*) or metathetic errors (transposition of adjacent sounds, as in *tevelision* for *television*).
- Consonant errors are more frequent than vowel errors.

Consistency of Errors Darley, Aronson, & Brown (1975), Wertz and associates (1984), Kearns & Simmons (1988) and others have identified articulatory inconsistency as one of the hallmarks of apraxia of speech. This inconsistency is seen (heard) as correct articulation of given phonemes at one time and incorrect articulation of the same phonemes at another time. Inconsistency in articulation often is related to variations in the context in which the phonemes are produced. A given phoneme may be articulated correctly in one phonemic context (such as when the same phoneme is repeated in words or phrases, as in *"**D**on did the **D**isbes."*), and misarticulated in another (such as when contrasting phonemes occur in words or phrases, as in *"**D**on bought the **p**ot."*).

Apraxic patients' articulation characteristically is better in natural situations than in artificial ones. An apraxic patient's production of *"See you later."* usually is better when she or he is actually leaving than when she or he is asked by a clinician to say it in the middle of a treatment session. This phenomenon is related to what Darley and associates (1975) referred to as *islands of fluent, error-free speech,* in which the patient produces occasional fluent words, phrases, or sentences in the midst of effortful, struggling speech. Such periods of fluent speech in an overall context of nonfluency help to differentiate apraxia of speech from the dysarthrias, in which such intermittent periods of correct articulation do not occur.*

Apraxia of Speech versus Aphasia
Apraxia of speech in its pure form, unaccompanied by aphasia, is very rare. Apraxia of speech usually occurs in association with nonfluent (Broca's) aphasia, and, in fact, descriptions of the speech output of patients with Broca's aphasia usually resemble those for apraxia of speech (Goodglass & Kaplan, 1983; Wertz and associates (1984). When apraxia of speech accompanies Broca's aphasia, the patient's speech often is *agrammatic* as well as apraxic; most function words are left out and the patient's speech consists primarily of content words, giving his or her speech a telegraphic character.

---

* The primary exceptions being dysarthrias accompanying cerebellar ataxia and some dysarthrias caused by extrapyramidal disease, wherein speech may be intermittently dysarthric and normal.

Agnosia

Agnosia is a generic label for a group of perceptual impairments in which patients are unable to recognize, through an intact sensory modality, stimuli they recognize in other modalities. Patients with *visual agnosia* are unable to recognize objects visually, even though they can see, which they can prove by matching identical objects or forms, and even though they are familiar with the visually unrecognized objects, which they can prove by recognizing them when they feel them or hear the sounds they make. Visual agnosia characteristically is caused by damage (usually bilateral) in the occipital lobes, in the posterior parietal lobes, or in the fiber tracts connecting the visual cortex to other areas in the brain. Visual agnosias usually are incomplete, intermittent, and inconsistent, and patients with visual agnosias usually function reasonably well in daily life. Because they can see, they do not bump into things and grope their way about and they usually recognize and respond appropriately to familiar visual cues in their daily life environment.

Patients with *auditory agnosia* do not appreciate the meaning of sounds, in spite of adequate hearing acuity. Patients with auditory agnosia respond to sound by turning toward its source and they are startled by loud sounds. However, they cannot match an object with the sound it makes, even though they recognize the object when it is shown to them or when they are permitted to feel it. Auditory agnosia, like visual agnosia, may be incomplete or intermittent. Auditory agnosia suggests damage (usually bilateral) in the auditory association areas. Patients with auditory agnosia may occasionally respond appropriately to sounds or may respond appropriately to certain sounds or categories of sounds.

Patients who have brain damage separating Wernicke's area from the primary auditory cortex in both hemispheres sometimes exhibit *auditory-verbal agnosia* (sometimes called *pure word deafness*). These patients fail to appreciate the meaning of spoken words but respond appropriately to nonverbal sounds such as ringing telephones or sirens. They are aware of spoken words but do not understand their meaning although they comprehend them in their printed or written form. Patients with auditory-verbal agnosia often respond to speech as if their native language is unknown to them, but their speech usually is appropriate both in content and form.

Patients with *tactile agnosia* cannot recognize objects by touch and palpation, even though their tactile perception is intact. However, they immediately recognize the objects if the objects are presented in other sensory modalities. Tactile agnosia typically is caused by parietal lobe damage that isolates the somatosensory cortex from other parts of the brain. Patients with tactile agnosia can report touch, pinprick, and other simple stimulation of the cutaneous receptors in the hands but cannot name, describe, talk about, or demonstrate the use of objects palpated with the hands. Patients with tactile agnosia usually can draw or demonstrate the shape and size of palpated objects and they usually can choose matching objects from a group of objects when vision is blocked. The term *astereognosis* is a synonym for tactile agnosia but sometimes it is (erroneously) used in a broader sense, to denote loss of tactile recognition in the presence of sensory impairment.

True modality-specific agnosias are rare and some may not exist in spite of occasional descriptions in the literature. Some cases of agnosia reported in the literature may not be true agnosias, but perceptual or sensory discrimination deficiencies, comprehension or cognitive disorders, psychogenic symptoms, or multiple-modality recognition disorders. Therefore, in arriving at a diagnosis of agnosia, the clinician must exclude the following alternatives.

- *Sensory deficits in the affected modality* that interfere with perception. Agnosias can be diagnosed only when sensory function in the affected modality is adequate for perception of the unrecognized stimuli.
- *Comprehension disorders* that prevent the patient from understanding what is required in the test for agnosia.
- *Expressive disturbances* that prevent the patient from verbally identifying test stimuli.
- *Unfamiliarity with test stimuli* that prevents the patient from relating the stimuli to her or his knowledge and previous experience. If the patient recognizes the stimuli in another modality, one can conclude that unfamiliarity does not explain the agnosia.

■ LIMITATIONS OF CONNECTIONISTIC EXPLANATIONS OF APHASIA AND RELATED DISORDERS

With the advent of brain imaging technology (CT, MRI, PET) cerebral damage came to be localized with greater accuracy and in greater detail than ever before (except, of course, for postmortem examination of patients' brains). The use of brain imaging technology has created new insights into the relationships between brain damage and aphasia syndromes. Numerous reports on the relationships between aphasia and lesions located and measured with brain imaging technology have appeared in the literature during the last two decades (Cappa and associates, 1983; Cappa, Cavallotti, & Vignolo, 1981; Knopman and associates, 1983; Knopman and associates, 1984; Levine, Laughlin, & Geschwind, 1982; Naeser and associates, 1981; Naeser and associates, 1981; and others). These reports have caused several modifications to the original formulations of the relationships between brain damage and aphasia syndromes. Two of the most important modifications are: (1) *Damage confined to Broca's area or Wernicke's area usually does not produce chronic Broca's or Wernicke's aphasia.* (2) *Aphasia can be caused by damage deep in the brain, below the periSylvian cortex and its association fibers.*

Several reports have suggested that lesions confined to Broca's or Wernicke's area do not produce persisting Broca's or Wernicke's aphasia. Mohr and associates (1978) studied 22 cases of aphasia in which the site and extent of brain damage was documented and they reviewed 83 published reports in which the brains of aphasic patients came to autopsy. They concluded that lesions confined to Broca's area do not produce chronic Broca's aphasia but produce transitory mutism progressing to rapidly resolving articulatory targeting and sequencing impairments, with no significant persisting impairments in language. According to Mohr and associates, lesions must extend beyond Broca's area to produce persisting Broca's aphasia. Knopman and associates' (1983) findings are consistent with those of Mohr and associates. They reported that patients with lesions confined to Broca's area exhibit transient nonfluent speech without persisting Broca's aphasia. According to Knopman and associates, persisting Broca's aphasia requires a lesion extending from Broca's area into the primary motor cortex or parietal lobe.

Similar doubts have been raised concerning the relationship between damage confined to Wernicke's area and chronic Wernicke's aphasia. Selnes and associates (1983) measured recovery of language by 39 aphasic adults with single left-hemisphere lesions. They tested the patients' language comprehension once a month for 5 months. Patients with damage confined to Wernicke's area recovered near-normal language comprehension. Patients with persisting severe language comprehension deficits characteristically had damage extending beyond Wernicke's area into the inferior parietal lobe. Selnes and associates (1985) reported that the most striking persisting consequence of damage confined to Wernicke's area is impaired repetition. Of ten patients who were classified as having Wernicke's aphasia at one month post onset, eight were classified as having conduction aphasia at 6 months post onset. Patients with damage confined to Wernicke's area exhibited chronically poor repetition and relatively good (though not normal) comprehension.

Classical connectionist models attribute aphasia to damage in key regions of the cerebral cortex or in fibers connecting one key region with another and disregard the possibility of aphasia resulting from deep subcortical damage. However, it is now apparent that right-handed patients with damage in the left basal ganglia or left thalamus can develop aphasia (Mohr, Walters, & Duncan, 1975; Naeser and associates, 1982; Ojemann, 1975; Cappa & Vignolo, 1979; Alexandar & Lo Verme, 1980; and others).

Naeser and associates (1982) studied nine cases of aphasia caused by damage in and around the left basal ganglia and reported three subcortical aphasia syndromes based on the front-to-back location of damage. Patients with an *anterior syndrome* (caused by damage in the internal capsule, the lenticular nucleus, and extending into anterior white matter) exhibited hemiplegia, slow, dysarthric speech with good phrase length and prosody, good comprehension, good repetition, poor oral reading and writing, and poor confrontation naming. Patients with a *posterior syndrome* (caused by capsular-putamenal damage extending into posterior white matter) exhibited hemiplegia, fluent speech without dysarthria, poor comprehension, good single-word repetition but poor sentence repetition, impaired reading and writing, and poor confrontation naming. (This syndrome resembles Wernicke's aphasia except for the presence of hemiplegia in the subcortical syndrome.) An *anterior-posterior syndrome* (caused by capsular-putamenal damage with both anterior and posterior extension) is characterized by a mixture of symptoms consistent with both Broca's and Wernicke's aphasias, "although they did not completely resemble cases of Broca's, Wernicke's, global, or thalamic aphasia in CT scan lesion sites, or language behavior (p. 2)."

Cappa and associates (1983) described an anterior aphasia syndrome and a posterior aphasia syndrome caused by damage in the internal capsule and adjoining basal ganglia. Their patients had smaller lesions than those of Naeser and associates, and their patients' aphasias were milder but resembled those of the patients studied by Naeser and associates. The current evidence suggests that patients with aphasia caused by damage in the basal ganglia exhibit a variety of disruptions in speech and language (Robin & Sheinberg, 1990), and that the three syndromes described by Naeser and associates do not account for all the varieties of aphasia that can be caused by lesions in the basal ganglia.

Aphasia caused by lesions in the left thalamus also has been described, and the role of the thalamus in language has received considerable attention (Mohr and associates, 1975; Ojemann, 1975; Cappa and Vignolo, 1979; and others). Patients with aphasia caused by thalamic lesions are almost always hemiplegic (because of damage to pyramidal tract fibers in the internal capsule). They have difficulty initiating spontaneous speech and their spontaneous speech is sparse, echolalic and neologistic. Their vocal intensity tends to decrease progressively during utterances. Their auditory comprehension and reading usually are good. Their writing usually is impaired, and word-finding problems are common. Patients with left thalamic damage tend to be perserverative, and their performance tends to fluctuate from task to task and moment to moment. Murdoch (1990) has commented that aphasia syndromes resulting from thalamic lesions resemble transcortical motor aphasia, in that repetition and comprehension tend to be preserved but self-initiated speech tends to be reduced. According to Murdoch, the language impairments of patients with left subcortical damage usually are mild, and patients with subcortical aphasia have a better prognosis for recovery than patients with aphasia caused by cortical damage.

Naeser and associates (1989) reported that two left-hemisphere fiber tracts—the *medial subcallosal fasciculus* (deep in the anterior frontal lobe) and the *periventricular white matter* (beneath the sensory and motor cortex for the mouth)—are important determinants of aphasic adults' recovery of spontaneous speech. They studied the relationship between recovery of speech by 27 aphasic adults and the location of their brain damage as indicated by CT scans. They reported that destruction of the subcallosal fasciculus and periventricular white matter always caused permanent severe impairment of spontaneous speech.

Even though aphasia syndromes follow subcortical damage, it is not clear that the damaged subcortical structures are directly involved in language. In many of the patients studied, damage was not confined to subcortical structures but extended to the cortex. Dewitt and associates (1985) asserted that MRI scans of patients with subcortical aphasias usually reveal involvement of cortical tissue not visualized by CT scans. Metter and associates (1983) reported that PET studies of patients with subcortical aphasia almost always reveal decreased cortical metabolism in areas of the left hemisphere without observable structural damage. Alexander, Naeser, & Palumbo (1987) studied 18 patients with only subcortical damage and retrospectively reviewed the cases of 61 more patients. They reported that damage confined to the thalamus does not cause persisting aphasia but may cause mild word-retrieval impairments. They suggested that subcortical lesions causing aphasia must involve deep nerve fiber tracts connecting subcortical regions with one another or nerve fiber tracts connecting subcortical regions to cortical regions.

The Explanatory Power of Connectionist Models In spite of the apparent objectivity of connectionist explanations of aphasia, they do not and probably cannot provide a complete explanation of brain-behavior relationships. As Jackson (1874) pointed out, symptoms appearing after brain damage identify the brain location in which damage produces a *symptom* and do not necessarily identify the location in the brain of the underlying *function* or *process* to which the symptom relates. Kertesz (1979) extends Jackson's assertion: "only lesions causing impairments are localizable, not the impairment itself (p. 142)."

When symptoms are produced by destruction of association fibers and not by destruction of functional regions of cortex, localizationist interpretations are likely to go astray. For example, damage in the left hemisphere at the parieto-occipital-temporal junction (the angular gyrus region) is known to cause reading impairments. From this evidence a strict localizationist might conclude that the parieto-occipital-junction in the left hemisphere is a center for reading. The conclusion would be ill-advised because reading is a complex process that requires the participation of at least several brain regions. Reading impairments and damage in the region of the angular gyrus of the left hemisphere tend to co-occur because damage there disrupts communication between the visual cortex and Wernicke's area (not because the angular gyrus region is a center for reading). Few would argue that the lesions producing transcortical motor aphasia do so by destroying a center for initiation of speech, but most would agree that these patients' reticence is caused by isolation of regions responsible for speech from regions responsible for activation and arousal.

According to Goodglass (1993) connectionist syndromes represent "the result of modal tendencies for the functional organization of language in adult human brains (p. 218)." Goodglass believes that adult human brains are to some extent "hard-wired" but that as the individual matures, her or his brain develops its own most efficient neural organization for carrying out the processes involved in language. According to Goodglass, there are common (modal) patterns of brain organization toward which brains gravitate (presumably these common patterns are the result of the hard wiring).

These modal patterns produce enough consistency in brain organization to produce, in turn, relationships between brain damage and language impairments that are sufficiently predictable to make connectionistic explanations of brain-behavior relationships useful. However, according to Goodglass, individual differences in how the brain has organized itself for language may be superimposed on these modal patterns. These individuals differences produce exceptions, contradictions, or incomplete representations of the classic connectionist syndromes in individual patients.

Because of these individual differences, connectionist explanations of aphasia work better at the group level than at the individual level. If a large group of right-handed adults with left temporal lobe damage were to be tested, their overall pattern of performance would almost certainly match the classic pattern for Wernicke's aphasia. Their comprehension would be substantially impaired, they would produce paraphasic speech errors (especially verbal paraphasias), they would produce inordinate numbers of vague and indefinite words, and they would say more than necessary to communicate a given amount of information. However, there would undoubtedly be some in the group who produced few or no paraphasic errors, some who produced few vague and indefinite words, some who did not exhibit press of speech, and perhaps a few whose comprehension was relatively good.

The uncertainty of connectionist models increases not only as one moves from groups of aphasic patients to individual patients, but as one moves from global characteristics (such as speech fluency) to more specific aspects of language (such as the behaviors seen as a consequence of word-retrieval failure). The fuzziness of connectionist models with regard to specifics is apparent when aphasia test batteries designed expressly to classify aphasic patients into connectionist syndromes prove unable to classify unambiguously from 15% (Poeck, 1983) to 40%

(Benson, 1979) or up to 80% (Goodglass & Kaplan, 1983) of patients into classic connectionist syndromes based on their language behaviors.

In spite of these shortcomings, connectionist aphasia syndromes and their terminology can be useful to the clinician who wishes to communicate efficiently or to make an educated guess about the location and perhaps the extent of a patient's brain damage from the patient's observed symptoms. Goodglass (1993) has commented that classic patterns of Wernicke's or Broca's aphasia usually point unambiguously to damage in the temporal lobe (in the case of Wernicke's aphasia) or the posterior inferior frontal lobe (in the case of Broca's aphasia), but when the classic patterns are mixed or incomplete, predicting the location of the brain damage underlying the symptoms becomes much less certain. Those who employ the connectionist model will frequently be surprised by patients who do not fit the model but their predictions will be supported by enough patients who do fit the model to make it a convenient tool.

The connectionist model is in many respects fictional but it remains a useful model for the speech-language pathologist who wishes to understand the basic relationships between symptoms of aphasia and their source in the nervous system. The speech-language pathologist who understands the relationships between connectionist aphasia syndromes and various patterns of language impairments can use the presence of a connectionist aphasia syndrome to help him or her plan assessment of the patient's communication impairments. Knowledge of the connectionist model also helps speech-language pathologists communicate with neurologists and other professionals who make referrals and talk in the language of the model.

The next section discusses how speech-language pathologists go about the business of assessing brain-damaged adults' language and communication. As described in Chapter 3, the assessment process begins when the referral appears on the speech-language pathologist's desk and proceeds through several phases before formal testing begins. Formal testing often begins with administration of a comprehensive language test to get a general sense of the patient's linguistic and communicative impairments, followed by administration of one or more free-standing tests to analyze in more detail the patient's specific impairments. This is the general organizing theme for what follows. Some widely used comprehensive language tests and some popular free-standing tests of specific abilities are described, and some ways in which comprehensive language tests and free-standing tests of specific abilities complement each other in assessment of brain-damaged adults are discussed.

■ ASSESSING LANGUAGE AND COMMUNICATION

Comprehensive Language Tests

Comprehensive language tests permit clinicians to measure patients' communication performance in the two primary language input modalities (vision and audition) and three output modalities (speech, writing, and gesture) at various levels of difficulty within modalities or combinations of modalities. The tests permit clinicians to identify and describe communication impairments and to estimate their severity. Some tests permit prediction of a patient's recovery and most help clinicians make a diagnosis.

Albert and associates (1981) described a model for designing comprehensive language tests that provides for assessment of all stimulus input and response output modality combinations related to language (Table 4-2). Most comprehensive language tests include subtests for assessing the stimulus-response combinations shown in the unshaded sections of Table 4-2 but none have subtests assessing verbal or gestural responses to tactile stimuli or a subtest in which patients pantomime the names or functions of objects.*

---

* The BDAE and the *Western Aphasia Battery* (WAB; Kertesz, 1982) include such subtests as supplemental tests.

T A B L E   4 - 2

A schema for constructing comprehensive language tests

Stimulus	Response			
	Point	Say	Write	Do
See objects	**Visual matching**	**Naming**	**Written naming**	**Pantomime**
Hear words (sentences)	Word discrimination, sentence comprehension	Word repetition, sentence repetition, answering questions	Writing from dictation	Follow commands
See words (sentences)	Word-object matching	Oral reading	Copying	Follow written commands
Feel objects	Visual-tactile matching (stereognosis)	Tactile naming	Tactile-written naming	Pantomime

Data From Albert and associates, 1981.

Although the subtests contained in most comprehensive language tests can be partitioned according to Albert and associates' schema, clinicians (and patients) are more likely to divide communicative activities into the traditional *speaking, listening, reading,* and *writing* categories. The following list of subtests found in most comprehensive language tests is arranged according to those categories:

Speech
- Reciting days of the week, months of the year, and counting aloud
- Naming objects or pictures indicated by the examiner
- Completing incomplete phrases or sentences spoken by the examiner
- Repeating words, phrases, and sentences spoken by the examiner
- Formulating and producing single sentence utterances
- Formulating and producing multiple sentence utterances

Auditory comprehension
- Answering spoken questions
- Pointing to objects or pictures named by the examiner

- Following spoken directions
- Understanding spoken discourse

Reading
- Matching pictures, letters, or geometric forms
- Matching printed words to pictures
- Answering printed questions
- Reading aloud printed numerals, letters, words, and phrases
- Silently reading and answering questions about printed sentences and paragraphs

Writing
- Copying letters, geometric forms, and words
- Writing letters, words, and sentences spoken by the examiner
- Formulating written narratives

Comprehensive language tests for adults are designed for assessment of adults with aphasia but most can be used to assess language performance of adults with other linguistic or communication impairments. In fact, several aphasia tests provide norms for other populations, such as adults with right-hemisphere damage or dementia. The major comprehensive language tests are similar in content but there are important differences in intent, scoring, and interpretation. The descriptions that follow illustrate some of these differences.

The Minnesota Test for Differential Diagnosis of Aphasia

The *Minnesota Test for Differential Diagnosis of Aphasia* (MTDDA; Schuell, 1972) is the longest and most detailed comprehensive language test with 47 subtests divided among five sections: *auditory disturbances* (9 subtests), *visual and reading disturbances* (9 subtests), *speech and language disturbances* (15 subtests), *visuomotor and writing disturbances* (10 subtests), and *disturbances of numerical relations and arithmetic processes* (4 subtests). The MTDDA is heterogeneous with regard to the number of items in subtests and the pattern of difficulty within subtests. The number of items within subtests ranges from 5 to 32. In some subtests, items increase in difficulty as the subtest progresses, and in others the items are of approximately equal difficulty. Because of its length and the time it takes to administer and score the entire MTDDA (3 to 6 hours), clinicians tend not to administer the complete test.

Schuell (1957) suggested a *baseline-ceiling* procedure for shortening the test. In this procedure, the examiner estimates the patient's probable level of performance in each performance category (listening, speaking, reading, writing, and calculating) before beginning the test. The examiner then begins testing in each performance category with the most difficult subtests he or she thinks the patient can complete with no more than one error. If the patient makes more than one error on a subtest the examiner administers progressively easier subtests until the patient performs one without error (this defines the patient's *baseline*). Then the examiner administers progressively more difficult subtests until the patient makes 90% errors, at which point testing in that subtest ends (the *ceiling*) and the examiner begins the baseline-ceiling procedure in another subtest. (Clinicians some-

times use this procedure or a similar one to shorten other lengthy tests.)

The patient's performance on the MTDDA is recorded in a test booklet. Most responses are scored plus-minus (correct-incorrect) with some longhand notation, although errors made in two subtests (matching printed words to pictures and matching printed words to spoken words) can be categorized as *semantic confusions, auditory confusions, visual confusions,* or *irrelevant responses.* As the MTDDA is administered, the examiner records the number of errors made by the patient adjacent to each subtest in the test booklet. After the test is completed, the user transfers the subtest scores to a *summary of test scores* section on the face sheet of the test booklet where they are entered as number correct. (This change in record keeping can create transcription errors for the unwary. Many users prevent transcription errors by writing the number correct next to the number of errors for each subtest, as in *12/15.*)

The MTDDA provides few standardized procedures for interpreting patients' performance. The test manual provides mean scores, standard deviations, and subtest-by-subtest percentages of subjects making errors for a group of 50 nonaphasic adults and 6 groups of aphasic adults representing 5 major categories of aphasia and 1 minor syndrome. (The norm group of aphasic adults ranges from 31 to 157 patients, depending on the subtest. Most subtests are normed on 75 aphasic adults.) The MTDDA manual provides no procedures for profiling patterns of impairment and no percentiles, either for individual subtests or the MTDDA as a whole. However, the test manual does provide a list of "signs" and "most discriminating tests," which enable the user to assign patients to one of five major categories and two minor categories of aphasia:

- Simple aphasia
- Aphasia with visual involvement
- Aphasia with sensorimotor involvement
- Aphasia with scattered findings compatible with generalized brain damage

- Irreversible aphasic syndrome
- Minor syndrome A: aphasia with partial auditory imperception
- Minor syndrome B: aphasia with persisting dysarthria

The MTTDA manual provides no standardized prognostic procedures although general descriptions of the patterns of expected recovery for the seven categories are included. The subjective nature of procedures for assigning patients to diagnostic categories gives users of the MTDDA considerable latitude in making these decisions, which may contribute to unreliability. The MTDDA test manual provides no information about either interexaminer reliability or the reliability of its patient categorization procedures.

The Porch Index of Communicative Ability

The *Porch Index of Communicative Ability* (PICA; Porch, 1981a) differs from other comprehensive language tests in several ways. It is relatively quick to administer (about 1 hour for most patients). The PICA has 180 test items in 18 subtests. Unlike other comprehensive language tests, the PICA uses the same 10 test stimuli (*pen, pencil, matches, cigarette, key, quarter, toothbrush, comb, fork, knife*) in all 18 subtests. Administration procedures are highly constrained. The exact instructions given to the patient are specified for each subtest, and the circumstances under which the examiner can repeat a test instruction or offer a prompt or cue are stipulated. Each patient response is scored with a 16-category, binary-choice (yes/no) system (Table 4-3). A set of diacritic markings (circles, squares, and triangles around scores, marks through scores, superscript letters) can be used to augment the 16-category system, thereby increasing the descriptiveness of PICA scoring. (For example, drawing a square around a score shows that the response was produced with motoric distortion or awkwardness.) The complexities of administration and scoring procedures for the PICA require that new users get 40 hours of formal training to become reliable in administering and scoring the PICA. Training,

together with tightly controlled administration and scoring procedures, ensure high reliability across clinicians and clinics.

Each response to a PICA item is scored with the 16-category scoring system, and the score is written on a score sheet. A mean score for the entire test (*overall score*) and modality mean scores for *writing, copying, reading, pantomime, verbal, auditory,* and *visual* subtests can be calculated. Profiles may be plotted on a *rating of communicative ability* form (Figure 4-7), which groups subtests according to each of the modalities, or plotted on a *ranked response summary* graph (Figure 4-8), which plots subtest scores in order of decreasing subtest difficulty across the page. Changes in a patient's performance over time can be recorded on an *aphasia recovery curve* form (Figure 4-9), on which the overall percentile score and the peak-mean difference score (a measure of intrasubtest variability) can be plotted.

The PICA is normed on 357 left-hemisphere-damaged adults, 96 right-hemisphere–damaged adults, and 100 bilaterally damaged adults. Duffy and associates (1976) have published norms for a group of 130 non-brain–damaged adults. Volume I of the test manual contains information about the development of the PICA, interscorer and test-retest reliability, and internal consistency. Volume II contains percentiles for overall scores, subtest scores, and various combinations of subtests within modalities.

The PICA manual provides procedures for predicting the recovery of aphasic patients by plotting a recovery curve, which allows predictions about eventual recovery of communicative ability based on the patient's performance 1 month or more after onset of aphasia. Porch calls this method *HOAP* for *high overall prediction*, which was described in Chapter 3.

The Boston Diagnostic Aphasia Examination

The *Boston Diagnostic Aphasia Examination* (BDAE; Goodglass & Kaplan, 1983) was the first

T A B L E   4 - 3

The 16-category, binary-choice scoring system used in the *Porch Index of Communicative Ability* (PICA)

Score	Level	Description
16	Complex	*Spontaneous, accurate, fluent elaboration* about the test item.
15	Complete	*Complete, accurate, fluent* response to test item.
14	Complete-distorted	*Complete, accurate,* response to test item but with *reduced facility of production.*
13	Complete-delayed	*Complete, accurate* response to test item but *significantly slowed or delayed.*
12	Incomplete	Accurate response to test item but *lacking in completeness.*
11	Incomplete-delayed	*Accurate, incomplete* response to test item that is *significantly slowed or delayed.*
10	Corrected	Accurate response to test item *self-correcting a previous error* by request or after a prolonged delay.
9	Repeated	An accurate response *after a repetition of instructions, by request* or *after a prolonged delay.*
8	Cued	*Accurate* response to test item *stimulated by a cue, additional information, or another test item.*
7	Related	An *inaccurate* response to test item that is *closely related* to a correct response.
6	Error	An *inaccurate* response to the test item.
5	Intelligible	An *intelligible* response that is *not associated with the test item,* such as perseverative or automatic responses or an expressed indication of inability to respond.
4	Unintelligible	Differential responses to the test item that are *unintelligible.*
3	Minimal	*Undifferentiated, unintelligible* responses.
2	Attention	Patient *attends* to the test item *but gives no response.*
1	No response	Patient exhibits *no awareness* of the test item.

Data From Porch, 1981a.

comprehensive language test designed to enable users to assign patients to classical neurodiagnostic syndromes such as Broca's aphasia and Wernicke's aphasia based on their performance on the test. Goodglass and Kaplan believed the nature of a patient's aphasia to be jointly determined by the organization of language in the patient's brain and the location of the brain damage causing the patient's aphasia. According to Goodglass and Kaplan, the BDAE permits clinicians to:

- Determine the presence of aphasia and the type of aphasia syndrome and make inferences concerning cerebral localization
- Measure a patient's level of performance over a wide range
- Assess a patient's assets and liabilities in all language areas as a guide to treatment

The BDAE is a relatively long test. Administering the complete BDAE requires from 1 to 5 hours. (The average for aphasic adults is about 2 hours.) The BDAE has 26 subtests plus a sepa-

Porch Index of Communicative Ability
Rating of communicative ability

Name _____ 50th %ile _____ No. _____ Onset _____

Description: _____

Test date ____ ____ ____ Lo ____ Target ____ Var ____

Response levels		1 2 3 4 5 6 7 8 9 10 11 12 13 14 15
Overall	10.89	
Writing	6.32	
Copying	12.00	
Reading	11.80	
Pantomime	10.80	
Verbal	10.77	
Auditory	14.25	
Visual	15.00	
Gestural	12.96	
Graphic	8.22	

Modalities

Subtest scores		1 2 3 4 5 6 7 8 9 10 11 12 13 14 15
A. Writes function in sentences	5.0	
B. Writes name of objects	6.0	
C. Writes names when heard	6.8	
D. Names, spelling dictated	7.5	
E. Names, copies	11.0	
F. Geometric forms	13.0	
II. Demonstrates function	10.2	
III. Demonstrates function, ordered	11.4	
I. Describes function	8.2	
IV. Names objects	10.2	
IX. Sentence completion	10.8	
XII. Imitative naming	13.9	
V. Reads function and position	11.6	
VII. Reads name and position	12.0	
VI. Point to object by function	14.1	
X. Point to object by name	14.4	
VIII. Matching pictures with object	15.0	
XI. Matching object with object	15.0	

Write / Copy / Pant / Verbal / Read / Aud / Vis — Output / Input

Figure 4-7 ■ A *Porch Index of Communicative Ability (PICA) Rating of Communicative Ability* form for a patient with moderate aphasia. Mean scores (on the 16-category PICA scoring system) are written in the middle column and graphed in the cells on the right. (From Porch BE: *Porch Index of Communicative Ability.* Palo Alto, Calif, 1981, Consulting Psychologists Press.)

Porch Index of Communicative Ability
Ranked response summary

Name _____ 50th %ile _____ Case No. _____

Description: _____ Onset _____

Test dates: Test 1 _____ Test 2 _____ Test 3 _____

MPO _____ h

1 _____ 10.89 6.32 12.00 11.90 10.80 10.17 14.25 15.00 12.96 8.22

2 _____

3 _____

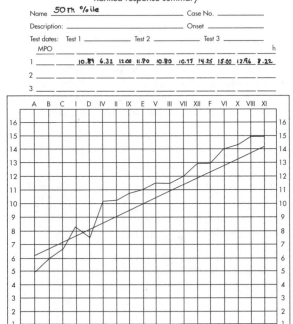

A B C I D IV II IX E V III VII XII F VI X VIII XI

Figure 4-8 ■ A *Porch Index of Communicative Ability (PICA) Ranked Response Summary Form* for a patient with moderate aphasia. The diagonal line represents the hypothetical performance of a group of patients whose PICA performance places them at the fiftieth percentile of a large group of aphasic adults. The PICA subtests are arranged from left to right in order of decreasing difficulty. (From Porch BE: *Porch Index of Communicative Ability.* Palo Alto, Calif, 1981, Consulting Psychologists Press.)

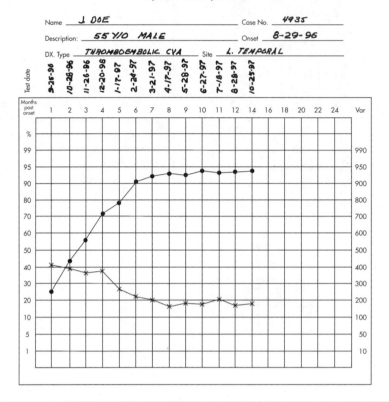

Figure 4-9 ▪ A *Porch Index of Communicative Ability (PICA) Aphasia Recovery Curve* for a hypothetical aphasic patient with a left temporal-lobe stroke. The circles denote the patient's overall mean percentile on the PICA and the Xs denote the patient's overall response variability on the PICA. The patient's overall PICA performance increases for the first 6 months and then plateaus. The patient's overall response variability gradually decreases during the first 8 months, after which it stabilizes. (From Porch BE: *Porch Index of Communicative Ability.* Palto Alto, Calif, 1981, Consulting Psychologists Press.)

rate section for elicitation of conversation and expository speech. The BDAE test manual also describes additional tests for evaluating basic musical ability, parietal lobe functions (drawing, visuospatial abilities, calculations), comprehension and expression, appreciation of spatial relationships, and apraxia.

Norms for the BDAE are based on a sample of 242 patients, most of whom apparently had aphasia caused by a single vascular lesion.* Data from several intercorrelation analyses, factor

---

* Norms for the 1972 version of the BDAE, based on 207 patients, are also provided in the manual.

analyses, and reliability coefficients among subtests are included in the test manual. A patient's BDAE subtest scores can be entered in a *subtest summary profile* from which percentile ranks for each subtest score can be read (Figure 4-10).

The BDAE is a comprehensive test of language and associated processes that permits clinicians to compare the performance of any aphasic patient with the performance of a large group of aphasic adults and to assign aphasic patients to neurodiagnostic aphasia syndromes based on their BDAE performance. However, as mentioned previously, users should be aware that many patients cannot be unambiguously classified on the basis of their BDAE performance. Duffy (1979), writing about the 1972 version of the BDAE, cautioned that the BDAE normative sample included many patients with isolated symptoms and small brain lesions. According to Duffy, this means that the norms may not accurately represent the population of patients seen in many programs, which typically include more patients with large lesions and severe aphasia.

The Western Aphasia Battery

The *Western Aphasia Battery* (WAB; Kertesz, 1982) is shorter and psychometrically more sophisticated than the BDAE, which it resembles in many respects (including an emphasis on classifying patients according to classic neurodiagnostic syndromes). The WAB employs what Kertesz calls a *taxonomic* approach to classification, in which patients are assigned to diagnostic categories (such as Broca's aphasia and Wernicke's aphasia) according to their scores on four language subtests *(spontaneous speech, auditory comprehension, repetition,* and *naming).* The WAB also includes subtests for evaluating reading and writing, one apraxia subtest, and several subtests for assessing constructional, visuospatial, and calculation abilities.

No normative information is provided in the WAB test manual. The reader is referred to Kertesz (1979) and Shewan and Kertesz (1980) for information on standardization of the 1977 version of the WAB. Subtest mean scores and their standard deviations are reported in Kertesz (1979) for 365 aphasic adults and 162 nonaphasic adults from two standardizations of the WAB. The first, in 1974, included 150 aphasic and 59 control subjects. The second, in 1979, added 215 aphasic and 63 control subjects. Information on the reliability and validity of the WAB are provided in Kertesz (1979).

A patient's score on each WAB subtest is entered on a score sheet, which is the last page in the test booklet. A patient's scores on the auditory comprehension and speech subtests can be used to calculate an *aphasia quotient,* and both language and nonlanguage subtest scores are used to calculate a *cortical quotient.* The *aphasia quotient* is said by Kertesz to be a reliable measure of the severity of language impairment. The *cortical quotient* is said to be a measure of cognitive functions. Shewan and Kertesz (1984) described an additional summary score, called the *language quotient.* The *language quotient* is based on the WAB oral language subtest scores that contribute to the *aphasia quotient* plus scores from the WAB reading and writing subtests.

The accuracy and reliability of WAB procedures for classifying patients has been questioned. Swindell, Holland, & Fromm (1984) compared the WAB classifications of 69 aphasic adults to subjective classifications made by clinicians who were trained to identify neurodiagnostic aphasia syndromes. They reported that the clinicians' judgments matched the WAB classification only 54% of the time. Wertz, Deal, & Robinson (1984) compared WAB and BDAE classifications for 45 aphasic adults. The two tests showed agreement on patients' classification only 27% of the time. Twenty-eight patients were unclassifiable with the BDAE, but only 5 patients were unclassifiable with the WAB. (The WAB has been criticized for forcing patients

Subtest summary profile

Name: **R. W.**   **9-17-96**

Category	Subtest	0	10	20	30	40	50	60	70	80	90	100
	Percentiles:	0	10	20	30	40	50	60	70	80	90	100
Severity rating			0	1				2		3	4	5
Fluency	Articulation rating		1	2	✗3	5	6	7				
	Phrase length			2	3	4	5	6	7			
	Melodic line		✗	2	4		6	7				
	Verbal agility		0	2	✗4	6	8	9	11	13	14	
Auditory comprehension	Word discrimination	0	15	25	37	46	53	60	64	67	70	72
	Body-part identification	0	1	5	10	13	15	16	17	18		20
	Commands	0	3	4	6	8	10	11	12	14	15	
	Complex ideational material		0	2	3	4	5	6	8	✗	11	12
Naming	Responsive naming			0	1	5	10	15	20	24	27	30
	Confrontation naming		0	9	28	43	64	72	84	94	105	114
	Animal naming			0	1	2	3	4	6	✗	23	
Oral reading	Word reading			0	1	3	7	15 ✗	21	26	30	
	Oral sentence reading				0	1	✗	4	7	9	10	
Repetition	Repetition of words		0	2	5	✗	8	9		10		
	High-probability			0	1		✗3	4	5	7	8	
	Low-probability					✗0	1		2	4	6	8
Paraphasia	Neologistic	40	16	9	4	2	1		✗0			
	Literal	47	17	12	9	6	5	3	2	1	✗	
	Verbal	40	23	18	15	12	9	7	4	3	✗	0
	Other	75	12	5	3	1	✗0					
Automatic speech	Automatized sequences			0	1	2	3	4	✗7		8	
	Reciting				0	✗					2	
Reading comprehension	Symbol discrimination	0	2	5	7	8	9		✗10			
	Word recognition	0	1	3	4	5	6	7		✗		
	Comprehension of oral spelling				0	1		✗	4	6	7	8
	Word-picture matching			0	1	4	6	8	9 ✗			
	Reading sentences and paragraphs			0	1	2	3	4	5	6	7	8 ✗
Writing	Mechanics	1		2		✗3		4		5		
	Serial writing		0	7	18	25	✗30	33	40	43	46	47
	Primer-level dictation		0	1	✗	6	9	11	13	14	15	
	Spelling to dictation					0	✗	2	3	5	7	10
	Written confrontation naming				0	1	2	✗5	6	7	9	10
	Sentences to dictation					✗0		1	3	6	8	12
	Narrative writing		✗	1			2			3	4	5
Music	Singing		0	✗		2						
	Rhythm		0	✗			2					
Spatial and computational	Drawing to command	0	6	7	8	9	10	11	12	✗		
	Stick memory	0	3	4	6	7	8	9	10	11	13	✗
	3-D blocks		0	2	4	5	6	7	8	9	✗	
	Total fingers	0	54	70	81	93	100	108	120	130	141	✗150
	Right-left	0	1	3	4	6	8	9	✗	16		
	Map orientation	0	2	5	6	9	11	✗		14		
	Arithmetic		0	2	4	8	11	14	✗	21	27	32
	Clock setting	0	3	4	6		8	9	10	✗12		
		0	10	20	30	40	50	60	70	80	90	100

Figure 4-10 ■ A *Boston Diagnostic Aphasia Examination Subtest Summary Profile* for a patient with Broca's aphasia. (From Goodglass H, Kaplan E: *The Boston Diagnostic Aphasia Examination.* Philadelphia, 1983, Lea and Febiger.)

into diagnostic categories. This may be one reason for the lack of agreement between WAB and BDAE classifications.)

Other Comprehensive Language Tests

The BDAE, the MTDDA, the PICA and the WAB are the most widely used comprehensive language tests for brain-damaged adults in the United States. Several other tests, though less widely used, are marketed in the United States and are the tests of choice for some clinicians. They include *The Neurosensory Center Comprehensive Examination for Aphasia* (NCCEA; Spreen & Benton, 1977); *Examining for Aphasia* (EFA; Eisenson, 1954); and *The Aphasia Language Performance Scales* (ALPS; Keenan & Brassell, 1975).

Screening Tests of Language and Communication

Assessment of brain-damaged patients' language and communication does not always begin with a comprehensive language test. Most patients are first seen at bedside, where the speech-language pathologist conducts a brief interview and may administer a quick screening test of speech, language, and communicative abilities. The interview gives the speech-language pathologist a general sense of the patient's background, problems, and concerns. The screening test gives the speech-language pathologist a general sense of the nature and severity of the patient's speech, language, and communicative impairments and sets the stage for more comprehensive testing that may follow.

Several screening tests for assessing adults' communication performance are on the market. Most are designed for adults with aphasia (Crary, Haak, & Malinsky, 1989; Fitch-West & Sands, 1987; Keenan & Brassell, 1975; Sklar, 1973). A few are designed for adults in other diagnostic categories such as traumatic brain injury (Helm-Estabrooks & Hotz, 1990), right-hemisphere syndrome (Pimental & Kingsbury,

1989; Ross, 1986), or motor speech impairments (St. Louis & Ruscello, 1987). Davis (1993) suggests that published screening tests are not needed for screening communicative abilities at bedside:

> We do not need one of these tests to evaluate a patient's language abilities at bedside. All we need is a concept of what needs to be assessed, a few common objects, a pen, and some paper. We have the patient answer some yes/no questions, point to things, and name and describe some other things. If the patient cannot converse, we want to see if he or she can count or recite the days of the week (p. 215).

However, Davis subsequently comments that published screening tests have advantages over informal ones because of their standardized administration, which contributes to consistency in measurement and interpretation. Although it is no doubt true that a skilled clinician can improvise a satisfactory bedside screening examination with a few common objects, something to write with, and something to write on, such an unsystematic approach may lead the examiner to miss important signs and may invalidate comparisons of the patient's performance with that of other patients or with the same patient on subsequent tests.

Many experienced clinicians forego published screening tests in favor of locally or personally designed tests but few are content with informal, unstructured, and unsystematic tests. Most large speech and language clinics have formalized protocols for screening patients with impaired communication (usually with separate protocols for screening patients with probable aphasia, motor speech disorders, right-hemisphere syndrome, traumatic brain injury, and dementia). The use of standard screening protocols ensures that everyone in the clinic does the screening in the same way and that the results obtained by one clinician are equivalent

Language screening assessment

Date:	Reason for referral, significant history

Orientation, memory

What year is it? _____ [__]   What day of the week is it? _____ [__]

What time is it right now? _____ [__]   What city are we in? _____ [__]

Three-word recall: _____ _____ _____ [__]   **Number Correct [__ /5]**

Auditory comprehension

Single-word ("Point to the. . .")

Chair[__]   Ring[__]   Shoe[__]   Key[__]   Pencil[__][__]   **Number correct [__ /5]**

Yes-no questions

Personal information: (1) Is your first name (correct name)? [__]   (6) Is your last name (incorrect name)? [__]

Immediate environment: (4) Are we in a bus station right now? [__]   (2) Is it nighttime right now? [__]

Factual information: (5) Is a dime worth ten cents? [__]   (3) Do carrots grow on trees? [__]

                                                                Number correct [__ /6]

Sentence comprehension ("Point to the one that best matches what I say.")

A   shoe. [__](shoe)   A   standard   comb. [__](comb)   Children   play   with   this   one. [__](ball) It has rubber on one end and a point on the other. [__](pencil)   The flat surface of this one is ideal for doing a jigsaw puzzle. [__](table)   **Number correct [__ /5]**

Reading comprehension

Word to picture matching (choices are in parentheses)

Fox (box, coat)[__]   Frog (flag, fish)[__]   Cup (spoon, cap)[__]   Letter (city, ladder[__] Television (thermometer, camera)[__]   **Number Correct [__ /5]**

Patient identification:

Speech Pathology: language screening assessment
(Page 1 of 2)

Figure 4-11 ■ A Language Screening Assessment form.

Automatized sequences

Counting: 1[__] 2[__] 3[__] 4[__] 5[__] 6[__] 7[__] 8[__] 9[__]
10[__]

Days of week: Sunday[__] Monday[__] Tuesday[__] Wednesday[__]
Thursday[__] Friday[__] Saturday[__]   **Number correct [__ /17]**

Repetition

Words: Boy[__] Dog[__] Cowboy[__] Gingerbread[__] Artillery[__]
Number correct [__ /5]

Sentences: It was raining.[__] Bill went to the store.[__] Please put the groceries in the
refrigerator.[__] Arthur was an oozy, oily sneak.[__]
Number correct [__ /4]

Confrontation Naming: Pictures

dog[__] broom[__] airplane[__] Igloo[__] tambourine[__] **Number correct [__ /5]**

Oral Reading

Words: Man[__] Book[__] Forever[__] Understanding[__] Conventional[__]
Number correct [__ /5]

Sentences: It was raining.[__] Mary baked a pie.[__] Under the table in the dining room. [__]
The little girl was happy to see the new puppy. [__]   **Number correct [__ /4]**

Rating of connected speech

Fluency: Fluent[__] Nonfluent[__]

Average phrase length (words): 1-2[__] 3-4[__] 5-6[__] >6[__]

Literal paraphasia: Absent[__] Infrequent[__] Frequent[__]

Verbal paraphasia: Absent[__] Infrequent[__] Frequent[__]

Word-finding in connected speech: Normal[__] Moderate impairment[__]
Severe impairment[__]

Writing

Name[__]
Letters to dictation: F[__] M[__] D[__] X[__] Q[__] **Number correct [__ /5]**
Words to dictation: Man[__] Today[__] Carrot[__] Venture[__]
Number correct [__ /4]

Comments and impressions:

_____   _____
Speech-language pathologist   Date
Speech pathology: language screening assessment
(Page 2 of 2)

Figure 4-11, For legend see opposite page.

to the results obtained by any other clinician in the clinic.

Table 4-4 shows a protocol for screening patients with suspected language impairments (aphasia). It takes 10 to 20 minutes to administer and provides a general sense of the patient's orientation and memory, auditory and reading comprehension, production of automatized sequences, repetition, naming, oral reading, and writing, together with a rating of the patient's conversational connected speech.

Screening protocols such as the one in Table 4-4 serve several purposes. Sometimes they help identify patients for whom no additional testing is appropriate—patients with no significant impairments, patients who have complicating conditions (such as dementia, confusion, and illness) that would make formal assessment impossible or meaningless, patients with severe and irreversible impairments, and so on. More often they help the clinician plan which tests to administer and the level of difficulty at which formal testing will begin. Finally, they provide the clinician with enough information about the nature and severity of the patient's linguistic or communicative impairments to permit her or him to write an initial response to the consultation request and to place a progress note containing initial impressions, diagnoses, and recommendations in the patient's medical record. (Some screening forms such as the one in Figure 4-11 are themselves progress notes that can be placed in the patient's medical record.)

Assessment of adults with neurogenic language impairments does not always begin with a screening test and end with a comprehensive language test. When a comprehensive language test has confirmed the presence of language impairments, the clinician usually administers supplemental tests to obtain a more detailed picture of the impairments. The following material provides an overview of how brain-damaged adults' speech, auditory comprehension, reading, and writing are assessed, beginning with subtests in comprehensive language tests and progressing to free-standing supplemental tests of specific abilities.

■ ASSESSING AUDITORY COMPREHENSION

Impairments in auditory comprehension have for many years occupied a central place in conceptualizations of aphasia. Schuell (1965) considered impaired auditory comprehension and shortened auditory retention span the essence of aphasic impairments, and numerous other writers since that time have, like Schuell, given auditory impairment special status in defining the nature of aphasia and special attention in treatment programs.* All comprehensive language tests include auditory comprehension subtests, and several free-standing tests devoted exclusively to assessment of auditory comprehension have been published. Some assess comprehension of single words either in isolation or at the end of short carrier phrases. Some assess comprehension of single-sentence questions or instructions and a few assess comprehension of spoken narratives.

Single-Word Comprehension

Single-Word Comprehension Subtests in Comprehensive Language Tests The most common procedure for testing single-word comprehension is a *select-from-an-array* procedure, in which the examiner places an array of drawn or printed stimuli (usually line drawings of objects) or real objects before the patient, says the names of the items in the array one at a time, and the patient points to or touches each item after the examiner names it.[†] Figure 4-12 shows an array of drawn objects from the MTDDA.

---

* *Auditory comprehension* includes both *comprehension* of spoken materials and their *retention* in memory.

[†] In most of these tests the examiner delivers the test word at the end of a short carrier phrase, such as "*Point to the* _____ ." Because the carrier phrase quickly becomes redundant, these tests qualify as tests of single-word comprehension rather than as tests of sentence comprehension.

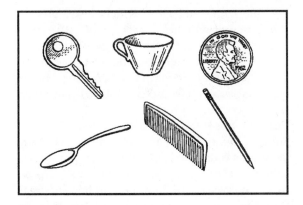

Figure 4-12 ■ **A single-word comprehension response card from the *Minnesota Test for Differential Diagnosis of Aphasia*. The patient points to the pictured objects as the examiner names them.** (From Schuell H: *The Minnesota Test for Differential Diagnosis of Aphasia.* Minneapolis, 1965, University of Minnesota Press. Drawings by Lawrence Benson.)

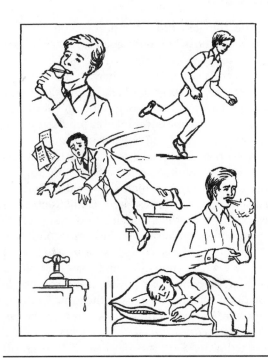

Figure 4-13 ■ **A verb comprehension response card from the *Boston Diagnostic Aphasia Examination*. The patient points to the pictured actions as the examiner names them.** (From Goodglass H, Kaplan E: *The Boston Diagnostic Aphasia Examination.* Philadelphia, 1983, Lea and Febiger.)

Arrays of drawings are not always drawings of objects. Sometimes they include drawings representing actions, printed letters or numbers, geometric forms, or color swatches. Figure 4-13 shows an array of drawings used to test comprehension of action names in the BDAE. Sometimes single-word comprehension is tested by asking the patient to point to objects in the environment and sometimes by asking the patient to identify body parts, either on his or her own body or the examiner's body.

The inclusion of tests for comprehension of color, form, number, and body-part names in some comprehensive language tests may be a response to a study by Goodglass and associates (1966), who tested aphasic adults' comprehension of the names of objects, actions, numbers, colors, and letters. They reported that aphasic adults are best at comprehending the names of pictured objects and actions and worst at comprehending the names of numbers, colors, and letters.

The presence of colors, letters, and geometric forms in some comprehensive language tests may also reflect the influence of several published case reports describing patients with unusual impairments in comprehending specific categories of words (color names, for example). However, the clinical value of assessing comprehension of color, letter, and form names seems limited because comprehension of spoken color, letter, and form names has minor importance in daily life. Although it may be clinically interesting and theoretically important to find a patient who comprehends color or letter names better (or worse) than the names of objects and actions, the relevance of such a finding to treatment planning or to estimation of the patient's daily life communicative competence seems enigmatic.

The single-word comprehension performance of most brain-damaged adults who are tested using select-from-an-array procedures is not strongly affected by whether the items in the array are pictures or objects, although brain-damaged adults with impairments in visual perception or visual discrimination tend to do better when arrays of real objects are used.

A study by Helm-Estabrooks (1981) suggests that aphasic adults may be affected by the nature of the array in which single-word comprehension stimuli are presented. Helm-Estabrooks tested aphasic adults' single-word comprehension in three conditions. In the *array* condition, 12 familiar objects (*book, spoon, cup,* etc.) were shown as individual line drawings on 12 cards arranged in three rows. In the *composite* condition, smaller versions of the same 12 drawings were presented on a single card. In the *environment condition,* the 12 objects were distributed around the testing room. As a group the aphasic adults performed significantly better when pointing to pictured objects than when pointing to the real objects. Their performance was not significantly affected by whether the drawings were presented on individual cards or in a composite array. However, many subjects showed differences among conditions that were not consistent with group performance. Some adults were better in one of the picture conditions than the other and some did better with real objects than they did with pictures.

Helm-Estabrooks commented that patients' difficulty *finding* objects distributed around the room rather than difficulty *comprehending* their names may, at least in part, have accounted for the differences between the pictured-object and real-object arrays. Helm-Estabrooks's report did not include the group's scores by conditions. Consequently, we cannot judge whether the statistically significant differences are also clinically significant. Nevertheless it seems important that clinicians keep in mind the potential effects of escalating demands on visual scanning and search as response arrays become larger and more widely distributed in the test environment.

Free-standing Tests of Single-Word Comprehension No free-standing tests of single-word auditory comprehension for brain-damaged adults have been published, although picture vocabulary tests such as the *Peabody Picture Vocabulary Test—Revised* (PPVT-R; Dunn & Dunn, 1981) are, in a way, tests of single-word comprehension. However, picture vocabulary tests differ in content and purpose from single-word auditory comprehension tests for aphasic adults. Picture vocabulary tests include infrequent and unusual words (such as *lancinate, bumptiously*), some of which are known by only a small proportion of normal adults, whereas single-word comprehension tests for aphasic adults focus on common words that should be familiar to most normal adults (*fork, spoon, airplane,* etc.). The early, most common words in picture vocabulary tests may be equivalent to those in single-word comprehension tests for aphasic adults.

The norms for picture vocabulary tests are based on the entire test, and norms for performance on the more common items alone cannot be extracted, making partially completed picture vocabulary tests of limited use to clinicians who wish to compare an individual patient's performance with that of a norm group. A patient's performance on the early part of a picture vocabulary test could, however, serve as a baseline measure against which to measure his or her response to treatment, and the patient's performance on the complete test provides an estimate of his or her available listening vocabulary, including a school grade level.

To carry the issue of how single-word comprehension may relate to daily life communicative competence a bit further, one might question the potential relevance of *any* test of single-word comprehension to daily life, given that in daily life one usually hears words in phrases or sentences and not in isolation. When one-word messages occur in daily life, they usually are embedded in situational or linguistic context, and it is well known that brain-damaged adults' comprehension of spoken messages is enhanced by context. Consequently, it seems unlikely that brain-damaged adults' performance on tests of single-word comprehension relates very strongly to daily life comprehension. Add to this the strangeness, in a daily life sense, of pointing to pictures or objects in response to their spoken names, and the potential relevance of tests of single-word comprehension to daily life comprehension becomes even more questionable.

Nevertheless, most clinicians assess single-word comprehension as part of their testing protocol for brain-damaged adults. Basic tests of single-word comprehension are quick and easy to administer. The results of single-word comprehension tests may suggest unusual patterns of impaired performance, leading the clinician to revise a diagnosis or a treatment plan. For patients whose single-word comprehension is unimpaired, testing single-word comprehension can provide a comfortable lead-in to more challenging sentence- and paragraph-level tests. For patients with severely impaired sentence comprehension, the results of testing at the single-word level may be the only indicator of the patient's ability to comprehend spoken language.

Variables That May Affect Brain-Damaged Adults' Single-Word Comprehension

Frequency of Occurrence A word's *frequency of occurrence* in the language affects the ease with which aphasic listeners comprehend it (Schuell, Jenkins, & Landis, 1961). This effect can be seen in aphasic adults' performance on listening vocabulary tests such as the PPVT-R, wherein most aphasic adults have inordinate difficulty with infrequently occurring words. (However, see the previous paragraph for comments on the potential implications of frequency of occurrence for comprehension in daily life.)

Semantic or Acoustic Similarity Between Target Words and Foils Semantic similarity usually has a much stronger effect on aphasic patients' accuracy in single-word comprehension tasks than acoustic similarity. Schuell and Jenkins (1961), for example, reported that semantic confusions (such as *mother* for *father*) are far more frequent than either acoustic confusions (such as *dime* for *time*) or random errors (such as *motorcycle* for *cigarette*) when aphasic patients match spoken words to pictures.

Part of Speech Part of speech affects some aphasic adults' single-word comprehension, although the effect appears highly variable across individual aphasic adults. Miceli and associates (1988) studied aphasic adults' comprehension of nouns and verbs and found all possible patterns of noun versus verb comprehension in a group of 75 brain-damaged adults. Some did better on nouns than verbs, some had greater difficulty with verbs than nouns, and some performed equally well (or poorly) on nouns and verbs. Consequently clinicians can anticipate that part of speech is likely to affect an aphasic adult's single-word comprehension, but the nature of the effect can only be determined by testing the patient.

Referent Ambiguity Referent ambiguity (ambiguity in pictured referents for spoken words) may affect aphasic patients' performance in matching spoken words to pictures. If pictorial referents are ambiguous or unclear, patients may respond inaccurately, not because they fail to comprehend the words, but because they are unable to deduce what the pictures represent. (See Chapter 5 for more on referent ambiguity and stimulus uncertainty.)

Fidelity The fidelity of spoken messages (from words to discourse) can have important effects on aphasic listeners' comprehension (and if the loss of fidelity is serious on that of non–brain-damaged listeners, too). Most aphasic adults' comprehension of spoken materials deteriorates in noisy listening environments or when speech is acoustically distorted. For this reason, answering the telephone can be a challenge for many aphasic adults. Most telephones are low-fidelity instruments and many produce background noise. (Comparison shopping to find a telephone with good fidelity and a good signal-to-noise ration may be advisable if there is an aphasic person in the family.)

Many audiotape recorders/players (especially inexpensive ones) have poor fidelity and create objectionable levels of background noise on playback. The distortion and interference can compromise aphasic adults' performance when these machines are used to play tapes in testing and treatment activities. Clinicians can minimize this problem by using high-quality tape recorders and high-quality audiotapes to record and play materials used in testing and treatment.

Sentence Comprehension

Sentence Comprehension Subtests in Comprehensive Language Tests All the major comprehensive language tests include sentence comprehension subtests. Most require patients to perform gestural or manipulative responses to spoken commands. In some the patient points to one or more items in a set of pictures, objects, or body parts. *("Point to the (pictured) dog, garage, and ladder." "Point to the ceiling and then to the floor." "Show me the one used for fixing hair." "Point to your left ear and your right knee.")* In others patients manipulate objects or body parts. *("Ring the bell, close the box, and give me the key." "Tap each shoulder twice with two fingers keeping your eyes shut.")*

Most comprehensive language tests include subtests for assessing patients' comprehension of spoken yes-no questions. The yes-no questions in these tests assess comprehension of different kinds of information. Some questions test personal information *("Is your last name Smith?")*. Some test the patient's perception of the surroundings *("Are the lights on in this room?")*. Some test knowledge learned in school *("Was Abraham Lincoln the first President of the United States?")*. Some ask for opinions, inferences, or abstractions *("Should children disobey their parents?" "Is it possible for a good swimmer to be drowned?")*. Some test general knowledge *("Do apples grow on trees?")*. Questions that test general knowledge can be further divided into questions that test comprehension of temporal relationships *("Does March come before June?")*, numerical relationships *("Are there seven days in a week?")*, and comparative relationships *("Are towns larger than cities?")*.

Free-standing Tests of Sentence Comprehension The *Token Test* (DeRenzi and Vignolo, 1962) and its variants are among the most widely used free-standing tests of sentence-level auditory comprehension. In the original DeRenzi and Vignolo version, 62 spoken commands direct the patient to touch or manipulate 20 tokens (5 large circles, 5 small circles, 5 large rectangles, and 5 small rectangles in each of 5 colors: red, yellow, green, white, and blue). There are 5 levels in the original *Token Test,* and the length and complexity of commands increases from level 1 to level 5 (see Table 4-4 for examples of commands at each

TABLE 4-4

Examples of commands from the five levels of the *Token Test*

Level	Command
1	Touch the red circle
2	Touch the large blue square
3	Touch the red square and the blue circle
4	Touch the large white circle and the small green square
5	When I touch the green circle, you take the white square

Data From DeRenzi and Vignolo, 1962.

level). Responses are scored correct or incorrect and the maximum score is 62. No norms are provided in DeRenzi and Vignolo (1962), although norms for adults and children can be found elsewhere (Gaddes & Crockett, 1973; Noll & Lass, 1972; Spreen & Benton, 1977; and Wertz, Keith, & Custer, 1971).

Several modified versions of the *Token Test* have been published. One is a subtest of the NCCEA (Spreen & Benton,1977). It contains 39 test commands similar to those in the original *Token Test*, divided among six levels of length and complexity.* The easiest level in the Spreen and Benton version contains commands such as *"Show me a square."* and *"Show me a red one."*, which permits testing patients at a lower level than provided for in the original *Token Test* and also permits identification of patients with specific impairments in comprehension of color or shape names. The Spreen and Benton version of the *Token Test* allows users to score patients' responses according to how accurately they represent the critical elements in test commands. For example, the command *"Point to the small white circle."* is worth 3 points, one each for *small, white,* and *circle.* A perfect score on the Spreen and Benton version of the Token Test is 163 points. Norms for aphasic, nonaphasic but brain-damaged, and non–brain-damaged adults are provided in the NCCEA manual.

The Spreen and Benton version of the *Token Test* appears to be as sensitive to the presence of impairments in auditory comprehension as the original DeRenzi and Vignolo version (Orgass & Poeck, 1966), has shorter administration, scoring and interpretation times, and has a scoring system that provides partial credit for responses that reflect some but not all of the critical elements in test commands. Consequently, the Spreen and Benton version is somewhat more widely used in the United States.

---

* Spreen and Benton replaced rectangles with squares, which brings the *Token Test* shape names closer together in terms of their frequency of occurrence in English.

The Revised Token Test (RTT; McNeil and Prescott, 1978), is a longer and more elaborate version of DeRenzi and Vignolo's test. The RTT has 10 subtests, each with 10 equally difficult test commands. The first four subtests in the RTT are similar to the first four parts of the original *Token Test.* Tests 5 through 8 each consist of 10 items that test comprehension of positional relationships *(in front of, behind, above, below, to the right of).* Tests 9 and 10 test comprehension of complex grammatical relationships *(instead of, unless, if, either).* Patients' responses to RTT items are scored with a multidimensional system similar to that for the PICA. Profiles for five "auditory processing deficits" are provided in the test manual. Several procedures for scoring and analyzing patients' responses are provided.

The RTT takes longer to administer, score, and interpret than the other versions (usually over an hour). Its comprehensiveness and its psychometric integrity make it a powerful research tool but its length and complexity may preclude its use in routine clinical evaluation of brain-damaged adults' sentence comprehension.

The *Token Test* and its variants are sensitive measures of sentence comprehension. Even patients with very mild comprehension impairments are likely to have difficulty on higher-level token test commands. However, this sensitivity makes the token tests difficult or impossible for persons with severe comprehension impairments. A few patients have inordinate difficulty with token tests, compared with their performance on other tests of auditory comprehension. Some have specific difficulty with color, shape and size descriptors. Others have temporal sequencing impairments that prevent them from maintaining the temporal order of the responses required by token test commands. (These patients typically point to the correct tokens but in the wrong order.) A few patients may have motor planning impairments (limb apraxias), which prevent them from making the required pointing responses even though they understand the commands.*

To rule out problems with comprehension of color, shape, and size descriptors, patients can be pretested by asking them to point to *"a red one, a circle, a small one"* and so on (a procedure included as the first level in the Spreen and Benton version of the *Token Test* and as a pretest for the RTT). To rule out temporal sequencing impairments and limb apraxias as the cause of deficient performance, the patient can be asked to imitate sequences of pointing responses modeled by the examiner. If the patient is successful, temporal sequencing impairments and limb apraxia become unlikely explanations for the deficient performance.

Some patients with poor comprehension improve their performance on tests like the token tests by visually fixating on items in the array as they are named by the examiner, thereby compensating for impaired auditory memory with visual strategies. These patients' performance deteriorates if the target items are covered while the commands are spoken. To ensure that patients' performance on such tests reflects only auditory comprehension and retention and not visual strategies, examiners can cover the target items while test commands are spoken.

For patients with subtle comprehension and retention impairments, examiners can increase the difficulty of sentence comprehension tests by imposing a delay interval between test sentences and the opportunity for the patient to respond. A 10 or 20-second delay usually reveals even the most subtle auditory retention impairments.[†]

The *Token Test* and its variants test comprehension of a limited range of syntactic structures and a limited vocabulary. A few freestanding tests of sentence comprehension permit testing a greater variety of syntactic structures and a greater vocabulary range.

The *Auditory Comprehension Test for Sentences* (ACTS; Shewan, 1979) tests comprehension of 21 spoken sentences differing in length, vocabulary difficulty, and syntax. The ACTS (and the other tests described in this section) use a *verification format,* in which patients indicate their comprehension of each sentence by pointing to one of several pictures on a page (Figure 4-14). Patients' responses to ACTS sen-

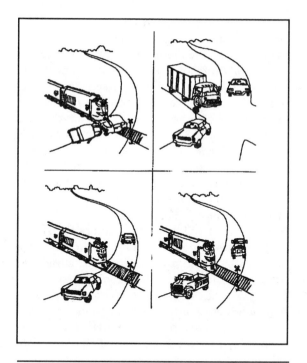

Figure 4-14 ■ A response plate from the *Auditory Comprehension Test for Sentences.* The stimulus sentence for this plate is *"Cars were not hit by the train."* (From Shewan CM: *The auditory comprehension test for sentences.* Chicago, 1979, Biolinguistics Clinical Institutes.)

---

* Few patients have such severe limb apraxia that they cannot point sequentially to test tokens. However, it should be kept in mind as a potential cause of poor performance on token tests and other tests requiring sequential pointing responses.

[†] However, testing patients using nonstandard procedures precludes comparison of their performance with norms based on the standard procedures.

tences can be analyzed to determine if their errors are related to the position of words in the sentences, the grammatical form of words, the syntactic complexity of sentences, or the grammatical function of words.

Some sentence comprehension tests designed for children can be used to test adults with suspected comprehension impairments. Most tests do not provide norms for either normal or brain-injured adults, but permit detailed analysis of the effects of various grammatical and syntactic variables on comprehension. For this reason they occasionally are used to evaluate how brain-injured adults are affected by those variables, even though no comparisons of brain-injured patients with an adult norm group can be made. However, the content and form of these tests can be child-like, and consequently some adults may consider them demeaning.

The *Northwestern Syntax Screening Test* (NSST; Lee, 1971) is a screening test of sentence comprehension for use with children. The NSST contains 20 sentences and ten four-choice picture pages. The 20 sentences evaluate comprehension of various grammatic and syntactic forms (such as locational prepositions, negation, subject-verb agreement, and tense).

The *Test for Auditory Comprehension of Language-Revised* (TACL-R; Carrow-Woodfolk, 1985) is a sentence comprehension test designed for use with children although it contains guidelines for use with adults. The test uses the verification format and assesses three categories of materials: *word classes and relations* (nouns, verbs, adjectives, adverbs), *grammatical morphemes* (noun-verb agreement, number, tense, and case), and *complex sentence constructions* (embedded sentences, partially connected sentences).

Variables That May Affect Brain-Damaged Listeners' Sentence Comprehension

Length and Syntactic Complexity Although several variables can affect brain-damaged listeners' comprehension of spoken sentences, two of the strongest variables are *length* and *syntactic complexity*. As spoken sentences become longer or syntactically more complex, they become more difficult for aphasic listeners to comprehend, provided other sentence characteristics do not change. Syntactic complexity seems to have stronger negative effects on comprehension than either sentence length or vocabulary difficulty (Shewan & Canter, 1971; Goodglass and associates, 1979; Nicholas & Brookshire, 1983).

For example, Goodglass and associates (1979) presented two sets of spoken sentences to aphasic listeners. The sentences in one set were syntactically complex *("The man greeted by his wife was smoking a pipe.")*, and the sentences in the other contained syntactically simpler forms of the same sentences *("The man was greeted by his wife and he was smoking a pipe.")*. Aphasic listeners comprehended the syntactically simpler sentences better than the syntactically complex ones, even though the simple sentences were longer than the complex ones. (Sometimes increasing sentence length facilitates aphasic adults' comprehension if the increased length also adds redundancy.)

Active sentences *("The dog bit the boy.")* usually are easier for aphasic listeners to comprehend than passive sentences *("The boy was bitten by the dog.")*. Conditional sentences *("If the cup is blue, give it to me.")*, negative sentences *("The dog is not chasing the rabbit.")*, sentences containing locational or directional prepositions *("Put the cup behind the box.")*, and comparative or relational sentences *("The boy is taller than the girl.")* are difficult for many aphasic listeners. Embedded clause sentences *("The letter the girl wrote is on the table.")* are very difficult for almost all aphasic listeners (and for many nonaphasic listeners). The relative difficulty of sentences with various syntactic structures appears to be similar, if not identical, for aphasic and nonaphasic adults. Aphasic adults take longer to comprehend sentences and make more errors but usually exhibit the same pattern of difficulty across sentence types as non–brain-damaged adults do.

Reversibility and Plausibility Reversible sentences, in which subject and object can be transposed without creating an implausible sentence (*"The man is hugging the woman."* reverses to *"The woman is hugging the man."*), are more difficult than sentences for which transposition generates an implausible sentence (*"The man is carrying the book."* reverses to *"The book is carrying the man."*). Sentences that are improbable (but not implausible) when subject and object are transposed (*"The dog is chasing the cat."* reverses to *"The cat is chasing the dog."*) are likely to be of intermediate difficulty.

Caramazza and Zurif (1976) investigated the effects of reversibility on aphasic listeners' comprehension of embedded clause sentences (*"The apple that the boy is eating is red."*). They concluded that the sentence comprehension of aphasic patients was poorer when sentences were reversible than when they were not, although their major finding was that their aphasic subjects relied heavily on plausibility to comprehend syntactically complex sentences.

Predictability Some sentences are predictable, in that they create expectations in the listener's mind, then violate the expectations. For this reason they are sometimes called *garden-path sentences.** Most garden-path sentences rely on the listener's (or reader's) more-or-less automatic syntactic processing to lead them down the garden path (as in *"The horse raced past the barn fell."* (Caplan, 1987), in which the listener/reader first assumes that *raced* is the sentence's main verb, but later discovers that *fell* is actually the main verb, whereas *raced past the barn* is a phrase modifying *horse*). Normal listeners' comprehension of garden-path sentences has been intensively studied (Bever, Garrett, & Hurtig, 1973; Foss &

Jenkins, 1973; Lackner & Garrett, 1972; Mackay, 1966; and others), primarily to construct or validate models of sentence processing. Not surprisingly, non–brain-damaged adults take more time to comprehend garden-path sentences than straightforward ones and they sometimes miscomprehend them.

Nicholas and Brookshire (1981) tested non–brain-damaged and aphasic adults' comprehension of spoken comparative sentences such as *"A fish is smaller than a whale."* Half of the sentences were nonsurprising in that their initial words created expectations that were subsequently confirmed, as in *"A brick is harder than a pillow."* The other half of the sentences were surprising in that their initial words created expectations that were subsequently refuted, as in *"A brick is harder than a diamond."* Both the non–brain-damaged adults and the aphasic adults made more errors on surprising sentences than on nonsurprising ones, the aphasic adults were more strongly affected by surprising endings, and, as expected, the aphasic adults made more errors overall than the non–brain-damaged adults.

Personal Relevance The personal relevance of questions affects their difficulty for most aphasic listeners. Gray and associates (1977) and Busch and Brookshire (1982) evaluated aphasic adults' responses to three categories of spoken yes-no questions: *(1)* questions that referred to nonpersonal factual information (*"Do apples grow on trees?"*), *(2)* questions that referred to information about the immediate environment (*"Are we in a hospital?"*), and *(3)* questions that referred to personal information about the patient (*"Is your name _____?"*). In both studies, aphasic subjects' responses to personal information questions were more accurate than their responses to questions about the immediate environment and their responses to questions about the immediate environment were more accurate than their responses to questions about nonpersonal factual information. Although similar studies

---

* "To be led down the garden path" is an idiomatic phrase meaning "to be led astray."

have not been carried out with open-ended questions, it seems reasonable to expect that their difficulty would be affected similarly by personal relevance.

Semantic Variables Brain-damaged adults may get into trouble when factual questions are falsified by substituting a semantically related word for a word that makes the sentence true. (*"Does the sun rise in the west?"* from the MTDDA confuses many patients, whereas *"Does the sun rise in the living room?"* would mislead only those with severely impaired comprehension (or who have very large living rooms).

Reasoning and Inferences Questions that require reasoning or inferring (*"Is it possible for a good swimmer to be drowned?"*) are more difficult than questions in which reasoning or inferring are not required, if the length, vocabulary, and syntactic structure of the sentences are equal. Answering inferential questions adds to the processing load in comprehension by requiring that the patient *(1)* recognize that relevant information is not in memory in verbatim form, *(2)* search memory and identify the relevant information, and *(3)* establish relationships between the question and existing knowledge. Brain-damaged adults may perform poorly on questions requiring inferences because they do not realize that an inference is called for, are unable to identify or retrieve from memory information relevant to the inference, or are unable to construct the inference. Questions such as *"Why should children attend school?"* also require longer and more complex responses so that verbal formulation and production problems may compromise brain-damaged adults' responses to them.

Rate Slowing the rate at which commands are spoken or placing pauses in test commands facilitates the performance of many aphasic patients (Parkhurst, 1970; Liles & Brookshire, 1975). Unfortunately, it is not clear which patients are most sensitive to rate or pause manipulations, and the effects are not always consis-

tent from test to test, even for the same patient (Brookshire & Nicholas, 1984a).

A study by Salvatore, Strait, and Brookshire (1978) showed that changes in the rate at which clinicians speak comprehension test sentences can have clinical consequences. Salvatore and his associates had experienced and inexperienced examiners administer a token test to two groups of patients. One group had mild comprehension impairments and the other had severe comprehension impairments. The experienced examiners spoke test commands at a slower rate than the inexperienced examiners. Both experienced and inexperienced examiners spoke test commands at a slower rate when they tested severely impaired patients than when they tested mildly impaired patients. Both experienced and inexperienced examiners spoke test commands at a slower rate following patient errors than following correct responses.

Because examiners' variability in delivering token test commands can affect patients' performance and because even experienced clinicians change their delivery of token test commands in response to patients' performance, clinicians who incorporate a token test into their testing routine may choose to record the test commands with uniform speech rate and consistent intonation, stress, and pauses and use the recording to test patients, rather than delivering the test commands live voice.

Redundancy The redundancy of spoken directions also affects their comprehensibility for aphasic adults. West and Kaufman (1972) evaluated aphasic listeners' comprehension of token–test-like commands, in which some commands contained repeated elements (as in, *"Show me the big **blue circle** and the little **blue circle**."*), and some contained no repeated elements (as in, *"Show me the big blue circle and the small red square."*). The redundant commands proved to be easier for aphasic adults than the nonredundant ones.

Gardner, Albert, and Weintraub (1975) reported that aphasic listeners comprehended semantically redundant sentences *("You see a cat that is furry.")* better than semantically neutral sentences *("You see a cat that is nice.")* although the statistical analyses did not strongly support their conclusion.

Number, Similarity, and Nature of Response Choices The *number of choices* available for pointing or manipulation and *similarity among the choices* can affect the difficulty of tasks in which aphasic listeners point to or manipulate tokens, objects, or pictures in response to spoken directions. In general, increasing the number of choices increases the difficulty of the task. *"Point to the red circle."* is less difficult if there are three choices (red circle, blue square, yellow circle) than if there are six choices (red circle, blue circle, yellow circle, red square, blue square, yellow square). Increasing the similarity among choices also increases the difficulty of the task. *"Point to the knife."* is more difficult for aphasic listeners if the targets are semantically related *(fork, knife, spoon)* than when they are not *(fork, umbrella, hippopotamus)*.

There is some evidence that brain-damaged adults' performance on point-to tests of spoken-sentence comprehension is slightly better when the choice stimuli are real objects rather than tokens (Kreindler, Gheorghita, & Voinescu, 1971; Martino, Pizzamiglio, & Razzano, 1976; La-Pointe, Holtzapple, & Graham, 1985). However, the differences between performance on token tests and picture or object tests generally are small and when results for individual subjects are reported, the performance of individual subjects often does not match that of the group. For most brain-damaged adults it probably makes little difference whether tokens, pictures, or objects are used in point-to tests of sentence comprehension. On average, their scores on token tests are likely to be slightly worse than their performance on picture or object tests. This makes token tests slightly more sensitive to the presence of subtle comprehension impairments, but also causes them to underestimate the patient's actual comprehension performance in daily life.

Sentence Comprehension and Comprehension in Daily Life

The items in most sentence comprehension tests are not very representative of what most adults are likely to encounter in daily life. In most sentence comprehension tests the patient hears a series of one-sentence minimally redundant utterances with no relationship between utterances in the series. The patient must remember the information from each sentence long enough to answer a question or point to tokens or a picture but then can forget it because each sentence is unrelated to the preceding ones. In this respect sentence comprehension tests are similar to immediate-memory tests in which the examiner reads lists of numbers or words and the patient must recognize or reproduce them after a few seconds' delay. In daily life, adult listeners rarely hear strings of nonredundant sentences with no relationship to each other or to the listener's prior knowledge. They usually need only remember the gist of the sentences and not their verbatim form and they usually have to remember the gist for more than a few seconds.

In daily life, speakers create ties between new information and what they assume the listener already knows, and they relate the new information to preceding utterances and to a topic, thereby creating a semantic context for individual utterances. Single-sentence comprehension tests eliminate that context, no doubt to the detriment of the patient being tested, because brain-damaged listeners, like non–brain-damaged ones, use context to help them comprehend what they hear (Stachowiak, Huber, Poeck, & Kerschensteiner, 1977; Waller & Darley, 1978: Pierce 1989; and others). Consequently, it seems unlikely that a brain-damaged patient's performance on sentence comprehension tests will predict her or his comprehension of what is said in typical daily life communicative interactions.

The results of several studies suggest that performance on sentence comprehension tests is not a dependable indicator of patients' comprehension of multiple-sentence spoken discourse (Stachowiak and associates, 1977; Brookshire & Nicholas, 1984a; Wegner, Brookshire, & Nicholas, 1984, and others). These studies have shown that sentence comprehension test scores do reasonably well in predicting scores on other sentence-level tests of comprehension, but they are poor at predicting scores on tests of discourse comprehension. Consequently, clinicians should be cautious in making inferences about aphasic listeners' daily life comprehension competence based on their performance on single-sentence comprehension tests, because aphasic listeners are likely to perform better in daily life than their single-sentence comprehension test scores suggest that they should.

Comprehension of Spoken Discourse

Discourse Comprehension Subtests in Comprehensive Language Tests Some comprehensive language tests include subtests to assess comprehension of spoken discourse, albeit in a limited way.* The materials in these subtests are paragraphs that the examiner reads aloud, followed by spoken questions about the paragraphs, as in the following example, which is part of a paragraph comprehension test item from the MTDDA.

Gold was first discovered in California by a millwright named James Marshall. Marshall was building a sawmill on the banks of the American River. One morning in January, 1848, as he was walking along the millrace, he saw some bright flakes at the bottom of a ditch. Marshall picked up a handful and took them back to the fort to show his partner, John Sutter. They turned out to be pure gold. Marshall and Sutter tried to keep the discovery a secret.

In this story, did Marshall discover gold on the Rio Grande?
Did Marshall and Sutter try to spread the news of the discovery?

The BDAE discourse comprehension subtest includes four short paragraphs, two of which are factual narratives similar to the one in the MTDDA and two of which are humorous vignettes such as the following.

A customer walked into a hotel carrying a coil of rope in one hand and a suitcase in the other. The hotel clerk asked, *Pardon me, sir, but would you tell me what the rope is for? Yes,* responded the man, *that's my fire escape! I'm sorry, sir,* said the clerk, *but all guests carrying their own fire escapes must pay in advance.*

Was the customer carrying a suitcase in each hand?
Did the clerk trust this guest?[†]

The BDAE and the MTDDA stories differ in several ways. The BDAE story seems more interesting, does not contain as much detailed information, and has an overall point (the punch line). It also resembles stories (or jokes) that are common in person-to-person interactions and on radio and television programs. Factual passages such as the MTDDA paragraph are more likely to be encountered in written form in educational settings than in everyday spoken interactions.

A Free-Standing Test of Discourse Comprehension The *Discourse Comprehension Test* (DCT; Brookshire & Nicholas, 1993) is the only free-standing standardized test of spoken discourse comprehension for assessment of brain-damaged adults. The DCT contains 10 tape-recorded narrative stories that are controlled for number of words and sentences, mean sentence length, speech rate, number of unfamiliar words, listening difficulty, and grammatical complexity. The word-choice patterns of the stories in the DCT closely resemble patterns of word choice in adult-to-adult conversations (Hayes, 1988), suggesting that the vocabu-

---

* Only the BDAE and the MTDDA of the major comprehensive language tests include such subtests.

[†]As mentioned earlier, each question is asked in two forms and the patient must answer both forms correctly to get credit.

lary used in the DCT stories closely approximates that used by normal speakers in daily life conversations.

Eight questions test the patient's comprehension and retention of information from each story in the DCT. Four questions for each story test main ideas and four test details. Two of the main-idea questions and two of the detail questions for each story test information that is directly stated in the story. The other two main idea and detail questions test information that is implied by information in the story so that patients must make inferences to answer them correctly. A story and questions from the DCT are reproduced in the box below.

The DCT manual provides performance data for 40 non–brain-damaged adults, 20 aphasic adults, 20 adults with right-hemisphere damage, and 20 adults with traumatic brain injuries. Cutoff scores for normal performance are provided for the full 10-story version of the DCT and for two 5-story short versions. Materials for administering the DCT as a silent-reading test are included, and performance data for 20 non–brain-damaged adults for the reading version of the DCT are included in the test manual.

Variables That May Affect Brain-Damaged Adults' Comprehension of Spoken Discourse

Many of the variables mentioned earlier as affecting sentence comprehension also affect discourse comprehension but not necessarily to the same degree as they affect comprehension of isolated sentences. Because discourse permits listeners greater use of heuristic processes, variables such as word frequency and syntactic complexity, which can have strong effects on listeners' comprehension of sentences do not have equally strong effects on their comprehension of discourse. However, several variables can have important effects on listeners' comprehension of discourse. Two of the most important are *salience* and *directness*.

A Story and Questions from the Discourse Comprehension Test (DCT).

One day last Fall, several women on Willow Street decided to have a garage sale. They collected odds and ends from all over the neighborhood. Then they spent an entire day putting prices on the things that they had collected. On the first day of the sale, they put up signs at both ends of the block and another one at a nearby shopping center. Next they made a batch of iced tea and sat down in a shady spot beside the Anderson's garage to wait for their first customer. Soon a man drove up in an old truck. He looked around and finally stopped by a lumpy old mattress that was leaning against the wall. He gestured to it and asked how much they wanted for it. Mrs. Anderson told him that it wasn't for sale. Then she added that they were going to put it out for the trash collectors the next day. The man asked if he could have it. Mrs. Anderson said that he could. Then she asked, "Why do you want such a terrible mattress?" "Well," he said, "My no-good father-in-law is coming to visit next week and I don't want him to get too comfortable."

Questions

1. Did several women *have a party?* (No) [Stated main idea]
2. Were there a *large number of things* at the garage sale? (Yes) [Implied main idea]
3. Did the women put up a sign *at a shopping center?* (Yes) [Stated detail]
4. Was it *cold* the day of the garage sale? (No) [Implied detail]
5. Was the man driving *a car?* (No) [Stated detail]
6. Was the mattress *in terrible condition?* (Yes) [Stated main idea]
7. Was the man *married?* (Yes) [Implied detail]
8. Was the man *fond of his father-in-law?* (No) [Implied main idea]

Data From Brookshire and Nicholas, 1993.

Salience Speakers (and writers) make information salient by means of devices such as repetition, elaboration, and paraphrase and by establishing syntactic and semantic relationships among parts of the discourse. In this way speakers make some of the information stand out as the *main ideas* and de-emphasize other information that is more peripheral to the overall sense of the discourse *(the details)*. Normal listeners and listeners with brain damage consistently comprehend and remember the main ideas in discourse better than the details (Meyer, 1975; Meyer & McGonkie, 1973; Kintsch, 1974; Brookshire & Nicholas, 1984b; Wegner, Brookshire & Nicholas, 1984; Nicholas & Brookshire, 1995; and others).

Directness Normal speakers do not always specify all the information needed for listeners to understand the speaker's meaning and intent (Clark & Haviland, 1977) but leave informational gaps and expect the listener to construct inferences and make assumptions to fill in the gaps. For example, a speaker might say:

> When I looked out the window, I saw that the garage was on fire. It took the firemen 20 minutes to get here and by then it was too late.

The speaker expected the listener to infer *(1)* that the speaker called the fire department right away, and *(2)* that the garage was destroyed.

Several studies have assessed the effects of directness (whether information is directly stated or implied) on brain-damaged adults' comprehension of information in spoken discourse (Nicholas & Brookshire, 1986; Nicholas & Brookshire, 1995; Katsuki-Nakamura, Brookshire, & Nicholas, 1988). In these studies, brain-damaged adults, like those without brain-damage, had more difficulty with questions that tested implied information from discourse than they did on questions that tested stated information. The differences between questions about stated information and questions about implied information were greatest when the inferences required went beyond simple paraphrase of information in the discourse and required listen-

ers to retrieve relevant information from memory and connect it with information provided by the speaker (Nicholas & Brookshire, 1986).

Redundancy Repetition, elaboration, and paraphrase increase the redundancy of discourse and highlight important information, making it easier for the listener to establish the overall theme or point of the discourse, organize it in memory, and recall it later. Repetition, elaboration, and paraphrase also contribute to the relatedness of information in discourse (its cohesion) and to the overall unity of the material (its *coherence*).

Cohesion and Coherence Cohesion denotes the degree to which the semantic units within discourse relate to each other. Cohesion is produced by linguistic devices called *cohesive ties*. Many kinds of cohesive ties have been described in the literature (Halliday & Hasan, 1976), but a few examples will suffice. *Pronominal* ties are created by pronouns that refer back to a previously mentioned referent *("The boy was lost. **He** stood in the center of the plaza crying.")*. *Conjunctive* ties are created by conjunctions *("The horse was fast, **but** lost the race.")*. *Lexical repetition* ties are created by repeating words (or their synonyms) in nearby propositions *("The man and the woman got on the train. The **man** carried a large black suitcase. The **woman** carried flowers.")*.

Coherence denotes the overall unity of discourse. Multiple variables, which are not readily quantified, contribute to coherence. Cohesion and coherence contribute to heuristic, top-down processes. Consequently cohesive and coherent discourse is much easier to comprehend and retain in memory than noncohesive or noncoherent discourse.

Speech Rate and Emphatic Stress Both of these variables can affect aphasic listeners' comprehension of discourse. Pashek and Brookshire (1982) presented spoken paragraphs at slow speech rate (120 wpm) or normal speech rate (150 wpm), with either normal stress or exaggerated stress (extra prosodic emphasis on important words). They found that *(1)* both slow rate and exaggerated stress facilitated aphasic listeners' comprehension of the paragraphs, *(2)* slow rate was slightly more effective than exaggerated stress in improving comprehension, and *(3)* comprehension was best when slow rate and exaggerated stress were combined.

Kimelman and McNeil (1987) replicated Pashek and Brookshire's study and reported similar results. However, Nicholas and Brookshire (1986) reported that not all aphasic listeners' comprehension of discourse improves when speech rate is slowed, and sometimes an aphasic listener benefits from slowed speech rate at one time and not at another. They presented narrative stories to aphasic listeners at slow (120 wpm) and fast (200 wpm) speech rates and tested their comprehension twice, with a week or more between tests. In the first session, slow speech rate improved comprehension of the aphasic listeners as a group. However, the facilitating effects of slow speech rate at the group level essentially disappeared by the second session, and there were many instances in which individual subjects failed to demonstrate rate effects exhibited by their group.

■ ASSESSING READING

Comprehensive Language Tests All comprehensive language tests contain subtests to assess reading. A few include *visual matching subtests,* in which the patient is shown a series of cards with a printed geometric form, a letter of the alphabet, or a word on each card. The patient then chooses the matching form, letter, or word from a card containing the test stimulus plus several foils. The test stimuli and target choices in these subtests are visually identical, permitting selection of the correct target based on visual form alone. When the test stimuli are letters or words, the patients can make correct choices by matching the visual form of stimuli and targets without translating either into alphabet letters or words. Consequently, such letter-matching or word-matching subtests are best characterized as tests of visual perception and

discrimination rather than as reading tests. Figure 4-15 shows a geometric–form-matching test item and response plate from the MTDDA.

Most comprehensive language tests assess *oral reading of printed words and sentences.* The patient is given a card on which a word or a sentence is printed and reads it aloud. These subtests provide an indication of patients' ability to convert the graphemic forms of words into their phonologic equivalents and to encode and produce those phonologic representations. They do not necessarily test reading comprehension because grapheme-to-phoneme conversion can be accomplished without accessing the semantic representations of the words involved in the conversion. In addition, errors on oral reading tests may be due to speech-production difficulties rather than reading impairments.

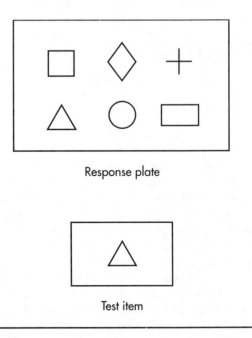

Response plate

Test item

Figure 4-15 ■ A geometric form-matching test item and response plate from the *Minnesota Test for Differential Diagnosis of Aphasia.* (From Schuell HM: *The Minnesota Test for Differential Diagnosis of Aphasia.* Minneapolis, 1965, University of Minnesota Press. Drawings by Lawrence Benson.)

Subtests in which patients *match printed words to pictures or objects* are the simplest reading *comprehension* tests in comprehensive aphasia tests. These subtests come in several forms. In one form the patient is shown a card on which a word is printed and then is shown a card containing several drawings, one of which represents the printed word. The patient points to the drawing representing the printed word *(word-to-picture matching)*. Most often the drawings are of objects but sometimes they portray verbs, colors, numbers, and geometric forms. In another form the patient is shown the printed name of an object and then chooses the named object from a set of real objects *(word-to-object matching)*.

Some comprehensive tests opt for a mirror-image version of the word-to-picture matching format by showing the patient a drawing of an object and asking him or her to choose the object's printed name from a card containing the name of the object plus the names of several other objects *(picture-to-word matching)*. For most brain-damaged adults it makes little difference which format is used. Word-to-picture and picture-to-word matching usually give equivalent results, and most patients perform similarly regardless of whether the printed words are matched to pictures or to real objects. (The exception being patients with impaired visual perception and discrimination.) However, as is true for spoken-word comprehension, brain-damaged adults generally do better at matching printed object names to pictures or objects than at matching the printed names of colors, numbers, or letters to their pictorial representations.

The MTDDA differs from the other comprehensive language tests in how it goes about testing single-word reading comprehension. The patient is shown a series of cards each of which contains a drawing beneath which are two printed words; one identifies the drawing (Figure 4-16). Patients' errors can be classified as semantic confusions *(cat/dog)*, auditory confusions *(hair/wear)*, visual confusions *(horse/house)*, and irrelevant responses *(bridge/paint)*.

Another unique aspect of the subtest is that patients can get half of the items correct by chance because there are only two response choices for each item.

Subtests in which patients *match printed words to spoken words* are somewhat more difficult than picture-to-word matching subtests for most brain-damaged adults. Like picture-to-printed word and printed word-to-picture subtests, printed word-to-spoken word subtests come in different forms. The most common form is one in which a card with several printed words is placed before the patient; the examiner says the words in random order and the patient points to each word as the examiner says it.

The format of the printed-to-spoken word subtest in the MTDDA resembles that of the MTDDA printed word-to-picture subtest. The patient is shown a series of cards, each of which contains two printed words. As each card is shown the

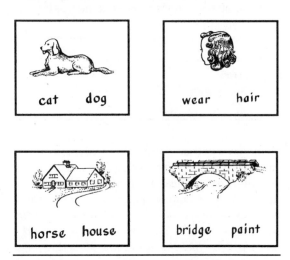

Figure 4-16 ■ **Four single-word reading test stimuli from the *Minnesota Test for Differential Diagnosis of Aphasia*. The top left card tests for semantic confusions; the top right card tests for auditory confusions; the bottom left card tests for visual confusions; and the bottom right card tests for unrelated errors.** (From Schuell HM: *The Minnesota Test for Differential Diagnosis of Aphasia*. Minneapolis, 1965, University of Minnesota Press. Drawings by Lawrence Benson.)

examiner says one of the two words and the patient points to the word on the card. As in the
MTDDA printed word-to-picture subtest, patients'
errors can be categorized as semantic, auditory, or
visual confusions, or as irrelevant responses, and
patients can get half the items correct by chance.

Tests for assessing *comprehension of printed
sentences* also come in several forms. In one form
the sentences are yes-no questions *("Do eggs
come from chickens?")*. Like the spoken yes-no
questions previously described, printed yes-no
questions may relate to personal information,
general knowledge, knowledge acquired in
school, or opinions, inferences, and abstractions.
And, like the spoken yes-no questions previously
described, the general-knowledge questions can
be separated into questions that test comparative,
temporal, and numeric relationships. In another
form of printed-sentence comprehension tests,
patients choose from a list of words the one that
best completes an unfinished sentence, as in:

A soldier carries a . . . *gun   shoot   fun
groceries*
(from the WAB).

In yet another form, the patient is given
cards with printed instructions for manipulating
test objects (or, less frequently, pictures). In
the PICA, for example, patients are given cards
with instructions such as, *"Put this card to the
left of the cigarette.",* or *"Put this card under the
one used for picking up food."* Sometimes the
printed instructions in comprehensive language
tests are similar to those in spoken-sentence
comprehension tests *("Pick up the pencil,
knock three times, and put it back.").*

Several comprehensive language tests provide subtests for assessing *comprehension of
printed texts.* In the most common form, the
patient is given several short, printed passages
to read. The final sentence in each passage is in-

complete, and several phrases that might complete the passage are printed below it, as in the
following item from the BDAE.

In the early days of this country, the functions
of government were few in number. Most of
the functions were carried out by local town
and county officials, while centralized authority was distrusted. The growth of industry and
of big cities has so changed the situation that
the farmer of today is concerned with. . . .

Local affairs above all
The price of lumber
The actions of the government
The authority of town officials

A few comprehensive language tests contain
expository test passages similar to those found in
primary-school and secondary-school reading materials. The following is a portion of the passage
that makes up the MTDDA paragraph-reading
subtest. The patient circles, underlines, or points
to her or his choice of *yes* or *no* for each question.

Lawrence Griswold, a writer and scientist who
lives in Minnesota, states that dragons really exist. In 1934, he and a classmate camped for 8
months on Komodo, an island in Indonesia.
Here they found dragons eighteen-feet long
who walked on their hind feet like the ancient
dinosaurs. They lived in mountain caves and
came down to prey upon animals and people
in the lowlands.

Did Griswold go to
    Komodo in 1943?. . . . .*Yes No*
Did he find dragons
    in Indonesia?. . . . .*Yes No*

The Discourse Comprehension Test (DCT) includes a reading comprehension subtest to assess brain-damaged adults' reading comprehension of 10 stories, together with normative information for 20 non–brain-damaged adults who were tested with the reading version of the DCT.

Free-Standing Tests of Reading Comprehension One free-standing test of brain-damaged adults' reading comprehension is currently on the market. As the title suggests, the *Reading Comprehension Battery for Aphasia* (RCBA, LaPointe and Horner, 1979) is designed for evaluating aphasic adults' reading abilities. The RCBA contains 10 subtests with 10 items in each subtest. Subtests 1, 2, and 3 assess single-word reading from preschool to Grade 3 vocabulary levels. The foils in these subtests permit clinicians to identify visual confusions *(leaf/leap),* auditory confusions *(anchor/tanker),* and semantic confusions *(guitar/violin).* Subtest 4 tests functional reading of signs, labels, menus, calendars, recipes, and other such daily life material (Figure 4-17).

Subtest 5 is a reading vocabulary subtest in which the test taker chooses synonyms for five common verbs and five common nouns, half of which are abstract and half of which are concrete. In Subtest 6 the test taker reads each of 10 five-word sentences and chooses, from sets of three pictures, the one that best illustrates the meaning of each sentence (Figure 4-18). The sentences are controlled for vocabulary level, imageability, and concreteness.

Subtest 7 contains 10 two-sentence (average = 25 words) paragraphs, in which the second sentence directs the test-taker to choose, from a set of three pictures, the one identified by the paragraph (Figure 4-19).* The reading level of the paragraphs in Subtest 7 ranges from Grade 2.7 to Grade 4.8.

Subtests 8 and 9 present five longer (average = 52 words) paragraphs. The reading level of the paragraphs ranges from Grade 2.9 to Grade 6.7. The test taker reads each paragraph and completes four statements about each paragraph by selecting a word or phrase from three choices for each statement (Figure 4-20). The first two questions for each paragraph assess comprehension of stated information and the last two assess comprehension of implied information. Scores on the 10 questions testing stated information are assigned to Subtest 8, and

---

* According to the RCBA manual, correct answers are not obvious from the command sentence alone. However, in several items (including the one in Figure 4-18) the correct answer seems obvious from the final (command sentence) alone.

Weather forecast
Turning much colder beginning today
Wednesday fair and cold
High today low 60s
Low tonight near 30
Chance of rain: 70%

Point to the part that tells how cold it will get tonight.

Figure 4-17 ▪ A functional reading test from the *Reading Comprehension Battery for Aphasia.* (From LaPointe LL, Horner J: *Reading Comprehension Battery for Aphasia.* Tigard, Ore, 1979, Pro-Ed, Inc.)

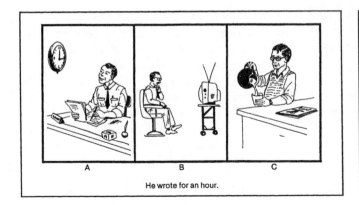

Figure 4-18 ■ A sentence comprehension test item from the *Reading Comprehension Battery for Aphasia.* (From LaPointe LL, Horner J: *Reading Comprehension Battery for Aphasia.* Tigard, Ore, 1979, Pro-Ed, Inc.)

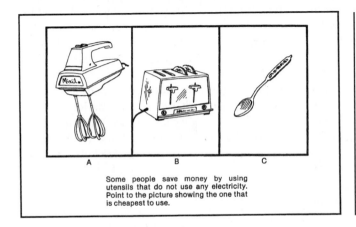

Figure 4-19 ■ A two sentence-paragraph comprehension item from the *Reading Comprehension Battery for Aphasia.* (From LaPointe LL, Horner J: *Reading Comprehension Battery for Aphasia.* Tigard, Ore, 1979, Pro-Ed, Inc.)

scores on the 10 questions testing implied information are assigned to Subtest 9.

Subtest 10 is a sentence-to-picture matching task in which the subject chooses (from three sentences) the one that best describes a picture (Figure 4-21). The choice sentences differ in syntax, ranging from active declarative (*"The player is hitting the ball."*) to object embedded (*"She threw the boy's dog the leash."*).

Individual responses to RCBA test items are scored correct/incorrect, and the time taken to complete each subtest is recorded. The number of correct responses for each RCBA subtest can be plotted to create a graphic profile of a given patient's RCBA performance. The RCBA test manual contains information about test construction, instructions for test administration and interpretation, and instructions for re-

sponse scoring together with a short list of references on reading impairments in aphasia. The test manual contains no normative information or documentation of the RCBA's reliability and validity, but some psychometric information is available elsewhere (VanDemark, Lemmer, & Drake, 1982; Pasternack & LaPointe, 1982).

Reading Tests for Non–brain-damaged Adults and Children Reading tests designed for brain-damaged adults are good screening tests to identify patients with moderate to severe reading impairments. However, most do not provide enough detail to enable clinicians to detect subtle reading impairments or describe the nature of a patient's reading impairment. For these purposes clinicians usually turn to standardized reading tests, which provide a comprehensive look at the severity and nature of a pa-

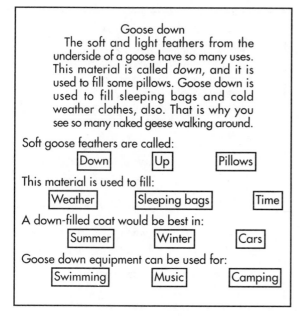

Goose down
The soft and light feathers from the underside of a goose have so many uses. This material is called *down*, and it is used to fill some pillows. Goose down is used to fill sleeping bags and cold weather clothes, also. That is why you see so many naked geese walking around.

Soft goose feathers are called:

Down   Up   Pillows

This material is used to fill:

Weather   Sleeping bags   Time

A down-filled coat would be best in:

Summer   Winter   Cars

Goose down equipment can be used for:

Swimming   Music   Camping

Figure 4-20 ▪ A longer paragraph comprehension item from the *Reading Comprehension Battery for Aphasia.* (From LaPointe LL, Horner J: *Reading Comprehension Battery for Aphasia.* Tigard, Ore, 1979, Pro-Ed, Inc.)

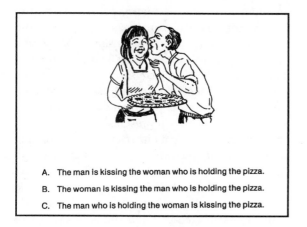

A. The man is kissing the woman who is holding the pizza.

B. The woman is kissing the man who is holding the pizza.

C. The man who is holding the woman is kissing the pizza.

Figure 4-21 ▪ A sentence-comprehension item from The *Reading Comprehension Battery for Aphasia.* (From LaPointe LL, Horner J: *Reading Comprehension Battery for Aphasia.* Tigard, Ore, 1979, Pro-Ed, Inc.)

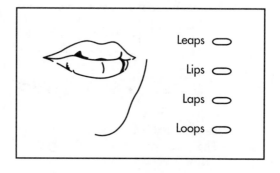

Leaps ⬭

Lips ⬭

Laps ⬭

Loops ⬭

Figure 4-22 ▪ A vocabulary item from the *Gates-MacGinitie Reading Test: Primary A.* (Copyright 1979 by Riverside Publishing Company.)

tient's reading impairments and permit the clinician to compare the patient with normal readers. Because brain-damaged adults' reading abilities range from single-word reading to college-level reading, clinicians who assess brain-damaged adults' reading need tests that span a range from primary-grade level to college level.

The Primary A and Primary C levels of the *Gates-MacGinitie Reading Tests* (Gates, 1978) are appropriate for testing brain-damaged adults who are reading at primary-grade levels. The *Primary A* version tests at approximately Grade 1 reading level, and the *Primary C* version tests at approximately Grade 3.* Both have vocabulary and comprehension sections. The vocabulary section of the *Primary A* version contains 45 items, each consisting of a picture and four words, one of which names or describes the picture (Figure 4-22). The person taking the test marks his or her choice for each item. The comprehension section of the *Primary A* version contains 40 items, each with four pictures and a sentence or short paragraph that defines or describes one of the pictures (Figure 4-23). The test taker marks or points to the picture that best matches the sentence.

---

* The *Primary B* version tests at Grade 2. *Primary B* and *Primary C* overlap sufficiently that brain-damaged adults who are testable with *Primary B* also are testable with *Primary C.*

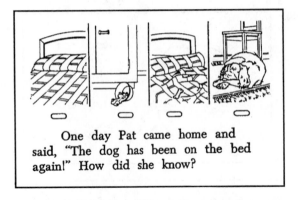

One day Pat came home and said, "The dog has been on the bed again!" How did she know?

Figure 4-23 ▪ A comprehension item from the *Gates-MacGinitie Reading Test: Primary A.* (Copyright 1979 by Riverside Publishing Company.)

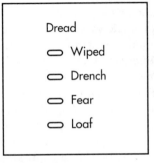

Dread

⟶ Wiped

⟶ Drench

⟶ Fear

⟶ Loaf

Figure 4-24 ▪ A vocabulary item from the *Gates-MacGinitie Reading Test: Primary C.* (Copyright 1979 by Riverside Publishing Company.)

The vocabulary section of the *Primary C* version contains 45 items, each of which consists of a stimulus word and four words or phrases, one of which is synonymous with the stimulus word (Figure 4-24). The test-taker marks the word or phrase that best defines the stimulus word. The comprehension section of the Primary C version contains 22 short paragraphs, each followed by two multiple-choice questions about the paragraph (Figure 4-25). The test-taker marks the word or phrase that best answers each question.

Children rode their bicycles on the sidewalk to avoid the buses and cars in the street. Some boys were playing catch in the lot, laughing and yelling at each other. As it grew later, one by one the children left for home, and the lot was quiet again.

A. Where were the boys playing catch?

⟶ In the lot   ⟶ In the street

⟶ On the sidewalk   ⟶ On the way home

B. They left for home when

⟶ It got late   ⟶ School was over

⟶ The bus came   ⟶ It got quiet

Figure 4-25 ▪ A comprehension item from the *Gates-MacGinitie Reading Test: Primary C.* (Copyright 1979 by Riverside Publishing Company.)

The reading comprehension subtest of the *Peabody Individual Achievement Test* (Dunn and Markwardt, 1970) can be used to test the sentence-reading comprehension of brain-damaged patients representing a range of reading impairments. The clinician shows a page containing a printed sentence to the patient and then covers it with another page that contains four pictures, one of which represents the meaning of the sentence. The patient responds by pointing to one of the pictures. Sentences increase in length (from 5 to 30 words) and difficulty of vocabulary as the test progresses. Norms (grade equivalents and percentiles) are provided for non–brain-damaged children and adults up to 18 years old. Most brain-damaged patients can complete this test in less than 30 minutes, making the test useful for moderately to severely impaired patients who might not tolerate longer tests.

The *Nelson Reading Skills Test* (NRST; Hanna, Schell and Schriener, 1977) is suitable for testing higher-level brain-damaged adults' comprehension of words and printed paragraphs. It permits measurement of reading levels from Grade 3 to Grade 9. Like the Gates-MacGinitie reading tests, the NRST contains a vocabulary section and a paragraph comprehension section for each of three reading levels. Level A tests at Grades 3 to 4.5, Level B tests at Grades 4.5 to 6, and Level C tests at Grades 7 to 9. Vocabulary section test items consist of a test word followed by four choices, one of which is a synonym for the test word. The test taker points to, underlines, circles, or otherwise indicates his or her choice. The paragraph comprehension section of the NRST contains five narrative or expository paragraphs at each of the three Levels (A, B, and C). Each paragraph is followed by several questions, as in the following example, which is from Level B.

A useful characteristic of the paragraph comprehension section of the NRST is its provision

---

Long ago, people believed in monsters. The manticore was thought to have the head of a man, the body of a lion, and three rows of sharp teeth. It ate people if it caught them. The centaur, which lived in the forest, was believed to have the body of a horse but the shoulders, arms, and head of a man. Its voice sounded like the whinny of a horse.

1. *Whinny* means:
A. Cry
B. Growl
C. Neigh
D. Roar

2. How did people probably feel about these monsters?
A. Afraid
B. Angry
C. Friendly
D. Puzzled

---

for assessing readers' comprehension of several kinds of information from the paragraphs. *Literal items* are items in which the information in the test item appears in the same form as it appears in the paragraph. *Translational items* are items in which the information in the test item is reworded from the way the information appears in the paragraph. *Higher-level items* are items that require inferences from information in the paragraph. Higher-level items require readers to identify cause and effect relationships, make judgments about events or the attitudes of characters, and make inferences and assumptions about information that is implied but not directly stated in the paragraph.

For patients who are reading at higher levels than those covered by the NRST, the *Nelson-Denny Reading Test* (NDRT; Brown, Bennet, & Hanna, 1981) provides reading materials graded at high-school through college levels. Like the NRST, the NDRT has vocabulary and paragraph comprehension sections. The NDRT permits users to classify test items according to whether they test *literal* (stated) *information* or *interpretive* (implied) *information,* and according to whether they test *details* (specific facts), *evaluations* (noting relationships, style, and mood; drawing conclusions, making generalizations and deductions), or *purpose* (the writer's purpose and central ideas).

Assessing Reading Rate and Capacity

In their standard administration, reading tests are given with a time limit, and norms for the test are based on scores obtained within the time limit. Clinicians who are interested in brain-damaged patients' reading usually want to know how much a patient can accomplish within the time limit so that their performance can be compared with the performance of the norm group. They also wish to know how much a patient can do if she or he is permitted to work without time constraints. This way of testing provides estimates of patients' *reading rate* and *reading capacity.* Reading rate tells the clinician how much the patient can read and understand under normal time constraints and allows comparison of the patient with norm groups, whereas reading capacity tells the clinician how much the patient can read under optimal conditions. Most brain-damaged adults' reading rate is slower than their premorbid rate even when their vocabulary, word recognition, and single-word comprehension seem intact. Estimates of reading rate and reading capacity are important in planning treatment programs and in counseling the patient and family about the patient's probable daily life reading competence.

Reading rate and capacity are measured in the following way. The patient begins the test and works for the amount of time prescribed by the test manual. At the end of that time the examiner marks the last item completed by the patient, and the patient continues until he or she complete the test or can go no farther. The examiner records the time at which the patient finishes the test and marks the last item completed.

Measuring Component Skills One weakness of most reading comprehension tests for adults is that they do not measure component skills that may be necessary for different aspects of reading comprehension (e.g., sound-to-letter conversion, getting main ideas, using context). After administering most adult reading comprehension tests the examiner has a test score, perhaps a percentile rank, and a reading grade level but no real sense of which component skills are compromised and which are preserved.

There is no universal list of component skills for reading, but the *Specific Skill Series* of remedial reading materials (Boning, 1990) provides materials suitable for getting a look at some of the more important ones: *working within words* (symbol-to-sound correspondences), *following directions, using context, locating answers, getting facts, getting main ideas, drawing conclusions, recognizing sequences,* and *identifying inferences,* with materials at 10 levels of graded difficulty within each skill. The box on p. 191 gives examples of items from the *following directions, getting main ideas, drawing conclusions,* and *identifying inferences* series.

The reading materials in the *Specific Skill Series* cover a wide range of reading levels (preschool to Grade 8). A set of placement tests enables users to place learners at the appropriate level within each skill. Some of the reading selections have juvenile themes, but the incidents and situations portrayed are sufficiently interesting so that most adult readers should not find them demeaning. With its compartmentalization of the reading process into component skills and its wide range of reading levels within each skill, the *Specific Skill Series* provides an excellent selection of materials for assessing and treating brain-damaged adults' reading impairments.

Reading Test Format Those who design standardized reading tests for normal adults and children assume that potential test takers have essentially normal (for their age) memory, organizational skills, problem-solving skills, and visual perception and are able to attend to and follow spoken directions. These assumptions permit users of the tests to conclude that impaired test performance signifies reading impairment and not impairment of some underlying or related ability. Because reading tests for normal children and adults were designed with these assumptions in mind, their format may make some of them unsatisfactory for testing brain-damaged adults who have memory impairments, impaired organizational or problem-solving skills, visual perceptual impairments, or difficulties in following instructions.

Most standardized reading tests for normal adults and children do not require written answers to test items but allow the test taker to check off, circle, or underline his or her choice from a multiple-choice array of possible answers. Consequently, brain-damaged adults are likely to have little difficulty with the responses required. Tests with machine-scorable answer sheets, in which the person taking the test must read a stimulus item, choose the correct answer from a group of possible answers,

---

Examples of Reading Items From the Specific Skill Series

Following Directions

Directions:
There are four words in the left-hand column. To the right of each word are two more words. Choose the one that is opposite in meaning to the word at the left. Circle it.

Listen	Speak, hear
Below	Beside, above
Everyone	Lately, nobody
Many	Few, some

Getting the Main Idea

There is a plant in our country that doesn't have any green leaves. This plant grows about 8 inches tall. At the end of each stem is a white flower. The stem is also white. The plant looks like many clay pipes. It is called the Indian Pipe.

The story tells mainly:
(A) Why American Indians smoke pipes
(B) Why American Indians named plants
(C) What the plant called the Indian Pipe looks like

Drawing Conclusions

Horses don't live as long as people. A horse that lives to the age of 30 is very old. One year of a horse's life is equal to 3 years of a person's. A 30-year-old horse is as old as a person who is 90 years old.

A horse of 10 is equal in age to a:
(A) 10-year-old child
(B) 30-year-old person
(C) 3-year-old baby

Identifying Inferences

"That's a pretty jewel you have in your ring," said Karen.

"Thank you," said Martha, "It was given to me as a present. I have other rings but this is my favorite. My mother always gives me things that I really like."

Martha has more than one ring.
True False Inferred*
The ring was given to Martha by her mother.
True False Inferred
Karen didn't like Martha's ring.
True False Inferred

From Boning RA: *The Specific Skill Series,* New York, 1990, Macmillian/McGraw-Hill.
True items are facts that are directly stated in the story. *False* items are not true, based on information in the story. *Inferred* items are items that are probably true, based on the story and the reader's experience.

remember the number of the test item and the number or letter of the correct choice, find the corresponding set of response choices on the answer sheet, and blacken the appropriate area on the answer sheet, often cause transcription and bookkeeping errors even for adults with no brain damage. Consequently, they should not be used to test brain-damaged adults unless the response format can be changed to eliminate demands on abilities other than reading.

The Passage Dependency of Reading Tests Passage dependency is a term coined by Tuiman (1974) to reflect the extent to which readers must rely on information from reading test passages to correctly answer items that test comprehension of the passages. Items that are answerable without reading the passages to which the items refer are *passage independent* because they do not depend on the test-taker's comprehension of the passage. When reading test items have low-passage dependency, the test is more likely a test of single-sentence reading skills than a test of multiple-sentence reading comprehension.

Nicholas, MacLennan, and Brookshire (1986) reported that the validity of most multiple-sentence reading tests for testing brain-damaged adults is compromised by low passage dependency. They evaluated the performance of non–brain-damaged adults and aphasic adults on reading-test items from the multiple-sentence reading subtests from the *Boston Diagnostic Aphasia Examination* (BDAE), the *Minnesota Test for Differential Diagnosis of Aphasia* (MTDDA), *Examining for Aphasia* (EFA), the *Western Aphasia Battery* (WAB), and the *Reading Comprehension Battery for Aphasia* (RCBA). First they had subjects respond to the test items without having previously read the passages to which the items referred. On the average, aphasic adults correctly answered beyond chance level 58% of the test items from these reading tests without having read the test passages, and non–brain-damaged adults correctly answered 64% of the items. Only the items from one of the two RCBA subtests had acceptable passage dependency. However, this subtest contained only two-sentence passages and would be unlikely to predict performance on longer passages that are more frequently encountered in daily life.

Nicholas and Brookshire (1987) subsequently evaluated aphasic and non–brain-damaged adults' ability to answer the questions in the paragraph comprehension section of the *Nielson Reading Skills Test* (NRST) (Level B) with and without having read the paragraphs to which the questions related. On average, aphasic adults correctly answered 40% of the NRST items beyond chance level without having read the passages, and non– brain-damaged adults correctly answered 58% of the items. Nicholas and Brookshire concluded that the NRST has acceptable passage dependency when used to test aphasic adults.* However, they also identified several NRST test items that had poor passage dependency and suggested that those test items

are likely to represent aphasic adults' general knowledge or test-taking skills rather than their reading performance.

It seems inappropriate to remove comprehensive language tests' multiple-sentence reading comprehension subtests and the RCBA multiple-sentence test items from clinicians' test protocols because they have questionable passage dependency. These tests are no doubt sufficiently sensitive and have sufficient validity to make them acceptable screening tests of multiple-sentence reading comprehension. They appear well suited for identifying patients with reading impairments who can then be tested with a more comprehensive free-standing reading test, if necessary.

■ ASSESSING SPEECH PRODUCTION

Subtests for assessing speech production are prominent parts of all comprehensive language tests, and several free-standing tests of speech production for brain-damaged adults are available. They cover a wide range of content, from repetition of syllables and words to self-generated connected speech. Patients with severely compromised communication usually can do the easiest tests reasonably well, whereas the most difficult tests may challenge even patients with extremely mild impairments.

Simple Speech Production Tests

The simplest speech production subtests are found in comprehensive language tests. They are useful in assessing patients with moderate to severe aphasia and permit assessment of patients' *production of rhymes, recitations, and automatized sequences, sentence completion,* and *speech repetition.**

Recitations, Rhymes, and Automatized Sequences These tests are among the easiest speech production tests for most brain-damaged

---

* Tuiman (1974) suggested that passages for which test takers can answer no more than 40% to 50% of test items without reading the passages have acceptable passage dependency.

---

* *The Porch Index of Communicative Ability* (PICA) does not provide for assessment of recitations, rhymes, and automatized sequences.

adults. They require the patient to produce highly practiced material, such as counting, reciting the days of the week, the months of the year, the alphabet, or familiar sayings.

Sentence Completion Sentence completion tests usually are more difficult than tests calling for recitation, rhymes, and automatized sequences but they are still within the capability of most brain-damaged adults. The stimuli in these tests are short, syntactically simple sentences, minus the final word, which is highly predictable from the rest of the sentence *("I like bread and _____." "Roses are red, violets are _____.")*.

Speech Repetition These tests span a range of difficulty, from repetition of monosyllabic words to repetition of phonologically complex phrases and sentences. The longer and more phonologically complex the phrase or sentence, the more difficult it is for the patient to produce.

Naming

Naming Subtests in Comprehensive Language Tests Naming tests are found in all the major comprehensive language tests and provide useful information about patients across the aphasia severity continuum. They take several forms. The most common is *picture naming or object naming* (sometimes called *confrontation naming*), in which the patient is shown a series of pictures or objects and is asked to say the name of each. The stimuli in most confrontation naming subtests are drawings or objects, but naming subtests in which the stimuli are geometric shapes, colors, numbers, or body parts are included in some comprehensive aphasia tests.*

Two variants on confrontation naming subtests are seen in some comprehensive language tests. In *responsive naming tests* the examiner asks a question that can be answered with a one- or two-word phrase *("What do you write with?,*

What do you do with soap?, or *What color is snow?")*. In *generative naming,* (sometimes called *category naming*), patients are asked to say within a specified time interval (usually one minute) as many words as they can think of that either begin with a particular letter or represent certain semantic categories (such as animals or tools).

Free-Standing Tests of Naming Several free-standing tests for assessing brain-damaged adults' naming have been published or described in the literature. One of the oldest is a generative naming test called the *Word Fluency Measure* (Borkowski, Benton, & Spreen, 1967), which was originally published as a research report and was subsequently included as a subtest of the *Neurosensory Center Comprehension Examination for Aphisia* (NCCEA). In the *Word Fluency Measure,* the patient is asked to say, in one minute, as many words that begin with a specified letter of the alphabet as she or he can think of. The letter (either *F, A,* or *S*) is specified by the examiner. The patient's score is the total of all appropriate words spoken in the 1-minute interval.[*]

The *Word Fluency Measure* is a sensitive indicator of brain injury but does not discriminate among aphasia syndromes or between aphasia syndromes and other neurogenic impairments of communication or cognitive functions. A patient's performance on the word fluency measure has marginal value for planning treatment because the task is an unusual one, with little relationship to daily life communication. Some clinicians make up informal generative naming tests in which the patient is asked to produce words within functional categories (such as furniture, foods, or flowers). Although no norms are available for these informal tests, they can provide useful insights into a patient's word re-

---

* Letter-naming tests are also found in some comprehensive aphasia tests. However, they can be categorized as low-level *oral reading* tests.

---

[*] The letters *F, A,* and *S* yield the largest numbers of correct responses from non–brain-damaged adults (Borkowski, Benton, & Spreen, 1967). No equivalent information is available for semantic categories.

trieval, speech production, and the state of the patient's semantic system.

Generative naming is, in one respect, easier for aphasic adults than confrontation naming. They are not restricted to a single word as a correct response to each stimulus, and if a single word would suffice, most aphasic adults would get higher scores in generative naming tasks than in confrontation naming ones. However, one word is not enough in generative naming, and aphasic adults almost always produce far fewer appropriate words than non–brain-damaged adults (and fewer also than adults with right-hemisphere brain damage). One potential problem for clinicians who wish to use generative naming tasks in treatment is that there is great variability in the number of names non–brain-damaged adults produce in generative naming tasks. For example, one group of non–brain-damaged adults produced, on the average, 23 animal names in a 1-minute interval, but productions of individual subjects ranged from 9 to 41 words (Goodglass & Kaplan, 1983).

The *Boston Naming Test* (BNT; Kaplan, Goodglass, & Weintraub, 1983) is a picture-naming test in which the examiner shows 60 line drawings one at a time to the person being tested and asks him or her to name each drawing. Word familiarity (the frequency of occurrence of target names) decreases as the test progresses. Each response is scored for latency, correctness, and whether a cue was given. Norms (means, standard deviations, and range of scores) are provided for 30 children (Kindergarten to Grade 5), 84 normal adults (age 18-59), and 82 aphasic adults (at six levels of aphasia severity). The BNT manual provides brief instructions for administering the BNT and scoring responses, but neither administration nor scoring instructions appear to be explicit enough to ensure interexaminer or test-retest reliability, and the manual does not report either. Nicholas and associates (1989) published more explicit procedures for administering and scor-

ing the BNT, together with intrajudge and interjudge reliability results for their more explicit procedures.

Variables That May Affect Naming Accuracy

Frequency of Occurrence A word's frequency in the language can affect the ease and accuracy with which aphasic patients name objects or pictures (Wiegel-Crump & Koenigsknecht, 1973; Rochford & Williams, 1965; Tweedy & Schulman, 1982; and others). More frequent words are easier to name than less frequent words. However, in most studies of the effects of word frequency, confounding variables, such as length, abstractness, age of acquisition, phonologic complexity of words, and ambiguity or uncertainty of pictures were not controlled (making conclusions about the effects of word frequency by itself somewhat ambiguous).

Length and Phonologic Complexity also affect aphasic adults' naming. Goodglass and associates (1976) found that aphasic adults' naming success decreased as the length (in number of syllables) of words increased. Articulatory complexity also may affect aphasic adults' naming, probably because the number of syllables in a word is related to the ease with which it can be articulated. Word length and articulatory complexity affect the mechanical production of words, unlike variables such as word frequency or stimulus uncertainty, which are more likely to affect accessing words and retrieving them from memory.

Semantic Categories The semantic characteristics of items to be named may slightly affect how readily some aphasic adults name pictures and objects. Goodglass and associates (1966) evaluated aphasic adults' ability to name (and comprehend) words representing five semantic categories: objects, actions, colors, numbers, and letters. They reported that object pictures were hardest to name and letters were easiest. (Interestingly, the spoken names of objects were easiest to comprehend and spoken letter names were hardest to comprehend.) However, the difference between object naming and letter naming was only 2 points of a possible 18, and it is almost certain that not every subject's performance pattern matched that of the group. Consequently, clinicians will undoubtedly choose to evaluate the strength of the effects of semantic categories on individual patients' naming before incorporating manipulations of semantic categories into their treatment procedures.

The Form of Visual Stimuli During the 1970s several investigators set out to determine if the *form* of visual stimuli (whether they are objects, pictures, photographs, or line drawings) affects the naming performance of brain-damaged patients. Benton, Smith, and Lang (1972) asked aphasic adults to name real objects and line drawings of real objects and found a small but statistically significant difference in favor of real objects. Bisiach (1966) asked aphasic adults to name either realistically colored pictures or line drawings of common objects. He reported a small but significant difference in favor of realistically colored pictures. Corlew and Nation (1975) reported conflicting results. They asked aphasic adults to name either real objects or line drawings representing the objects. They found no meaningful difference between their subjects' naming of objects and their naming of line drawings of the objects.

Most brain-damaged adults are unlikely to perform much differently if they are asked to name objects, colored photographs, or line drawings. However, as in the case of comprehension tests, differences in the form of visual stimuli used in naming tests may be important for severely impaired patients or for patients with visual perceptual impairments. For these patients, real objects may elicit better naming performance than pictures or drawings, and realistic photographs may elicit better performance than line drawings.

Context Context seems to have stronger effects on naming performance than the nature of the stimuli to be named. For many aphasic adults, naming of drawings, pictures, or objects improves when they are portrayed in a natural context. For example, an aphasic adult who cannot name a drawing of a horse portrayed in isolation may name it if it is shown harnessed to a cart. A patient who has difficulty naming cups, plates, knives, and forks presented in isolation or in an array of unrelated items may name them more easily if they are arranged in a place setting like those experienced in daily life.

Williams and Canter (1982) reported conflicting findings with regard to the effects of context on groups of aphasic adults' naming. They asked aphasic adults to name line drawings of objects that were shown either in isolation or in a pictorial context. Adults with Broca's aphasia were better at naming the drawings of objects in isolation, and adults with Wernicke's aphasia were better at naming them in contexts. Other groups of aphasic adults exhibited no group preference for contextual or acontextual pictures, although Williams and Canter reported that individual aphasic adults in all groups showed marked differences in performance between the two conditions.

The presence of context can have negative effects on the naming performance of some patients with right-hemisphere brain damage, traumatic brain injuries, or dementia. These patients may focus on trivial or tangential details of the context, with consequent negative effects on their naming performance. For these patients highly structured test procedures with minimally contextual stimuli may yield better performance than less-structured procedures with contextually rich stimuli.

Sentence Production

Sentence Production Subtests in Comprehensive Aphasia Tests Sentence production subtests are included in all comprehensive language tests. They take several forms. In *word definition* tests, the examiner provides a word and asks the patient to tell what the word means

("Tell me what _____ means."). In *make-a-sentence-from-a-word* tests, the examiner says a word and asks the patient to respond with a sentence containing the word. In *expressing ideas* tests, the examiner asks the patient to produce a sentence or two in response to the examiner's instructions. For example, in the MTDDA expressing ideas subtest the examiner says to the patient, *"Tell me three things you did today.",* and in the PICA expressing ideas subtest the examiner says to the patient, *"As completely as possible, tell me what you do with each of these."* ("these" being the PICA test objects).

Free-Standing Tests of Sentence Production The *Reporter's Test* (DeRenzi & Ferrari, 1978) is a reversal of the *Token Test* (DeRenzi & Vignolo, 1962). In the *Token Test* the examiner asks the patient to manipulate large and small circles and squares. In the *Reporter's Test* the examiner manipulates the tokens and the patient describes the examiner's actions.

There are five levels in the *Reporter's Test* similar to the five levels in the *Token Test*. In Level 1 (four items) only large tokens are present and the examiner touches a single token *("You touched the green circle.")*. In Level 2 (four items) large and small tokens are present and the examiner touches one of them *("You touched the small white circle.")*. In Level 3 (four items) only large tokens are present, but the examiner touches two in succession *("You touched the red circle and the green square.")*. In level 4 (four items) all tokens are present, and the examiner touches two in succession *("You touched the large red circle and the small green square")*. In Level 5 (10 items) only the large tokens are present and the examiner manipulates them in several ways *("You put the red circle on the green square. You touched all the circles except the green one. You put all the circles into the box.")*.

Responses to *Reporter's Test* items are scored either with a three-category system *(correct on first try, correct after a repeated demon-* *stration, incorrect)* or with a weighted scoring system, which takes into account some of the qualitative characteristics of responses. Mean scores and standard deviations are included for normal and aphasic (Italian) adults. DeRenzi and Ferrari assert that the *Reporter's Test* is a sensitive indicator of the presence of aphasia and that it is more sensitive to the presence of language impairment than confrontation naming, word fluency, picture description, or sentence repetition tests.

Wener and Duffy (1983) compared the *Reporter's Test* with other measures of speech production and language comprehension for English-speaking aphasic adults. Their results support DeRenzi and Ferrari's assertions about the test's sensitivity to language impairments. However, Wener and Duffy concluded that the *Reporter's Test* in combination with other tests is more sensitive to the presence of language impairments than the *Reporter's Test* alone.

Discourse Production

Discourse Production Subtests in Comprehensive Language Tests The most common test format for eliciting discourse in comprehensive language tests is *picture description,* in which the examiner shows the patient a drawing depicting several characters engaged in activities that should be familiar to most adults and asks them to describe the picture. The BDAE, the MTDDA, and the WAB include picture description subtests. Figure 4-26 shows the pictures that are used to elicit connected speech in those three tests.

Story retelling is sometimes used to elicit connected speech from aphasic adults. The patient reads (or less frequently, hears) a narrative and then retells it to the examiner. The MTDDA is the only major comprehensive language test to provide a story retelling subtest. The examiner reads aloud a 107-word paragraph (a factual paragraph about quicksand) and the patient recounts as much of it as he or she can remember. The patient's narrative is scored with a seven-

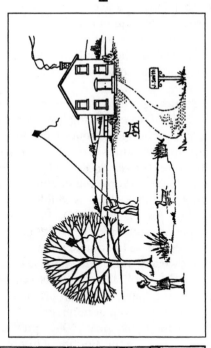

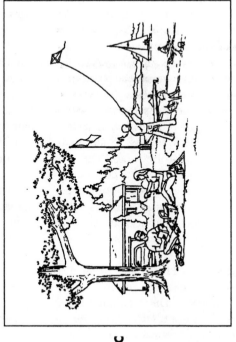

Figure 4-26 ■ The connected-speech elicitation pictures from **(A)** the *Boston Diagnostic Aphasia Examination* (From Goodglass H, Kaplan E: *The Boston Diagnostic Aphasia Examination.* Malvern, Pa, 1983, Lea and Febiger.), **(B)** the *Minnesota Test for Differential Diagnosis of Aphasia* (From Schuell HM: *The Minnesota Test for Differential Diagnosis of Aphasia.* Minneapolis, 1965, University of Minnesota Press.), and **(C)** *The Western Aphasia Battery* (From Kertesz A: *The Western Aphasia Battery.* New York, 1982, The Psychological Corporation.).

category system for number of ideas and amount of irrelevant material.

Story retelling makes heavy demands on comprehension and verbal memory. Consequently, poor performance on story retelling tasks may not always be attributable to impaired speech formulation or production. Other connected-speech tasks, which do not make such demands on comprehension and memory, usually are a better choice if the clinician's concern is with speech formulation and production and not with comprehension and memory.

Interviews and conversations are important parts of the BDAE and the WAB. The BDAE and the WAB base judgments regarding patients' aphasia type primarily on the characteristics of the speech produced in an interview. The examiner asks the patient for personal information such the patient's name and address and inquires into the patient's complaints or problems *("How are you today? Tell me a little about why you are here.")*. Then the interview proceeds to a conversation about topics familiar to the patient *("What kind of work did you do before you became ill?,"* and so on). The BDAE provides a scale for rating melodic line, phrase length, articulatory agility, grammatical form, paraphasia, repetition, and word finding in the patient's connected speech (from the interview/conversation and picture-description tasks) with a *Rating Scale Profile of Speech Characteristics* (Figure 4-27). Voice loudness, voice quality, and speech rate can also be rated. The rating scale is subjective, but can be used to construct a speech profile that can be compared with profiles for major aphasia syndromes. The examiner also considers connected speech when rating the patients' overall aphasia severity (Table 4-5).

The WAB provides two 11-point (0-10) scales for rating the speech elicited in the WAB connected-speech subtests. The examiner rates *information content* with one scale and *fluency, grammaticality, and paraphasias* with the other. Speech fluency is important in Kertesz's taxonomic approach, in which patients are assigned

to diagnostic categories (such as Broca's or Wernicke's) according to their performance on the WAB. Trupe (1984) questioned the reliability of the WAB's procedures for scoring spontaneous speech, as well as the validity of assigning patients to diagnostic categories based on those scores.

Free-Standing Tests of Discourse Production Several free-standing procedures for eliciting and scoring discourse produced by language-impaired adults have been described in the literature (Glosser & Deser, 1990; Glosser, Wiener, & Kaplan, 1988; Golper and associates, 1980; Hier, Hagenlocker, & Shindler, 1985; Nicholas and associates, 1985). Because standard elicitation and scoring procedures were not published, these are not actually *tests* of discourse. However, their materials and procedures may be useful for clinicians concerned with measuring (and treating) brain-damaged adults' discourse production impairments.

Yorkston and Beukelman (1980) published a system for measuring the amount of information conveyed by aphasic adults as they described the *"cookie theft"* picture from the (BDAE; Figure 4-25). The central measure in their system is what Yorkston and Beukelman called *content units,* which they defined as groupings of information that were always expressed as a unit and were mentioned by at least 1 of 78 non–brain-damaged adults who described the BDAE picture.

Yorkston and Beukelman reported that *content units per minute* differentiated the speech of aphasic adults from that of non–brain-damaged adults. (The aphasic adults produced fewer content units per minute.) Results reported by Yorkston and Beukelman for one aphasic adult suggested that both *number of content units* and *content units per minute* are sensitive measures of change in connected speech as a result of treatment.

Others have modified or expanded on Yorkston and Beukelman's content unit measures (Golper and associates, 1980; Shewan, 1988). However, the content units measure and its

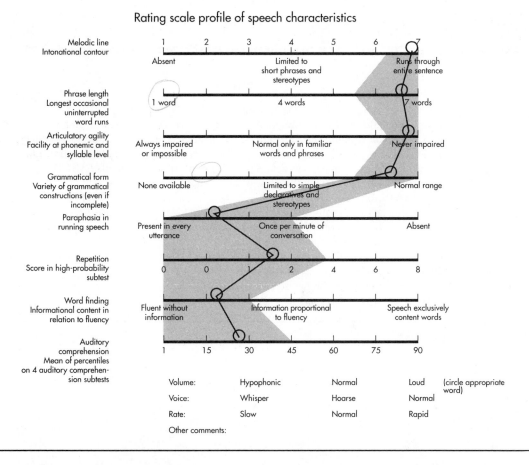

Rating scale profile of speech characteristics

Figure 4-27 ■ A *Rating Scale Profile of Speech Characteristics* from the *Boston Diagnostic Aphasia Examination* for a patient with Broca's aphasia. (From Goodglass H, Kaplan E: *Assessment of Aphasia and Related Disorders.* Boston, 1983, Lea and Febiger (p. 77).)

variants are limited in application because they can only be used to analyze speech elicited with the BDAE *"cookie theft"* picture.

Nicholas and Brookshire (1993, 1995) published a standard protocol for eliciting and scoring discourse from brain-damaged adults. Their speech elicitation stimuli include:

- The speech elicitation pictures from the BDAE and the WAB (Figure 4-26).
- Two *single pictures* depicting story-like situations with a central focus and interactions among picture elements (Figure 4-28).
- Two *picture sequences,* each of which contain

six pictures portraying a short story (Figure 4-29).
- Two *requests for personal information* ("Tell me what you usually do on Sundays." and "Tell me where you live and describe it to me.").
- Two *requests for procedural information* ("Tell me how you would go about doing dishes by hand." and "Tell me how you would go about writing and sending a letter.").

Nicholas and Brookshire (1993, 1995) provided rules for scoring *words, correct information units,* and *main concepts* in speech samples elicited with the protocol. *Correct information units* are words that are accurate, relevant, and

	T A B L E 4 - 5

Aphasia severity rating scale from the *Boston Diagnostic Aphasia Examination* (BDAE).

Rating	Description
0	No usable speech or auditory comprehension.
1	All communication is through fragmentary expression. There is great need for inference, questioning and guessing by the listener. The range of information that can be exchanged is limited, and the listener carries the burden of communication.
2	Conversation about familiar subjects is possible with help from the listener. There are frequent failures to convey the idea, but the patient shares the burden of communication with the examiner.
3	The patient can discuss almost all everyday problems with little or no assistance. However, reduction of speech and/or comprehension make conversation about certain material difficult or impossible.
4	Some obvious loss of fluency in speech or facility of comprehension, without significant limitation on ideas expressed or form of expression.
5	Minimal discernible speech handicaps; the patient may have subjective difficulties that are not apparent to listener.

Data from Goodglass and Kaplan, 1983.

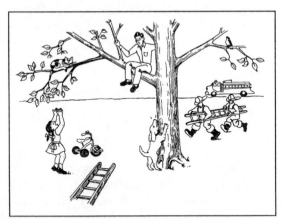 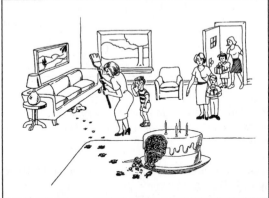

Figure 4-28 ▪ Connected-speech elicitation pictures. (Copyright, Brookshire RH, Nicholas LE, 1993.)

informative relative to the eliciting stimulus. *Main concepts* are statements that convey the most important information about a stimulus.

Nicholas and Brookshire (1993) reported that *words per minute, correct information units per minute,* and *percent of words that are correct information units* reliably discriminate aphasic adults from those without aphasia, but suggested that combining a speech rate measure *(words per minute)* with an informativeness measure *(per-*

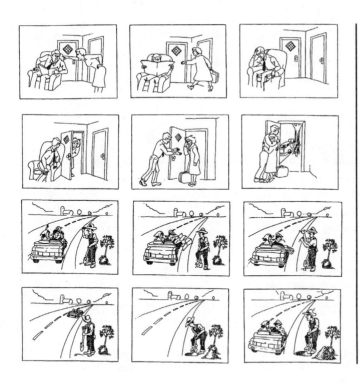

Figure 4-29 ▪ Prompted story-telling pictures. (Copyright, Brookshire RH, Nicholas LE, 1993.)

cent of words that are correct information units) provides a better description of aphasic adults' connected speech than any single measure. They also reported that it was not the number of main concepts that subjects failed to mention that best distinguished aphasic speakers' performance from that of non–brain-damaged speakers, but rather the accuracy and completeness of the main concepts they did produce (Nicholas & Brookshire, 1995). Normative information for 20 non–brain-damaged adults and 20 aphasic adults are provided in Nicholas and Brookshire (1993, 1995) and for 40 non–brain-damaged adults in Brookshire and Nicholas (1995).

Brookshire and Nicholas (1995) also described a rule-based system for scoring what they called *performance deviations* in the speech of adults with aphasia and reported the frequency of performance deviations in speech samples from 40 non–brain-damaged adults, 10 adults with fluent aphasia, and 10 adults with nonfluent aphasia. They defined performance deviations as "features that make the connected speech of aphasic adults distinctive (e.g., inaccurate or vague words, revised utterances) . . . (p 118)," and described nine categories of those features (Table 4-6).

Several categories of performance deviations distinguished non–brain-damaged speakers from those with aphasia. Non–brain-damaged adults produced fewer inaccurate words, false starts, and part words or unintelligible productions than the aphasic adults. The non–brain-damaged adults also produced fewer instances of unnecessary exact repetition than fluent aphasic adults and produced fewer instances of the word "*and*" and less nonword filler than nonfluent aphasic adults. There were no differences between non–brain-damaged adults and adults with aphasia in the frequency with which they produced nonspecific words, filler words, or off-task words.

Brookshire and Nicholas suggested that measuring performance deviations in brain-damaged adults' connected speech provides a useful

T A B L E   4 - 6

Performance deviation categories.

Performance deviation	Definition	Examples
NonCIU Categories		
Inaccurate	Not accurate with regard to the stimulus and no attempt to correct.	. . . on a *chair* (for stool)
False start	False start or abandoned utterance.	. . . on *a chair . . no,* a stool
Unnecessary exact repetition	Exact repetition of words, unless used purposefully for emphasis or cohesion.	. . . on a *on a* stool
Nonspecific or vague	Nonspecific or vague words or words lacking an unambiguous referent.	. . . on a *thing* . . . on *it* (with no referent for "it")
Filler	Empty words that do not communicate information about the stimulus.	. . . on a . . *you know* . . stool
The word "and"	All occurrences of the word "and."	. . . a boy *and* a stool
Off-task or irrelevant	Commentary on the task or the speaker's performance.	*I've seen this one before. I can't say it.*
Nonword Categories		
Part word or unintelligible production	Word fragment or production that does not result in a word that is intelligible in context.	. . . on a *st . . sk* . . stool . . . on a *frampi*
Nonword filler	Utterances such "uh" or "um."	. . . on a . . *um* . . stool . . *ub*

Data From Brookshire and Nicholas, 1995.
Note. In the examples, only nonwords and words printed in boldface italics are scored as performance deviations.

supplement to other measures of communicative informativeness and efficiency. Although Brookshire and Nicholas studied only aphasic adults, their categories of performance deviations and and their scoring systems may be appropriate for quantifying the connected speech of brain-damaged adults in other diagnostic categories.

Speech Fluency Several methods for assessing brain-damaged adults' speech fluency have been described in the literature. None have been standardized, and their reliability remains to be documented, but they do provide procedures with which speech fluency can be assessed in more-or-less systematic fashion.

Wagenaar, Snow, and Prins (1975) described 30 measures for quantifying various characteristics of aphasic adults' connected speech. Among their conclusions were the following:

- The most useful measure for classifying aphasia patients on the basis of their speech production is *fluency.*
- Patients can be classified as fluent or nonfluent on the basis of *speech tempo* (words per minute) and *mean length of utterance.*
- Telegraphic speech and empty speech are separate syndromes.
- Grammatic and articulatory errors are separate factors and are not directly related to fluency.

Wagenaar and associates' procedures are too cumbersome for routine clinical use, but their list of measures and their findings may help clinicians develop systematic and practical procedures for analyzing aphasic patients' spontaneous speech.

Assessment of Intelligibility The speech of most patients with neurogenic *language* disorders caused by unilateral brain damage is intelligible. Consequently, assessment of intelligibility is not an important component of the evaluation of these patients. When intelligibility is a concern, *Assessing Intelligibility of Dysarthric Speech* (Yorkston & Beukelman, 1981) permits measurement of percent intelligibility of connected speech. Yorkston and Beukelman's procedure is described in Chapter 10.

■ ASSESSING WRITTEN EXPRESSION

Writing Subtests of Comprehensive Language Tests All the major comprehensive language tests include subtests for assessing written expression at several levels, but no standardized free-standing tests designed for assessment of brain-damaged adults' writing are currently available. The writing subtests in comprehensive language tests permit clinicians to assess written expression at four levels: *generating automatized sequences, copying, writing to dictation,* and *writing self-formulated material.* However, there are minor differences in test content within levels, and some comprehensive language tests include writing subtests not seen in the others. For example, the MTDDA includes a subtest in which patients *orally* spell words dictated by the examiner in the *Visuomotor and Writing Disturbances* section even though no written output is required.

In *generating automatized sequences* subtests, the patient is asked to write overlearned sequences (usually the alphabet and numbers from 1 to 20 and sometimes the patient's name). Scoring of patients' responses differs across tests but usually involves counting misspellings, omissions, transpositions, and illegible productions. Producing automatized sequences usually is the easiest writing subtest for most brain-damaged adults. Many can write strings of consecutive numbers and letters when they can produce little else in the way of written material. Signing one's name is a highly automatized activity for most adults, and many brain-damaged adults who cannot generate strings of letters or numbers can write their name fluently and with little effort.

Copying subtests require patients to copy geometric forms, symbols, letters, printed words, or printed sentences. Adults with posterior brain damage often have unusual difficulty with copying subtests, perhaps because of impairments in visual perception and discrimination. Aphasic patients usually do well at copying simple stimuli, such as forms, symbols, and letters, but their performance deteriorates when they copy words and sentences, wherein spelling errors, syntactic errors, and word substitutions may appear. Nonfluent aphasic patients who are weak or paralyzed in their preferred hand and arm usually produce distorted representations of stimuli in copying tests because of the mechanical difficulty of producing forms or letters with their nonpreferred hand and arm.

The *writing to dictation* subtests in comprehensive aphasia tests follow a letter-word-sentence progression. Patients are asked to write letters, then words, then sentences to dictation.

In *letter transcription* subtests the patient writes letters or numbers dictated by the examiner, not in alphabetic or numeric sequence. The PICA includes a subtest in which the examiner spells the names of the PICA test objects aloud, first at a moderate rate, pausing between syllables. If the patient fails at that level, the examiner spells each word letter-by-letter, pausing while the patient writes each letter. The latter procedure is equivalent to the letter-transcription and number-transcription procedures in the other comprehensive language tests. Spelling words aloud without pausing between letters makes heavy demands on auditory memory and spelling ability, and for many brain-damaged adults writing words dictated letter-by-letter is more difficult than writing words to dictation.

All major comprehensive language tests include subtests in which patients *write words to dictation.* The examiner may say a phrase containing the target word and then repeat it, as in the MTDDA *("I went to the dentist. Write went."),* but most often the examiner simply explains the procedure to the patient, then says the target words one at a time. *("Now I'll say some words one at a time. I want you to write each word after I say it. Say _____.").* Some comprehensive language tests provide backup procedures when the patient cannot write a word. In the BDAE the examiner asks the patient to spell orally the words he or she cannot write or to spell them manually using anagram letters. When a patient misses a word in the spelling subtest of the WAB the examiner orally spells the word while the patient writes it letter by letter, and if the patient still fails, the examiner provides anagram letters with which the patient can manually spell the word. Tests in which patients write words to dictation are primarily tests of spelling ability, although performance may also be affected by impairments in auditory retention and visuomotor abilities.

The BDAE, the MTDDA, and the WAB each provide a subtest in which patients' ability to *write sentences to dictation* is assessed. In the BDAE the (three) sentences relate to the *"cookie theft"* picture: *("She can't see them. . ." The boy is stealing cookies. . ." "If he is not careful the stool will fall.)."* The MTDDA subtest includes seven sentences ranging in length from two words *("Come in.")* to thirteen words *("There is a church, a drugstore, and a filling station on the corner.").*

All major comprehensive aphasia tests include subtests in which patients write material for which the examiner provides no spoken model. For most brain-damaged adults the easiest of these subtests are *written confrontation*

naming subtests in which the patient is shown a drawing or an object and asked to write its name. (The WAB provides an object-based subtest as a backup for the *writing words to dictation* subtest. When a patient fails to write the name of an object in the writing-to-dictation subtest, they are shown the object and asked to write its name.)

The MTDDA and the PICA include subtests that require *writing self-formulated sentences.* In the MTDDA the patient is asked to create and write a sentence containing each of six printed words. In the PICA the patient is asked to write the functions of each of the 10 PICA test objects *("As completely as possible, write here what you do with each of these.").*

The BDAE, the MTDDA, and the WAB each contain a written version of the picture-description subtest described earlier. In each test, the patient is asked to write a paragraph about the picture he or she has previously described orally. (See Figure 4-25 for the pictures used in these subtests.)

Free-Standing Tests of Written Expression Few free-standing writing tests are commonly used in evaluation of brain-damaged adults' writing abilities, perhaps because the subtests in comprehensive aphasia tests are sufficient for most clinical purposes. However, written spelling tests such as the spelling subtest of the *Wide Range Achievement Test* (Jastak & Wilkinson, 1984) sometimes are used to evaluate brain-damaged adults' written spelling.

■ THE EFFECTS OF MANAGED CARE ON ASSESSMENT OF NEUROGENIC COMMUNICATION DISORDERS

The foregoing description of tests and procedures for assessment of brain-damaged adults' language and communication is consistent with clinical practice during the past several decades. It may be a somewhat less-accurate description of clinical practice in the next 10 years because changes in the way health care is paid for are having strong effects on how health care is provided and promise to affect the future delivery of health-care services in important ways. Some of the most striking effects are likely to be on the scope and complexity of assessment and diagnostic procedures.

In *managed care,* organizations or institutions who pay for health care *(third-party payors)* pay a fixed price for the health care of a patient or, more frequently, a group of patients. For example, a corporation with 1,000 employees might contract with a health-care provider (a group of physicians, allied health practitioners, and administrators) to provide 1 year of health care for its employees for, say, $850,000. In return for the $850,000 the provider agrees to provide comprehensive medical care (office visits, examinations, tests, medical and surgical procedures, rehabilitation services, and so on) for the corporation's 1,000 employees and their dependents. Because most providers are in business to make a profit, they expect their actual cost per employee to be less than $850. If the provider can care for the corporation's employees for an average cost of $600 per employee, they make $250,000 profit on the contract, but if their average cost is $950 per employee the provider loses $100,000. Thus managed care has a built-in incentive for keeping down the cost of medical care (which is one of the primary purposes of managed care).

The positive side of managed care is that it rewards efficiency. Efficient providers make a profit and inefficient ones go out of business. The negative side of managed care is that its emphasis on reducing costs can compromise the quality of care provided to patients served by the managed-care provider. Physicians may be encouraged to forego expensive tests that might provide potentially important information about the nature of a patient's medical problems, to substitute cheaper, but less effective, treatments for more expensive and more effective ones, to postpone elective procedures, or to change their traditional way of caring for patients to better fit the financial imperatives of the provider.

The effects of managed care are not confined to physicians. Psychologists, social workers, occupational and physical therapists, speech-language pathologists, and other allied-health practitioners also are affected. Shortened in-hospital lengths of stay can make evaluation something of a race, with practitioners competing for the limited number of appointment times available during a patient's stay. Evaluations that at one time could be spread across several sessions may now have to be completed in a single test session. Comprehensive evaluation of a patient's impairments may be replaced by selective testing of a patient's most obvious deficits. Treatment options may be reduced. Some groups of patients who traditionally have received treatment may not receive it and patients who do receive treatment may get it in less-frequent and shorter treatment sessions.

For the speech-language pathologist concerned with assessment and diagnosis of brain-damaged adults' linguistic and communicative impairments, test administration time is likely to become increasingly important, given contemporary pressures from employers and health-care funding agencies to increase efficiency and decrease costs. In a health-care system that emphasizes economy and efficiency, tests requiring 2 to 6 hours to administer, score, and interpret will be at a significant disadvantage relative to shorter and quicker tests.

Maintaining quality of care under these conditions will pose a major challenge. Sensitive and reliable screening tests to detect communication impairments and give a general sense of the pattern of those impairments will become increasingly important. Comprehensive test batteries may have to be shortened and made more efficient, perhaps by providing norms for individual subtests or combinations of subtests.* Most contemporary comprehensive language tests could stand (and perhaps benefit from) some pruning. The danger is that the pruning will lop off too much, leaving clinicians with incomplete or inaccurate descriptions of their patients' impairments.

The days of comprehensive language testing may be numbered. If they are, speech-language pathologists and other practitioners must work to ensure that gains in economy and efficiency do not come at the expense of their understanding of their patients' impairments and do not compromise their ability to provide the most efficacious treatment for those impairments.

■ KEY CONCEPTS

- The left hemisphere of right-handed adults (and most left-handed ones) has the primary responsibility for speech and language processes. Aphasias caused by damage in the anterior language-dominant hemisphere typically are characterized by nonfluent speech and relatively preserved comprehension. Aphasias caused by damage in the posterior language-dominant hemisphere typically are characterized by fluent speech and moderately to severely impaired comprehension.

- Localizationist models of speech and language processes emphasize the importance of the central zone of the language-dominant hemisphere. This zone encompasses *Broca's area* in the posterior inferior frontal lobe, *Wernicke's area* in the temporoparietal-occipital region, and the *arcuate fasciculus,* a band of nerve fibers that connects Broca's and Wernicke's areas. Broca's area is considered responsible for planning and organizing speech

movements, and Wernicke's area is considered responsible for comprehension of spoken or printed verbal material and for formulation of verbal output via speech or writing.

- Various nonlinguistic disorders may accompany aphasia. They include *disconnection syndromes,* in which communication between cortical areas is disturbed, *agnosias,* in which individuals fail to recognize stimuli in a given modality in spite of intact perception in the modality, and *apraxia,* in which the patterns or plans for volitional movement sequences are disrupted.

- Some aphasia syndromes have been linked to subcortical pathology, although the relationships between subcortical structures and language processes are not well understood.

- Comprehensive language tests provide an overall impression of general language performance and are the starting point for assessment of language and related abilities. The primary purpose of assessment is to identify the deficient processes that account for the patient's comprehension and production impairments. Another important purpose is to identify unimpaired or minimally impaired linguistic and cognitive processes. Freestanding tests often are administered after a comprehensive language test to describe a patient's individual pattern of impairments and preserved abilities in more detail.

- Assessment of listening and reading comprehension requires measurement of the patient's comprehension of single words, sentences, and discourse. The vehicles for assessment include subtests from comprehensive language tests and freestanding tests of listening and reading comprehension.

- Assessment of speech production requires measurement of syllable, word, sentence, and discourse production. Assessment of speech production at the word and sentence level depends primarily on speech production subtests from comprehensive language

---

* Some existing comprehensive language tests already provide subtest-by-subtest norms. Because they permit subtest-by-subtest comparisons of a patient with norms, these comprehensive language tests should prove particularly appealing to clinicians who wish to shorten their testing protocol.

tests. In-depth assessment of naming and discourse production requires administration of freestanding tests designed for these purposes.

- Assessment of writing usually has a somewhat lower priority than assessment of listening comprehension, reading, and speech production, perhaps because impaired listening, reading, and speaking have more serious daily life consequences than impaired writing. For most aphasic adults, assessment of writing is limited to word and sentence writing.

The Context for Treatment of Neurogenic Communication Disorders

■ THE TREATMENT TEAM

Contemporary medical care is oriented around the concept of the treatment team. Under the treatment team concept, the responsibility for a patient's overall care rests with a group, rather than with one person or with independently operating professionals, although one member of the team usually has primary responsibility for coordinating the team's activities. Which professions are represented on a patient's treatment team depends on the nature of the patient's physical and medical problems. For example, the treatment team for a patient with chronic obstructive pulmonary disease might include a pulmonary physician, a cardiologist, a respiratory therapist, an occupational therapist, a nurse, and a social worker. The treatment team for a stroke patient might include a neurologist, a nurse, a speech-language pathologist, a neuropsychologist, a physical therapist, an occupational therapist, and a dietitian. Each member of the team has primary responsibility for a given aspect of the patient's care, but responsibilities often overlap so that planning, coordination, and communication among team members is crucial if the treatment program is to be efficient and effective.

Speech-language pathologists who participate in the care of brain-damaged adults are likely to serve on teams with an assortment of other professionals, and, as noted above, the composition of the team for any given patient depends primarily on the patient's needs. Even though one cannot always predict who will be on a given patient's treatment team, speech-language pathologists who work with brain-damaged adults often serve on teams with representatives of the following professions.

Neurologists As described previously, neurologists have primary responsibility for the medical care of patients with brain damage or other nervous system pathology. Because their role in patient care has been described in detail earlier in this book, it will not be repeated here.

Physiatrists (Rehabilitation Medicine Physicians) Physiatrists have primary medical responsibility for patients admitted to rehabilitation wards. They help physically disabled patients regain the use of impaired muscles and, when restitution of function is not possible, they help the patient compensate for the muscular impairments. Physiatrists examine the patient, determine the patient's medical and rehabilitation needs, design comprehensive rehabilitation programs, and oversee the activities of physical, occupational, corrective, vocational, and recreational therapists.

Physical Therapists Physical therapists evaluate the patient's muscle strength and range of limb movement. Under the supervision of a physiatrist they also carry out programs to help patients retain or regain muscle strength and limb movement. When a patient is confined to bed, a physical therapist may see the patient at bedside and teach the patient how to turn over in bed, sit up, and transfer from the bed to a chair or wheelchair. Physical therapists carry out passive range-of-movement exercises, in which bedbound patients' limbs are moved and muscles are stretched to prevent contractures (permanent shortening of muscles resulting from spasticity) and to preserve muscle strength and tone. Other physical therapy activities take place in the physical therapy clinic and include teaching patients how to transfer to and from a wheelchair, how to use braces, canes, and crutches, and how to get dressed, together with muscle strengthening and range-of-movement activities. If a patient is about to be discharged

home or to a nursing home, the physical therapist may help the family or nursing home staff prepare the living environment for the special needs of the patient and may provide the patient with exercise programs to be done at home.

Occupational Therapists Occupational therapists help patients regain abilities necessary for activities of daily living (ADLs), such as cooking, dressing, and grooming. Although both occupational and physical therapists work on muscle strengthening, occupational therapists usually work on muscles in activities that resemble those of daily living. A patient who needs to strengthen hands and arms might sand boards, saw wood, or weave on a loom. A patient with visuospatial impairments might perform craft activities requiring eye-hand coordination. An important part of occupational therapists' responsibilities is to help the patient resume daily life activities, such as cooking, cleaning, and making beds. They teach compensatory strategies, provide special tools and appliances, and modify standard tools and appliances to help patients compensate for their disabilities. Occupational therapists help patients develop leisure activities and hobbies and they sometimes test and treat patients for sensorimotor and visuospatial disorders. Because occupational therapists often deal with visual perception and reading or writing, speech-language pathologists often collaborate with them on improving these aspects of the patient's daily life communication.

Vocational Therapists Vocational therapists provide vocational testing and evaluation. They administer work-aptitude tests and real or simulated on-the-job evaluations to determine if the patient can go back to work. Vocational therapists sometimes arrange appropriate job placements or modify a patient's work environment and responsibilities to enable them to perform a job successfully. In some medical facilities, occupational therapists provide vocational testing and evaluation.

Corrective Therapists Corrective therapists are primarily responsible for ambulation training. They collaborate with physical and occupational therapists to help the patient regain the strength, balance, and endurance needed for walking and may teach the patient how to use crutches and canes and how to climb and descend stairs.

Recreation Therapists Recreation therapists provide therapeutic recreational activities (usually arts and crafts) and may get the patient started in leisure activities that can be continued by the patient following discharge from the medical facility.

Neuropsychologists Neuropsychologists administer tests of cognitive functions (attention, memory, mental flexibility, intellect, and so on), which may help to discriminate between psychiatric and neurologic conditions, distinguish between different neurologic conditions, and predict the course of a patient's recovery. Neuropsychologists provide the treatment team with information about the patient's adjustment to his or her disabilities and his or her present and future cognitive and behavioral abilities and limitations. They participate in planning and carrying out a plan of care for the patient and may have primary responsibility for assessing the effects of treatment on the patient's cognitive abilities. Neuropsychologists often collaborate closely with speech-language pathologists in planning the patient's care and in assessing brain-damaged patients' cognitive and communicative status. The neuropsychologist takes the lead in evaluating cognitive functions, such as perception, attention, and memory, while the speech-language pathologist takes primary responsibility for evaluating communicative and linguistic abilities.

Clinical Psychologists Clinical psychologists administer and interpret tests of intelligence, cognition, and personality, and provide the patient-care team with information about the patient's intellectual, cognitive, and emotional state. A clinical psychologist may help the

patient and family deal with the emotional and psychologic effects of the patient's brain damage on the family. When a patient is depressed or anxious, the clinical psychologist may help the patient and family deal with the feelings.

Psychiatrists Some brain-damaged patients develop symptoms of depression, psychosis, neurosis, or other personality aberrations. A psychiatrist may provide diagnostic, referral, and treatment services for these patients (especially when medications to control the patient's psychiatric symptoms are appropriate).

Dietitians Dietitians evaluate patients' nutritional needs and recommend dietary adjustments to remediate nutritional deficiencies. Dietitians work with the other members of the treatment team to ensure that the patient's food and liquid intake are sufficient to meet nutritional and hydration needs. Dietitians often collaborate with speech-language pathologists to set up special diets and feeding programs for patients with *dysphagia* (swallowing disorders) caused by neurologic or structural damage that affects the mechanics of chewing and swallowing.

Speech-Language Pathologists Speech-language pathologists provide assessment, treatment, and referral services for communication disorders and related impairments. Speech-language pathologists often play a prominent part on treatment teams for brain-damaged patients with communication disorders because they are experienced in communicating with these patients. Because the speech-language pathologist's work with communicatively impaired patients often touches on the patient's personal concerns, they often learn a great deal about the needs and concerns of the patient and family. Consequently, the speech-language pathologist often plays an important part in communicating the needs and concerns of the patient and family members to the treatment team.

Social Workers Social workers coordinate and manage communication between medical facility staff and the patient and family. Social workers keep families informed about treatment and discharge plans. They suggest, initiate, and coordinate referrals to medical, financial, and social-service agencies and programs. They may provide patients and families with information about nursing homes, county and state medical and family services, and other social and community resources that help the patient and family adjust to altered financial, vocational, and social conditions in daily life. Social workers ensure that physicians' orders for wheelchairs and other prosthetic appliances to be provided at discharge are carried out, and the social worker may make arrangements for programs such as meals on wheels or public health nurse visits to the patient's home. Social workers coordinate evaluations of legal competence for patients whose competence is questionable and make referrals to psychological and mental health services, chemical dependency programs, social security or veterans administration counselors, financial advisors, vocational counselors, or family and marriage counselors. Social workers play a key role in coordinating interactions among the medical facility staff, the patient, the patient's family, and community and state agencies. Social workers help the patient and family adjust to changed life styles and ensure that the patient's post-hospital placement represents the needs, wishes, and current circumstances of the patient and the family.

The treatment team approach can significantly improve both the quality and the efficiency of patient care by ensuring that a comprehensive treatment plan addressing all important aspects of the patient's care is created and followed, by maximizing communication among members of the team, and by delegating important components of care to team members who are professionally qualified to assume responsibility for them. The remainder of this chapter will address how speech-language pathologists carry out their treatment responsibilities for brain-damaged patients, beginning with an overview of patient characteristics that

may indicate whether a patient is likely to benefit from treatment.

■ CANDIDACY FOR TREATMENT

The process of deciding which patients with neurogenic communication disorders should get treatment has received little attention in the literature; due perhaps to the number of factors that enter into the process as well as the subjective nature of the decisions. Although there are no immutable rules that permit clinicians to separate the good treatment candidates from the poor ones, there are several general principles that can be used to guide the decision-making process.

The amount and location of a patient's brain damage are important determinants of her or his potential response to treatment. The greater the brain damage and the more the damage includes areas of the brain involved in communication, the less likely it is that the patient will recover communication abilities, with or without treatment. The size and location of a patient's brain damage can be estimated directly from laboratory measures such as CT or MRI scans, or estimated indirectly from behavioral measures, such as tests of speech, language, memory, and cognition. However, the relationship between lesion size, lesion location, and behavioral deficits may be weak immediately following strokes or traumatic brain injuries when temporary bilateral reduction of cerebral blood flow, neurotransmitter release, cerebral edema, and diaschisis are present. For this reason, clinicians may choose to wait several weeks before deciding not to treat a patient because of the severity of her or his brain injury.

A patient's medical and physical condition almost always affect the outcome of treatment. Ill, depressed, or physically weak patients may not profit sufficiently from treatment to justify its cost. Patients who cannot sit up and attend to a task for 30 minutes may not be strong enough to tolerate intensive treatment, and the clinician may elect to forego treatment or at least to defer it until the patient recovers sufficient health and strength to benefit from treatment.

A patient's enthusiasm and motivation to recover often have powerful effects on the outcome of treatment. Some highly motivated and resourceful patients may benefit from treatment in spite of severe impairments. Some unmotivated or unconcerned patients may fail to benefit from treatment even though their impairments are not severe. A patient's life situation may also affect the outcome of treatment. A supportive, motivated, and caring family can enhance the effects of treatment programs, while a nonsupportive, unmotivated, and uncaring family may compromise them.

Clinicians often resolve their doubts about the appropriateness of treatment for questionable treatment candidates by offering a short interval of trial treatment. If the patient responds well to the trial treatment, treatment continues, and if the patient responds poorly to the trial treatment, treatment is terminated. Most clinicians would offer trial treatment to all questionable treatment candidates if they were free to do so, to minimize the chances of missing patients who are good treatment candidates. Given unlimited professional and financial resources, every patient with a neurogenic communication disorder would get at least a trial period of treatment. However, health-care funding is increasingly limited, and health-care providers face increasingly severe restrictions on who receives treatment and how much the treatment costs. This means that identifying those patients who are likely to benefit most from treatment will become an increasingly important part of the clinician's responsibilities. Limitations on resources will require that treatment be provided to those who are likely to receive the greatest benefit at the least cost. The issues of how benefit is defined and what constitutes a reasonable cost-benefit ratio are complex, and one's attitude depends greatly on the direction from which one looks at the problem.

The issue is one that every clinician must eventually face, although few feel they have satisfactorily resolved it.

Patients have the right to refuse treatment, even though a clinician may feel that treatment is indicated. If the patient understands the nature of his or her communication disabilities, his or her potential effects on the patient and family, and the nature and potential benefits of treatment, and nevertheless refuses treatment the patient's refusal must be accepted. If a patient is confused, intellectually impaired, or otherwise not competent to refuse potentially beneficial treatment, family members or others with the right to represent the patient may decide for the patient.

■ GENERAL CHARACTERISTICS OF TREATMENT SESSIONS

Frequency and Duration How frequently brain-damaged adults are seen for treatment and how long their treatment lasts are affected by several variables. One variable is the patient's medical and physical condition. Immediately after brain injury, and for intervals that last anywhere from a few days to several weeks, many patients' physical and mental endurance are compromised by the physiologic effects of their brain injury. For these patients, 15-minute to 30-minute treatment sessions may be best, with the length of sessions increasing as they recover their physical and mental stamina.* To increase short-time-post-onset patients' exposure to treatment while keeping the length of treatment sessions within a patient's tolerance, a patient may be scheduled for multiple daily treatment sessions (e.g., one session in the morning and one in the afternoon.)

_____

* Many facilities bill for speech-language pathology services in 15-minute increments, making 15-minute treatment sessions a possibility. However, unless the patient is seen at bedside, the logistics of getting the patient to and from the speech pathology clinic usually make 15-minute sessions impractical.

The complexity of a treatment program also affects the length of treatment sessions needed to carry it out. Some simple treatment programs may have only a single objective that can be accomplished by one or two treatment tasks (e.g., speech production drills to increase a dysarthric patient's speech intelligibility). Thirty-minute sessions may be sufficient for such programs. Complex treatment programs with several objectives typically need more time (e.g., treatment of a right-hemisphere–damaged patient to facilitate affective expression, improve abstract thinking, diminish tangentiality in spontaneous speech, and improve turn-taking behavior in conversations).

Logistics often play an important part in determining a patient's treatment schedule. Close by and accessible patients can reasonably be scheduled for shorter and more frequent appointments than those who are farther away or less accessible. Ambulatory hospitalized patients who can get themselves up, dressed, and to the clinic are logistically easier to schedule for multiple appointments than patients for whom a journey to the clinic requires that ward personnel get the patient up, dressed and into a wheelchair, and that an escort bring the patient to the clinic and return him or her to the ward. It usually is not practical for outpatients to come to the clinic more than once a day and most end up with twice-a-week or three-times-a-week appointments. Outpatients who attend other clinics (such as physical therapy) on a regular schedule often can have their appointments scheduled so that they can keep both appointments with one trip to the treatment facility.*

For patients who are approaching discharge, making treatment sessions shorter and increas-ing the time between sessions can provide a transition between intensive treatment and discharge. As patients approach discharge, the emphasis is on consolidation of the patient's current performance and extension of that performance to daily life. As the patient approaches discharge, the content of treatment sessions moves away from training new strategies and behaviors to enhancing generalization of already-learned strategies and behaviors to the patient's daily life. Shorter and more widely spaced sessions can contribute to the generalization process.

Format Treatment sessions tend to have a consistent format. Most begin with a period of conversation (the *hello segment*), in which the clinician and the patient talk about what has happened since the last session. The patient recounts achievements, significant happenings, and problems, and the clinician applauds the achievements, discusses the happenings, and helps with the problems. The clinician also uses this time to evaluate the patient's performance relative to previous sessions, to estimate the extent to which treated behaviors are generalizing to conversational interactions, and to appraise the patient's mood and energy level. The hello segment gives the patient time to settle in, get comfortable, get problems and concerns out of the way, and helps to establish and maintain personal rapport between the patient and the clinician.

The hello segment leads into a short interval of work on easy tasks in which the patient's performance is nearly error free (the *accommodation segment*). The tasks in the accommodation segment usually are tasks that the patient has mastered in previous sessions. The accommodation segment gets the patient into the sequence and timing of treatment procedures and provides him or her with a warm-up for the more difficult tasks that follow in the *work segment*.

The work segment is the heart of the treatment session. Tasks become more challenging and are focused on specific treatment objec-

---

* The policies of the agencies who pay for treatment are another important determinant of appointment schedules. For example, some agencies will pay for only a predetermined number of speech pathology appointments for patients with a particular communication disorder. Speech-language pathologists frequently must work within such limits when setting up appointment schedules for their patients.

tives. The clinician instructs, explains, delivers treatment stimuli, provides feedback, and records the patient's performance. The patient works at or near her or his maximum capacity in each treatment task. The interaction between the clinician and the patient is governed by the treatment protocol—the clinician's contributions and the patient's responses are task directed. There is little purely social interaction except for transitions between tasks.

Many clinicians follow the work segment with some work on familiar tasks in which the patient is highly successful (the *cool-down segment*). The patient's successful performance in cool-down tasks can contribute to a sense of accomplishment that generalizes to the session as a whole. Many clinicians end treatment sessions with a short interval of conversation about what happened in the session, what the patient plans to do before the next session, and what the clinician and patient plan to do in the next session (the *goodbye segment*).

The foregoing generic format described how the focus of typical treatment sessions changes within the sessions. Not every clinician follows this format and those who do may not follow it in every session, but may deviate from it or abandon it altogether, depending on what he or she perceives as the patient's needs. In the next section, the generic content of treatment sessions will be discussed beginning with how clinicians manipulate the characteristics of treatment tasks to provide them with maximum therapeutic power. Adjusting treatment tasks to the patient's level of performance is a key element of these manipulations.

After more than a century of study, treatment of adults with neurogenic communication disorders remains as much art as science. Hundreds of data-based studies of neurogenic communication disorders have been published but only a small fraction of studies are directly relevant to treatment. Many treatment procedures have been described in the literature but most are little more than descriptions of the procedures,

with anecdotes or the authors' opinions substituting for empirical evidence of their efficacy. Consequently, most decisions about how to approach a given patient's communication impairments rely more on the clinician's experience and intuition than on empirical evidence. Beginning clinicians are not, however, condemned to trial and error as their only guide while they accumulate the experiences and intuitions that create clinical expertise. The clinical and research literature reveals regularities in how adults with neurogenic communication disorders respond to manipulations of the clinical environment and shows that most patients with a particular pattern of communication impairments respond to the manipulations in predictable ways, although idiosyncratic responses are common. For example, the performance of most brain-damaged adults is adversely affected by noisy or distraction-loaded environments but a few may perform as well in noisy and distracting conditions as they do in quiet ones. The following section summarizes some regularities that permit clinicians to manipulate certain aspects of treatment to accomplish their clinical objectives. The section begins with a brief discussion of resource-allocation models of cognition and the application of these models to treatment of brain-damaged adults.

■ ADJUSTING TREATMENT TASKS TO THE PATIENT
Resource-Allocation Models and the Clinical Process

Many adults with brain damage have perceptual, attentional, cognitive, and performance impairments that compromise their ability to perceive and discriminate sensory input, diminish the flexibility and efficiency of their cognitive processes, and compromise the speed and accuracy of their responses to stimulation. Clinicians who work with brain-damaged adults are obliged to deal with the effects of these impairments on the patient's performance throughout assessment and treatment. Fortunately, there are many ways in which clinicians can manipulate the characteristics of assessment and treatment procedures to lessen the effects of these impairments. However, knowing which characteristics of the procedures to manipulate requires that the clinician have an idea of why the patient is having trouble. If the clinician knows *why* the patient is having trouble, *how* to treat the patient becomes more apparent.

Resource allocation models of cognitive processes provide a convenient metaphor for organizing the search for the causes of impaired performance, which in turn contributes to an organized approach to improving performance. Several resource allocation models of cognitive processing have been described in the literature (Friedman & Polson, 1981; Holtzman & Gazzaniga, 1982; Kahneman, 1973; Norman & Bobrow, 1975). McNeil and associates (McNeil & Kimelman, 1986; McNeil Odell, & Tseng, 1990) have described a resource-allocation model for adult aphasia. Although the models differ in details, they share a common theme, which is that every human has a finite amount of cognitive resources available for carrying out mental operations such as perceiving incoming stimuli, comprehending messages, storing information in memory, and formulating responses. In resource allocation models the mental operations are called *cognitive processes,* and the mental energy, which is contained in a *central pool,* is called *processing resources.*

Activation of any cognitive process depends on transfer of resources from the pool to the process. Processes of greater complexity require more resources than processes of lesser complexity. If several cognitive processes are simultaneously active, each draws resources from the pool. Consequently, the amount of processing resources drawn from the pool depends both on the number of active cognitive processes and their complexity. As more processes are activated and as the complexity of the active processes increases, more resources are drawn from the pool. If the demand for resources exceeds the amount available in the pool, some processes may be shut down or shortchanged, and the performance of the system suffers. Because there is only one resource pool for all cognitive processes and because the resources in the pool are limited, increasing the resources allocated to one cognitive process diminishes the amount available for others. When processing demands are low this is not a problem, because the pool contains enough resources to keep all the active cognitive processes in business. However, as processing demands reach the capacity of the pool, either calls for more resources from individual processes are ignored, or resources are diverted from other active processes to the one making the call. In either case, performance deteriorates.*

Many resource-allocation models propose that the availability of resources in the central pool is not constant but varies in quasi-random fashion across time. The reasons for this variability are unknown, but the individual's emotional state, level of fatigue, the metabolic activity of the individual's brain, and other such changeable conditions may contribute to it. By incorporating cyclical, quasi-random patterns of resource availability, resource-allocation models attempt to explain the variability in performance that customarily is seen when individuals are working at or near their processing capacity (e.g., comprehension of a lecture by a university student waxes and wanes across 20 or 30 minutes, even though the complexity of the lecture does not change).

When resource-allocation models attempt to explain the performance of brain-damaged adults, most assume that brain damage reduces the

---

* In contemporary resource allocation models, separate pools for different categories of cognitive processes are postulated. In these models, increasing the call for resources from one pool does not affect the resources available from the other pools, and the effects of shortages in a pool will be seen only on cognitive processes that depend on that pool. To keep it simple, this discussion will assume a single-pool model.

amount of available processing resources in the pool.* Consequently, the pool runs out of resources at lower-than-normal levels of processing workload, causing the brain-damaged person to perform poorly on many tasks that she or he could easily do before acquiring brain damage, and to perform poorly relative to adults without brain damage. Resource-allocation models assume that when a brain-damaged person is performing tasks in which the need for processing resources is well below the capacity of the person's resource pool, her or his performance should be essentially normal. As the number or complexity of processing demands approach the capacity of the pool, the brain-damaged person's performance begins to deteriorate, becoming progressively worse as the processing demands reach and exceed the available resources. Importantly, if some elements of the tasks are simplified, thereby diminishing their demands on the pool, the brain-damaged person's performance improves. The following example shows how this works.

A brain-damaged aphasic patient who also has a visuoperceptual impairment is asked to point to black-and-white line drawings of objects when the clinician describes them by function (*Point to the one used for writing and erasing*). After 10 trials he has made 8 errors. When the clinician pauses after the tenth trial, the patient complains that he is having trouble making out what the drawings represent. The clinician trades the drawings for colored photographs and does 10 more trials. The patient makes only 3 errors in those 10 trials.

---

* Whether the brain damage reduces the amount of resources in the pool or compromises access to the resources in the pool without diminishing the volume of the pool is not known. In either case, the effects on performance would be similar, though not identical in all situations.

This patient had trouble with two aspects of the task: auditory comprehension and visual perception of the line drawings. In resource-allocation terms, the patient's problems perceiving and comprehending the auditory and visual inputs increased the processing workload to a level at which it exceeded the resources available. By changing the stimuli from line drawings to more realistic colored photographs, the clinician reduced the complexity of the visual processing required to perform the task, freeing resources that could be redirected to auditory comprehension, which then improved. If the treatment focus had been on perception and recognition of line drawings, the clinician could have facilitated the patient's identification of the line drawings by reducing the difficulty of the auditory comprehension aspects of the task, thereby freeing additional resources for visual processing.

This *quid pro quo* (one thing in return for another) characteristic of resource-allocation models has important implications for clinicians working with brain-damaged adults. The general principle is that clinicians can focus treatment on a targeted process by controlling the processing load associated with incidental task variables that are not related to the treatment objectives. This is what happened in the preceding example when the clinician facilitated the patient's comprehension (the targeted process) by lowering the processing load associated with perceiving and recognizing the visual stimuli (an incidental task variable). Resource-allocation concepts help to sensitize clinicians to the potential unintended effects of incidental task variables when they design treatment tasks. Clinicians who are aware of these effects can control for them, so that treatment tasks focus on the intended processes and are not complicated by heavy processing demands associated with incidental task variables.

Because cognitive processes are internal, they cannot be directly manipulated. However, clinicians can indirectly manipulate processing workload by manipulating the characteristics of task stimuli and by changing the specifications for the responses expected from the patient. Stimulus manipulations permit clinicians to regulate the amount of resources the patient needs for perception, discrimination, and interpretation of task stimuli. Changing the specifications for the patient's responses permits clinicians to regulate the amount of resources needed for formulating and producing the responses. First we will consider how clinicians can regulate patients' workload by manipulating stimulus input. Then we will see how clinicians can adjust the patient's workload by manipulating response specifications.

Stimulus Manipulations

Clinicians can manipulate the difficulty of treatment tasks by adjusting several characteristics of treatment task stimuli. These adjustments affect the workload associated with perception, discrimination, and comprehension of the task stimuli and move the task stimuli up or down a continuum of workload. These adjustments permit clinicians to design tasks that force the patient's processing system to operate at or near its maximum but do not overwhelm it. Clinicians can manipulate processing workload by adjusting the *intensity and salience,* the *clarity and intelligibility,* the *redundancy and contextual support,* or the *novelty and interest value* of task stimuli.

Intensity and Salience Increasing the intensity or salience of stimuli helps many brain-damaged patients perceive, discriminate, and comprehend them better. *Intensity* as used here, refers to the perceived magnitude or strength of a stimulus. *Salience* refers to the perceived prominence or conspicuousness of a stimulus—how clearly it stands out from its surroundings. In some ways intensity and salience are related because making a stimulus more intense (louder, brighter, bigger) usually makes it more salient. However, intensity and salience differ in that intensity is a property of the stimu-

lus itself, whereas salience expresses a relationship between the stimulus and its surroundings. A loud auditory stimulus presented against a noisy background may be less salient than a soft auditory stimulus presented against a silent background, and a brightly colored visual stimulus presented against a brightly colored and cluttered background may be less salient than a stimulus with more subdued colors presented against a plain and colorless background.

Increasing the intensity or salience of treatment stimuli can help brain-damaged patients whose impaired perceptual or attentional processes compromise their perception, recognition, or comprehension of the stimuli. For example, a patient with problems focusing and maintaining attention in the presence of distracting or competing stimuli may perform poorly in structured conversations when a radio is playing in the background. In resource-allocation terms, the effort required for the patient to maintain attention creates a need for increased processing resources. If resources are diverted from other processes (comprehension, for example) to shore up attention, attention gets better and the processes from which resources are diverted get worse (the patient attends but fails to comprehend). If the conversational partner increases the intensity of his or her contributions (by talking louder, moving in closer, adding gesture) or increases the salience of what he or she says (by turning down the radio or moving away from it) the patient's conversational performance improves, presumably because the resources needed to overcome the distracting effects of the background noise can be redirected to comprehension and other conversational operations.

Clinicians sometimes increase the salience of treatment stimuli by presenting them in more than one stimulus modality (most commonly auditory plus visual, as when a clinician simultaneously says the name of an object and shows the patient a picture of it). Several studies have reported slight-to-moderate improvements in brain-damaged adults' performance with multi-modality stimulation (Gardiner & Brookshire, 1972; Halpern, 1965; Lambrecht & Marshall, 1983). However, in almost every study in which positive effects of multimodality stimulation have been reported for groups of brain-damaged adults, not all of the subjects in the groups exhibited those effects. This suggests that clinicians only will know if multimodality stimulation will help a particular patient by trying it with that patient and observing its effects on the patient's performance.*

Clarity and Intelligibility Vague or ambiguous stimuli are notoriously difficult for almost all brain-damaged patients, and making stimuli clearer and more intelligible usually helps them (especially those with impaired perception, recognition, or discrimination of sensory stimuli). The negative effects of vagueness and ambiguity often are seen when treatment stimuli are line drawings representing common objects or situations. For patients with visual processing impairments, line drawings that seem unambiguous to the clinician may be ambiguous to the patient. For example, brain-damaged adults sometimes call the drawing of a harmonica in the *Boston Naming Test* (Kaplan, Goodglass, & Weintraub, 1983) a *building* or a *factory* (Figure 5-1).

Mills and associates (1979) studied the effects of what they called *stimulus uncertainty* on aphasic adults' naming of line drawings of common objects. Their measure of uncertainty for each drawing was the number of different names a group of 14 normal adults gave to the drawing. The more different names given to a drawing, the higher its uncertainty. When Mills and associates subsequently had a group of non–brain-damaged adults and a group of apha-

---

* This is true for almost all group studies involving manipulations of treatment stimuli. Although some manipulations seem to have relatively consistent effects across patients in the groups, exceptions are almost always encountered. Consequently, clinicians typically verify the effects of a manipulation by trying it with the patient.

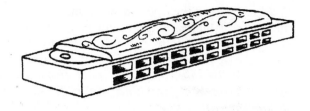

Figure 5-1 ▪ An example of a stimulus that sometimes proves ambiguous for brain-damaged adults with visual perceptual impairments, who frequently misidentify it as a building or factory. (From Kaplan E, Goodglass H, Weintraub S: *The Boston Naming Test.* Philadelphia, 1983, Lea & Febiger.)

sic adults name the drawings, they found that both groups took longer to name and were more likely to misname drawings with high uncertainty values. The effects of uncertainty on response times and error rates were greater for the aphasic subjects than for the non–brain-damaged subjects. Mills and associates recommended that item uncertainty be added to the list of variables that affect the speed and accuracy of aphasic adults' naming performance. (The operational definition of uncertainty provided by Mills and associates provides a way for clinicians or investigators to determine uncertainty values for stimuli used in their clinical activities or research.)

Redundancy and Context The words *redundancy* and *context* denote similar and sometimes overlapping concepts. *Redundancy* refers to the presence of information in a stimulus beyond that needed to specify the target response. For example, a clinician doing auditory comprehension drill might increase the redundancy of a command such as "Show me the small red cup," by saying, "I want you to show me a *cup* that is *red* and *small*. Show me the *small, red cup*." Redundancy almost always facilitates the performance of brain-damaged patients. For example, some patients perform poorly on point-to tasks in which they must point to objects named by the clinician (*"Point to the cup.")*, but their performance improves if the clinician increases the redundancy of the commands by asking the patient to point to objects the clinician describes by function. *("Point to the one you drink coffee from.")** *Repetition, paraphrase, and multi-modality stimulation are common ways of adding redundancy to task stimuli*

Context refers to the presence of a background or setting for a stimulus that provides information about the stimulus not found in the stimulus itself. For example, the clinician doing the auditory comprehension drill mentioned above might provide contextual support for the patient by changing the array of response choices from a group of randomly chosen objects to a group in which the cup is portrayed in its usual location: in a place setting on a table.

The context in which responses are elicited often has potent effects on brain-damaged patients' response accuracy. One of the most striking characteristics of the behavior of brain-damaged adults is that responses that are difficult or impossible in one context can be astonishingly easy in another. Most brain-damaged adults say more and say it better when they talk in natural communicative interactions than when they talk in acontextual and unnatural situations. Similar effects of context on performance are seen in listening, reading, and writing. The major exceptions are some distractible or impulsive right-hemisphere–damaged patients, some traumatically brain-injured patients, and a few aphasic patients who cannot handle unstructured natural situations as well as they handle structured situations in which distractions are minimized and the focus of the interaction is carefully controlled.

---

* However, some brain-damaged patients cannot handle the added information and do less well when task stimuli are made more redundant by adding information. The only way to find out who will profit from redundancy and who will not is to try adding redundancy on a few trials and see what happens.

Treatment tasks usually are carried out in supportive contexts. The clinician's instructions and directions are cohesive and complete. Task stimuli are carefully selected and consistent from trial to trial. The pace of stimulus delivery and responses is constant across treatment tasks. Background noise, distractions, and intrusions are minimized. Patients who perform flawlessly in such supportive contexts often break down when they leave the treatment room and have to deal with the less controlled and more chaotic situations of daily life. Clinicians sometimes help patients learn to deal with these less-than-ideal situations by adding negative context to treatment tasks. For example, when a patient's auditory comprehension reaches normal levels in the clinician's quiet office environment, the clinician may add background noise or move the activity into a noisy commons room to give the patient practice at comprehending in noisy environments such as those he or she may be faced with in daily life. Such replication of the elements of daily life environments helps to ensure that skills learned in the clinic will generalize to daily life by letting the patient practice the skills in situations that match those he or she is likely to encounter outside the sheltered clinic environment.

Novelty and Interest Value The novelty and interest value of treatment stimuli have less-obvious effects on brain-damaged patients' performance, and clinicians sometimes overlook these stimulus characteristics when they select stimuli for treatment tasks. This can be an important oversight because making treatment stimuli more novel and interesting often helps the patient perform better. For example, Faber and Aten (1979) asked aphasic adults to talk about drawings portraying common objects in their normal state and other drawings portraying the objects in broken or altered states (a pair of eyeglasses with a broken lens, a shirt with a torn sleeve, etc.). The aphasic adults produced significantly more appropriate words and significantly longer utterances when they talked about the drawings of broken or altered objects than when they talked about the drawings of intact objects.

An item in the *Communicative Abilities in Daily Living* measure (*CADL*; Holland, 1980) further illustrates the striking effects of novelty on brain-damaged adults' attention and comprehension. The item is contained in a role-playing section of CADL, in which the clinician plays the role of a physician who is giving the patient instructions on lifestyle. The clinician says, (*"Okay, Mr./Ms. _____, before our next visit I want you to smoke three packs of cigarettes and drink a bottle of gin a day. Okay?"*) Few brain-damaged patients fail to do a double-take in response to this item and most respond appropriately to it with more amusement, laughter, and commentary than is seen in their responses to the more prosaic CADL items.

The experience of many clinicians matches what Faber and Aten reported and replicates what occurs when patients respond to the doctor's lifestyle instructions in the CADL. Most brain-damaged patients attend, comprehend, and respond more accurately and with less effort when treatment materials are novel and/or personally interesting than when the materials are mundane or have limited personal relevance to the patient. A patient whose speech output is limited to single-word utterances when obliged to talk about cups and spoons, keys, and combs, produces full sentences when asked to talk about his or her family, hobbies, or profession. A patient who struggles to comprehend commands such as *"Show me the white cup."* easily gets the sense of longer and more complex utterances when he or she is personally relevant, as in *"Tell me what the weather was like on the day you got married."*

Cues and Prompts Clinicians usually manipulate the stimulus characteristics described above in a preplanned way. They specify the levels of the stimulus characteristics when they design the treatment task and they keep the levels constant across trials within the task. How-ever, most clinicians also manipulate some stimulus characteristics in a trial-by-trial impromptu fashion, most often when the patient appears to be having trouble. For example, a clinician might intervene to facilitate a struggling patient's production of the word *pen,* by saying, *"It starts with puh, it rhymes with ten,"* or *"It has ink and you write with it."* These clinician behaviors are called *cues* (Barton, Maruszewski, & Urrea, 1969; Li & Williams, 1990; Rochford & Williams, 1965; Stimley & Noll, 1991; and others).

Cues are hints a clinician gives when a patient is having difficulty getting a response out. The cues provide the patient with additional information that leads him or her in the direction of the target response without giving away the response itself. Strategic use of cues gives the clinician control over the pace of treatment tasks and permits him or her to adjust the processing load associated with an individual treatment trial. More importantly, cues give the clinician a dependable way to intervene and get the patient back on track when she or he is momentarily defeated by a treatment trial, thereby breaking up strings of error responses and keeping error rates at optimal levels. Cues are discussed in greater detail subsequently, when treatment of specific communication impairments is addressed.

Response Manipulations

As noted earlier, the second major way in which clinicians can control the processing demands of treatment tasks is by manipulating the characteristics of the responses required from their patients. By easing response requirements clinicians diminish the demands for resources associated with formulation and production of responses, and by requiring more complex and effortful responses clinicians escalate the processing workload associated with those aspects of treatment tasks. The two most obvious contributors to response workload are the *length* and *complexity* of the responses required from the patient. Less obvious contributors are *familiarity and naturalness, response delay,* and *redundancy.*

Length and Complexity Length and complexity tend to interact, in that longer responses also tend to be more complex, although each can be manipulated separately. (Responses of the same length can differ in their level of complexity, and responses of different lengths can have the same overall level of complexity.) The length of responses usually is defined by measuring how many units (usually syllables or words) they contain or, less often, how much time it takes the patient to perform the responses.

The complexity of responses can be defined in many ways, most of which are more subjective than counting units or measuring time. In treatment tasks for brain-damaged adults, complexity may be defined in motoric terms (e.g., the number of different articulatory movements per word or per unit of time), in linguistic terms (e.g., the number of syntactic operations needed to determine the meaning of sentences), or in cognitive terms (e.g., the presumed amount of abstraction or inference needed to produce appropriate responses to spoken messages). As a general rule, increasing the length or complexity of responses increases their call for processing resources, and if resources are in short supply, increasing the length or complexity of responses causes performance to deteriorate. Importantly, the deterioration need not be limited to the adequacy of the responses themselves but may extend back to input processes, such as perception, discrimination, and comprehension, depending on how the patient's system attempts to compensate for the shortage of resources.

Familiarity and Meaningfulness The familiarity and meaningfulness of responses is related to the frequency with which a patient has performed the responses in the past. Highly practiced and socially meaningful responses (e.g., social greetings and farewells) almost always are easier for brain-damaged adults than infrequently practiced ones produced in unnatural contexts (e.g., naming objects or pictures), and many brain-damaged patients who can say little else can get out highly practiced social verbalizations such as *"hello"* and *"goodbye"* in the appropriate settings. The effects of familiarity go beyond speech. Brain-damaged patients with language comprehension impairments usually comprehend personally relevant material (e.g., questions about home and family) better than impersonal material (e.g., questions about the relative sizes of bicycles and locomotives). Brain-damaged patients with impaired vocabulary typically are more successful at accessing frequently occurring words (such as *house* and *woman*) than infrequently occurring words (such as *scholar* and *piccolo*).

Delay Many brain-damaged adults have impairments in immediate memory that interfere with their ability to maintain information or action plans in memory for more than a few seconds. One consequence of these impairments is that the patient's performance deteriorates when the clinician imposes delay intervals between the clinician's presentation of treatment stimuli and the opportunity for the patient to respond. A patient whose responses to spoken commands are quick and accurate when she or he is permitted to respond as soon as the clinician finishes saying each command may falter, equivocate, and make mistakes when the clinician requires a 5- or 10-second wait before the patient can respond. A patient who flawlessly repeats phrases after the clinician under no-delay conditions may stumble, struggle, and grope about when forced to retain the clinician's model in memory for 10 or 20 seconds before producing it.

Sometimes imposing (or permitting) delays between stimuli and responses improves rather than detracts from brain-damaged patients' performance. Most brain-damaged adults experience some general slowing of language processes. It takes them longer to retrieve the words they need to express their ideas. It takes them longer to combine words into meaningful strings. It takes them longer to recognize complex or unfamiliar stimuli. It takes them longer to deduce the meaning of incoming messages. Their need for increased processing time causes them to respond slowly, creating delays between treatment stimuli and the patient's responses. Most brain-damaged patients are excruciatingly aware of their slowness and feel obligated to get responses out as quickly as possible. Encouraging these patients to respond more quickly simply adds to their problems, whereas teaching them to resist the tyranny of the clock usually helps.

Some brain-damaged patients try to compensate for their immediate memory problems by responding quickly before the memory traces of the stimulus have time to decay. This strategy often leads them to "jump the gun," or to begin their response before the clinician has finished delivering the stimulus. This strategy rarely solves the patient's problems and often makes things worse, because the patient almost invariably misses the material that comes in after he or she has begun to respond. Imposing short delays between stimuli and responses often improves the performance of these hyperresponsive patients (Yorkston, Marshall, & Butler, 1977).

Although it is not always obvious which patients will be hurt by response delay and which will be helped by it, the following general guidelines may help. When a patient's immediate memory is compromised and when a treatment task makes demands on immediate memory, imposing response delays is likely to cause worsened performance. When a patient's internal processing is slow or inefficient and the treatment task calls upon those processes, permitting response delays may lead to improved performance.

What does the clinician do when a patient suffers both from immediate-memory impairments and slow or inefficient internal processes? If the clinician's purpose is to target immediate memory, then he or she might take slow processing out of the picture by slowing the rate at which stimuli are presented (thereby compensating for the patient's slowness and inefficiency in processing). The clinician might also set the delay between stimulus delivery and the time at which the patient is permitted to respond so as to put the appropriate amount of load on retention. If the clinician's purpose is to target the slow processing, then he or she might minimize memory demands by permitting the patient to respond immediately and adjust the rate at which the stimuli are presented to put an appropriate amount of load on the patient's processing speed and efficiency.

Response Redundancy The redundancy of responses sometimes can have important effects on the speed and accuracy of brain-damaged patients' responses. Response redundancy comes in two forms. In one form, elements are repeated within responses *(within-trials redundancy)*. In another form responses are repeated across trials *(across-trials redundancy)*. Within-trials redundancy is a prominent feature of many speech articulation drills in which the patient is asked to generate strings of words in which the same articulatory positions are repeated within each string (as in *baby—bible—bobbin—beanbag*). Across-trials redundancy is prominent in many different treatment tasks in which some characteristics of the responses are invariant across trials. (e.g., the pointing or gesturing responses called for on every trial of some auditory comprehension tasks). The ultimate in redundancy between task stimuli and the patient's responses happens when the clinician and patient produce responses in unison. One step down in redundancy are repetition tasks in which the patient's responses are direct copies of the clinician's productions, produced immediately after the clinician's productions.

■ HOW CLINICIANS DECIDE WHAT TO TREAT

A clinician's decisions regarding what to treat come from the clinician's conclusions about the nature of the patient's communicative impairment, the clinician's attitudes about the nature and purpose of therapy, and from the clinician's previous clinical successes and failures. There are no rules and few guiding principles, but a few general approaches to deciding what to treat have been described in the literature.

Perhaps the most commonly used approach to planning treatment is the *relative level of impairment* approach, in which the patient's performance on various tests is analyzed to identify "peaks" and "valleys" in the patient's performance profile. These peaks and valleys are then given special attention in treatment. Clinicians sometimes choose to treat in the valleys (areas of relative impairment) but are more likely to treat at the peaks (areas in which impairments are less pronounced). The relative-level-of-impairment approach has been most clearly explicated with reference to aphasia, but the principles apply equally well to treatment of patients with other neurogenic communication disorders.

Porch (1981b) described a relative-level-of-impairment approach based on variability in patients' performance within and across subtests of the *Porch Index of Communicative Ability* (*PICA*). Porch calls his measure of across-subtest variability the *high-low gap.* The high-low gap is calculated on the 18 subtests of the PICA. The average for the nine subtests with the highest scores and the average for the nine subtests with the lowest scores are calculated. The difference between the two averages is the *high-low gap.* According to Porch, the high-low gap represents, in part, the amount of change that can be expected from treatment. Porch suggests that when the high-low gap is closed (a difference at or near zero), the patient has achieved maximum treatment benefits and may be ready for discharge.

Porch calls variability in performance within subtests *intrasubtest variability (ISV).* He defines intrasubtest variability as the number of different scores within a subtest. A 10-item

PICA subtest in which a patient receives 8 scores of *13* (with the PICA 16-category scoring system) and two scores of *15* would have low ISV, while a subtest in which a patient's 10 responses included scores of *7, 9, 10, 13,* and *15* would have large ISV. According to Porch, intrasubtest variability is related to a patient's potential for change in the task represented by the subtest, with greater potential for change on subtests with high ISV than on subtests with low ISV. According to Porch, intrasubtest variability decreases as the patient approaches the limits of his or her recovery potential.

In the *fundamental processes approach* to treatment, clinicians attempt to identify impairments in underlying processes that are thought to contribute to several related linguistic or communicative abilities. Treatment focuses on those processes, with the expectation that improving a process will improve the abilities that depend on the process. For example, Schuell and associates (1965) have claimed that impaired auditory comprehension is a central problem in aphasia and that improving auditory comprehension leads to improvement in other language abilities. Clinicians who agree with Schuell and associates are likely to test auditory comprehension in detail and to make auditory comprehension disabilities the focus of treatment, expecting that as auditory comprehension improves, so will general linguistic and communicative abilities. Gardner and associates (1983) and Myers (1991) have suggested that impaired capacity to make inferences is a central problem for many right-hemisphere–damaged persons. Those who subscribe to this view might focus treatment on inference-making, expecting that improvements there would generalize to other communicative abilities.

Clinicians who use a *functional abilities approach* to treatment direct treatment toward skills or abilities that are likely to be important in patients' daily life communication. For example, a clinician might train a nonverbal patient to produce gestural *"yes"* and *"no"* responses, because the patient's acquisition of dependable yes-no responses should enhance communication with others in the patient's natural environment. Clinicians using the functional abilities approach often invite patients and family members to help decide what is to be worked on in treatment. Because the focus of treatment is on communication in daily life, families and caregivers often participate directly in treatment procedures.

Most clinicians combine elements of the three approaches and most consider functionality (the relevance of a skill, process, or ability to the patient's daily life) when deciding on a treatment approach. Clinicians rarely focus on fundamental abilities that have little relationship to a patient's daily life, and clinicians employing the "relative level of impairment" approach usually consider how important a process or ability is in daily life when making decisions about what to treat.

■ TASK DIFFICULTY

Most clinicians structure treatment tasks so that patients are working at or just below their maximum performance level. In easy tasks (those that are well below a patient's maximum performance level), all (or nearly all) responses are prompt and accurate. As tasks become more difficult, responses become hesitant, tentative, or delayed; false starts, revisions, self-corrected errors, and uncorrected errors appear. As task difficulty continues to increase, errors also increase, but cues or repetition of the stimulus by the clinician may elicit correct responses. When the difficulty of the task goes beyond the patient's maximum performance level, strings of uncorrected errors appear, and cues or repetition of stimuli have no beneficial effects.

Although there is considerable agreement that treatment tasks should target performance levels that challenge but do not overwhelm the patient, not everyone agrees on the precise level of difficulty at which treatment tasks should be pitched. Porch (1981b) asserts that treatment tasks should begin at levels where patients make no outright errors, but produce combinations of immediate, correct responses and correct responses that are delayed, self-corrected, distorted, or correct after the clinician repeats the stimulus. He also declares that clinicians should not change tasks or response criteria until 100% of a patient's responses are immediate and correct, because responses trained to less-than-perfect levels will deteriorate in real-life situations or in more difficult treatment tasks.

Brain-damaged patients differ in their tolerance for errors just as they differ in many other ways. Some fret, fuss, and brood over every misstep, while others remain serene and undisturbed in the face of repeated failure. Sensitive clinicians take such patient characteristics into account when deciding how hard to push a patient in treatment tasks. For the hypersensitive patient who is troubled by every mistake, the clinician may pitch treatment so that immediate, correct responses outnumber delayed, self-corrected, or prompted ones by a good margin. For the patient who is constructively challenged by failure, the clinician may permit greater proportions of delayed, self-corrected, and prompted responses, and even some uncorrected errors.

For the mythical average patient, a good general rule is to keep patient performance at 60% to 80% immediate and correct responses during the beginning of a given task and to increase the difficulty of the task when immediate, correct responses exceed 90% to 95% over two or three administrations of the task. Generally, if less than 10% of the average patient's responses are delayed and self-corrected across many trials, then the clinician should consider making the task more difficult. One important exception to this principle is patients near discharge from treatment whose performance is plateauing. For these patients, clinicians may elect to stay with treatment tasks until all the patient's responses are immediate and correct, to give the patient extended experience in tasks calling for sustained effort at maximum performance levels, to give the patient a strong sense of what successful performance at this level of effort feels like, and to build the patient's confidence in his or her ability to handle situations that call for this level of performance.

Another reason for structuring treatment tasks to minimize the frequency of error responses is that error responses on one trial increase the probability of errors on subsequent trials. Brookshire (1972) found that when aphasic adults made an error in a picture-naming task, they had a strong tendency to misname following items, even when those items ordinarily were easy for them to name. Brookshire (1976) later found the same effect in a sentence comprehension task. Brookshire and associates (1979) also found a similar effect in videotaped aphasia treatment sessions involving a variety of tasks. Regardless of the treatment task, when a patient made an error on one trial, the probability of errors on subsequent trials went up significantly. Strings of error responses proved to be especially disruptive to performance. When strings of error responses occurred, the probability of a correct response diminished with each error in the string, so that by the time three or four consecutive errors had occurred, the probability of a correct response on the next trial was near zero, unless the clinician changed the task or loosened response requirements.

As a general rule, it is a good idea to keep most brain-damaged patients' percentage of uncorrected error responses at no more than 10% to 20% of all responses. However, clinicians (and patients) can sometimes tolerate higher error rates if the patient moves closer to the intended response with each attempt. Rosenbek and associates (1989) comment that a stimulus may be adequate even if it does not elicit a correct response, as long as it leads to problem-solving or if a series of incorrect responses moves in the direction of adequacy. However, if there is no improvement across sequences of off-target responses (especially if the patient emits the *same* response on every trial), the patient is not learning much beyond tolerance for failure, and the clinician should make the task easier.

■ INSTRUCTIONS, EXPLANATION, AND FEEDBACK

Clinicians organize and regulate brain-damaged patients' performance in treatment activities (and in assessment too) by *instructing* and providing *feedback*. *Instructions* tell the patient what he or she is to do in an upcoming activity. *Feedback* tells the patient *how* he or she did on a single treatment trial or a collection of trials. Although there is some functional overlap between them, each serves a different purpose. Clinicians who keep these purposes straight keep treatment activities focused and running smoothly. Clinicians who give feedback when they should be instructing or instruct when they should be giving feedback may confuse the patient and compromise the effectiveness of their treatment procedures.

Instructions are the lead-in to treatment activities. They tell the patient what he or she will be doing and (sometimes) why he or she will be doing it. Good instructions are clear and concise and are delivered at a rate the patient can handle, using language the patient can understand, and saying everything the patient needs to know (but no more). Many beginning clinicians (and some experienced ones) overdo instructions by providing more information than the patient needs or by unnecessarily repeating or paraphrasing until the patient is confused. Instructional excess can be avoided or at least minimized by monitoring the patient's apparent understanding and by backchecking with the patient to see if she or he understands. Most brain-damaged patients (including those with severe impairments) indicate their understanding or confusion by facial expression, gesture (especially head nods), and demeanor. Clinicians who attend to these sometimes subtle signs tend not to stray into instructional excess.

Experienced clinicians know that a little demonstration and a few practice trials can take the place of large amounts of verbal instruction and are a good way to check a patient's understanding of instructions. Clinicians start with a concise explanation of the upcoming activity and when they think the patient understands, they demonstrate the task and do a few practice trials to see if the patient has gotten the point. If the patient's performance on the practice trials shows that he or she knows what is expected, the clinician proceeds into the treatment activity. If the patient's performance shows that he or she does not know what he or she is to do, the clinician provides more demonstration or explanation, guided by what the patient did during the practice trails. If the patient's performance suggests that he or she missed something in the instructions, the clinician restates the missed information perhaps with added emphasis on key elements and does some more practice trials. If the patient's performance suggests that the clinician has failed to provide some important information, the clinician adds it and may do some additional demonstration and practice.

A clinician is starting a new treatment activity with Mrs. Adair, an aphasic woman with a moderate languge-comprehension impairment and serious word-retrieval difficulties, both of which cause her great concern. **Clinician:** *Okay Mrs. Adair, now we'll be doing something different.* (The clinician alerts Mrs. Adair to the upcoming change and gives her some time to make whatever mental adjustments are needed.) *I'm going to show you some pictures, one at a time. They're pictures of things you have in your kitchen at home and they're the same ones you've been naming for me.* (The materials are familiar to Mrs. Adair and relevant to her daily life. The clinician relates the new activity to one with which Mrs. Adair has had experience.) *I know that you can name them, because you got all their names right last time and this time. Now let's see what else you can say about them.* (The clinician tells Mrs. Adair the purpose of the new activity and provides her with more time to process and make mental adjutments.) *Here's what I want you to do. I want you to tell me what you do with each one as I show it to you.* (The clinician highlights the upcoming instruction with an alerting phrase.) *Are you ready?* (The clinician monitors Mrs. Adair's facial expression, eye movements, and other indicators of her understanding and readiness.) Mrs. Adair nods, and the clinician puts a picture of a broom on the table. **Clinician:** *See this one? Tell me what you do with it.* (The clinician provides a lead-in question to highlight the request.) **Mrs. Adair:** *Broom.* **Clinician:** *No, that's not what I had in mind. Tell me what you do with it.* **Mrs. Adair:** *Sweep.* **Clinician:** *Here's another one.* (Puts down a picture of a food mixer.) **Mrs. Adair:** *Mixer.* **Clinician:** *No, that's not what I'm looking for. Tell me what you do with it. I'll show you what I mean.* (Turns over the next card—a picture of a knife.) **Clinician:** *This is something I'd use to cut things up. See what I mean? I didn't name it. I told you what I do with it. Now you try one. Remember, tell me what you do with it.* (Turns over card showing a kettle.) **Mrs. Adair:** *Well, it's a kettle— and I'd boil potatoes or make a stew in it.* **Clinician:** *Great! Let's do another one.*

Several things about the clinician's behavior with Mrs. Adair are noteworthy. The clinician uses repetition, paraphrase, and lead-in phrases liberally to highlight important information and to give Mrs. Adair extra processing time. She asks Mrs. Adair if she is ready before beginning the first trial. (For experienced clinicians this behavior is so routine as to be almost automatic. This is not so for beginners who often move too fast and present stimuli before the patient is ready.) When Mrs. Adair responds to the first practice item with its name, the clinician gives her appropriate feedback, does not correct her, and repeats the instruction. When Mrs. Adair continues to name on the second practice trial, the clinician adds demonstration to repetition of the task instructions, at which point Mrs. Adair responds appropriately.

Mrs. Adair's clinician combines instruction and explanation with response-contingent feedback to coach her into a new treatment activity with minimum fuss and confusion. When Mrs. Adair's responses to the first two practice items are not what the clinician intends, the clinician combines negative feedback ("no") with explanation *("That's not what I had in mind")* that elaborates on the feedback and also helps to soften its hard edges. Importantly, the clinician does not *correct* Mrs. Adair's unacceptable responses as in *("No. You sweep with a broom."* or *"No. You mix food with a mixer."),* because the problem is not with the correctness of Mrs. Adair's responses, but either with her understanding of the new activity or her ability to change her response set from naming-to-describing function. After two practice trials in which feedback and explanation fail to elicit the intended responses, the clinician moves on to demonstration combined with explanation. The switch in tactics succeeds and the clinician and patient continue into the new activity.

Knowing when to provide feedback and what kind to provide, and knowing how to combine feedback, explanation, and demonstration are important clinical skills. Brookshire

(1973) addressed the *"what kind"* question. He identified two major categories of response-contingent feedback in treatment activities: *incentive feedback* and *information feedback. Incentive feedback* can maintain (or eliminate) behaviors whose only purpose is to elicit (or avoid) the feedback. If the feedback stops, the behavior stops. The food pellets that drop into the hopper when the pigeon pecks a key are incentive feedback (sometimes called *positive reinforcement),* which keeps the pigeon pecking the key. The quarters that drop down the chute of the slot machine are incentive feedback, which keeps the customer putting in coins and pulling the lever. If the key is disconnected from the pellet dispenser, the pigeon loses interest in the key. If the slot machine is programmed to keep the customer's coins and return none, the customer (eventually) stops putting in coins and pulling the lever. The power of incentive feedback over behavior depends strongly on the subject's real or apparent state of deprivation for the feedback stimulus. If the pigeon is fed until it is no longer hungry, it loses interest in pecking the key. If the slot machine customer is given 40 million dollars, a new BMW, and a ticket to Fiji, he or she loses interest in putting coins in the machine and pulling its lever.

Increasing the magnitude of incentive feedback or increasing the subject's level of deprivation often increases its effect on behavior, at least within certain ranges. Increasing the payoff on the pecking key or the slot machine makes their users respond faster and stay at it longer (unless the payoff is large enough to reduce the subjects' deprivation levels).

Incentive feedback is used in the clinic when the objective is a change in the frequency of behaviors that a patient is capable of but doesn't do often enough (such as making eye contact with listeners) or does too often (such as shouting at doctors and nurses). Many different stimuli can be incentive feedback, and what works as an incentive for one person may not work for another. Some stimuli, such as food (to hungry people) water (to thirsty people), electric shocks (to most), and loud noise (except for patrons of rock concerts) seem intrinsically rewarding or punishing—they serve as reward or punishment for most of the adult population. Other stimuli seem less intrinsically rewarding or punishing, and they work for smaller segments of the population—For example verbal approval and reproof are not intrinsically rewarding or punishing but have rewarding and punishing properties for some individuals but not for others.

Information feedback provides information about the appropriateness, correctness, or accuracy of the responses they follow. Information feedback comes in many forms, ranging from a tracing on an oscilloscope that tells a patient how close her or his vocal intensity is to a target, to the clinician's smile and spoken *"good"* that tells the patient that she or he has successfully communicated an intended message. Incentive feedback can also function as information feedback, as when the young traumatically brain-injured patient gets an M & M (his favorite candy) contingent on each successful detection of a target in a visual-monitoring task. However, information feedback need not possess incentive characteristics to be effective in regulating the performance of most brain-damaged adults who are motivated to get better and for whom the payoff is not in the feedback but in the improved performance that comes with progress in treatment. For these patients it is the information about the appropriateness, correctness, or accuracy of the behaviors leading to the feedback that is important.

There are no specific rules for how and when feedback should be used in treatment of brain-damaged adults, because patients differ in their need for feedback and clinicians differ in their preferences with regard to what kind of feedback to deliver and when to deliver it. However, the following observations may help beginning clinicians get at least a general sense of how feedback functions in treatment activities for brain-damaged adults.

Incentive feedback does not play an important part in treatment of most brain-damaged adults. Most brain-damaged adults are motivated and willingly do what is needed to get better without the need for external incentives. For these patients, progress is its own reward. Conversely, severely impaired, depressed, agitated, or confused patients who do not recognize progress in treatment activities or who are not rewarded by it may need incentive feedback. Incentive feedback often is needed in treatment of traumatically brain-injured patients in the early stages of recovery. These patients often are minimally responsive to their environment and have little tolerance for tasks that require mental or physical effort. Incentives for responding may be the only way to get these patients' cooperation in treatment tasks. Incentive feedback also may be needed when clinicians are working with patients in the late stages of dementia (when social rewards and penalties no longer function to maintain or change behavior).

Most brain-damaged adults appreciate *general encouragement* in treatment activities. General encouragement may be response-contingent positive feedback or it may be occasional positive statements that are not contingent upon any given response *("You're doing fine."* or *"You're doing much better today.")*.

The positive effects of encouraging comments by the clinician and the negative effects of discouraging ones were shown in a study by Stoicheff (1960). Stoicheff studied three groups of aphasic adults who performed picture-naming and word-reading tasks in three instructional conditions. One group received encouraging instructions *("I'm very satisfied with what you have been able to do. I think that you will find the going much easier today. I expect that you will do just as well today if not better.")*. One group received discouraging instructions *("As I expected, you did even more poorly last time than the time before. I am dis-*

appointed in how much you have slipped behind. This seems to be harder for you each time instead of easier."). One group received neutral instructions *("I want you to do the same kinds of things as last time. We'll be working on different/words/pictures.").* The clinician also made encouraging comments *("Good! You're doing fine!")* to the *encouragement* group and discouraging comments *("You missed that one! That's wrong!")* to the *discouragement* group during the tasks.* After three sessions, the *discouragement* group performed significantly worse than the *encouragement* group. The performance of the *neutral* group fell between the other two groups but did not differ significantly from either. Stoicheff commented that subjects in the *discouragement* group were withdrawn, tense, and not smiling by the end of the third session, whereas those in the *encouragement* group were spontaneous, friendly, and smiling.[†]

Many clinicians tend to avoid negative feedback, perhaps because they do not wish to discourage their patients. Brookshire and associates (1977) evaluated clinicians' use of feedback in 40 videotaped treatment sessions. They reported that clinicians provided negative feedback for only about 10% of unacceptable patient responses and they were as likely to provide positive feedback as negative feedback following unacceptable responses. It is not clear why clinicians have this seeming aversion to negative feedback. Perhaps they wish to avoid discouraging their patients, as Stoicheff did with her negative instructions and comments. However, it is important to remember that Stoicheff's negative instructions and comments were not contingent on poor performance. It is not surprising that her subjects were tense and hostile following three sessions of negative instructions and criticism unrelated to their performance. Brain-damaged adults, like the rest of us, are likely to become tense and hostile when subjected to gratuitous negative commentary from another, but few are so sensitive that they cannot deal with negative feedback if it is delivered contingent on off-target responses, and if the overall mood created by the clinician is supportive and reassuring.

It is true, however, that most clinicians (including this writer) deliver negative feedback in diluted form but deliver positive feedback full strength. One seldom hears clinicians say *"Wrong!"* or *"No!"* in response to inaccurate patient responses. They are more likely to say *"close"* or *"not quite"* and they sometimes sweeten the negative feedback even more by blending it with weak positive feedback, as in *"Good try, but that's not quite it."* Positive feedback tends to be more emphatic. Exclamations such as *"Good! Great! Super!"* or *"Wonderful!"* are commonly heard in treatment sessions. By manipulating the strength of positive and negative feedback in this way, clinicians put more emphasis on the positive aspects of their patients' performance, contribute to their patients' self-confidence, and maintain an encouraging and supportive atmosphere in treatment activities.

As the patient and clinician become more familiar with each other and with treatment activities, feedback can become quite subtle. Once a treatment activity has achieved a consistent pace or rhythm, in which the clinician's delivery of stimuli and the patient's responses have fallen into a regular temporal pattern, the clinician need only interrupt the pattern by withholding delivery of the next stimulus for a few seconds to signal to the patient that his or her response was off target. Similarly, clinicians

---

* The comments were not delivered contingent on acceptable or unacceptable responses.

[†] At the end of the study, Stoicheff explained to the subjects that they had participated in a study and reassured those in the *discouragement* and *neutral* groups to counteract any detrimental effects of their treatment on subsequent performance. It is unlikely that Stoicheff could have done this study today because of rules requiring that subjects be told, in advance, about the purposes and general conduct of any study in which they participate.

who acknowledge on-target responses with a consistent head nod need only withhold it to signal to the patient that a response was off target. Most moderately to mildly impaired brain-damaged patients quickly become attuned to these subtle cues, but those with more severe impairments may need more conspicuous feedback and they may need it after every response, rather than intermittently. However, patients with mild or moderate impairments may need feedback after each response when new treatment tasks are introduced and they are faced with determining the point of the task and the criteria that determine what constitutes on-target responses. Feedback schedules tend to be more nearly continuous (feedback after every response) and feedback stimuli tend to be more overt and more intense at the beginning of new treatment tasks. As the patient gains experience with the task, the feedback schedule becomes more intermittent and feedback stimuli often become more subtle.

Delivering overt feedback contingent on every response is rarely necessary once a treatment activity has become a familiar routine with a consistent pace. Then, intermittent positive feedback plus negative feedback for all (or nearly all) off-target responses usually is sufficient (unless the patient is aware of all off-target responses, in which case negative feedback can also be delivered on an intermittent schedule). Feedback schedules in which every patient response gets overt feedback soon become tiresome for clinician and patient, and the effectiveness of the stimuli used as overt feedback usually is diminished by frequent use. However, as noted above, most clinicians provide subtle indications of response acceptability even when they don't provide overt feedback, so in this sense it might be said that most clinicians provide some form of feedback for every patient response.

Keeping the purposes of *feedback* separate from the purposes of *instruction* is important. Feedback tells the patient whether his or her re-

sponses were acceptable. Instruction tells the patient what she or he is to do. Instructions usually come at the beginning of treatment tasks. If error responses seem to be caused by incomplete understanding or misunderstanding of the task, the clinician gives more instruction on how to do the task. If error responses represent simply off-target responses caused by performance limitations, the clinician provides information feedback regarding how or why the responses were off target. Providing negative feedback when deficient performance is caused by the patient's incomplete understanding or misunderstanding of task instructions is a procedural error on the part of the clinician, as is providing instruction when the patient already understands the task but makes off-target responses because of performance limitations.

■ RECORDING AND CHARTING PATIENTS' PERFORMANCE

Documenting what goes on in treatment by keeping organized and accurate records of patients' performance is an important clinical responsibility. Accurate records of performance permit clinicians to establish stable baseline levels of performance to document the effects of treatment. Sensitive measures of changes in a patient's performance over time or in response to treatment procedures permit clinicians to modify treatment procedures or introduce new ones to maximize treatment effectiveness. Good record keeping can contribute to the orderliness and efficiency of treatment, because accurately and concisely recording a patient's performance in a treatment task requires that the task itself be orderly and easily described. Finally, those who pay for speech-language pathology services (insurance companies and governmental units) and health-care accrediting agencies require that clinicians keep accurate and objective records of patients' performance and their response to treatment. Clinicians need to be careful, however, that response scoring and record-keeping procedures do not become so elaborate, cumbersome, and intrusive that they disrupt the rhythm of treatment, compromise the naturalness of the interaction between the clinician and the patient, and divert the attention of the patient and the clinician from the primary objectives of treatment.

Record-keeping methods cover a range of complexity and sophistication, from simple paper-and-pencil routines devised by individual clinicians to elaborate standardized methods marketed commercially. Both personal and commercial record-keeping methods provide a way of labeling or describing the treatment activity, space for listing treatment stimuli (usually trial by trial), and space for entering the patient's responses to treatment stimuli. Figure 5-2 shows an example of a personalized record sheet for a treatment session, in which the clinician has recorded a patient's responses to 10 test stimuli across 3 trials in each of 6 treatment activities.

LaPointe's (1977) *Base-10 Programmed Stimulation* is an example of a commercially marketed system for task specification and response recording, which formalizes the personalized record-keeping systems used by many clinicians. In Base-10 Programmed Stimulation, scores for patients' responses to treatment stimuli are entered in a *Base-10 Response Form* (Figure 5-3), on which the clinician also includes information about the treatment task, target performance criteria, the scoring system used, and the stimuli presented. The form also provides a graph on which a patient's performance can be charted over several treatment sessions. A different response form is used for each treatment task so that several are needed to record what happens in treatment sessions with several tasks.

When doing treatment in Base-10 format, the clinician selects treatment tasks for the patient and writes a description of each task on a response form. A target behavior and a target level of performance are selected for each task and entered on the response form. Ten stimuli are selected (hence the label *Base-10*) and described on the response form. When the treatment task is carried out, the patient's response to each stimulus is entered on the response form. After several sessions the clinician may graph the patient's performance to assess changes in performance over time.

In most didactic treatment tasks (such as pointing to pictures named by the clinician or writing words dictated by the clinician) the clinician controls the rate at which stimuli are delivered—the clinician does not deliver the stimulus for a new trial until he or she has scored the patient's response to the last trail. Consequently, it is relatively easy for the clinician to score every patient response as it occurs (*online scoring*). The scoring situation is different in less-structured treatment tasks, such as conversations, in which target behaviors occur unpredictably and the clinician no longer controls the rate at which scorable responses occur. In such tasks, target responses often occur so rapidly that the clinician cannot score every response and get the score down on a record form without falling behind. In these situations the clinician has two options: *off-line scoring* and *sampling*.

In *off-line scoring* the clinician records the treatment activity on audiotape or videotape and does the scoring later, stopping and rewinding the tape as necessary to score every response. The advantage of off-line scoring is that every response can be scored without the need for the clinician to hurry transcription and scoring to keep up. There are some disadvantages to off-line scoring. It requires the use of videotape or audiotape recording equipment, which may not always be available. When it is available, its presence can distract the patient or make him or her uneasy or tense. The time it takes to do off-line scoring may make it impractical for clinicians with busy schedules and pressing demands on their time.

Sampling provides an alternative to off-line scoring. Sampling permits clinicians to score a

Patient: J. Smith Date: 7/12/96 Clinician: M. Johnson

Task / Stimulus	Name			Point by name			Point by function			Imitation			Sentence completion			Point by two's		
Trial	1	2	3	1	2	3	1	2	3	1	2	3	1	2	3	1	2	3
Pencil	15	13	15	13	15	15	13	15	15	15	15	15	15	15	13	13	13	15
Bell	15	15	15	15	15	13	13	13	15	15	15	15	13	13	15	13	15	13
Comb	13	15	13	13	13	10	13	9	10	15	13	15	13	15	15	15	15	15
Knife	15	15	15	13	13	13	15	15	15	13	15	13	15	14	14	13	10	15
Flag	15	15	15	15	15	15	15	15	13	13	15	15	15	15	15	9	13	15
Knife	15	15	15	5	15	15	13	15	15	15	10	15	14	14	14	13	15	13
Horn	13	15	15	10	15	15	10	15	15	15	15	15	15	15	15	13	13	9
Lamp	15	15	15	15	15	15	15	13	15	15	15	15	15	15	15	15	15	15
Brush	10	15	15	13	15	15	15	15	15	15	15	13	15	15	15	10	15	15
Candle	15	15	15	13	15	15	15	15	13	15	15	15	13	13	15	15	10	15
Mean score	14.6			13.7			13.9			14.5			14.4			13.4		

Figure 5-2 ■ A record sheet for recording patient performance in treatment tasks. Treatment stimuli are listed in the left-hand column and treatment tasks are listed across the top. The clinician administered three consecutive trials, which elicited 30 patient responses within each treatment task.

BASE 10 RESPONSE FORM
PROGRAMMED SPEECH-LANGUAGE STIMULATION

TASK *Generate and verbalize sentences: function words (30 second limit)*

CRITERION *90% +, 3 consecutive sessions* SCORING *+ -*

Post Baseline Therapy
1. isolate errors
2. repeat 5 times
3. repeat 3 times after 5 sec delay

Chart (PERCENTAGE vs SESSION): plotted points — B: 50, 1: 70, 2: 60, 3: 60, 4: 75, 5: 90, 6: 100, 7: 90, 8: 100, 9: 90. "6 wk interval" marked between sessions 8 and 9.

STIMULI	B.	B.	B	1	2	3	4	5	6	7	8	9	10
1. on	+	—	—	+	+	+	—	+	+	+	+	+	
2. if	—	—	—	—	—	+	+	+	+	+	+	+	
3. with	—	—	—	—	+	—	+	+	+	+	+	+	
4. from	+	—	—	+	+	+	+	+	+	+	+	+	
5. to	—	—	—	+	+	—	—	+	+	+	+	+	
6. of	—	—	—	—	—	—	—	—	—	+	—	+	—	
7. which	—	—	—	+	+	—	—	+	+	+	+	+	+	
8. in	+	—	—	+	+	+	+	+	+	+	+	+	
9. about	+	—	—	+	—	+	+	+	+	+	+	+	
10. for	+	—	—	+	+	+	+	+	+	+	+	+	

MEANS   5 (Baseline)   7   6   6   7   8   10   9   10   9

Figure 5-3 ■ The Base-10 task specification and response recording form. The task is described at the top left, the treatment stimuli are described at the bottom left, and the patient's responses are recorded on the bottom right. The columns labeled *B* are for entering the patient's scores in *baseline* conditions before treatment begins.

percentage of patient responses, rather than every response, and makes it possible for them to score rapidly occurring responses on line.[*] Various formalized procedures for sampling have been described (Powell, Martindale, & Kulp, 1975; Thomson, Holmberg, & Baer, 1974; Repp and associates, 1976; Brookshire, Nicholas, & Krueger, 1978), but most clinicians opt for a less-formalized approach in which they score as many responses as they comfortably can. They score the first occurrence of the target response, taking as much time as needed to decide on a score and enter it on a record form, ignoring any scorable responses that occur

[*] Sampling also can be used in conjunction with off-line scoring to decrease the amount of time expended in documenting the events in a treatment task.

while they are doing this. After they enter a score for that response on the record form, they look for the next scorable response, score it, and go on to the next one. The proportion of a patient's responses that gets scored depends on the complexity of the scoring system and the rate at which scorable responses occur. Complex scoring systems and fast patient response rates reduce the proportion of responses that gets scored.

There is no absolute proportion of responses that must be sampled to generate an accurate representation of patients' performance in a treatment task. Clinicians using the "score-as-many-responses-as-you-can" approach can expect to get half or more of scorable patient responses on the record sheet in most treatment tasks. This proportion should (most of the time) yield accurate representations of patients' performance, if the scored responses are fairly evenly distributed across the task. Brookshire, Nicholas, and Krueger (1978) reported that scoring only 1 response in 5 yielded records that deviated from patients' actual performance by less than 10%, provided that sampling was uniform across treatment activities. Consequently, it seems likely that scoring, on the average, every other response should almost always yield highly accurate indicators of patients' actual performance.

■ ENHANCING GENERALIZATION FROM THE CLINIC TO DAILY LIFE

Treatment of communication disorders is not successful if the changes achieved in the clinic do not extend to the patient's daily life. Even though most clinicians recognize that extension of treatment gains to daily life is important, until the 1970s most aphasia clinicians seemed to operate largely on the *train-and-hope* principle (Stokes & Baer, 1977), in which generalization-of-treatment effects from the clinic to outside contexts are hoped for but are neither actively pursued nor objectively measured. It is probably true that most aphasia clinicians (at least the

better ones) either target communicative behaviors that are relevant to the patient's daily life environment or target underlying processes that are assumed to enhance daily life communicative behavior. (However, many do not pursue generalization in a systematic way nor measure it carefully).

In the 1970s psychologists and behavior analysts began to address the problem of extending changes obtained in the clinic to outside environments. Literature on generalization developed, and procedures for enhancing generalization gradually made their way into clinical aphasiology. These procedures generally resemble those articulated by Stokes and Baer (1977), the first of which *(train and hope)* was described in the preceding paragraph. The other procedures include the following:

Using Natural Maintaining Contingencies Stokes and Baer see this as "the most dependable of all generalization programming mechanisms" (p. 353). The easiest way to make use of natural contingencies is to target behaviors that will naturally elicit favorable consequences in the patient's daily life environment. For example, Thompson and Byrne (1984) trained patients with Broca's aphasia to produce various social conventions such as greetings; expecting that the patients' use of such social conventions would be naturally reinforced by others in daily life.

Sometimes natural contingencies are not present in the patient's daily life environment or are not consistent enough. Then one might redesign or restructure the daily life environment so that the targeted behaviors receive enough payoff to maintain them. An example of such restructuring is provided by an aphasic patient who learned to produce one- and two-word requests in the clinic but continued to communicate at home with grunts and gestures, by which he usually succeeded in getting family members to do what he wanted. The clinician taught family members to respond to spoken requests and to ignore or delay responses to grunts and gestures unaccompanied by speech. This soon brought the patient's clinic-learned spoken requests into his home environment, after which natural contingencies maintained them, both in the home and in other contexts with other listeners.

Training Sufficient Exemplars *(Exemplar* is technical jargon with various meanings. As used here it means, roughly, *stimulus-response–reinforcement triads.)* One way of training sufficient exemplars is to train a behavior in enough different settings that the behavior generalizes to all settings in which the behavior is desired. Once the behavior is dependably established in one context, the training is systematically extended to other contexts one or two at a time, with the expectation that at some point the behavior will generalize to all contexts of interest. Using social conventions as an example, this means that one might first train social conventions in the clinic, then extend the training to other rooms, other interactants, and to the patient's home or other community settings, expecting that at some point the patient's use of social conventions would generalize to all relevant communicative contexts. Another way of training sufficient exemplars is to train enough different representatives of a class of responses to ensure that a class of responses, rather than a specific response (or subset of responses), generalizes. Using social conventions as an example, one might successively train several social conventions of a given kind (such as several different greetings) with the expectation that increasing the frequency of greetings might naturally lead to increases in the frequency of other conventions, such as questions *("How are you?")* and self-disclosures *("I am fine.").*

Loose Training In loose training, stimulus conditions, response requirements, and reinforcement contingencies are permitted to vary (within limits), so as to increase generalization across responses within a response class and to increase generalization from the training environment to other environments. Loose training attempts to prevent a patient's responses from being tightly bound to specific contexts, which can often happen when treatment conditions are carefully controlled (as in many clinic treatment activities). In loose training (1) a variety of stimuli are employed to elicit targeted responses, sometimes in different situational contexts, (2) a range of responses within a predefined response class is considered acceptable, and (3) response contingencies vary both in kind and schedule.

Loose training is *not* unsystematic treatment. Specific response classes are targeted, eliciting stimuli and situational contexts are planned in advance, and response contingencies and their schedule are predefined. Well-done loose training is as carefully thought out and as carefully controlled as more traditionally structured treatment procedures.

Thompson and Byrne (1984) used loose-training procedures to train their aphasic patients to use social conventions. The social conventions were first established by asking the patients to imitate the clinician's production of them. Then the eliciting stimuli were systematically broadened to (1) requests by the clinician (e.g., *"Tell me hello."*), (2) naturalistic prompts given by the clinician (e.g., the clinician said *"hello"* and waited for a response from the patient), and (3) role-playing situations structured to resemble natural conversations. Verbal feedback (e.g., *nice job*) was provided contingent on responses, and the schedule of feedback was gradually loosened, from feedback for every response in the early stages of training to a variable schedule (feedback for an average of one response in four) in the later stages. Thompson and Byrne reported that loose training increased their patients' production of social conventions and that the increased production of social conventions generalized to novel social interactions. Although Thompson and Byrnes' procedures departed somewhat from prototypical loose training (they targeted specific responses for intervention), their study is a good example of how loose training can be incorporated into treatment procedures for brain-damaged adults.

Sequential Modification In sequential modification (Stokes & Baer, 1977), generalization across contexts is obtained by carrying out training in every context to which generalization is desired. For brain-damaged adults, sequential modification may be practical when a communicative behavior is appropriate (or important) in only a few contexts, when there are only a few contexts in which the brain-damaged person will be communicating, and it is practical to carry out training in each context. It usually is difficult to identify all potential communicative contexts for a given brain-damaged person and it is almost always impractical in terms of time and resources to carry out training in every context. Consequently, sequential modification usually has limited usefulness in treating neurogenic communication impairments. (Except, perhaps, for some patients with restricted communicative environments, such as those confined at home or in a nursing home, who have contact with only a few others, and whose communication is limited to a small range of topics.)

Using Indiscriminable Contingencies Stokes and Baer suggest that generalization to settings outside the treatment setting is enhanced if the response contingencies in treatment are gradually altered to make them more like those that can be expected in natural settings. These alterations may include (1) changing the schedule of contingencies from continuous (for every response) to intermittent (for every n^{th} response) to intermittent and variable (for every n^{th} response on the average, but varying around the average); (2) interposing delay between responses and their contingencies; and (3) choosing contingencies that resemble those expected in natural settings. Many clinicians routinely include such alterations in contingencies in their treatment procedures to increase the likelihood of generalization to natural contexts. Making

contingencies indiscriminable also is an important part of other techniques such as loose training.

Programming Common Stimuli Programming common stimuli means that the context in which behavior is trained is purposely made to resemble the context(s) to which the behavior is to generalize (the target context). Programming common stimuli manipulates *stimulus control* to enhance generalization across contexts. *Stimulus control* refers to how stimuli or stimulus complexes govern the occurrence of behavior. A laboratory rat that is reinforced with food pellets for pressing a bar when a green light is on but not when a red light is on soon presses the bar only when the green light is on. The rat has learned to *discriminate* the reinforcement condition from the nonreinforcement condition. To extend stimulus control to a patient's daily life environment, a clinician might incorporate stimuli from the environment into training, expecting that when the patient then encounters those stimuli in daily life, she or he will be more likely to emit the trained behavior. The greater the similarity between the training environment and daily life, the more likely it is that the trained behavior(s) will generalize to daily life. The extent to which the training environment and the target environment resemble each other usually is decided subjectively. In most cases certain key elements (such as eliciting stimuli, surroundings, and sometimes people) are selected to resemble elements in the target environment. As is true for alterations in contingencies, programming common stimuli can be incorporated into any treatment approach to increase the likelihood of generalization to natural contexts.

Mediating Generalization *Mediation* refers to the elicitation of one response by another response. Mnemonic devices are one example of mediation. One attaches easily remembered verbal labels (the mnemonic devices) to difficult-to-remember material and uses the mnemonic devices to retrieve the difficult-to-remember material (as in the rhyme for remembering the names of the cranial nerves in Chapter 1). In *mediated generalization* easier responses are used to elicit more difficult responses. For example, an aphasic person might be taught to retrieve words by thinking of their visual images. Most of the literature on mediated generalization has studied verbal mediation (Stokes & Baer, 1977), and verbal mediation may be inappropriate for many brain-damaged adults with language impairments. However, verbal mediation sometimes is useful in treatment programs for persons with right-hemisphere syndrome or traumatic brain injuries.

Training Generalization Sometimes patients spontaneously generalize during treatment activities. For example, a patient who is working on improving syntax in written work may begin using better syntax in spoken utterances. These spontaneous generalizations might themselves be targeted for reinforcement, and reinforcement contingencies might be gradually modified so that such responses receive a greater proportion of reinforcement than rote responses to training stimuli.

▪ SOCIAL VALIDATION

Social validation is a procedure for evaluating the clinical significance of changes created by a treatment program. Social validation attempts to determine whether the patient is better in a real-world sense than he or she was before treatment. It can be accomplished in two ways (Kazdin, 1982). One way is to compare the (socially relevant) behavior of the person receiving treatment with the behavior of a normal group of peers. The greater the progression toward normalcy, the more "clinically significant" the change in behavior. The other way is to obtain subjective evaluations of the behaviors of interest from persons in the patient's natural environment.

Although clinicians have for years carried out informal social validation by soliciting family members' opinions about how the patient is communicating at home, structured procedures for socially validating the effects of treatment on

neurogenically impaired patients' communication have only recently been described (Doyle, Goldstein, & Bourgeois, 1987; Thompson & Byrne, 1984). Doyle and associates trained four adults with Broca's aphasia to produce sentences with various syntactic forms in response to pictures. They all improved on measures of accuracy, grammar, and utterance length. Doyle and associates then evaluated the social validity of the improvements by playing audiotape recordings of the aphasic adults' picture descriptions to five adults who did not know the aphasic people and who knew nothing about the study. Some of the recordings were made before treatment began and others were made after treatment had ended and they were arranged so that pretreatment and posttreatment samples occurred in random order. The judges were asked to judge whether each sample was "adequate" or "inadequate." In spite of subjects' improvements on measures of accuracy, grammar, and utterance length during treatment, the social validation procedure revealed no general increase in judgments of adequacy by the judges (although there were significant increases in judgments of adequacy for some syntactic forms). Doyle and associates concluded that social validation measures are crucial for evaluating the effectiveness of treatment programs, and that they may be useful as pretreatment measures for selecting behaviors to treat.

Thompson and Byrne (1984) used a peer-group-comparison method to assess the social validity of changes in the use of social conventions (such as greetings, farewells, introductions) by their aphasic subjects. They had each aphasic subject participate in a conversational interaction with a normal adult whom the subject had not met before. Then they compared the aphasic subjects' use of social conventions with that of the normal adults. Before treatment the aphasic subjects' use of social conventions was well below the range of the normal subjects, but at the end of treatment it approximated that of the normal subjects.

Social validation in clinical management of adults with neurogenic communication disorders is in its infancy but it promises to become an increasingly important aspect of management as structured, reliable procedures for assessing and quantifying it are created, improved, and validated.

■ KEY CONCEPTS

- Speech-language pathologists customarily participate in a patient's care as a member of a treatment team that has overall responsibility for the patient's care. The treatment team includes members from the major disciplines involved in caring for the patient.

- There are no standard criteria for deciding if a patient will benefit from treatment of his or her communicative impairments. The location and severity of a patient's brain damage, his or her medical and physical condition, and his or her motivation to recover are important indicators of the potential benefit of treatment. When a decision cannot be made based on patient characteristics, a short interval of trial treatment may help the speech-language pathologist make the decision.

- The frequency and duration of treatment sessions depend on several variables, including the patient's medical and physical condition, the complexity of the treatment program, logistics, and how close the patient is to the end of treatment.

- Treatment sessions usually have a consistent format, with challenging treatment activities sandwiched between less challenging warm-up and cool-down activities.

- Resource-allocation models of cognitive processes provide a useful metaphor on which to base the search for the causes of a patient's deficient performance on a task. Resource-allocation models assume that every individual possesses a finite amount of cognitive processing resources (the *pool*), and that

active processes draw resources from the pool. If processing demands exceed the capacity of the pool, or if allocation of resources is faulty, performance deteriorates.

- Clinicians may adjust the difficulty of treatment tasks by adjusting any of several characteristics of treatment stimuli (intensity, salience, clarity, intelligibility, redundancy, context, novelty, interest value, cues and prompts); by adjusting the length, complexity, familiarity, meaningfulness, or redundancy of the responses required of patients; or by imposing delays between stimulation and the patient's responses to stimulation.

- Clinicians' treatment decisions are a product of their insights into the nature of a patient's communicative impairment, their philosophy concerning the nature and purpose of treatment, and their previous experiences with similar patients. Clinicians' treatment plans may reflect a *relative level of impairment* approach, a *fundamental abilities* approach, or a *functional abilities* approach.

- Clinicians usually structure treatment so that patients work at a level at which performance is impaired but does not completely break down.

- Judicious and appropriate use of instructions, explanation, and feedback makes an important contribution to the outcome of treatment. Knowing when to provide feedback and knowing when information feedback or incentive feedback are appropriate are important clinical skills.

- Keeping accurate records of patients' performance in treatment activities permits clinicians to establish pretreatment baselines, measure the effects of treatment, and make decisions about what to treat, how to treat it, and when to stop.

- Helping patients transfer gains made in treatment to their daily lives is a crucial aspect of treatment, and clinicians are responsible for ensuring that the transfer takes place. Several more-or-less formalized procedures for enhancing generalization are available.

Treatment of Aphasia and Related Disorders

This chapter provides an overview of how clinicians go about treating adults with aphasia and related communication impairments. Some of the principles and procedures presented in this chapter may also apply, in whole or in part, to treatment of communication impairments other than aphasia. They are presented here because they occupy a central place in treatment of aphasia, whereas their applicability to treatment of adults with other neurogenic communication disorders may be more peripheral. The chapter begins with a discussion of some general issues and concepts relating to treatment of aphasic adults' language and communication impairments. The first section relates to a basic concern—whether what speech-language pathologists do in treatment of aphasic adults is effective.

The Effectiveness of Treatment for Aphasia

The question of whether or not treatment of aphasic adults' communication is worthwhile has been a source of controversy for many years. Some have argued that there is no convincing evidence for the effectiveness of aphasia treatment, while others have argued that the effectiveness of aphasia treatment is supported both by experimental evidence and by clinical experience. A number of investigators have concluded that treatment for aphasia provides no significant improvement in speech and language beyond what would be generated by spontaneous recovery (Vignolo, 1964; Sarno, Silverman, & Sands, 1970; Lincoln and associates, 1984). Other investigators have reported positive effects of treatment (Butfield & Zangwill, 1946; West, 1973; Deal & Deal, 1978; Basso, Capitani, & Vignolo, 1979; Wertz and associates, 1981; Wertz and associates, 1984).

In spite of numerous attempts to evaluate scientifically the effects of aphasia treatment, the evidence generated has not been conclusive because most of the studies contain scientific, procedural, or logical flaws that compromise the interpretation of their results. Few have included control groups against which the effects of treatment programs can be measured. When control groups have been included, the validity of the control groups often has been compromised by flaws in sampling procedures and subject assignment. The treatment procedures in most studies and their appropriateness to the aphasic subjects studied is largely undocumented. The frequency of treatment sessions and the duration of treatment programs sometimes has been so limited that treatment had no chance to generate meaningful changes in patients' performance. In many cases the measures used to document changes (or lack of changes) in response to treatment were nonstandardized, with undocumented reliability and dubious validity.

Wertz and associates (1981, 1984) reported two studies of the efficacy of aphasia treatment that satisfy most requirements for scientific quality, replicability, and dependability of results. Both were large multicenter studies in which patients were carefully selected and randomly assigned to groups, patients' neurologic and speech and language status was measured at regular intervals with standardized and reliable tests, the content of treatment was controlled and documented, and the possibility of experimenter bias was eliminated. In both studies the results supported the investigators' conclusion that treatment of aphasic adults has significant positive effects beyond the changes that would be expected from spontaneous recovery.

Poeck, Huber, and Willmes (1989) also concluded that aphasia treatment is efficacious, based on the results of a well-designed study in which they provided 6 to 8 weeks of intensive treatment to 68 aphasic adults. Ninety-two aphasic adults in a control group received no treatment but were tested on the same schedule as the treated subjects. Poeck and associates reported that both the treated group and the untreated group improved significantly on measures of speech and language, but subjects who received treatment improved significantly more than those who did not.

In addition to group studies of the effects of aphasia treatment, a number of single-case design studies (e.g., Kearns & Salmon, 1984; Thompson & Byrne, 1984) have demonstrated that carefully controlled treatment programs produce meaningful changes in targeted aspects of aphasic patients' performance and that generalization of the changes to patients' daily life environments can be obtained. The weight of the evidence at this time clearly supports the efficacy of treatment for aphasia, provided that several conditions are met:

- The treatment is delivered by qualified professionals.
- Patients with irreversible aphasia are excluded.
- The content, duration, and timing of treatment are appropriate for those receiving treatment.

This does not mean, however, that speech-language pathologists are off the effectiveness hook, because the emphasis has shifted somewhat from *efficacy* (whether treatment yields a significant change on one or more tests) to *effectiveness* (whether treatment causes meaningful changes in daily life communication performance). When the concepts of efficacy and effectiveness are separated, it becomes clear that most existing studies of aphasia treatment are efficacy studies (their measures of the effects of treatment were changes on one or more tests of communication ability). Consequently, the evidence supports the *efficacy* of aphasia treatment but not necessarily its *effectiveness*. The issue of effectiveness has now taken center stage, and investigators are at work developing measures of treatment effectiveness and planning

studies to determine if aphasia treatment is *effective* as well as *efficacious*.

Timing of Intervention

Another question that has dogged clinical aphasiology relates to the timing of intervention; namely whether intervention begun weeks or months post onset of aphasia is as efficacious (or effective) as treatment begun within the first days and weeks after a patient becomes aphasic. Scientific studies of early versus late intervention have yielded equivocal results. Several investigators have reported that delaying treatment by 2 months or more after the onset of aphasia has significant negative effects on patients' eventual recovery (Butfield & Zangwill, 1946; Wepman, 1951; Vignolo, 1964; Sands, Sarno, & Shankweiler, 1969). Vignolo (1964), for example, studied the recovery of 69 aphasic patients. Some received treatment and some did not. Vignolo concluded that it is important that treatment begin while physiologic recovery is most rapid. "Only the period which extends from 2 to 6 months after the onset of aphasia seems to provide a ground where intrinsic capacity for recovery can be highly enhanced by the intervention of planned training" (p. 366).

Poeck and associates (1989) reported that neither age nor time post onset of aphasia significantly affected aphasic adults' *recovery of language*. However, time post onset appeared to affect the magnitude of patients' *response to treatment*. Of those patients who began treatment within the first 4 months post onset of aphasia, 78% improved significantly on a standardized aphasia test, while 46% of those who began treatment from 4 to 12 months post onset improved significantly on the same test, even when subjects' test scores were corrected for the effects of spontaneous neurologic recovery. Poeck and associates' results suggest that delaying treatment negatively affects aphasic adults' recovery of communicative abilities.

Others have concluded that delaying treatment has no major effects on outcome. Wertz and associates (1986) randomly assigned aphasic patients to two groups. The patients in each group were from 2 to 24 weeks post onset of aphasia. One group received 12 weeks of treatment that began as soon as they qualified for the study and the other group (matched with the first group on numerous variables) waited 12 weeks and then received treatment equivalent to that given to the immediately treated group. At 12 weeks (when the immediate-treatment group had received 12 weeks of treatment and the deferred-treatment group had received none) the immediate-treatment group had improved significantly more (on aphasia test scores) than the delayed-treatment group. However, when the delayed-treatment group then received 12 weeks of treatment while the immediate-treatment group received none, the delayed-treatment group made significant improvement and eventually caught up with the immediate-treatment group. Wertz and associates concluded that delaying treatment for 12 weeks had no irreversible effects on aphasic patients' eventual recovery.

Even if it were to be shown that delaying treatment has few or no significant effects on patient's scores on standardized tests of language and communication (the criterion used in the published studies), it may not be legitimate to conclude that delaying treatment has no negative effects on the patient or the patient's family. Clinicians do more than treat specific speech and language behaviors in the first weeks following the onset of a patient's aphasia. They educate patients and families about the causes of the patient's aphasia and provide them with strategies for dealing with communication breakdown. They make referrals to other disciplines and help the patient and family make use of community resources. They provide reassur-

ance, advice, and support to patients and families.

Education, counseling, and support may not affect an aphasic patient's scores on standardized tests, yet they are important to patients and families immediately after onset of aphasia. Consequently, it cannot be said that clinicians have nothing to contribute to aphasic patients during the first 10 or 12 weeks post onset that cannot just as well be done later. It may be that delaying treatment of aphasic adults has no significant and irreversible effects on their test scores. However delaying or eliminating the counseling, education, and support provided during the first weeks after the patient becomes aphasic may have important and irreversible negative effects upon the patient and the family.

The Goals of Treatment

Most adults who remain aphasic for more than a month or so post onset do not completely regain their premorbid communicative ability. Some with very mild aphasia at a month or so post onset may eventually approximate their premorbid communicative abilities but they are a small proportion of the aphasic population. Consequently, clinicians formulating treatment objectives usually expect that the patient will be left with residual communication impairments at the end of treatment. The objective of treatment usually is to enable the patient to communicate with maximum effectiveness in the face of these residual communication impairments. Schuell, Jenkins, and Jimenez-Pabon (1965) asserted that:

> The primary objective in treatment of aphasia is to increase communication. What the aphasic patient wants is to recover enough language to get on with his life (p. 333).

Holland (1977) observed that traditional didactic treatment approaches tend to focus on:

Activities such as matching, naming, and helping aphasics to comprehend utterances defined by their linguistic structure, instead of their likelihood of being heard in everyday communication. . . . Most therapy is disproportionately centered on the propositionality of an utterance, not on its communicative value (p. 171).

Holland went on to recommend that treatment focus on *communicative competence,* which is a person's use of language in naturalistic contexts.

During the 1980s many clinicians moved away from traditional linguistically oriented, didactic treatment, which had predominated until that time, toward treatment that emphasized functional communication in naturalistic contexts. The functional communication treatment programs typically relied on within-the-clinic analogues to naturalistic communicative interactions (e.g., conversations), with the expectation that communicative skills acquired in those situations would generalize to daily life. These treatment approaches downplayed traditional didactic drills and emphasized natural communication with natural materials in natural contexts. Patients were encouraged (or taught) to communicate nonverbally with gestures and facial expression, and to enhance their comprehension by using the information provided by others' gestures and facial expressions and by situational contexts. Functional approaches to treatment recognized that aphasic persons need not be perfect speakers or perfect listeners to communicate adequately.

There is no strong empirical evidence that functional approaches to treatment are more successful in creating improvement in daily life communication than traditional approaches, although an advantage for functional approaches seems intuitively reasonable. However, it also seems intuitively reasonable that traditional didactic approaches might lead to comparable improvements in daily life communication if the

behaviors targeted for treatment are important in daily life communicative interactions. That the *procedures* employed in treatment resemble natural communicative interactions may be less important than that the *behaviors* (or processes) targeted for treatment are relevant to daily life communication. For example, it seems reasonable that placing an aphasic person in activities in which she or he must quickly adjust to changes in stimuli or response requirements might enhance his or her comprehension in daily life interchanges in which topics and speakers change abruptly and without warning, even though the activities do not mimic daily life interchanges.

The important issue here is that of *generalization* (the transfer of what is accomplished in the clinic to the aphasic person's daily life). Regardless of how one approaches treatment, generalization to daily life often does not occur unless procedures for enhancing generalization to daily life are part of the treatment program. Because improvements in communicative ability that do not extend outside the clinic are of little value, it behooves the clinician to plan for, work for, and test for generalization of skills, strategies, and behaviors acquired in the clinic to the patient's daily life. (See Chapter 4 for more on generalization.)

Candidacy for Treatment

Not all adults with aphasia receive treatment for their aphasia and not all should. Some have such mild impairments that neurologic recovery alone leaves them with no significant linguistic or communicative impairments. Some are too ill or too weak to tolerate treatment sessions. Some are so severely impaired that existing treatment procedures offer no hope of recovery sufficient to justify the cost of treatment. Some who would otherwise be candidates for treatment refuse it. And, regrettably, some who are treatment candidates do not have the money or the insurance coverage to pay for it. Because patient refusal and financial coverage usually are not the clinician's to control, the clinician's decision about offering treatment to a patient customarily depends on her or his best guess as to whether treatment will produce improvements in the patient's communication performance sufficient to justify its cost.

There is no substitute for trial treatment as an indicator of a patient's potential response to treatment. Within a few sessions of trail treatment the clinician can tell if the patient's performance improves in treatment tasks, if the improvement lasts from session to session, if improvements in treatment tasks generalize to other tasks or other contexts, and if the patient can (or will) expend the time and effort needed to make these things happen. However, trial treatment is an expensive way to tell if a patient will benefit from treatment, both in terms of the cost of the treatment itself and the potential diversion of treatment from those who will benefit from it to those who will not. Consequently, for some patients, clinicians may forego trial treatment and decide not to treat, based on negative indicators observed during their evaluation of the patient.

Schuell (1965) described the test performance of a group of aphasic adults who exhibited what she called *irreversible aphasic syndrome,* which she characterized as "almost complete loss of functional language skills in all modalities" (p. 14). These patients made frequent errors pointing to common objects named by the examiner. They could not follow simple spoken directions, could not read aloud nor comprehend simple printed sentences, could not name objects or give simple biographic information, and could not write simple words, either spontaneously or to dictation. A few of these patients could match some simple words to pictures, some produced a few automatic and overlearned speech responses such as counting or profanity, and some could copy simple drawings. Schuell commented that some patients with irreversible aphasic syndrome

made limited gains in auditory comprehension but she asserted that none recovered functional language in any modality.*

What Schuell called *irreversible aphasic syndrome* others call *global aphasia.* Collins (1991) characterizes global aphasia as follows:

> Global aphasia is a severe, acquired impairment of communicative ability across all language modalities, and often no single communicative modality is strikingly better than another. Visual nonverbal problem-solving abilities are often severely depressed as well and are usually compatible with language performance. It (global aphasia) usually results from extensive damage to the language zones of the left hemisphere but may result from smaller, subcortical lesions. (p. 6).

Collins noted that global aphasia can be acute, evolving, or chronic. According to Collins, many aphasic patients (perhaps the majority) are globally aphasic at and immediately following onset. Some (the acute ones) evolve to less severe forms within the first week or so post onset. Others (the evolving ones) are globally aphasic at onset but over a period of months or years slowly evolve to less-severe forms of aphasia. The remainder (the chronic ones) are left with profound impairments for the rest of their lives.

Goodglass & Kaplan (1983) described global aphasia as follows:

> In global aphasia, all aspects of language are so severely impaired that there is no longer a distinctive pattern of preserved versus impaired components. It is only articulation that is sometimes well preserved in the few words or stereotyped utterances that are preserved. Global aphasics sometimes produce stereotyped utterances that may consist of real or nonsense words. Some patients produce a continuous output of syllables that employ a limited set of vowel-consonant combinations that make no sense, even though they are ut-

---

* Presumably Schuell was referring to verbal language (auditory comprehension, reading, speaking, writing) and not gestural communication, body language, or other nonverbal means of communication.

tered with expressive intonation. . . . Auditory comprehension of conversation concerning material of immediate personal relevance may appear fairly good in comparison to the patient's poor performance on all the formal auditory comprehension subtests (p. 97).

The foregoing descriptions are remarkably consistent. They portray the globally aphasic adult as one who has limited comprehension of personally relevant spoken language but little usable expressive language beyond a few stereotyped utterances.

The healing effects of time apparently have little effect on the language capabilities of most patients who remain globally aphasic beyond the immediate post-onset period. The results of studies by Brust and associates (1976), Kertesz and McCabe (1977), and Prins, Snow, and Wagenaar (1978) show that the prognosis is grim for patients who are globally aphasic at one month or more post onset.

Brust and associates reviewed the medical records of 177 aphasic stroke patients. Of those who were diagnosed as globally aphasic at onset, 75% remained globally aphasic at 1 to 3 months post onset. Kertesz and McCabe reported that 83% of patients who were globally aphasic at 1 month post onset remained globally aphasic at 1 year post onset. Prins, Snow, and Wagenaar found that 80% of patients who were globally aphasic at 3 months post onset remained globally aphasic at 1 year post onset.

There seems little doubt that the presence of global aphasia at 1 month post onset is an ominous prognostic sign. Only about one-in-five patients achieve functional use of language and most of those who do remain markedly aphasic, with functional verbal communication limited to communication of basic needs, and comprehension limited to bits and pieces of simple conversational interactions on highly familiar topics.

There are several indicators of severe global aphasia that suggest that a patient may not have the capacity to become a functional verbal communicator. The presence of one indicator in a neurologically recovered patient is ominous, and the presence of more than one indicator should make clinicians extremely cautious about the functional outcome of speech and language treatment.*

Verbal Stereotypies or Repetitive Utterances and Severely Impaired Comprehension The presence of repetitive, stereotypical, perseverative utterances (such as *"me-me-me-me"* or *"oh boy- oh boy-oh boy- oh boy")* in combination with severely impaired language comprehension in neurologically recovered patients suggest severe and irreversible aphasia. Few neurologically recovered patients with these symptoms become functional verbal communicators, even with treatment. Some may eventually learn to communicate a few basic needs using single words and gestures and some may learn to communicate basic needs with alternative communication systems such as communication boards or communication books.

Inability To Match Identical Objects or Pictures and Objects If neurologically recovered patients cannot match common objects (such as forks, pencils, keys) or cannot match common objects to pictures, they are unlikely to regain functional verbal communication, even with treatment. Inability to match objects to objects or objects to pictures frequently (some would say always) is associated with bilateral brain damage and is unusual even in severely aphasic patients with unilateral brain damage.

Unreliable Yes-No Responses Neurologically recovered aphasic patients who cannot reliably indicate (or learn to indicate) *"yes"* and

---

* The adjectives "neurologically recovered" will be used herein to denote patients for whom "spontaneous" physiologic recovery is mostly complete. For most patients with occlusive strokes, physiologic recovery is essentially complete within 4 to 6 weeks, although slow improvement beyond that time is common. For patients with hemorrhagic strokes and for those with traumatic brain injuries, physiologic recovery may last longer, but usually is essentially complete by 3 to 6 months.

"no" verbally, by gesture or head nod, or by pointing to cards showing words or symbols representing *"yes"* and *"no"* usually are not good candidates for treatment. A neurologically recovered patient's failure to develop dependable yes-no responses with training suggests severe aphasia. If such a patient cannot be taught reliable yes-no responses to simple *nonverbal* stimuli within an hour or two, the prospects for positive effects of treatment are poor.

Jargon and Empty Speech Without Self-Correction Some patients with severe comprehension disabilities produce jargon (nonwords such as *"kalimfropper"*) or meaningless strings of words such as *"That's Sheila's aunt in a full subscription."* without recognizing that there is anything wrong. Neurologically recovered patients who exhibit these behaviors usually are not good candidates for treatment directed toward speech and language disabilities.

The signs in the foregoing list are prognostically ominous because treatment for aphasia, unlike medication, is not something that can be given to a passive patient with good therapeutic effects—it requires the active participation of the patient. Patients whose cognitive impairments, confusion, agitation, depression, or distractibility prevent them from participating in an interview or test session are unlikely to be capable of participating in treatment in any meaningful way. Patients who cannot learn even simple nonverbal tasks (such as matching identical objects, pictures, or forms, or sorting them into categories based on salient characteristics) are unlikely to have the attentional and cognitive capacity to participate in or benefit from treatment. Patients who can learn a simple task but cannot generalize the learning from that task to other similar tasks are unlikely to progress through a treatment program at an acceptable rate and will almost certainly fail to generalize what they learn in the clinic to their daily life environment.

Prolonged treatment to reinstate functional verbal communication for such patients is rarely successful. The speech-language pathologist's primary role with most such patients is to help the family or other caregivers structure the patient's daily life environment to take advantage of the communicative abilities that the patient has retained.

During the last decade, several investigators have developed treatment programs for severely aphasic persons (Alexander & Loverso, 1993; Collins, 1991; Helm & Barresi, 1980; Helm-Estabrooks, Fitzpatrick & Barresi 1982; Salvatore & Thompson, 1986; Steele and associates, 1989). If the effectiveness of these new treatment programs can be demonstrated, what Schuell called "irreversible" aphasia may become at least partially reversible.

The Focus and Progression of Treatment

Aphasia test batteries typically partition communication among verbal processes (listening, speaking, reading, and writing) and provide tasks within each process that test various input and output modalities (auditory, visual, and sometimes tactile input; oral, gestural, and graphic output). Such partitioning of communication can prove attractive to novice clinicians who are searching for a rationale to guide their treatment and may lead them to adopt a *treat-to-the-test* approach to treatment, in which the clinician identifies tests in which a patient's performance is deficient and constructs treatment tasks that mimic the content and structure of those tests. The clinician may distribute the tasks across processes or modalities to increase the generality of treatment and may select tasks in which the patient's performance is somewhat deficient but not completely erroneous to ensure that the treatment tasks are at an appropriate level of difficulty. If a simple *treat-to-the-test* approach to treatment is to be effective (which means that it has positive effects on the patient's daily life communication) the tasks in the test that serve as the model for treatment must be valid representations of daily life communication. If the approach is not effective, the treatment may improve a patient's test scores, but have little effect on their daily life communication. (The treatment is *efficacious,* but not *effective.*)

A more sophisticated version of the *treat-to-the-test approach* is the *selective treat-to-the-test approach.* Clinicians using this approach consider deficient performance in some tests more important than deficient performance in other tests. For example, those who believe that impaired auditory comprehension is a central problem in aphasia pay particular attention to patients' performance on tests that assess auditory comprehension and design treatment materials and procedures that mimic those of the auditory comprehension tests on which a patient exhibits impaired performance. The *selective treat-to-the-test approach* assigns greater importance to some tests than others, based on some underlying rationale, but the tasks included in treatment are identical to, or closely resemble, the tests that led to their inclusion in the treatment program.

The major problem with *treat-to-the-test* approaches is that the tasks in aphasia test batteries may have little to do with patients' daily life communication needs. Consequently, *treat-to-the-test* approaches run the risk of wasting the clinician's and the patient's time, energy, and resources in treatment tasks that have little or no positive effect on the patient's life and well being beyond escalation of the patient's test scores (an escalation that often proves temporary—when treatment stops, the patient's test scores decline).

The *treat underlying processes approach* orients clinicians away from structuring treatment tasks to replicate tests on which a patient performs poorly and toward underlying cognitive processes that are assumed to be responsible for the impaired performance. Most clinicians and investigators agree that aphasia is not a loss of language (either vocabulary or rules) but is the result of impairments in processes necessary for comprehending, formulating, and producing spoken and written language. For example,

comprehension impairments in aphasia may be caused by reduced speed and efficiency in attaching meaning to words, rather than loss of word meanings, or they may be caused by reductions in the speed, efficiency, or accuracy of retrieval from memory, rather than loss of vocabulary. Similarly, speech production problems may be caused by disruptions of word retrieval or phonologic selection and sequencing, rather than loss of words or syntactic rules.

For those who believe that aphasia represents a reduction in the speed and efficiency of processes underlying language, rather than loss of language, treatment focuses on *reactivating* or *restimulating* language processes, rather than on *teaching* specific responses (Schuell, Jenkins, & Jimenez-Pabon; 1965). For example, if an aphasic patient has a reading problem, the clinician might attempt to determine whether the problem is related to *(1)* eye movements and visual search, *(2)* single-word comprehension, *(3)* use of syntactic rules, *(4)* ability to deduce main ideas, make inferences, or draw conclusions, or *(5)* storage and recall of information gained from printed materials. After the determination is made, treatment focuses on the processes identified as deficient. One of the major advantages of a process-directed approach to treatment is that treating a general process may affect several specific communicative abilities that depend on the process.

■ TREATMENT OF AUDITORY COMPREHENSION

Schuell, Jenkins, and Jimenez-Pabon (1965) considered impairments in auditory comprehension and auditory retention span a central problem in aphasia. Since that time, treatment of auditory comprehension impairments has had a special status for many clinicians who believe that improving auditory comprehension is the most efficient way to improve aphasic adults' general language competence. This belief has not been empirically supported by experimental evidence, but treatment of auditory comprehension impairments continues to play a central role in many approaches to aphasia treatment.

For many years auditory comprehension was thought to proceed through a series of stages, beginning with analysis of the acoustic characteristics of spoken messages and culminating in derivation of the meanings of utterances. Listeners were thought to identify the phonemes in the message, combine the phonemes into representations of words, retrieve the meanings of the words, determine the relationships among words, and construct a mental representation for the meaning of the utterance, in that order. Such models of comprehension eventually became known as *bottom-up* models, because listeners start with the physical characteristics of the message and work their way up through a series of levels until the meaning of the utterance becomes apparent.

During the 1960s and 1970s other models of comprehension were proposed, in which listeners' general knowledge and expectations played an important part in their comprehension of spoken material. These models made it clear that comprehension is not simply the result of a series of computations by which listeners deduce the meaning of what they hear. For listeners in naturalistic situations, the words seem only to provide a starting point from which listeners go on to identify the speaker's intent, construct presuppositions, develop expectations, decide what is important and what is not, and relate what they hear to what they already know. These models became known as *top-down* models, because listeners start out with general expectations about what a speaker is likely to say and confirm or change the expectations based on what the speaker actually says.

Listeners seem to use lexical and syntactic processes primarily to establish what the speaker is talking about and to identify how what the speaker is saying relates to what he or she has previously said. These lexical and syntactic processes are sometimes called *text-based processes* because they depend strongly on the words and syntax of what is said, in contrast to processes in which the listener invokes general knowledge, intuition, and guessing to deduce the meaning of spoken material. These latter processes are sometimes called *knowledge-based* or *heuristic processes*.

Text-based processes require more mental effort than knowledge-based (heuristic) processes. Heuristic processes lighten the processing workload by allowing the listener to deduce a speaker's general meaning and intent without the need for continuous word-by-word lexical and syntactic analysis. Normal listeners usually emphasize heuristic processes over text-based ones and rely heavily on text-based processes only when forced to so do by the absence of extralinguistic sources of information, unusual vocabulary, or complex syntax.

Scripts provide a good example of heuristic processes and how they can facilitate comprehension. Scripts are mental representations of sequences of events that an individual has repeatedly encountered in daily life. For example, if a speaker is describing what went on at a party the previous night, a listener can call upon his or her knowledge of what typically happens at parties to construct a set of expectations about what most likely took place at the party attended by the speaker. Once the listener has mentally activated her or his party script, she or he can predict much of what the speaker is likely to say:

- That a number of people were there
- That food and drink were served
- That there was a host or hostess
- That the party was at the host or hostess' home
- That social conversations took place

Numerous studies of discourse comprehension show that normal listeners use such mental representations to organize information from discourse and to form expectations about what is likely to be conveyed in a particular sample of discourse (Adams & Collins, 1979; Bower, Black, & Turner, 1979; and others). Armus,

Brookshire, and Nicholas (1989) have shown that aphasic adults' knowledge of scripts for common situations is preserved and have suggested that preserved script knowledge may at least partially account for some aphasic adults' good comprehension of spoken discourse in the face of substantially impaired performance on tests of single-sentence comprehension.

Memory and Listening Comprehension

Listening comprehension and memory cannot be separated. Listeners cannot comprehend spoken language unless they can retain it in memory long enough to carry out whatever processes are necessary to arrive at its meaning and they must retain the mental representation of its meaning long enough to respond appropriately. That listening comprehension and memory are related is clear. However, the relationships between memory and listening comprehension have not yet been well described.

During the 1960s several models of memory were proposed, which conceptualized memory in terms of the transfer of information among several storage components or stages. The traditional model postulated three stages through which information passes from perception to long-term storage. These stages were given different labels in different models, and different models assigned slightly different responsibilities to stages, but the differences among models were mainly in the details and not in their general form. The first stage in most models is a *sensory register* (sometimes called *sensory memory*) in which traces of incoming stimuli are briefly stored in modality-specific form (auditory, visual, or tactile after images). The sensory register has limited capacity and its contents decay within 1 or 2 seconds, after which the information is lost unless it is transferred to another stage. Information in the sensory register cannot be maintained by rehearsal.

The second stage is commonly called *short-term memory* (or *primary memory*). Short-term memory also has limited capacity, and information within it decays but at a slower rate than in the sensory register (within several seconds to several minutes). Information can be maintained in short-term memory by rehearsal. Short-term memory capacity is often quantified as *retention span,* or the number of items of discrete information (numerals, letters, words) that can be held in memory at one time. For many years short-term memory was considered a passive storage space through which information passes on its way to *long-term memory* (or *secondary memory*). Long-term memory has very large (perhaps infinite) capacity, and information in long-term memory decays slowly, if at all. Long-term memory is conceptualized as a static repository for memories of our experiences and for our knowledge. The meanings of sentences are integrated into permanent memory at this stage.

In the late 1960s and early 1970s some investigators (Warrington & Shallice, 1969; Shallice & Warrington, 1970; Baddeley, 1986) formulated the concept of *working memory* to denote a mental space wherein active processing of information coming from the sensory register or retrieved from long-term memory takes place. Working memory was conceptualized as a limited-capacity processing space in which cognitive processes (such as sentence comprehension) can be carried out. Working memory has many of the characteristics of what others call short-term memory, except that short-term memory is conceptualized as a static repository for information on its way to long-term storage, whereas working memory is a place where active mental processing goes on.

Some contemporary models of memory (such as Craik & Lockhart, 1972) reject the *stages* concept of memory in favor of a continuous *depth of processing* explanation. However, the general concept of how comprehension proceeds in depth of processing models is similar to that for stages models.

The exact role of memory in aphasic adults' comprehension impairments is not well understood. Most aphasic adults have impairments in short-term verbal memory that interfere with comprehension and recall of spoken material. In fact, Schuell and associates (1965) identified deficient short-term retention and recall as one of the defining characteristics of adult aphasia. There is little doubt that short-term verbal memory impairments affect comprehension of single-sentence messages such as those in the *Token Test* (De Renzi & Vignolo, 1962) and other tests of single-sentence comprehension in which test takers must comprehend and retain unrelated sentences such as, *"Touch the large yellow square and the small green circle."* or *"The thin girl with a bow in her hair chases the small, black dog with no collar."* Aphasic adults' performance on such tests has been shown to correlate strongly with their performance on tests of short-term memory (Lesser, 1976; Martin & Feher, 1990).

Short-term memory impairment apparently does not account for aphasic adults' problems in comprehending syntactically complex sentences (such as *"The dog that the cat chased was white."*), because nonaphasic adults with impaired short-term memory usually have little difficulty with comprehension of such sentences (Vallar & Baddeley, 1984), and aphasic adults' performance on tests of short-term memory is not meaningfully related to their performance on tests that assess comprehension of syntactically complex sentences (Martin & Feher, 1990). That aphasic adults comprehend longer sentences such as *"The man was greeted by his wife and he was smoking a pipe."* better than shorter but syntactically more complex sentences such as *"The man greeted by his wife was smoking a pipe."* (Goodglass and associates, 1979) also suggests that short-term memory does not account for aphasic adults' difficulties with syntactically complex sentences.

■ TREATMENT OF SINGLE-WORD COMPREHENSION

The prototypical treatment for impaired single-word comprehension is pointing drill in which the clinician places an array of pictures or (less frequently) objects before the patient, names the objects one at a time in essentially random order, and asks the patient to point to each item as it is named.* The clinician manipulates the difficulty of the task by manipulating the familiarity or abstractness of the stimulus words. Single-word comprehension drills are appropriate for patients with severe comprehension impairments who cannot comprehend phrase-length or sentence-length materials. Single-word comprehension drills usually serve as a starting point for a succession of drills in which the length, information density, and complexity of the treatment stimuli increase as the patient's comprehension improves.

If a patient does not progress beyond single-word comprehension within a reasonable number of treatment sessions (5 to 10), continuing single-word comprehension drills usually is not worthwhile. Improved single-word comprehension, by itself, rarely creates meaningful changes in the daily life communicative competence of severely aphasic patients. Even if such patients acquire rudimentary single-word listening vocabularies, most cannot use them in daily life contexts, in which single-word messages are infrequent and speakers do not adjust their output to fit these patients' limited linguistic capacities.

Single-word comprehension drills also are not appropriate for patients who can comprehend short phrases or sentences, but have mild to moderate single-word comprehension impairments. These patients' single-word comprehension impairments involve primarily low-frequency words, and low-frequency words usually do not play an important part in daily life conversations. According to Hayes (1988) 83% of

---

* Most clinicians put the stimulus word at the end of a short carrier phrase, such as "Point to the _____" or "Show me the _____." Although the clinician's utterances technically are sentences, the redundancy of the carrier phrase makes it irrelevant to successful performance.

the words used in daily life adult-to-adult conversations in the United States are within the 1,000 most frequent words in English, and 94% are within the 5,000 most frequent words.* Consequently, comprehension of most daily life spoken material seems unlikely to depend much on comprehension of low-frequency words. Furthermore, the context in which words occur often gives strong hints about their meanings, and the aphasic listener who can make use of context to deduce the meaning of uncomprehended words is unlikely to have much difficulty comprehending most daily life spoken material, even when it contains some low-frequency words.

A small number of patients with mild or moderate aphasia experience remarkable difficulties in attaching meanings to words they hear (or read). They behave (usually intermittently) as if they do not know the meanings of spoken or printed words, even when the words are common in the language. Their performance is not word-specific—sometimes they comprehend a given word and at other times they do not. Sometimes they behave as if they are hearing words from a foreign language. They may repeat an unrecognized word over and over and they may even spell the word while attempting to associate it with a meaning. When these patients are given a clue to the meaning of an unrecognized word (such as a synonym or antonym), they often recognize the word.

Treatment for these patients usually consists of drills in which they match spoken words to pictures or give definitions, synonyms, or antonyms for spoken words. Unfortunately, such drills rarely yield meaningful improvements in single-word comprehension. However, these patients' single-word comprehension sometimes can be treated indirectly by improving their short-term auditory memory and sentence comprehension and by teaching them

---

* The 1,000th most frequent word in English is *pass* and the 5,000th most frequent word is *vibrate*. Carroll, Davies, and Richman (1971).

to use context to arrive at the meaning of unrecognized words.

■ UNDERSTANDING SPOKEN SENTENCES

Impaired sentence comprehension commonly is targeted in treatment programs for aphasic adults, not only because it seems to be important in daily life, but because of the central role played by auditory comprehension in some models of aphasia. Treatment to improve comprehension of spoken sentences typically is accomplished by means of drills in which patients answer questions, follow directions, or verify the meaning of sentences.

Answering Questions

The questions in question-answering drills can be either yes-no questions to which patients can respond with spoken or gestural indicators of *"yes"* or *"no"*, or open-ended questions which call for longer and more complex responses.

Yes-No Questions   Yes-no questions can emphasize general knowledge (*"Is Mason City the capital of Iowa?"*), verbal retention span (*"Are monkeys, horses, cows, and pigs animals?"*), semantic discriminations (*"Do you brush teeth with a comb?"*), phonemic discriminations (*"Do you wear a shirt and pie?"*), syntactic analysis (*"Do you wear feet on your shoes?"*), or semantic relationships (*"Is a banana a vegetable?"*).

Yes-no questions are suitable for treating comprehension in severely impaired patients who cannot produce enough speech to answer open-ended questions. Most of these patients can indicate *"yes"* and *"no"* either verbally, by nodding and head-shaking, or by pointing to words or symbols signifying *"yes"* and *"no."*

Open-Ended Questions   Open-ended questions such as *"Why do people put locks on their doors?"* permit clinicians to sample a greater variety of information and permit greater flexibility in the structure of the questions, but their validity as comprehension training items may be compromised by the need for patients to formulate and produce longer verbal responses. Because of this, most clinicians use open-ended questions as vehicles for work on word retrieval and speech formulation, rather than as items in comprehension drills.

Following Spoken Directions Treatment tasks in which patients follow spoken directions require sequential pointing or manipulative responses to directions spoken by the clinician, as in *"Put the spoon beside the pencil, the quarter beside the comb, and give me the key."* In following–spoken-directions drills, the length and complexity of the spoken directions are controlled so that the patient is continuously working at a level that taxes, but does not exceed, her or his processing capacity. As the patient's comprehension improves, treatment progresses along a hierarchy of increasingly longer and/or syntactically complex sentences such as the one described by Kearns and Hubbard (1977). Their hierarchy is empirically determined, based on the average difficulty of 13 levels of spoken directions for a group of 10 aphasic adults. The group's average scores (on a 16-point scale) for the 13 levels, from easiest to most difficult, were:

- Point to one common object by name. (14.30)
- Point to one common object by function. (14.02)
- Point in sequence to two common objects by function. (12.90)
- Point in sequence to two common objects by name. (12.67)
- Point to one object spelled by the examiner. (12.51)
- Point to one object described by the examiner with three descriptors *("Which one is white, plastic, and has bristles?")*. (12.23)
- Follow one-verb instructions *("Pick up the pen.")*. (12.05)
- Point in sequence to three common objects by name. (10.74)
- Point in sequence to three common objects by function. (10.72)

- Carry out two-object location instructions *("Put the pen in front of the knife.")* (10.20)
- Carry out, in sequence, two-verb instructions *("Point to the knife and turn over the fork.")*. (9.77)
- Carry out, in sequence, two-verb instructions with time constraint *("Before you pick up the knife, hand me the fork.")*. (8.60)
- Carry out three-verb instructions *("Point to the knife, turn over the fork, and hand me the pencil.")*. (7.53)

Kearns and Hubbard's 13-level hierarchy may be useful for setting up a hierarchy of task difficulty for individual patients, although the hierarchy for a given patient may not match Kearns and Hubbard's, which was based on group average performance. Consequently, clinicians may elect to personalize a hierarchy for individual patients by assessing their performance across the hierarchy and selecting the level(s) at which the patient's performance has the appropriate proportions of correct, nearly correct, and incorrect responses.

Following–spoken-directions drills primarily target patients' verbal retention span. Many clinicians believe that if an aphasic patient's verbal retention span improves, his or her language comprehension in general will improve. At this time there is no empirical evidence to support this assumption, and evidence from studies of normal language comprehension suggest that comprehending language in natural situations does not depend strongly on verbal retention span. Given that most utterances in daily life conversations are less than 8 words long (Goldman-Eisler, 1968), and given that most utterances in daily life are not as informationally dense as the sentences in verbal retention span drills, it seems likely that improving aphasic patients' verbal retention span beyond 6-word to 8-word moderately redundant utterances may have weaker effects on daily life comprehension than many clinicians believe.

This does not mean, however, that following-spoken-directions drills may not *indirectly* improve daily life comprehension by improving the operation of other processes that support comprehension. One likely candidate for such a supporting role is *attention*. Successful performance in following-spoken-directions drills requires that the patient focus attention quickly and maintain it for the duration of the incoming message. Patients who cannot quickly focus attention miss information at the beginning of messages and those who cannot maintain it miss information at the end. Consequently, it seems reasonable that following-spoken-directions drills might enhance auditory comprehension in general by enhancing attentional skills that support the comprehension process.

Sentence Verification In sentence verification drills, the patient listens to a series of spoken sentences and makes a judgment about the relationship of each sentence to one or more pictures. In one form of verification, the patient sees a picture as he or she hears each sentence and indicates whether or not the picture accurately portrays the meaning of the sentence.

Each sentence is presented several times (not consecutively), sometimes with a picture that matches the sentence's meaning and sometimes with a foil. The foil pictures usually are chosen to contrast with the stimulus sentence in specified ways (e.g., differing from the stimulus sentence in subject, verb, or object, as in Figure 6-1).

In a second form of sentence verification (called *match to sample*), each time the patient hears a sentence he or she is shown a page containing several (usually four) pictures, one of which portrays the meaning of the sentence (Figure 6-2). The other pictures (the foils) usually contrast with the stimulus sentence in specified ways, as described above. The patient points to the picture that represents the meaning of the sentence.

In most match-to-sample tasks, foil pictures have systematic relationships to target pictures. Figure 6-2 shows a set of four pictures that might accompany the sentence *"The man is hugging the woman."* To respond correctly, listeners have to perceive subject, object, or verb mismatches between foil pictures and the stimulus sentence. The difficulty of an item such as this for aphasic listeners depends on the seman-

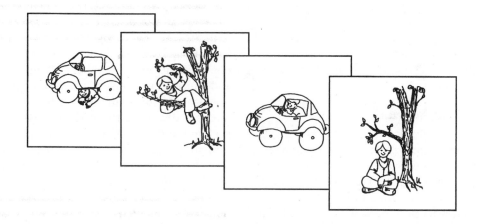

Figure 6-1 ▪ **Response cards that might be used in a sentence verification drill for the sentence *"The boy is in the tree."* These four cards would be mixed with other cards and the clinician would say the sentence whenever one of these cards came up.**

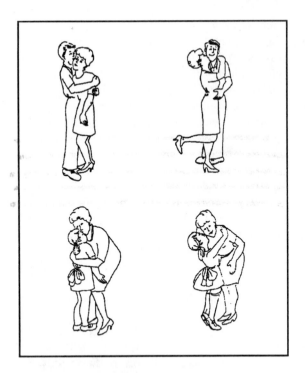

Figure 6-2 ▪ A sentence-to-picture match-to-sample response card that might be shown as the clinician says *"The man is hugging the woman."*

tic closeness of foils to the target. (*"The cat is chasing the dog."* as a foil for Figure 6-2 would be easily identified as a foil by most aphasic adults, whereas *"The man is hugging the girl."* would catch many.)

Task Switching Activities

Many aphasic adults are tripped up when they get into conversational interactions wherein they must maintain a sense of the overall purpose or theme of a conversation while simultaneously dealing with quick changes in topics, speakers, or conversational roles. Task-switching drills can help these patients. Task-switching drills are sentence-comprehension drills in which the form of the stimulus sentences and the nature of the responses expected from the patient change

unpredictably from trail to trail, as in the following sequence:

- Pick up the spoon.
- Point to the black one.
- Which one do you drink from?
- Does Thursday come after Wednesday?
- Make a fist and blink three times.
- Put the key in the cup.
- Is your name Fred?

▪ TREATMENT OF DISCOURSE COMPREHENSION

When planning treatment for patients with impaired discourse comprehension it is important to remember that the traditional concept of comprehension skills as progressing from words to sentences to extended texts is inappropriate (Pierce, 1989). Words and sentences in discourse are easier to comprehend than words and sentences in isolation. When sentences occur in discourse, their comprehension depends more on their relationship to the overall theme of the discourse and the degree to which the discourse relates to a given patient's knowledge and experience than on their length or syntactic complexity.

The difficulty of a discourse comprehension task is determined not only by the content and structure of the discourse, but by what the patient is asked to comprehend and remember from the discourse. If the patient is asked to comprehend and remember only the main ideas and the overall point of the discourse, the patient does better than if she or he is asked to remember details. If the patient is asked to comprehend and remember only directly stated information, the patient does better than if she or he is asked to comprehend and remember implied information.

Most adults with mild-to-moderate aphasia are likely to have retained at least some of their discourse comprehension abilities. Most should get the main ideas, providing the discourse is well structured and unambiguous. Most should be able to construct the major inferences suggested by discourse, especially inferences that relate to main ideas or the overall theme of the discourse. However, their comprehension suffers when discourse is not well structured, with clearly identified main ideas and an obvious topic or theme, or if the information is outside their experience.

The Format of Discourse Comprehension Treatment

The typical format for discourse comprehension treatment is for the clinician to read aloud or play a recording of a sample of discourse, after which the patient answers questions about information in the discourse. The questions typically are yes-no questions such as those in the *Discourse Comprehension Test* (Brookshire & Nicholas, 1993; previously described). Yes-no questions *("Did the women put up a sign at a shopping center?")* typically are used because they minimize the effects of patients' memory impairments and speech formulation and production problems on their discourse comprehension performance.

Yes-no questions test patients' *recognition* rather than *recall* of information from discourse. To move patients toward recall, yet keep memory, speech formulation, and speech production demands under control, yes-no questions can be replaced with *sentence completion* items, in which patients complete sentence fragments provided by the clinician. *("The women put up a sign at a _____ ")*. For patients who can handle the limited formulation and speech production demands, sentence completion provides a more demanding test of recall of information from discourse than yes-no questions.

Open-ended questions ("Where did the women put up a sign?") move the patient farther away from recognition and toward recall, but place even more demands on speech formulation and production.

Retelling, in which patients recount as much as they can remember from a sample of discourse, requires patients to retrieve and produce information from memory without help from the content of the clinician's questions. Retelling provides the strongest indicator of patients' ability to comprehend and store information from discourse and retrieve it later without prompting. However, it places great demands on speech formulation and production.

Variables That May Be Manipulated in Treatment of Discourse Comprehension

Clinicians can regulate the difficulty of discourse comprehension tasks by manipulating several variables, either one by one or in combination. The most important of these variables are *familiarity, length, redundancy, cohesion, coherence, salience, directness,* and *speech rate.*

Familiarity Treatment typically begins with material that is familiar to the patient. Familiar material permits the patient to call on his or her pre-existing knowledge to facilitate comprehension of new information in the discourse. As the patient's comprehension of familiar material improves, the clinician gradually introduces less familiar material, thereby forcing the patient to depend less on his or her preexisting knowledge and more on the content of the discourse itself.

Many familiar situations and routines (such as going to a restaurant, buying groceries, or taking a plane trip) can be represented by *scripts* (discussed earlier). As previously mentioned, scripts are mental devices by which individuals organize knowledge of common situations. They permit individuals to formulate expectations about what events are likely to occur in a situation and the order in which they are likely to occur. Armus and associates suggested that aphasic adults' knowledge of scripts be exploited to facilitate their comprehension of discourse by:

- Teaching patients and their families that some daily life spoken discourse is predictable, based on what the listener already knows about the topic or situation being talked about.
- Giving patients practice identifying scripts that underlie samples of discourse.

- Asking the patient to predict what is likely to happen next in samples of discourse that represent scripts.

Length Treatment usually begins with short samples of discourse and progresses to longer ones. However, as noted earlier in this book, the samples should be long enough to permit the patient to develop a sense of its macrostructure (at least 100 to 200 words). As the patient's comprehension improves, the length of the discourse materials in the treatment program may increase.

Redundancy, Cohesion, and Coherence Treatment typically begins with samples of discourse in which repetition, paraphrase, and elaboration create substantial redundancy and high levels of cohesion and coherence. Redundancy, cohesion, and coherence establish relationships among ideas and help the listener determine the topic and establish the macrostructure of the discourse. Establishing the macrostructure of discourse permits patients to substitute less effortful heuristic processes for more effortful lexical and syntactic processes. As the patient's comprehension improves, materials with less repetition, paraphrase, and elaboration are gradually introduced to increase the patient's ability to deal with less redundant and less coherent discourse.

Salience Treatment begins with material in which main ideas are easily identified and the focus of treatment is on identification of main ideas. As the patient's comprehension improves, the treatment focus gradually extends to comprehension of details.

Directness Treatment begins with materials in which the important information is stated, rather than implied, and questions relate to information that has been presented in verbatim form in the discourse. As the patient's comprehension improves, questions that require simple inferences are introduced, followed by questions that require more complex inferences.

Speech Rate For those whose comprehension declines when materials are spoken at normal rates, the rate at which samples of discourse are played may be slowed by placing pauses at strategic locations.* As the patient's comprehension improves, the rate at which samples of discourse are presented can be gradually increased until the patient is working with materials spoken at normal rate.

Nicholas and Brookshire suggested that increasing the salience (or redundancy) of information in discourse and stating information directly are more dependable ways to improve aphasic listeners' comprehension of discourse than slowing the rate at which it is spoken. However, they recommended that clinicians still advise those who communicate with aphasic patients to speak slowly, because negative effects of slow speech rate are rare, and because some aphasic listeners benefit from slow speech rate. Nicholas and Brookshire also recommended that if a clinician intends to manipulate speech rate in treatment of an aphasic adult's comprehension impairments, he or she should pretest the patient to determine how that patient is affected by the manipulations.

■ TREATMENT OF READING COMPREHENSION

Aphasic adults almost always have impaired reading comprehension, and for most reading comprehension is more impaired than auditory comprehension. Aphasic adults usually suffer from an assortment of problems when they are confronted by printed texts. Their letter recognition, word recognition, and semantic and syntactic processing are slower and less efficient than that of normal readers. Consequently aphasic readers' overall reading rate is slow, letters and words may be misperceived, and for many, complex syntactic structures must be decoded by laborious word-by-word analysis. Impaired semantic and syntactic processes may lead to

---

* Pauses after main ideas may help to highlight them and provide the listener with extra processing time for comprehending them and storing them in memory.

misinterpretations and failure to establish the overall sense of printed materials. Impaired short-term retention may prevent the aphasic reader from establishing the overall topic or gist of printed materials, or, having established it, cause him or her to lose it part-way through. Given the multiplicity of obstacles, it should not be surprising that reading comprehension is a major problem for most aphasic adults or that few become fluent recreational readers.

Processes in Reading

Word Recognition Recognizing and attaching meanings to words is a prerequisite for comprehending printed texts. Word recognition quickly becomes automatic as readers develop skill in reading, and only unskilled readers depend heavily on word-by-word reading. Skilled readers usually do not read sentences or texts word by word unless the material is complex or contains unfamiliar words.

When readers deduce the meaning of individual printed words they may do so in any of four ways:

1. In *whole-word reading,* words are recognized as units and the reader does not analyze letters or letter strings within words. Whole-word reading requires that words be in the reader's reading vocabulary.
2. In *phonemic analysis,* the reader separates the word into letters or letter combinations, translates the letters or letter combinations into the sounds they represent, blends the sound representations together, and identifies the word represented by the sequence of sounds. Word recognition by phonemic analysis requires that the unfamiliar word be in the reader's listening vocabulary, but not necessarily in his or her reading vocabulary.
3. In *word recognition by context,* the reader uses the meaning of the context in which a word appears to guess a word's meaning. Recognition by context does not require that the unfamiliar word be in the reader's listening vocabulary.

4. Skilled readers read most words as whole words and use phonemic analysis and recognition by context only when they encounter unfamiliar words. When these three methods fail, the reader may look up unfamiliar words in a dictionary.

Syntactic Analysis Syntactic analysis is the primary way in which readers deduce relationships among words. Syntactic analysis presupposes knowledge of syntactic rules and recognition of syntactic structures. Syntactic knowledge allows readers to combine word strings into units of meaning that can be stored in long-term memory. Failure to perform syntactic analysis overloads the reader's short-term memory, and errors in syntactic analysis lead to miscomprehension of sentence meanings. An important difference between failure to recognize a word and failure to recognize a syntactic structure is that readers usually know when they fail to recognize a word but may be unaware when they fail to recognize a syntactic structure.

There was once general acceptance of the idea that if a reader could translate letters into their corresponding words he or she could comprehend printed texts. This assumption is no longer considered valid because it neglects the role of syntactic analysis in reading. Reading depends on syntactic analysis more than listening does. In listening, syntactic information can be conveyed by pauses, intonation, word order, and syntactic markers. In reading, the reader depends completely on word order and syntactic markers to deduce syntactic structure. Furthermore, printed texts usually are syntactically more complex and more formal in style than spoken discourse, making most printed texts more difficult to analyze syntactically than most spoken discourse.

Semantic Mapping Semantic mapping is a process by which readers relate the writer's intended meanings to their own knowledge and experience. Semantic mapping is the stage at which a text can be said to make sense to the reader. It involves organizing the meanings conveyed by a text into a coherent and sensical whole and integrating those meanings into memory. A reader's failure to organize the information in a text leads to confusion about which elements of the text are important and which are unimportant and may contribute to difficulty in getting the information into memory and retrieving it later. A reader's failure to relate meanings from texts to his or her knowledge leads to problems in appreciating the true meanings of metaphor, idioms, and figurative language.

Most of the top-down processes that contribute to comprehension of spoken discourse also contribute to comprehension of printed texts. Readers, like listeners, use the lexical content and syntactic structure of printed texts to deduce relationships among units of information. From there they go on to use general knowledge and intuition to determine a text's overall meaning. Readers, like listeners, use heuristic processes to bypass continuous word-by-word lexical and syntactic analysis when permitted to do so by the structure and content of printed texts. Readers, like listeners, often emphasize heuristic processes over text-based ones and may rely upon text-based processes only when pushed to do so by unfamiliar subject matter, complex syntax, or ambiguity or uncertainty.

Surface Dyslexia and Deep Dyslexia

Two patterns of word-reading impairment that sometimes accompany aphasia have received considerable attention in recent years. They are *surface dyslexia* and *deep dyslexia* (Marshall & Newcombe, 1973). These syndromes come from a model of reading that envisions two routes from the visual form of words-to-word meanings. Readers who use the *direct* (lexical) route access the mental representations of words and their meanings directly, based on the visual form of the words. Readers who use the *indirect* (phonologic) route access the mental representations of words indirectly, by converting graphemes to phonologic equivalents and accessing meaning via these phonologic representations.

Individuals with *surface dyslexia* have lost (or are impaired in) the direct (lexical) route and depend on the indirect (phonologic) route, which requires letter-by-letter decoding to deduce the meaning of printed words (Figure 6-3). These individuals read regularly spelled words (such as *keep* and *banana*) accurately, but misread irregularly spelled words by regularizing their pronunciation (*neighbor* may be read as

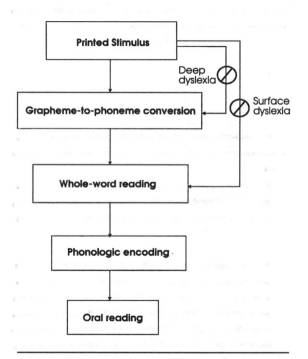

Figure 6-3 ■ A schematic diagram showing impaired processes responsible for surface dyslexia and deep dyslexia. In surface dyslexia the direct route from the printed stimulus to semantic representations is unavailable and the patient must depend on the indirect route (grapheme-to-phoneme conversion). In deep dyslexia the grapheme-to-phoneme conversion route is unavailable and the patient must depend on whole-word reading.

negbor). Individuals with surface dyslexia can read aloud phonologically legitimate nonwords (such as *tobada*) accurately. Because analysis is letter by letter, long words take longer to identify than short words.

Individuals with *deep dyslexia* have lost (or are impaired in) the indirect (phonologic) route and depend on the direct (whole-word) route that requires whole-word recognition to deduce the meaning of printed words (Figure 6-3). These patients cannot read phonologically legitimate nonwords *(tobada)* and their misreadings of real words lead to semantic errors rather than phonemic errors (e.g., reading *chair* as *table*). Individuals with deep dyslexia may substitute morphologically related or visually similar words for target words (e.g., *steal* for *stealth*, *wise* for *wisdom*). Individuals with deep dyslexia have more difficulty reading *closed-class* (function) words (articles, conjunctions, prepositions) than *open-class* (content) words (nouns, verbs, adjectives, adverbs). Semantically supportive context often helps these individuals recognize words that they otherwise would fail to recognize.

The various forms of acquired dyslexia have received much attention from investigators who are interested in how the brain recognizes printed words and how it connects the visual images of words to their semantic representations. The models of the reading process constructed by these investigators provide a systematic approach to differential diagnosis of acquired reading impairments. Nevertheless, it is important to keep in mind that descriptions of acquired dyslexia focus on single-word recognition, and reading comprehension (at least for normal readers) is largely a top-down process. Consequently, the effects of word-recognition impairments, as typified in the various forms of acquired dyslexia, may not be as striking when the individual is reading texts as when she or he is reading single words. It seems likely that mild to moderate word-recognition impairment would not dramatically affect an aphasic patient's comprehension of printed texts, if semantic and syntactic contexts give them clues to the identity of words that are erroneously recognized in isolation.

Survival Reading Skills

Treatment of aphasic adults' reading impairments is most appropriate for those with mild or moderate aphasia. For severely aphasic patients it usually is more important to improve speech production and listening comprehension than to improve reading comprehension, because few patients with chronic severe aphasia regain functional reading.

The first step in treating an aphasic adult's reading impairments is to obtain what Webb (1990) calls a *literacy history* by interviewing the patient and family members. The literacy history gives the clinician a sense of the patient's premorbid reading skills, habits, and interests and provides an indication of the potential outcome of treatment. Patients who were nonfunctional readers before they became aphasic will not become functional readers with treatment, and there is little point in attempting to make recreational readers of patients who were not interested in recreational reading before they became aphasic. However, these patients may profit from treatment to provide what have been called *survival reading skills* (Rosenbek and associates, 1989; Webb, 1990). Survival reading skills are the skills needed to read materials commonly encountered in daily life, such as signs, labels, bills, checkbook registers, addresses, telephone listings, and menus. The first step in teaching (or reactivating) survival reading skills is to determine which daily life reading activities are most important to the patient. Rosenbek, LaPointe, and Wertz (1989) suggest doing this by asking aphasic patients and family members to make two lists. One list specifies the materials that the patient most wants to be able to read and the other list identifies materials that the patient wishes to be able to read, but can do without. A list produced by one of Rosenbek and associates' patients is shown in Table 6-1. Rosenbek and associates focused treatment on the materials in the two lists, beginning with the items in the *most important* list, and when the patient could sight read those items, treatment moved on to the second list.

Parr (1992) compiled a similar list by asking 50 non–brain-damaged British adults to list daily life reading activities and to rate how important each activity was to them. Parr then calculated an index of importance for the group by multiplying the number of individuals who listed an activity by its average rating of importance. Table 6-2 shows Parr's ranked list.

Lists such as Rosenbek and associates' and Parr's provide a useful beginning point for the clinician who wishes to help a severely impaired patient regain basic functional reading abilities. The clinician cannot assume, however, that any given patient's needs will match those of groups of individuals who contributed to such lists. A patient with no bank account is unlikely to consider reading bank statements or checkbook registers important and a patient who has no television is unlikely to be very concerned with reading television program listings.

Consequently, the clinician must devise an individualized list of important daily life reading activities for each patient, perhaps by asking the patient and family members to generate a list and to rank the items on the list. Treatment can then begin with the highest-ranked activities and progress down the list as functional reading is achieved for each activity.

Functional reading for categories of everyday materials, such as those in Rosenbek and associates' and Parr's lists, depends on the patient's acquisition of a sight-reading vocabulary of commonly occurring words for each category. A core sight-reading vocabulary for reading the instructions on medicine labels might require only 15 or 20 words, whereas a core sight-reading vocabulary for reading advertisements in newspapers and magazines might require several hundred words. Once a category of materials has been identified as important to the patient,

TABLE 6 - 1

Lists of materials that an aphasic adult most wanted to read and wanted to read but could do without

Most want to read	Want to read but could do without
Mail	Messages
Checkbook	Signs
Medicine labels	Newspapers
Maps	Magazines
Phone book	TV Guide
Elevator	Menus
Calendar	Bible
Product labels	Playing cards

TABLE 6 - 2

Reading activities ranked by importance by a group of non–brain-damaged British adults

Activity	Index of importance
Personal letters	188
Bills	171
Forms	168
Official letters	162
Advertisements	144
Phone numbers	140
Newspaper	136
Television listings	131
Books	130
Bank statement	130
Address Book	125
Dosage instructions for medications	130
Personal letters	118
Menus	107

Adapted from Parr, 1992.

the clinician can test the patient with several examples of materials in the category to determine which commonly occurring words for the category are missing from the patient's sight-reading vocabulary. These words can then be incorporated into treatment activities.

Sight reading of core vocabulary words typically is trained with flash-card drills in which the patient is shown, one at a time, the printed words making up the core vocabulary and reads each aloud, with the clinician providing feedback and correction as appropriate. Such drills are a good way to give the patient intensive sight-reading practice, but they may not be the fastest or most efficient way to get the patient to the point at which she or he can incorporate newly acquired reading vocabulary into relevant daily life contents. This is because sight-reading drills in which vocabulary items are presented in isolation deprive the patient of contextual cues that may facilitate her or his acquisition of individual vocabulary items. For example, the meaning of the word *tablet* is likely to be appreciated quicker and more consistently in a context such as *"Take one tablet by mouth twice a day."* than when presented, by itself, on a flash card. Furthermore, generalization to daily life is likely to be quicker and more complete if the sight-reading vocabulary is acquired in naturalistic contexts.

Several computer-based programs to enhance sight reading of vocabulary considered important for general daily life activities have been designed. Such programs may prove useful in providing patients with intensive sight-reading drill without substantial demands on the clinician's time (Major & Wilson, 1985; Katz & Tong Nagy, 1983; Weiner, 1983; and others). However, their effectiveness has not been empirically demonstrated beyond a few case reports.

Treating Patients With Mild To Moderate Reading Impairments

Treatment for patients with mild to moderate reading impairments usually begins with mea-surement of reading vocabulary, sentence comprehension, and paragraph comprehension using standardized timed reading tests. These tests assess both *reading capacity* (the level of vocabulary and complexity that the reader can comprehend) and *reading rate* (how quickly the reader can progress through a text with acceptable comprehension). Reading test scores often are defined by *grade level*. Grade level quantifies the difficulty of the reading materials in terms of the school grade at which average students can comprehend them. Most newspapers, popular books, and magazines are at about Grade 6 in reading difficulty. Consequently, those reading at 6th-grade level or above are likely to comprehend most daily life reading materials (Chall, 1983).

Comprehension of Printed Words As noted earlier, many patients with acquired reading impairments have difficulty recognizing and assigning meaning to printed words. Problems in comprehending printed words can arise from several sources. Many aphasic patients exhibit *deep dyslexia*. They struggle with phonemic analysis of printed words and have difficulty blending individual sound representations into sound patterns for words. For these patients, grapheme-to-phoneme (letter-to-sound) conversion processes may be strengthened by exercises in which they orally sound out words and nonwords that have one-to-one grapheme-to-phoneme correspondence, discriminate between words with similar phonologic structure (e.g., *cabbage/cottage*), supply missing letters to complete regularly spelled partial words (e.g., *ban-na, anniver—ry*), and other activities that call for phonologic analysis and synthesis.

Some aphasic adults have visual impairments that interfere with their perception of printed words. They confuse words that look alike or they reverse or invert letters with similar configurations (such as confusing *b* and *d* or *m* and *w*). For these patients, the reading process may be strengthened by exercises in which they discriminate between visually similar words (e.g., *taxes, taxies*) or identify transposed or reversed letters within words (e.g., *birhtday, gadren*).* However, unless they are severe, misperceptions of individual letters may not dramatically affect reading comprehension beyond slowing the patient's reading rate, because the context provided by the remainder of the word in which the letter is misperceived and by other words in the sentence may permit accurate-word identification in spite of misperception of some letters.

Some aphasic patients can translate printed words into phonemic representations but are unable to attach meaning to the representations. These patients may become better readers if they are taught to use context to deduce word meanings. Vocabulary drills and word-association exercises also may help these patients read better.

Comprehension of Printed Sentences
Aphasic readers' comprehension of printed sentences is likely to be affected by the same variables that affect their comprehension of spoken sentences. These variables have been discussed previously. However, most aphasic patients' reading comprehension is worse than their comprehension of equivalent spoken materials, for several reasons. As mentioned earlier, most aphasic patients have difficulty translating printed words into their phonemic representations—a process that is important in reading, but not in listening. Reading depends more on syntactic analysis than listening does, and many aphasic patients have trouble with syntactic analysis. Many aphasic readers overlook or misread function words in sentences (words such as *to, but,* and *by*). Finally, printed sentences usually have less extralinguistic support than spoken sentences. When a listener fails to com-

prehend a spoken sentence, the speaker may repeat, paraphrase, or simplify to repair the miscommunication. The speaker's pauses, intonation, stress, reiteration, paraphrasing, and gestures all help facilitate comprehension. The time of day, the location of the interaction, the speaker's identity, and other situational characteristics of spoken interactions also reduce the listener's dependence on the linguistic content of the speaker's utterances.

Patients who can read at the sentence level should be reading at the sentence level in treatment, even though their reading rate may be slow and their comprehension imperfect. And, because reading comprehension, like auditory comprehension, is largely a top-down process for most patients, the sentences should have contextual support of some kind, rather than being free standing. However, tasks with free-standing sentences may be appropriate for some higher-level readers whose deficient syntactic skills lead them to miscomprehend information conveyed by the syntactic structure of printed materials. These patients' comprehension of individual sentences and of printed texts may be enhanced by exercises in which they are required to deduce the meaning of sentences with troublesome syntactic structures, such as passives (*"The woman was hugged by the man."*), center-embedded, (*"The dog the boy chased ran into the street."*) and comparatives (*"The policeman was shorter than the burglar."*). However, clinicians should keep in mind that heuristic (top-down) processes often can diminish or eliminate the need for syntactic analysis if the sentences appear in context.

Reading drills with free-standing sentences may be appropriate for patients whose comprehension of printed texts is so poor that the beneficial effects of context cannot operate. Improving the rate and accuracy with which these patients process individual sentences may diminish the overall processing workload to the point at which contextual influences can exert their beneficial effects.

---

* Sometimes patients are given practice in identifying inverted or reversed letters in isolation. For some patients this is a necessary preliminary to identifying them in context. However, the clinician should move into contextual stimuli as soon as possible.

Numerous workbooks containing sentence-level reading exercises that are appropriate for aphasic adults are on the market.

Some require the patient to complete sentences that have missing words: *For breakfast, John likes bacon and* _____. Others require the patient to choose a target word from a list of foils: *Brush is to teeth as comb is to* _____ (*Ear Hair Brush Rooster*). Some require the patient to rearrange scrambled words into a sentence: *School is day most happy last the time for of a students.**

Some are match-to-sample tasks, in which a printed sentence is presented along with several pictures, one of which matches the printed sentence, as in Figure 6-4.

Patients who can read and comprehend at least some information from printed texts should spend most of their reading treatment time reading printed texts that challenge but do not exceed their processing capacity. As a general rule, reading passages should be selected so that the patient can, at minimum, determine the overall theme or point of the passage, get most of the main ideas, and get at least some of the details. Clinicians can adjust the difficulty of reading materials by manipulating many of the variables that affect comprehension of spoken discourse (*familiarity, length, redundancy, cohesion/coherence, salience,* and *abstractness/directness*), plus variables that have a broader range in reading materials than in spoken discourse (*vocabulary* and *syntactic complexity*).

Variables That May be Manipulated in Treatment of Reading

Familiarity The familiarity of reading material has strong effects on how easily it can be comprehended. Familiar material helps readers establish context, separate main ideas

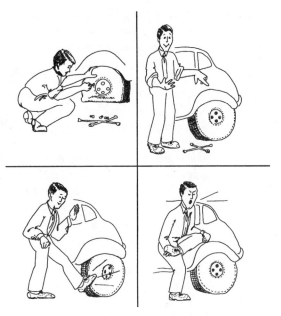

The man is kicking the tire.

Figure 6-4 ▪ A response card for reading comprehension of the sentence *"The man is kicking the tire."*

from details, and relate what they are reading to what they already know, all of which facilitates comprehension. Consequently, the reading materials used at the beginning of treatment deal with topics or themes that are highly familiar to the patient. As the patient's reading proficiency increases, the familiarity of the materials used in treatment gradually decreases, thereby increasing demands on lexical and semantic analysis, reasoning, intuition, and the ability to organize and retain unfamiliar material.

Length In general, making reading passages longer increases their difficulty by putting increased load on retention and memory, provided that the passages are made longer by adding new information and not by restating or paraphrasing existing information. (Increasing a passage's

---

* This sequence of words should challenge even patients with very mild impairments, and non–brain-damaged readers may find it a challenge.

length by restating or paraphrasing information may actually diminish passage difficulty by increasing the redundancy of the material.) Making passages shorter does not always make them easier. When a passage is drastically shortened, it becomes difficult for the reader to develop a sense of its overall topic or theme, and the context-based processes that permit top-down processing are curtailed or eliminated.

There is no absolute lower limit below which reading passages are too short to permit efficient use of top-down processes, because a passage's suitability for top-down processing depends on its structure as well as its length. However, as a general rule, passages less than about 100 words are likely to be too short to permit efficient use of top-down processes by most aphasic adults. Webb (1990) suggests that the minimum length for passages used in treating aphasic adults' reading should be 200 words, because it takes average readers that many words to develop a sense of the overall meaning of reading passages. Webb suggests that the average length of reading passages used in treating aphasic adults' reading should be about 500 words. However, 500-word passages may prove to be too long for aphasic adults with retention and memory impairments.

Redundancy As is true for spoken discourse, redundancy (repetition, elaboration, and paraphrase) in printed material makes it easier for the reader to establish the overall sense of the material, organize it in memory, and recall it later. Repetition, elaboration, and paraphrase also contribute to the cohesion and coherence of printed material in the same way that they contribute to the cohesion and coherence of spoken discourse. (See Chapter 4 for a discussion of cohesion and coherence in discourse.)

Salience and Directness Aphasic readers are likely to be affected by the salience and directness of information in printed texts in the same way that salience and directness affect their comprehension of spoken discourse.

Aphasic readers, like non–brain-damaged readers, comprehend and remember main ideas better than details and stated information better than implied information.

Vocabulary Increasing the proportion of uncommon words (those with low frequency of occurrence in the language) in a reading passage usually increases the reading difficulty of the passage.* However, most newspapers, magazines, books, and similar materials written for the general public do not contain large proportions of uncommon words. Hayes (1989) has shown that 75% of the words in typical books for adult readers are within the 1,000 most frequent words in English, and that 88% are within the 5,000 most frequent English words. Table 6-3 provides frequency-of-occurrence data for various reading materials in the United States. Only specialized technical manuals and books are likely to contain many uncommon words. If a patient's goal is recreational reading, it makes little sense to treat his or her reading impairments with materials containing large numbers of uncommon words.

Syntactic Complexity The syntactic complexity of reading materials affects their reading difficulty, and, as noted earlier, aphasic adults often are tripped up by complex syntax. Fortunately, most newspapers, magazines, and books are written with reasonably uncomplicated syntax. (The primary exceptions are some editorial and opinion pieces in newspapers and magazines and some novels.) Consequently, most recreational readers are unlikely to have to deal with syntactically complex materials, and when they must, context may permit them to substitute heuristic, top-down strategies for

---

* *Frequency of occurrence* of vocabulary may be less directly related to the ease with which readers recognize words than *familiarity*—the reader's previous experience with the words (Gernsbacher, 1984). However, for most words, frequency of occurrence and familiarity are strongly related. Therefore, for most adults, a word's frequency of occurrence is a reasonably good predictor of its reading difficulty.

T A B L E   6 - 3

Percent of words that are within the 500, 1,000, 5,000, and 10,000 most frequent English words for various reading materials

Material	Percent of words in the first:			
	500	1,000	5,000	10,000
Preschool books	73	81	94	97
Children's books	72	79	92	96
Comic books	68	75	89	93
Adult books	69	75	88	93
Popular magazines	62	69	85	91
Science abstracts	46	52	70	78

Data from Hayes, 1989.

more laborious syntactic analysis. The reader who can handle passive sentences *("The cat was chased by the dog."),* cleft-object sentences *("It was the cat that the dog chased."),* dative sentences *("The banker gave the money to the robber."),* and conjoined sentences *("The dog barked at the cat and chased the rabbit.")* should be able to handle the syntax of most commonly available reading materials, even when top-down processes cannot be substituted for syntactic analysis.

Readability Formulas

Readability formulas attempt to quantify reading difficulty by measuring specific characteristics of printed texts. Several dozen readability formulas have been published. (See Klare, 1984 for descriptions of the major ones.) Most include sentence length and number of uncommon words; some include counts of the number of long words (e.g., words of three or more syllables); and a few include grammatical measures such as number of prepositional phrases per 100 words. Cloze procedures have also been used to measure readability. In cloze procedures, words are deleted from a text and readability is based on the number of errors normal readers make filling in the missing words.

Although there is some variability in how well each of the published procedures predict actual reading difficulty, no one procedure stands out as particularly accurate. Consequently clinicians who wish to estimate the reading difficulty of printed materials might choose a formula that is easily calculated, such as the *Dale-Chall formula* (Dale & Chall, 1948) or the *Fog Index* (Gunning, 1952).

The *Dale-Chall formula* is based on the average number of words per sentence and the percent of words not on a 769-word list of common words. The *Fog Index,* in addition to having one of the more interesting names, is easy to calculate. It is based on the average number of words per sentence and the percentage of words three or more syllables long.

Even the simplest readability formulas require 10 to 20 minutes to calculate readability for a 100- to 200-word text. Some readability procedures have been computerized to lessen the time required to get a readability estimate, but the computerized procedures require that the text first be typed into an appropriately formatted computer text file, which may take longer than hand calculation.

Clinicians often bypass the time and effort of readability estimation by using commercially prepared materials with known readability. (The readability of these materials usually is specified in terms of grade levels.) If their content is suitable for adult readers, these materials provide a convenient way for clinicians to obtain materials of predetermined reading difficulty for use in treatment of adults with reading impairments.

Commercial Reading Programs

Basal readers, the most common vehicle for teaching reading comprehension in elementary schools, provide one source of materials with graded reading difficulty. Basal readers provide an integrated approach to reading instruction, with teachers' manuals, a collection of stories and expository passages for students to read, and a set of workbooks with exercises for students to complete. Most basal readers are designed to address specific reading and comprehension skills, but the number and type of skills differ from one basal reading program to another, and materials are not specific to any skill or subset of skills.

Objectives-oriented reading programs target specific reading skills (such as getting main ideas or using context). These programs provide materials that focus on specific skills at several levels of reading difficulty as well as tests to assess an individual's performance within each skill. Objectives-oriented programs differ in the number and kinds of skills addressed, as well as the reading levels for which they are appropriate. Most are designed for elementary-school use (Grades 1 through 6), so some may be inappropriate for use with adults because of their juvenile content. The *Specific Skills Series* of remedial reading materials (Boning, 1990) is an objectives-oriented set of materials that is appropriate for treatment of aphasic adults' reading impairments. (See Chapter 4 for a description of the *Specific Skills Series.*)

Rosenshine (1980) divided the skills addressed by objectives-oriented reading programs into three categories: *locating details* (recognizing, paraphrasing, and matching spe-

cific information), *simple inferential skills* (understanding words in context, recognizing sequences of events, recognizing cause-and-effect relationships, comparing and contrasting), and *complex inferential skills* (recognizing main ideas or topics, drawing conclusions, predicting outcomes). Carver (1973) has commented that only skills such as those subsumed under *locating details* are truly reading skills. He asserts that skills such as those subsumed under *simple or complex inferential skills* are not specific to reading but represent general reasoning ability. The implication is that one would not work on these skills only in reading if they represent general reasoning skills.

Treatment of aphasic patients' reading disabilities usually includes extensive homework. Patients often work on reading assignments at home and bring the completed assignments to the clinic, where the clinician goes over the completed work, corrects and discusses errors, and provides instruction and practice with new materials. Sometimes work on auditory comprehension is carried on simultaneously with work on reading to enhance generalization from one to the other.

■ TREATMENT OF SPEECH PRODUCTION

Most aphasic adults are more troubled by impairments in speaking than by impairments in reading, writing, or listening comprehension, and an aphasic adult's speech has important effects on how he or she is regarded by others in daily life interactions. Accordingly, most speech-language pathologists give treatment of speech production an important place in their plans for aphasic adults. Which aspects of speech production get treated and how much speech production is emphasized relative to other communication modalities depends, of course, on the nature and severity of the patient's communication impairments. For patients who can produce few, if any, volitional words, simple repetition tasks may be appropriate. For patients with some volitional speech the emphasis may be on efficient and accurate production of words, sentences or discourse.

Facilitating Volitional Speech

Sentence completion tasks can help get volitional speech from patients who on their own can produce little more than automatisms and stereotypic utterances. In sentence completion tasks, the clinician says a sentence that is missing the final word or the final few words and the patient supplies the missing word or words. Highly constrained sentences containing word combinations that occur frequently in daily life (e.g., *"A cup of _____."*) are the strongest facilitators of volitional speech. When a patient's responses to such highly constrained sentences are uniformly quick and accurate, treatment can move on to less-constrained sentences (such as, *"Put a stamp on the _____."* or *"We wear shoes on our _____."*) Stimulus sentences in which the missing elements are not constrained (*"Today Joe bought a _____."*) are not likely to be very effective in eliciting specific target words from aphasic speakers (or from nonaphasic speakers, for that matter). Such sentences can be incorporated into the late stages of sentence completion treatment tasks to put more emphasis on volitional vocabulary search, word retrieval, and speech production.

Completing phrases or sentences representing overlearned everyday expressions is almost always easier for aphasic speakers than confrontation naming (Barton, Maruszewski, & Urrea, 1969; Wyke & Holgate, 1973; Podraza & Darley, 1977) or providing words in response to definitions given by the clinician (Barton and associates, 1969; Goodglass & Stuss, 1979). Automatic sentence-completion tasks can be used to facilitate subsequent confrontation naming. That is, a clinician might elicit a set of object names with highly constrained sentence completion stimuli, then follow with confrontation naming of the same objects. Generally, confrontation naming improves when it follows automatic sentence completion.

Unfortunately, the facilitating effects of sentence completion on confrontation naming are not very durable (Kremin, 1993). If the clinician waits a day or two and retests the patient's confrontation naming of items previously facilitated by automatic sentence completion, they usually find that the patient's confrontation naming has returned to baseline. According to Kremin (1993), "This suggests that the deblocking of a word via an automatic expression, although immediately very effective, leaves but a faint trace over time. On the other hand, the active search for a words within the semantico-syntactic framework of a neutral sentence induces less immediate success but guarantees nonetheless the same level of performance on naming tasks after 24 hours (p.271)."

It seems apparent that highly constrained sentence completion tasks are best used as stepping-stones to tasks in which volitional vocabulary search and word retrieval are required. If a patient cannot move on to volitional word retrieval and speech production, automatic sentence completion tasks are dead ends and should be abandoned.

Word and phrase repetition provides a somewhat less powerful but fairly dependable way of getting volitional speech from patients who produce little or no volitional speech in less constrained contexts. Repetition drills are a common component of treatment for patients with articulatory selection and sequencing impairments (apraxia of speech) and patients with weakness, paralysis, or incoordination of muscle groups involved in speech (dysarthria). For these patients, the emphasis is on the mechanics of speech production. The use of repetition drills for these patients is discussed elsewhere.

Word and phrase repetition tasks are sometimes used early in treatment programs for some aphasic patients, when the ultimate goal is to enhance linguistic or quasi-linguistic processes such as word-retrieval and sentence formulation. Repetition drills are used to get the patient started and gradually are replaced by activities

that require vocabulary search and word retrieval, such as naming drills.

Confrontation naming drills require patients
to name pictures (usually) or objects (sometimes) designated by the clinician. Confrontation naming drills can be used to move patients
away from rote production of words and
phrases toward more purposeful retrieval, encoding, and production of words and phrases.
However, confrontation naming drills as an end
in themselves may provide little lasting benefit
to patients. Brookshire (1975) trained 10 aphasic adults to name pictures of common objects.
Their naming improved within training sessions, but there was no evidence that the improvements carried over to the next day, and
there was no generalization of improved naming from trained items to untrained items within
training sessions.

Naming objects or pictures is not a very useful
behavior, unless one is a child learning the
names of things, or an adult learning (or teaching) a new language. If the item is present, naming it usually is unnecessary (and often inappropriate) because its presence creates shared
knowledge between speaker and listener, making its name redundant. If an aphasic patient
wishes to communicate the name of an object or
picture that is present in the immediate environment, she or he can do so by pointing rather than
naming. Consequently, naming drills, like sentence completion and repetition drills, are best
thought of as stepping stones to more advanced
(and functional) speech communication.

Cueing Hierarchies   Clinicians have known
for decades that aphasic adults' retrieval and production of names can be facilitated if the clinician
provides prompts or cues to lead the patient in
the direction of the target words. Weigl (1968)
described what he called a "deblocking" approach to treatment, in which brain-damaged patients' inadequate responses to stimuli in one
modality are facilitated by prestimulating the patient with cues delivered in another modality.
For example, a patient who cannot name pic-

tured objects might be prestimulated with the
sound an object makes, or with a semantically related word prior to the presentation of each picture to be named. In deblocking, the idea is that
the prestimulus *primes* the patient's subsequent
response to the target stimulus.

Podraza and Darley (1977) studied the effects
of four kinds of prestimulation on aphasic adults'
picture naming: *(1)* prestimulation with the first
sound of the name plus a neutral vowel (as in
buh followed by a picture of a bee); *(2)* prestimulation with an open-ended sentence (*I got stung
by a bumble* _____"); *(3)* prestimulation with
the target word plus two unrelated foils (*line,
bee, goat*); and *(4)* prestimulation with three
words that were semantically related to the target (*sting, honey, hive*). Podraza and Darley reported that three of the four (first sound plus
neutral vowel, open-ended sentence, and target
word plus two foils) facilitated their subjects'
naming performance with no clear difference
among the three. Prestimulation with three semantically related foils worsened subjects' naming performance rather than helping it. The pattern of facilitation differed across subjects, leading Podraza and Darley to conclude, "The emergence of a slightly different hierarchy of
effectiveness for each of the subjects in the study
suggests that the use of these techniques or any
other technique in language therapy must be
based on a hierarchy determined individually for
each patient (p. 681)."*

---

* Podraza and Darley's procedures differ from those described by Weigl and his associates and, except for the
open-ended-sentence condition, differ from deblocking procedures typically used in the clinic. Prestimulating with the
target word plus several unrelated words seems strange, because stimulation with the target word alone would be more
effective in eliciting the target name. However, this changes
the picture-naming task into a word repetition task, which
should be very easy for most aphasic adults. That prestimulation with semantically related words worsened aphasic
adults' naming performance is not surprising, given that
aphasic adults' errors in confrontation-naming tasks often
are semantically related to the target words, as Podraza and
Darley mention.

Not all cues have equal power in facilitating aphasic adults' naming. Over the years, numerous studies of the relative power of various cues have been reported (Barton, Maruszewski, & Urrea, 1969; Love & Webb, 1977; Pease & Goodglass, 1978; Weidner & Jinks, 1983), and several cueing hierarchies for clinical use have been proposed (Brown, 1972; Davis, 1993, Linebaugh & Lehner, 1977). There is considerable overlap across the hierarchies, but reasonably good agreement about the relative power of various cues. The following hierarchy is an amalgamation of several reported in the literature, with cues arranged in approximate order of decreasing power.

Level 1: Imitation ("Say coffee.")

Level 2: First sound/syllable ("It starts with kuh" or "It starts with kof.")

Level 3: Sentence completion ("Pour me a cup of _____.")

Level 4: Word spelled aloud ("c-o-f-f-e-e")

Level 5: Rhyme ("It rhymes with toffee.")

Level 6: Synonym/antonym ("Folgers/decaf")

Level 7: Function/location ("You drink it at breakfast.")

Level 8: Superordinate ("It's something you drink.")

Standard hierarchies like this one can give clinicians a general idea of what to expect from a given aphasic patient, but exceptions are common. Therefore clinicians typically do a test run to determine the optimal cueing hierarchy for any given patient. They place the patient in a naming task and, when the patient misnames or fails to name a target item, the clinician provides a cue and observes its effect on the patient's naming. When a cue elicits the target word, the clinician works her or his way down the hierarchy, progressing from the potentially most powerful cues to the least powerful. The frequency with which each cue elicits the target words is then used to arrange the cues into a personalized hierarchy for the patient.

A patient's cueing hierarchy is used in word-retrieval tasks as follows. When the patient fails to retrieve a target word, the clinician provides the least powerful cue in the hierarchy. If this cue elicits an accurate response, the patient and clinician move on to the next item. If it does not, the clinician delivers the next more powerful cue. This continues until a cue elicits an accurate response. When the patient produces the target word in response to a cue, the clinician reverses course through the hierarchy and presents the next less powerful cue, continuing until the patient either makes an error or makes accurate responses to all cues, including the least powerful cue in the hierarchy. If the patient makes it all the way through the hierarchy with accurate responses, the patient and clinician move on. If the patient makes an error somewhere along the way, the clinician once again reverses course and delivers progressively more powerful cues until the patient responds accurately, at which time the clinician and patient move on to the next item. (This ensures that the patient always ends with successful production of each item.)

When word-retrieval drills yield a corpus of words that the patient can dependably produce, treatment procedures may be modified to diminish the patient's reliance on clinician-supplied cues and substitute patient-generated cues or retrieval strategies. For example, patients whose word retrieval has been facilitated by the clinician's provision of a rhyming cue might be trained to think of a rhyme on their own, and patients whose word retrieval is facilitated when the clinician provides a synonym or an antonym might be trained to think of synonyms or antonyms on their own to elicit target words without the clinician's help. If patients' gestures help them produce the words they want, the use of gesture may be encouraged (or trained).

Behaviors Associated with Word-Retrieval Failure

What aphasic adults do when they fail to retrieve a word sometimes gives the clinician clues to the nature of the patient's word-retrieval difficulties and may provide the clinician with indications of strategies the patient may be using to cope with word-retrieval failure. Marshall (1976) studied the spontaneous speech of 18 aphasic adults to determine what they did to cope with word-retrieval failures. He described five such coping behaviors—*delay, semantic association, phonetic association, description,* and *generalization.* In *delay* the patient produces a filled or unfilled pause or "some stalling tactic to let the listener know they did not want to be interrupted and needed more time to produce the word (p.446)." In *semantic association* the patient produces one or more words that are semantically related to the target word, including antonyms (front—*back*), class membership (fruit—*banana*), part-whole relationship (foot—*toe*), or serial relationship (Sunday—Monday—*Tuesday*). In *phonetic association* the patient produces words that are phonologically similar to the target word (hamper—clamper—*damper*). In *description,* the patient describes characteristics of the target ("It's round and red and it grows on trees—it's an *apple.*"). In *generalization,* the patient produces general words and phrases without specific meaning ("It's one of those *things.* It's a *thing* that I know. It's a *spider.*"). Semantic association was the most frequently-occurring behavior, followed by description, generalization, delay, and phonetic association.

Marshall evaluated the apparent success of these behaviors by calculating the percentage of times that each behavior led to the target word. Delay was followed by successful production of the target word about 90% of the time. Semantic association and phonetic association preceded correct production of the target about 55% of the time. Description and generalization were followed by their intended targets only 35% and 17% of the time, respectively.

It is tempting to assume a cause-effect relationship between behaviors that precede successful production of target words and the sub-

sequent production of the target words. Although it may be that at least some of the behaviors described by Marshall represent purposeful strategies on the part of the aphasic speakers, it seems likely that at least some represent symptoms of word-retrieval problems, rather than strategies used to access words. This is a crucial difference, because if the behaviors represent strategies, one might wish to encourage the patients to engage in those that have the greatest success. If the behaviors represent symptoms, one would probably not wish to increase their frequency and might even search for ways to eliminate them, because they may diminish communicative efficiency.

Enhancing Word Retrieval in Speech

Rosenbek and associates (1989) described a three-part program for enhancing aphasic adults' word retrieval in connected speech. The program begins with diagnosis, moves on to strategy development and practice in controlled environments, and ends with the patient's internalization of strategies and generalization of their use across words and environments. The following program is modeled on that of Rosenbek and associates.

Part 1: Diagnosis This part of the program focuses on *(1)* generating a list of words and semantic categories (e.g., foodstuffs, tools, personal care items) that are especially important to the patient and family, and *(2)* getting baseline measures of the patient's successful and unsuccessful word retrieval strategies. The clinician interviews the patient and one or more family members to develop a list of important words representing several semantic categories. The clinician also observes the patient in unstructured interactions and in structured drill activities to determine how reliably the patient produces various categories of words (with special attention to those on the list), to identify strategies the patient may be using to cope with word-retrieval failure, and to get a sense of which strategies work and which do not.

Part 2: Strategy Development and Practice In this part of the program the patient receives structured practice to expand and strengthen word-retrieval processes. If the patient is already using strategies that facilitate word retrieval, their use is reinforced. If the patient has few or no successful strategies, the clinician and patient work together to develop some. The primary vehicle for strategy development is the patient's use of self-cueing (such as saying a related word, a rhyme, or the first sound of a word) to facilitate word retrieval. The patient then practices the selected strategies in controlled drill activities with words from the patient's list of important words. When retrieval of a word has been strengthened, the clinician may introduce other forms of the word. For example, if the patient's retrieval of the word *chair* has been enhanced and stabilized, practice with words and phrases such as *armchair, chairman, wheelchair, easy chair,* or *high chair* may follow. (Rosenbek and associates caution against introducing semantically related prompts (such as *table,* or *couch* for *chair*) noting that semantically related words often interfere with retrieval of the previously-stabilized target words.)

Part 3: Stabilization and Generalization In this part of the treatment program the focus is on helping the patient extend her or his use of effective word-retrieval strategies to environments beyond the clinic and on moving the patient's word retrieval toward normalcy by replacing overt self-cueing strategies with covert ones. The emphasis is on self-correction and self-cueing by the patient, and on extension of improved word-retrieval from the tightly controlled elicitation conditions typical of the clinic to the less predictable conditions typical of daily life.

Activities to strengthen word associations and enhance semantic representations may be incorporated into this phase of treatment. These activities may include providing synonyms, antonyms, and rhymes for words presented by the clinician; providing lists of words that are in categories specified by the clinician; cloze procedures, in which the patient provides the words to fill in blanks in sentences or narratives; separating printed semantically related words from unrelated ones; or generating lists of words or word combinations with a common root (e.g., *wash-washer-washcloth, washing machine, car wash.* The expectation is that as the patient's internal semantic associations and organization move toward normalcy, her or his word retrieval will improve, diminishing the need for strategies to volitionally evoke the words the patient wishes to say.

Sentence Production

Sentence-length utterances can be elicited in several ways. The simplest is *imitation,* in which the clinician says a sentence and the patient repeats it. Sentence imitation drills are most commonly used to increase articulatory accuracy for patients with motor speech or motor programming impairments and are sometimes used to increase auditory retention span for patients with aphasia. Sentence imitation drills sometimes follow word-repetition drills for patients with speech production impairments. Word repetition gets them talking, then treatment moves them on to more difficult (and more natural) sentence production tasks.

The next step for many of these patients is *repetition/elaboration drill.* In repetition/elaboration drill, the clinician asks questions designed to elicit formulaic, stereotypical responses typical of those that frequently occur in social encounters and conversations.

Clinician: *How are you?*
Patient: *Fine. And how are you?*
Clinician: *What do you like for breakfast?*
Patient: *Bacon and eggs. What do you like for breakfast?*

Story completion provides patients with less contextual information to lead them in the direction of the expected response. In story completion the clinician provides a short two- or three-sentence narrative and asks the patient to provide a phrase or sentence to complete it.

Clinician: *It's ten o'clock and my children are still up. I want them to go to bed. So I say to them. . . .*
Patient: *Go to bed.*

Helm-Estabrooks (1981) developed a program for eliciting such utterances from aphasic adults, called the *Helm Elicited Language Program for Syntax Stimulation* (HELPSS).

Question-answer drill further diminishes supportive context. The clinician asks questions related to the patient's experiences, opinions, or general knowledge. The patient responds with a phrase or sentence.

Clinician: *What did you do last evening?*
Patient: *Watched TV and went to bed.*
Clinician: *What's your opinion of our governor?*
Patient: *If he was any dumber, they'd have to water him.*
Clinician: *What's the most important difference between cats and dogs?*
Patient: *You don't have to walk a cat.*

In *story elaboration* the clinician tells a short story and follows with a series of questions designed to elicit a phrase or sentence in response.

Clinician: *Fred and Ethyl decided to go out for dinner to celebrate Ethyl's birthday. They drove across town to a nice restaurant and had a nice meal. When the bill came, Fred reached for his wallet, only to discover that it was not there.*
—What do you think Fred and Ethyl did next?
Patient: *Maybe Ethyl paid the bill, if she had any money.*
Clinician: *Where do you think Fred left his wallet?*
Patient: *Probably at the bar.*

Story elaboration calls on several other processes in addition to sentence formulation and production. The patient must comprehend the stories and retain the information long enough to produce the appropriate responses. The patient also must call upon his or her general knowledge, make inferences, and foresee consequences to formulate a response that is consistent with the story.

Picture-story elaboration is similar to story elaboration, except that, instead of telling a story, the clinician shows the patient a picture depicting a situation with a salient theme and a predictable outcome (as in Figure 6-5) or a series of pictures depicting a sequence of events. Then the clinician asks the patient a series of questions to elicit phrase-length or sentence-length responses.

The clinician might ask the following questions about Figure 6-5:

- "What's the occasion?"
- "Why is the boy crying?"
- "What do you think will happen next?"

In *sentence construction* the clinician provides a spoken (or printed) word, phrase, or two or more related words, and asks the patient to produce a sentence containing the words.

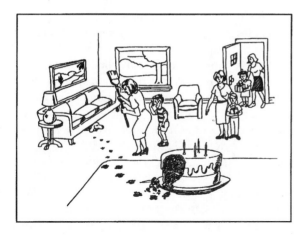

Figure 6-5 ■ **A picture that might be used to elicit connected speech. The picture has a central theme, a predictable outcome, and suggests events that happened before the events portrayed.** (Copyright from RH Brookshire, LE Nicholas, 1991)

Clinician: *Give me a sentence containing the word* boy.
Patient: *The boy is happy.*
Clinician: *Give me a sentence containing the words* man, drink, *and* coffee.
Patient: *The man drinks coffee.*

Sentence production drills permit considerable flexibility in manipulating task difficulty. When the eliciting stimulus is a single word, task difficulty depends primarily on the stimulus word's part of speech and frequency in English. Nouns usually are relatively easy for most aphasic adults to incorporate into a sentence, followed by verbs, pronouns, adjectives, adverbs, and function words. Frequently occurring and concrete words usually are easier to incorporate into sentences than infrequently occurring and abstract ones. When aphasic patients have to incorporate several words into a sentence, pro-

viding the words in noun-verb or noun-verb-noun order facilitates their performance because the order of the words in the stimulus matches the subject-verb or subject-verb-object order of the two most common sentence structures. Scrambling the order of the words in the stimulus (noun-noun-verb or verb-noun-noun) increases task difficulty by requiring the patient to rearrange them to create a syntactically correct sentence. Providing stimuli that represent common word combinations (such as *a piece of pie*) or express commonly-encountered relationships (such as *man-drink-coffee*) makes the task easier for most aphasic patients.

Sentence production tasks can sometimes entice clinicians into thinking that grammaticality is what they and the patient should be seeking, when for most patients, *communication,* not grammaticality, is the answer. Ungrammatic utterances often do an adequate job of communicating an aphasic speaker's thoughts, wishes, and intentions. The patient who responds to *"What did you do last evening?"* with *"TV—bed—sleep"* has successfully, though not elegantly, communicated the essentials. Clinicians who insist on grammatical utterances run the risk of wasting their own and the patient's time and energy. The principal exceptions are some high-level aphasic patients who, with a reasonable amount of coaching, are capable of speaking both informatively and grammatically.

Connected Speech

Connected speech is a generic label for speech in which a person produces several utterances in response to a stimulus, topic, or event. The utterances may be continuous, on a common topic, and not separated either by introduction of a new stimulus or by the contributions of another speaker *(monologue),* or they may be separated by questions, comments, or contributions from another speaker *(conversation, interview).* Monologues are more common in testing and treatment than conversation and interview, perhaps because they provide better control over the content and form of patients' responses and are easier to quantify.

Picture Description Picture description is one way of eliciting monologues. In picture description, target sentences are not constrained and the patient has free choice of the kinds of sentences that she or he will produce, as well as considerable latitude in word choice. However, the nature of the picture (or pictures) used to elicit descriptions may affect both the amount and kind of verbalizations elicited from the patient. Familiar occurrences or situations elicit more verbalization than unfamiliar ones. Pictures that suggest a past (events leading up to the situation or event depicted) and a future (events following the situation or event depicted) encourage those who describe them to go beyond the content of the pictures and talk about preceding and following events. Pictures depicting static situations often elicit enumeration from patients (naming items in the picture), whereas pictures depicting dynamic interactions usually elicit more elaborate descriptions.

Figure 6-6 shows two pictures. The one on the left is more likely to elicit enumeration than the one on the right.

Correia, Brookshire, and Nicholas (1990) empirically demonstrated that static speech elicitation pictures tend to elicit enumeration from aphasic adults. They had aphasic adults describe the speech elicitation pictures from the *Boston Diagnostic Aphasia Examination* (BDAE; Goodglass & Kaplan, 1983), the *Western Aphasia Battery* (WAB; Kertesz, 1982), and the *Minnesota Test for Differential Diagnosis of Aphasia* (MTDDA; Schuell, 1972). (See Figure 4-25, Chapter 4). The aphasic speakers' responses to the static WAB and MTDDA pictures contained greater percentages of enumerations (42% and 45% respectively) than their responses to the more dynamic BDAE picture (38%), although only the difference between the WAB picture and the BDAE picture was statistically significant.

Prompted Story Telling Prompted story telling elicits stories by means of sequences of pictures that represent events in a story (Figure

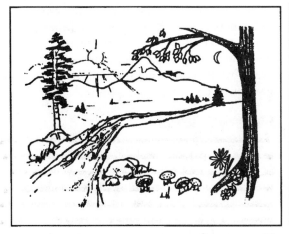 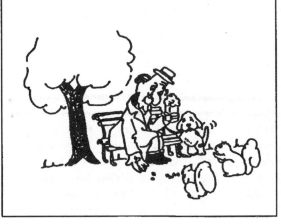

A   **B**

Figure 6-6 ■ Two pictures that might be used to elicit connected speech. The picture on the left (A) is more likely to elicit enumeration than the picture on the right (B). (*A* courtesy Howard E. Gardner, PhD.)

6-7). The amount of speech that a picture sequence elicits depends on the number of incidents pictured in the sequence, with more incidents generating longer speech samples. The picture sequence shown in Figure 6-7 elicited, on the average, slightly over 80 words from aphasic speakers, but the range was substantial (23 words for a nonfluent patient to 164 words for a fluent patient).

Procedural Discourse Procedural discourse is connected speech made in response to requests such as *"Tell me how you make pumpkin pie."* When they describe procedures such as making scrambled eggs, writing and mailing a letter, and doing dishes by hand non–brain-damaged adults usually produce from 75 to 125 words per procedure, depending on the procedure (more complex procedures usually elicit longer samples). The range for aphasic speakers is great. Some nonfluent aphasic speakers may generate 25 to 30 words per procedure, and some fluent aphasic speakers may generate nearly 300 words.

Procedural discourse usually is not syntactically complex. Ulatowska and associates (1983) evaluated procedural descriptions produced by nonaphasic adults and by aphasic adults and found that neither group produced many syntactically complex sentences. They commented that procedural descriptions do not require syntactically complex language, so that even many patients with relatively severe aphasia produce syntactically adequate procedural descriptions.*

Conversation Conversation sometimes is used as a vehicle for eliciting speech from aphasic patients in treatment activities. However, many of these interactions do not resemble natural conversations, because the clinician does most of the talking and the patient's responses do not go beyond providing what the clinician requests. The resulting interaction resembles an interview more than it resembles conversation. It consists of a series of requests for information from the clinician, with single-word, phrase, or short sentence responses by the patient, as in the following segment.

---

* Excepting, of course, those with Broca's aphasia who speak agrammatically.

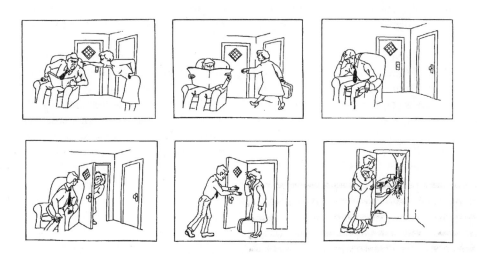

Figure 6-7 ■ A picture sequence that might be used to elicit prompted story telling in treatment activities. (Copyright from RH Brookshire, LE Nicholas, 1991)

Clinician: *What kind of work did you do before your stroke?*

Patient: *Foreman.*

Clinician: *A foreman. What company did you work for?*

Patient: *Amurcan.*

Clinician: *Amurcan? Do you mean American? American what?*

Patient: *Amurican Freight.*

Clinician: *American Freight. Is that a trucking company?*

Patient: *Yeah.*

Clinician: *And you were a foreman. Who did you supervise?*

Patient: *Dock.*

Clinician: *People on the dock?*

Patient: *Yeah.*

Clinician: *And what kind of jobs did they do?*

Patient: *Oh—most ever'thing.*

Unless carefully structured with pragmatic principles about conversational interactions firmly in place, such clinician-patient interactions are not effective in eliciting connected speech from the patient. They are more appropriately employed when the objective is to improve the patient's conversational behaviors (such as turn taking, eye contact, and topic maintenance).

■ TREATING APRAXIA OF SPEECH

Apraxia of speech can occur in isolation (a rare occurrence) but it usually occurs in combination with aphasia that ranges anywhere from mild to severe. Whether or not an apraxic patient will benefit from treatment depends both on the severity of his or her apraxia and the severity of any accompanying aphasia. The more severe the impairments are (beyond the

first 3 or 4 weeks post onset), the poorer the prognosis for recovery. As noted earlier, patients who, a month or more post onset, have no volitional speech, emit stereotypic speech responses and are severely aphasic are unlikely to recover functional speaking abilities, even with intensive treatment.

According to Rosenbek and Wertz (1972), treatment for patients with apraxia of speech should:

> . . . concentrate on the disordered articulation and, therefore, be different from the language stimulation and auditory and visual processing therapies appropriate to the aphasias.*
>
> . . . emphasize the relearning of adequate points of articulation and the sequencing of articulatory gestures.
>
> . . . provide conditions such that the apraxic patient can advance from limited, automatic-reactive speech to appropriate, volitional purposive communication. (p. 192)

Most apraxic speakers can produce individual sounds and one-syllable words correctly, but their problems arise when they must create sequential articulatory movements. As the number of syllables and the articulatory complexity of utterances increases, so does the effortfulness and struggle of the apraxic patient's speech behavior.

Apraxic speakers' problems are not caused by inability to hear or discriminate the sounds of speech. Consequently, it is unnecessary and unproductive to provide auditory discrimination training for patients with apraxia of speech. Early studies of apraxic speakers suggested that they often were deficient in oral sensation and oral form identification (Guilford & Hawk, 1968; Larimore, 1970; Rosenbek, Wertz, & Darley, 1973), but subsequent studies have failed to support these conclusions (Deutsch, 1981; Square

---

* Rosenbek and Wertz were addressing treatment of apraxia *per se.* This does not imply that "therapies appropriate to the aphasias" are not appropriate for patients who are both apraxic and aphasic.

& Weidner, 1976). The evidence suggests that sensory anomalies may coexist with apraxia of speech, but are not strongly related to its severity. Consequently, work on oral sensation is unlikely to be of much help to apraxic patients.

Severe Apraxia of Speech

Characteristics at Intake Patients with severe apraxia of speech usually have no volitional speech. Many emit stererotypic speech responses during the first month or two post onset. These stereotypic responses usually disappear by 2 months post onset, unless the patient is severely aphasic. Most patients with severe apraxia of speech also exhibit moderate to severe buccofacial and limb apraxia. They are almost always hemiparetic or hemiplegic, and most are at least moderately aphasic.

Progression of Treatment Treatment of severely apraxic patients begins at elemental levels. Many cannot phonate voluntarily. Most of those who can phonate cannot modify their phonation to produce vowels, and few can produce consonant-vowel syllables. Consequently, early stages of treatment usually are concerned with developing volitional vocalization and a small repertoire of vowels and consonant-vowel syllables. Treatment procedures make use of phonetic placement (mechanical positioning of the patient's articulators) and phonetic derivation (deriving a new sound from one that the patient can make). Severely apraxic speakers usually are poor imitators. Consequently, imitation drills may not be appropriate, although *integral stimulation* ("watch me and do what I do") may be useful for some patients.

Some severely apraxic speakers occasionally utter single words, but the words are likely to have little or no communicative value and are likely not to be under the speaker's volitional control. Helm and Barresi (1980) have suggested that such words can be brought under the patient's control and have described a program for incorporating such involuntary utterances into treatment.

Alternative communication devices (communication boards, communication books—see Chapter 10) frequently are necessary to provide a means of communication for patients with severe apraxia of speech, at least on a temporary basis. Severely apraxic patients' use of gestural communication may also be emphasized and trained. Education and counseling of those who care for the patient are crucial aspects of treatment for severely apraxic patients.

Outcome Only a small proportion of patients who remain severely apraxic at 3 or more months post onset develop even rudimentary functional speech. Patients with severe apraxia of speech who are also severely aphasic frequently are placed in nursing homes. For these patients, it may be particularly important to develop some form of rudimentary communication between the patient and those who care for him or her.

Moderate Apraxia of Speech

Characteristics at Intake Patients with moderate apraxia of speech usually have some volitional speech at 1 to 2 months post onset. These patients may emit stereotypic utterances for a short time immediately after onset, but the utterances disappear as the patient recovers. Many patients exhibit mild-to-moderate buccofacial and limb apraxia. Almost all are hemiparetic or hemiplegic. Mild-to-moderate aphasia often is present.

Progression of Treatment Because patients with moderate apraxia of speech usually have some volitional speech, treatment can begin at the syllable, word, or phrase level. These patients can be active participants in treatment—they are motivated to recover, they can work independently, and they can learn and generalize learning to new situations. They often collaborate with the clinician in setting goals and in designing and carrying out treatment procedures, and they take responsibility for independent practice. Patients with moderate apraxia of speech usually move quickly from single-syllable to multiple-syllable speech production. Consequently, treatment activities can emphasize volitional control of sequenced articulatory movements, together with manipulations of rate, pauses, and intonation.

Wertz, LaPointe, and Rosenbek (1984) recommend *contrastive stress drill* for the early phases of treatment for patients with moderate apraxia of speech, and suggest that oral reading may be suitable in later phases of treatment.* Relaxation training in conjunction with speech retraining may help many of these patients speak better and with less effort. Many patients with moderate apraxia of speech can learn a problem-solving approach to communication, in which they learn to anticipate difficult words and difficult speaking situations, recognize communication failure when it occurs, and respond to communication failure in a planned and systematic way.

Outcome Most patients with moderate apraxia of speech regain some functional speech. Many continue slow improvement in speech ability over many years (even after formal treatment has ended). Most return to their homes following discharge from the hospital and most function independently in common daily life activities. A few whose work does not depend heavily on speech may return to work, but most will not.

Mild Apraxia of Speech

Many patients with mild apraxia of speech at the end of the first month or so post onset spontaneously recover enough speech to be functional talkers in daily life. Most patients with mild apraxia of speech are only mildly aphasic,

if aphasic at all. Patients with mild apraxia of speech usually profit from articulation drills, instruction in strategic approaches to communication, and how best to deal with the inconveniences created by their communication disabilities. Treatment usually involves repetition drills and formulation and production of phrases, sentences, and extended speech. The emphasis is on improving articulatory agility and accuracy and on developing appropriate prosody and rate.

Outcome Patients with mild apraxia of speech almost always return home. Some may return to work. Almost all communicate independently in most daily life situations.

Stimulus Manipulations That May Affect Response Accuracy in Apraxia of Speech

Visibility, Length, and Articulatory Complexity Visible and motorically simple movements are easiest for apraxic speakers. Visibility and complexity interact to some extent, because more visible movements also tend to be less motorically complex. As word length increases, the probability of apraxic speech errors also increases (Shankweiler & Harris, 1966; Johns & Darley, 1970), although short words with complex articulatory sequences may be more difficult than long words without complex sequences. Apraxic errors tend to increase as the distance between successive points of articulation increases (Wertz and associates, 1984), although this last clinical observation has not been experimentally verified.

Rate, Delay In general, the faster the rate at which articulatory sequences must be produced, the more difficulty an apraxic speaker will have in producing the sequences. If delay intervals are imposed between the clinician's model and the apraxic speaker's opportunity to imitate the model, imitation usually is more difficult than if no delay is imposed.

Context The phonologic characteristics of the word or phrase in which a particular sound is located may affect the likelihood that it will be

---

* In contrastive stress drill the clinician says a sentence such as *"Bake a pie."* and then asks the patient questions such as **"Do what** *to a pie? Bake a* **what?",** and so on. The patient answers each question, putting emphatic stress on words that answer the question (**"Bake** *a pie."*) Contrastive stress drill also is useful in treating patients with dysarthria (see Chapter 10).

produced correctly by an apraxic speaker. There is some evidence suggesting that the first sound in a word is more likely to be produced correctly than subsequent sounds (Shankweiler & Harris, 1966; Trost & Canter, 1974). However, others have failed to confirm this effect (Johns & Darley, 1970; LaPointe & Johns, 1975; Dunlop & Marquardt, 1977).

The linguistic context in which a word is produced usually affects how difficult it is for an apraxic patient to say. Placing a word in a frequently occurring phrase usually makes it easier. For example, the word *coffee* usually is easier if it is elicited by a phrase such as *"I want a cup of _____ ."* than if it is elicited by a picture. Situational context may also affect apraxic speakers' success. Most speak better to friends and relatives (and clinicians) than they do to strangers. Most speak better face to face than on the telephone. Most speak better when they express their own knowledge, opinions, and wishes than they do when they must speak about things prescribed by others.

Cues The nature of cues provided to apraxic patients has strong effects on their success in producing speech. In general, the probability of successful responses increases as more information about target responses is provided by the cues. Love and Webb (1977) studied the effects of four different cues on picture naming by patients with Broca's aphasia (and apraxia of speech). The cues were *the complete target word, a sentence with the target word missing, the first sound of the target word,* and *the printed target word.* They found that, on the average, providing the complete word was most successful in eliciting the target word. Providing the initial syllable was next most effective, followed by sentence completion and printed words, in that order. Each of these differences was statistically significant except the one between sentence completion and printed words.

Love and Webb do not report whether individual subjects all generated the same hierarchy as the group (it is doubtful that they did). Fur-

thermore, Love and Webb's subjects' may have been both apraxic and aphasic, with word retrieval impairments complicating their attempts to produce spoken words (a probability to which Love and Webb allude). However, Love and Webb's results do show that cues can have strong effects on the accuracy of apraxic speakers' word retrieval and production of single words. Their hierarchy also may provide a starting point for clinicians who wish to construct a cueing hierarchy for an individual patient.

Rosenbek and associates (1973) proposed an eight-step continuum of cues for treatment of patients with apraxia of speech. The continuum gradually reduces the salience of cues while gradually increasing response requirements.

- The clinician and patient produce the target utterance in unison.
- The clinician produces the target utterance. The patient then produces the utterance while the clinician silently mouths the utterance with the patient.
- The clinician produces the utterance. The patient says the utterance.
- The clinician produces the utterance. The patient says the utterance several times in succession.
- The patient is given the target utterance printed on a card and reads it aloud.
- The printed utterance is given to the patient to study and then is taken away. The patient then says the utterance.
- The clinician asks a question that is answerable with the target utterance. The patient says the target utterance.
- The clinician and patient interact in a role-playing situation in which given target utterances are appropriate. The patient says the target utterances at appropriate times.

Stimulus Modality Most treatment programs for apraxic patients manipulate the modalities in which stimuli are delivered, although not all do so systematically. In spite of the frequently encountered claim that multimodality stimulation is better than unimodality stimulation, no experimental evidence exists to support it, and it almost certainly does not apply to every apraxic patient seen for treatment.

Visual stimulation in apraxia treatment consists primarily of two techniques: the ubiquitous *watch me and do what I do* technique, and the use of mirrors (or sometimes videotapes) in which the patient watches himself or herself speak, with or without the clinician alongside. The former is almost always helpful. The latter may be helpful with some patients, but may be counterproductive with others.

Emphasizing the patient's attention to *tactile and kinesthetic stimuli* during speech may in many cases improve the accuracy of apraxic patients' speech. (This does not imply that tactile stimulation by itself, outside of speech activity, is likely to be beneficial.)

Although the *auditory modality* is not usually written about in treatment of apraxia of speech (Wertz and associates, 1984 is an exception), most treatment programs depend heavily on the patient's ability to listen to his or her own speech. Most clinicians spend little or no time training auditory discrimination as a separate skill. However, most encourage apraxic patients to listen to themselves to tell when a given utterance is adequate (not necessarily *correct*).

Meaningfulness In general, the more meaningful a given speech response is, the easier it will be for an apraxic speaker. Consequently, most clinicians structure treatment around meaningful words, phrases, and sentences. However, Dabul and Bollier (1976) recommend that treatment for patients with apraxia of speech should begin by concentrating upon production of *nonmeaningful* articulatory sequences to teach the patient volitional control of speech production before she or he attempts meaningful words. There is no conclusive evidence for either position. Majority opinion at this time seems to favor using real words as soon as possible.

Automacity Overlearned sequences (counting, reciting the alphabet, reciting the days of the week) may be surprisingly easy for some patients who are severely apraxic. In such cases, repeated production of such sequences may increase oral agility and oral motor control in preparation for work on more volitional speech production.

Reorganization

Rosenbek, Collins, and Wertz (1976), and Rosenbek (1978) have discussed the use of *intersystemic reorganization* and *intrasystemic reorganization* in treatment of patients with apraxia of speech.

Intersystemic Reorganization In *intersystemic reorganization,* behaviors that are not ordinarily part of a given motor performance are introduced into the performance in order to improve it (e.g., tapping or pantomiming along with speech movements). Rosenbek and associates (1976) propose the following sequence of activities for intersystemic reorganization. First, a set of simple, meaningful, and easily recognizable gestures is compiled for the patient. The patient is taught to recognize each gesture and its verbal equivalent when they are produced by the clinician. Then the patient is taught to imitate the gesture. (Rosenbek and associates stress the importance of feedback from the clinician at this stage, because they have observed that many apraxic patients have difficulty judging the adequacy of their own gestures.) During this stage the clinician may manipulate the patient's hand and arm to bring about the gesture, or the patient may be given real objects to use in the movement. When the patient can produce each gesture without effort, he or she is taught to combine each gesture with a word or phrase.

When the patient can reliably and appropriately produce speech and gesture combinations both in and outside of the clinic, the gestures may be gradually deemphasized. However, Rosenbek and associates recommend that even at this stage patients should be encouraged to continue using gestures for self-cueing and self-correction of errors. According to Rosenbek and associates, patients who cannot learn gestures, patients who cannot learn to pair gestural and speech responses, and patients who are severely aphasic are not candidates for intersystemic reorganization. According to Rosenbek and associates, patients who are severely aphasic usually do no better when treated with intersystemic reorganization than when they are treated with other procedures.

Intrasystemic Reorganization Intrasystemic reorganization is accomplished by using different components of the same system to produce or enhance movements, usually by shifting the locus of control from one level of the system to another. The shift in control usually is from automatic to volitional. The typist who slows down and types words syllable by syllable when typing unfamiliar or complicated words is employing intrasystemic reorganization to decrease errors. (The typist who subvocally spells the word is using intersystemic reorganization.) Many treatment activities for apraxic patients qualify as intrasystemic reorganization, even though they are not labeled as such. Teaching patients to speak slowly and with consciously controlled articulatory movements is one example of intrasystemic reorganization. Teaching them to speak with exaggerated prosody and teaching them to concentrate on kinesthetic feedback during speech are two other examples.

There are no reliable data to support the efficacy of reorganization in eliciting speech from apraxic patients, or in reinstating speech that apraxic patients are likely to use in daily life communication, and there are no data comparing reorganization with other treatments. Anecdotal reports suggest that reorganization is effective in eliciting speech from many apraxic patients, and that it makes meaningful changes in the daily life communicative ability of some of them.

Melodic Intonation Therapy (MIT)

Melodic intonation therapy (Sparks, Helm & Albert, 1974; Sparks & Holland, 1976) was designed to elicit speech from severely aphasic (and apraxic) patients who have little or no volitional speech by increasing the participation of the non-dominant hemisphere in speech activities. MIT places the patient in structured drills in which phrases are produced with exaggerated stress, rhythm, and pitch, and the patient taps out the rhythm of each phrase as he or she produces it.

In MIT the patient is trained to utter propositional phrases and sentences, using sung intonation patterns that are similar to the natural intonation patterns of the spoken phrases or sentences. First the clinician intones sentences and helps the patient tap the stress patterns of the sentences in unison with the clinician's utterances. Then the patient and clinician intone the sentences and tap their stress patterns together. Then the clinician gradually fades his or her participation in production and tapping, until the patient is intoning and tapping them without assistance, in response to the clinician's intoned model.

When the patient's simultaneous intonation and tapping have stabilized, speech production moves away from melody toward more natural prosody. First, there is a transition from melodic intonation to *sprechgesang* (speech song), in which words are no longer sung, but are spoken with exaggerated inflection. The next transition is from *sprechgesang* to spoken prosody.

According to Sparks, Helm, and Albert (1974), MIT is appropriate for patients with the following characteristics:

- Auditory comprehension is better than verbal expression. (Spontaneous recognition and self-correction of errors by the patient is considered a favorable sign.)
- The patient is emotionally stable and has good attention span.
- The patient has severely impaired verbal output, and has little or no ability to name, repeat, or complete sentences.
- The patient makes vigorous attempts at self-correction.
- The patient emits clearly articulated, stereotyped utterances.

There are no controlled evaluations of the efficacy of MIT, either by itself or relative to other treatment approaches. Anecdotal reports suggest that MIT is effective in eliciting speech from patients who otherwise cannot produce volitional speech. The most significant problem with MIT appears to be generalization of speech learned in the clinic to daily life. Little generalization of what patients learn in MIT to other activities usually occurs until the patient is in the final stages of MIT, and many patients do not make it to the final stages. (A particularly difficult transition seems to be the transition from sung phrases to *sprechgesang*.)

Nonspeech Communication Systems
Many severely apraxic patients never regain enough volitional speech to permit them to communicate even simple messages by talking. Nonspeech communication systems may help some of them communicate with those around them. However, most severely apraxic patients also have significant aphasia, which may compromise their ability to use alternative communication systems that depend on verbal skills. Some patients with apraxia of speech may learn gesture and pantomime as part of reorganization (Rosenbek, 1978). The gestures and pantomime may function both as a substitute for speech and as a facilitator for the patient's production of speech. Some patients with apraxia of speech may learn to use sign languages, either temporarily as they are reacquiring speech or as a permanent substitute. Producing such signs may also facilitate speech through intersystemic reorganization. (See Chapter 10 for more on alternative and augmentative communication systems.)

■ WRITING

Many of the same processes used to produce spoken messages are used to produce written ones. It is only at the production stage that speaking and writing differ appreciably. Writers, unlike speakers, need a sense of how to spell. Writing requires visual-motor coordination and sufficient strength to produce written letters. Writers need better syntax than speakers, because speakers can compensate for deficient syntax by providing prosodic clues to meanings, while writers do not have this option. Written style is more formal and more grammatically complex than spoken style. Consequently, it should not be surprising that aphasic adults almost always write less well than they speak.

As discussed in the last chapter, aphasic patients' writing resembles their speech. Fluent speakers tend to be fluent writers. They write in cursive, produce well-shaped letters, and maintain horizontal and equally-spaced writing lines. Nonfluent speakers tend to be nonfluent writers (partly because they are using their nonpreferred hand). They produce distorted letters and their lines are uneven in contour and spacing. Nonfluent writers usually print, rather than writing in cursive. Agrammatic speakers are likely to be agrammatic writers, and aphasic speakers who generate "empty" speech (devoid of meaning) are likely to generate "empty" written materials.

Treatment of Writing Impairments

Most aphasic adults have disabilities in spelling and syntax that make it difficult or impossible for them to communicate effectively by writing. Consequently, most writing treatment programs concentrate on spelling, syntax, and grammar. Writing treatment programs for aphasic adults employ didactic procedures and rely heavily on homework. Sometimes commercially available spelling and writing workbooks are used. Teaching written spelling and syntax to aphasic adults may be an exception to the general assumption that treatment involves *stimulation* or *reactivation* rather than *teaching*. In most cases, procedures used in teaching aphasic adults to spell and write do not differ much from those used to teach beginning writers.

It may be fortunate that most aphasic adults do not really need advanced writing skills in daily life. If an aphasic adult can write short notes, fill out forms, and write checks, she or he can probably get by in most daily life environments. Consequently, treatment programs that can get aphasic writers to this level are likely to be sufficient for most of them. Writing one's name is no doubt the most frequent single daily life writing act, and often is the first treatment objective for patients who cannot write. Fortunately, writing one's name is a highly automatized writing activity. It is common to see adults with severe aphasia who can write their name when they can write nothing else.

Most of the linguistic variables that affect how easy it is to produce spoken sentences (length, word frequency, syntactic complexity, and so on) also affect how easy it is to write them. Context affects aphasic persons' writing in the same way that it affects their speaking. If part of a sentence is provided and patients have only to complete the sentence, success rates are higher than if they have to produce the same words without contextual support. Cloze procedures, in which single words are deleted from printed passages, sometimes help patients get started. Most aphasic patients write single words better when they fill in blanks in a sentence or paragraph than when they have to write them in isolation.

Survival Writing Skills For patients with substantially impaired writing, the concept of *survival writing skills* is a useful guide to treatment. The clinician and the patient (and sometimes family members) make a list of things that the patient would most like to be able to write. Treatment is then directed toward developing a core writing vocabulary and enough syntactic skills to enable the patient to perform the writing tasks on the list. The following list of writing skills was produced by a woman with moderately severe Broca's aphasia. The skills are listed in order of importance to the patient (from top to bottom):

- Signing forms
- Writing shopping lists
- Writing checks
- Writing personal notes
- Writing personal letters

A Writing Treatment Program Haskins (1976) suggested a progression of tasks for treating the writing impairments of aphasic patients who need more than survival writing skills. The progression begins with auditory stimulation and progresses to production of written materials A modified version of Haskins's progression follows.

1. The patient points to letters after the clinician says the sound of the letter (not the letter name).
   - -1 letter
   - -2 letters
   - -3 letters
   - etc.
2. The patient points to printed words after the clinician says the sound sequence for the word (for example, /k/-/a/-/t/).
3. The patient points to alphabet letters after the clinician names them.
   - -1 letter
   - -2 letters
   - etc.
4. The patient points to printed words after the clinician spells them.
5. The patient points to printed words after the clinician names them.
   - -1 word
   - -2 words
   - etc.
6. The patient traces letters of the alphabet.
7. The patient copies letters of the alphabet.
8. The patient writes letters of the alphabet to dictation.
   - -In serial order
   - -In random order
9. The patient writes words to dictation.
   - -The clinician spells words letter by letter and the patient writes each letter.
   - -The clinician spells words, 1 second per letter and the patient writes the words.
   - -The clinician says words and the patient writes them.

10. The patient copies structured sentences (such as *"I eat pie, I eat cake, I eat meat,"* and so on).
11. The patient writes structured sentences to dictation.
    -Word-by-word dictation
    -Sentence dictation
12. The patient writes sentences containing words provided by the clinician.

Haskins recommends that clinicians expand or reduce the complexity of the treatment program to meet the needs of individual patients. Some patients will not need the training provided in early steps of the progression. They would begin at a point at which their performance begins to break down.

It is unusual for an aphasic adult's treatment program to concentrate exclusively on writing. Treatment of writing impairments usually is an adjunct to other treatment, with considerable reliance on homework. If the clinician plans carefully, treatment of writing impairments can be coordinated with other treatment activities to create maximum generalization from writing to other communicative abilities, and vice-versa, and from the clinic to daily life.

■ GROUP ACTIVITIES FOR APHASIC ADULTS

Group activities for aphasic adults (and sometimes family members) may be provided either as adjuncts to or as replacement for one-to-one clinician-patient treatment. Some groups include only aphasic patients, and some include patients and family members. Group activities can be divided into four general categories, depending on their purpose: *treatment, transition, maintenance,* and *support.*

Treatment Groups The purpose of treatment groups is to provide structured experiences in communication among group members. For many patients, group treatment activities provide an environment in which they can try out new behaviors or new ways of communicating in a more natural situation than treat-

ment sessions with a clinician, but which is better controlled (and usually less threatening) than daily life social interactions. Activities for treatment groups tend to be clinician directed and clinician controlled, structured, and task oriented. The clinician ensures that each group member receives stimulation appropriate to her or his abilities and consistent with the therapeutic objectives for the group member. Sometimes group activities are didactic and resemble activities seen in one-to-one clinician-patient treatment. Sometimes group activities resemble daily life conversational interactions, with emphasis on communication among group members. Group treatment can provide patients with experiences that are not possible in one-to-one treatment activities. Group treatment is also cost effective (more patients can be treated in groups than in one-to-one treatment).

Transition Groups Activities for transition groups prepare patients for communication in daily life environments by giving them training and practice with strategies and problem-solving skills that are useful in daily life. Role-playing activities involving common experiences give patients a chance to try out new strategies or problem-solving methods in a protected environment resembling real life. Transition groups also provide patients with information and advice about how to find and make use of community services such as adult day-care centers, visiting nurse services, and senior citizens' centers. Transition group experiences are intended to provide a smooth transition between treatment and discharge from treatment. Patients usually participate in transition groups for specified periods of time (usually from 4 to 6 weeks).

Maintenance Groups Maintenance groups are made up of aphasic patients who have been discharged from individual treatment. Activities in maintenance groups are designed to keep participants' communicative abilities at optimum levels and to prevent the deterioration that might occur when patients no longer receive regular treatment. Maintenance groups usually meet no more than once a week and sometimes as infrequently as once a month. Activities in maintenance groups emphasize social interaction and communication in social contexts. Patients may stay in maintenance groups for several months or even years, depending on the needs of the patient and family and the resources of the facility offering the group activities.

Support Groups Support groups for patients and family members serve several functions. They provide information to patients and families about the nature of aphasia. They help patients and families understand the consequences of aphasia, and help them deal with the psychological, social, and vocational effects of aphasia. Support groups may help patients and families cope with long-term changes in life style caused by brain injuries and aphasia. They may provide emotional support and help patients and families find new friends and acquaintances. Support groups typically offer activities such as:

- Group discussions in which group members ask questions, exchange ideas and information, express attitudes, and discuss problems associated with aphasia and stroke.
- Lectures or speeches by resource persons about problems related to stroke and aphasia.
- Leisure and entertainment activities, either at the meeting site or at theaters, restaurants, or other such locations.

The Value of Group Activities It is difficult to measure the value of group activities, and the value of group activities has not received much attention in the literature. According to Eisenson (1973) most of the literature on group treatment for aphasia consists of favorable testimonials with little empirical support. Schuell and associates (1965), suggest that group treatment may help patients feel less isolated and may provide them with opportunities

to observe others with aphasia. However, Schuell and associates feel that group treatment should be offered only as an adjunct to one-to-one individualized treatment, and that group treatment should not be substituted for individual treatment.

> "treatment for aphasia must constantly be dovetailed to patient response. There are no mass methods, and none are possible. What reaches or helps one patient at one point in time loses another. For these reasons, we are unable to have confidence in group therapy as a basic method of treatment for aphasia (p.343)."

Eisenson (1973) agrees that group treatment is not a substitute for individual treatment, but suggests that group activities may improve aphasic patients' adjustment and reduce their anxiety. Eisenson feels that group activities should provide psychological support (according to Eisenson, their most important purpose), allow patients to practice communication in a permissive and nonthreatening setting, and provide some teaching about communication. According to Eisenson, group activities can provide patients with an opportunity for socialization, motivation from peers, awareness of their own speech habits, opportunities to observe the techniques with which other aphasic patients deal with communicative impairments, practice in responding to speakers with different ways of using speech and language, and an opportunity to ventilate feelings and air grievances.

Wertz and associates (1981) experimentally evaluated the effects of individual and group treatment on aphasic adults. Aphasic patients in *individual treatment* (Group A) received 8 hours of clinician-directed treatment per week for 44 weeks. Patients in *group treatment* (Group B) received 8 hours of group treatment and group recreational activities each week for 44 weeks. All patients' speech and language abilities were periodically assessed with several standardized measures. With minor exceptions, both groups made significant improvement on all speech and language measures between 4 weeks post onset (when they entered treatment) and tests at the end of 11, 22, 33, and 44 weeks of treatment. There were few significant differences between the two groups on any test occasion, although Group A almost always performed somewhat better than Group B. Both groups improved significantly between 26 and 48 weeks post onset (after 22 to 44 weeks of treatment, when, according to Wertz and associates, spontaneous recovery should no longer be taking place). Wertz and associates concluded that both individual and group treatment of the kind provided in their study were efficacious. They suggested that individual treatment may be "slightly superior" to group treatment. However, they also suggested that the cost-effectiveness of group treatment "should prompt speech-language pathologists to consider it for at least part of an aphasic patient's care (p. 592)."*

Kearns and Simmons (1985) surveyed 91 Veterans Administration Medical Centers to find out what kinds of group treatment activities they offered. Fifty-nine percent offered *treatment* groups and 54% sponsored *counseling* or *support* groups. Kearns and Simmons's report focused on treatment groups. The average treatment group size was 5.5 patients (89% of groups contained eight or fewer patients). Eighty-nine percent of groups met either one or two times a week. Average session length was about 1 hour. Seventy-eight percent of patients in treatment groups were more than 1 year post-onset, and 49% of group members received both individual treatment and group treatment.

Most respondents (84%) reported that the primary goal of their treatment groups was language stimulation. However, many respondents reported other goals which would be consistent with transition, maintenance, or support groups: *emotional support* (59%), *carryover* (47%), and *socialization* (45%). Treatment group activities fell into several categories: *general discussions about a given topic* (31%), *individualized structured tasks* (22%), *nondirected social interactions* (18%), *multimodality stimulation* (14%), and *teaching communicative strategies* (14%). Most respondents (73%) reported that the effects of group treatment were evaluated by periodic formal testing of group members, and 57% reported that periodic behavioral ratings were made. However, 20% reported that the effects of patients' participation in the treatment groups were not measured.

Kearns and Simmons suggested that eclectic, multipurpose groups may not be the most effective form of patient management, and that treatment and maintenance groups have different goals and require different procedures. They also urged that the effects of group treatment on individual group members be documented, and that standard criteria be used in selecting patients for groups and in discharging them from the groups.

■ KEY CONCEPTS

- Treatment of aphasia is efficacious if it is delivered by qualified professionals, if patients with irreversible aphasia are excluded, and if the content, timing, and duration of treatment are appropriate for those receiving the treatment. Whether treatment is *effective* as well as *efficacious* remains to be determined.
- Not all aphasic patients should receive treatment for their communication impairments. Patients with very mild aphasia are likely to recover essentially all of their premorbid communication abilities without treatment. Patients with very severe aphasia following

---

* However, Wertz and associates studied the *efficacy* of group treatment, not its *effectiveness*. (Their measure of treatment effects was changed on standardized aphasia tests.) See the section on *Effectiveness of Treatment for Aphasia* earlier in this chapter for more on efficacy versus effectiveness.

neurologic recovery rarely recover functional communication, even with treatment. However speech-language pathologists may provide support, education, and counseling for untreated patients, their families and caregivers, and may help them find ways to maximize the effectiveness of the communication abilities the patient has retained.

- Treatment directed toward underlying processes usually is more efficient and effective than treatment that mimics test tasks in which deficient performance has been observed.
- Auditory comprehension of verbal materials is a combination of text-based (bottom-up) processes and knowledge-based (top-down) processes. Treatment of auditory comprehension impairments should permit patients to use knowledge-based processes as well as text-based ones.
- Sentence comprehension and discourse comprehension are only weakly related. Consequently, focusing treatment on a patient's sentence comprehension is unlikely to have strong effects on her or his discourse comprehension.
- Text-based and knowledge-based processes that are important in auditory comprehension also are important in reading comprehension. Patients with mild-to-moderate aphasia may benefit from treatment directed toward sentence-level and discourse-level reading materials. Patients with moderate to severe aphasia may benefit from treatment directed toward survival reading skills.
- Treatment of aphasic adults' impaired speech production often focuses on word retrieval, usually by means of confrontation naming tasks in which prompts and cues are systematically manipulated to improve patients' word retrieval. However, confrontation naming drills, in themselves, are not likely to lead to improved word retrieval in

daily life interactions unless generalization-enhancing procedures are incorporated into the treatment program. Improvements in word retrieval are more likely to generalize to daily life if the word-retrieval drills responsible for the improvement focus on the same processes as are needed in daily life interactions.

- Treatment of patients with apraxia of speech is strongly affected by the severity of a patient's impairments. Treatment of patients with severe apraxia of speech is carried out at elemental single-sound levels. Treatment of patients with moderate apraxia of speech is carried out at word and simple-phrase levels. Treatment of patients with mild apraxia of speech is carried out at sentence or discourse levels.
- *Intrasystemic and intersystemic reorganization* (facilitating speech production by bringing motor systems that usually do not participate in speech production into the process) and *melodic intonation therapy* (facilitating speech production by incorporated exaggerated melody into speech) are two formalized procedures for enhancing apraxic patients' speech production.
- Treating aphasic adults' writing impairments typically relies on procedures similar to those used to teach beginning writers. Spelling, syntax, and word retrieval often are targeted in writing treatment for aphasic adults.
- Although little research has been directed toward determining the value of group treatment for aphasic adults, many facilities provide group treatment programs. The purposes of these programs may include, individually or in combination, providing direct treatment, preparing patients for discharge from treatment, maintaining communication abilities for patients who are no longer receiving individualized treatment, or providing emotional and psychologic support.

Right Hemisphere Syndrome

That the two hemispheres of the human brain serve different functions has been suspected since the late 1800s. In 1861 Paul Broca reported that eight patients with language disturbance secondary to brain damage all had lesions in the left hemisphere. Within the next few years the dominance of the left hemisphere for language had become widely accepted.* During the next decade most believed that the left hemisphere was dominant for most cognitive functions, with the right hemisphere responsible only for perceptual and motor functions and perhaps some rudimentary mental processes. Then, in 1874, John Hughlings Jackson, a British neurologist, asserted that the left hemisphere is responsible for language and that the right hemisphere is responsible for visual recognition, discrimination, and recall. During the next hundred years the right hemisphere's contribution to cognition and intellect was largely neglected, as investigators concentrated on exploring the allocation of responsibilities for language within the left hemisphere. It was not until the middle of the twentieth century that in-

---

* Statements about hemispheric specialization such as this may be misleading unless the qualifier "in right-handed adults" is added. Few writers add the qualifier, and I will not belabor the reader with it. However, the reader should keep it in mind whenever reading descriptions of right-hemisphere–damaged adults.

vestigators began to explore the organization and function of the right hemisphere in any concerted fashion. Consequently, our knowledge of what the right hemisphere does, and how it does it, remains imperfect, although we are slowly becoming more sophisticated.

Early theories of hemispheric function contended that the left hemisphere is specialized for language and reasoning while the right hemisphere is specialized for music and visual processes. This concept of hemispheric specialization gradually changed as investigators found that the two hemispheres appeared to operate in fundamentally different ways. Writers began to describe the left hemisphere as "rational and analytic" and the right hemisphere as "intuitive and holistic." Contemporary models of hemispheric functions depict the left hemisphere as specialized for processing sequential, time-related material, which requires linear (serial) processing, and the right hemisphere as specialized for processing nonlinear arrays, which require holistic, gestalt-like (parallel) processing. Because auditory information often comes in time-ordered sequences (syllables in a word, words in a sentence) the left hemisphere may have greater responsibility for auditory events, and because visual information often comes in multidimensional arrays (pictures, scenes, faces) the right hemisphere may have greater responsibility for visual events. However, these hemispheric differences reflect the nature of the information with which the brain must deal, rather than the modality through which it enters the brain.

Regardless of how one chooses to explain the right hemisphere's contribution to cognition and behavior, it is clear that only about half of adults who sustain right-hemisphere brain damage develop communication impairments (Joanette and associates (1983). The variables contributing to communication impairments following right-hemisphere brain damage are not well understood, although Joanette and associates (1983) suggest that patients with corti-cal lesions, a history of familial left-handedness, and low education levels are the most likely candidates. The relationship of the first two variables to right-hemisphere communication impairments makes intuitive sense. Because language and communication are cortical, rather than subcortical processes, it is not surprising that cortical lesions in the right hemisphere are more likely than subcortical lesions to produce communication impairments, as is true for left-hemisphere lesions. Because familial left-handedness is likely to be related to right-hemisphere dominance for language, it is not surprising that left-handers with right-hemisphere lesions are more likely to develop communication impairments than left-handers without such a family history. There is no obvious logical relationship between low education level and the development of communication impairments by adults with right-hemisphere brain damage. It may be that low education levels are associated with other patient variables that actually account for the relationship.

■ BEHAVIORAL AND COGNITIVE SYMPTOMS OF RIGHT HEMISPHERE BRAIN DAMAGE

Descriptions in the clinical literature of the perceptual, cognitive, and behavioral consequences of right-hemisphere brain damage usually describe a stereotypic collection of impairments that by implication is exhibited by all adults with right-hemisphere brain damage. Typically no mention is made of the fact that only about half of adults with right-hemisphere brain damage have communication impairments, and little attention is given to individual-to-individual variability in symptoms within groups of right-hemisphere–damaged adults who do have communication impairments, although it is well known that appreciable variability exists. Group studies of adults with right-hemisphere brain damage often contribute to misconceptions about the generality of stereotypic patterns of impairment by reporting results obtained by testing heterogeneous groups in which the location and severity of subjects' right-hemisphere brain damage have not been controlled for or reported. Results typically are reported as average group performance, with little consideration of the extent to which individuals in the group conform to the group average.

The interpretation of these studies is further compromised by the failure of most to include control groups with left-hemisphere damage to permit separating the effects of right-hemisphere brain damage from the effects of brain damage in general. Right-hemisphere-damaged patients with posterior lesions do not often have hemiparesis or hemiplegia. Consequently, most are discharged from the hospital quickly, so that groups of right-hemisphere-damaged adults enrolled in studies tend to contain disproportionately large numbers of patients with frontal-lobe damage.* When patients with posterior right-hemisphere damage are included, they tend to be in the immediate post-onset stage of recovery, when global effects of brain damage create symptoms that are caused by brain damage in general, rather than right-hemisphere brain damage.

Tompkins (1995) speaks to the heterogeneity of symptoms within the population of right-hemisphere-damaged adults as follows:

> One of the most important things to remember about adults with RHD [right-hemisphere damage] is one of the most important characteristics of any "category" of people; they are quite heterogeneous. Not all patients will have communicative impairments. Those who do will not have all symptoms, and individual patients will display dif-

---

* McDonald (1993) has pointd out the striking similarities between communication disturbances of groups of patients with frontal lobe damage and groups with right-hemisphere damage. McDonald comments that these similarities may arise, at least in part, from the inclusion of large proportions of patients with frontal lobe damage in groups with right-hemisphere brain damage.

ferent patterns of behavior. Complicating things further, it can be quite difficult to specify "disordered" status, because normative information is almost nonexistent for abilities and performance broken down by age, education, socioeconomic status, and cultural variables. It is part of the clinical challenge in working with brain-damaged individuals to identify the presence and absence of the deficits that result from neurologic insult, as well as those that are not necessarily due to the brain damage (pp. 15-16).*

The symptoms generated by right-hemisphere damage, like those generated by left-hemisphere damage, differ in their nature and severity, depending on the site and extent of the brain injury causing them, although, as noted above, our understanding of these relationships is imperfect. Although the relationships between damage in various regions of the right hemisphere and behavioral symptoms have yet to be dependably elucidated, many right-hemisphere–damaged adults exhibit distinctive cognitive and behavioral impairments. Some of the most striking are perceptual and attentional.

Perceptual and Attentional Impairments

Denial of Illness (Anosagnosia) Denial of illness is a frequent consequence of right-hemisphere brain damage, especially for patients with parietal lobe damage. Denial takes several forms. In its mildest form, patients acknowledge their disabilities but are indifferent to them. Patients with moderate levels of denial acknowledge their disabilities, but underestimate their severity and minimize their effects (e.g., a right-hemisphere–damaged patient with dense left hemiplegia who asserted that his paralyzed left arm and leg were "a little weak" and gave him problems only when he attempted to climb stairs). Patients with severe denial may disavow the existence of severe disabilities such as paralysis, sensory loss, and visual field blind-

---

* Tompkin's comments relate equally well to all other categories of adults with brain damage.

ness, and some even deny that their hemiplegic limbs belong to them. Patients with severe denial sometimes claim to perform activities that clearly are beyond their physical capabilities— for example, the patient with left-sided paralysis who claimed to be in training for the national speed-skating championships. Many right-hemisphere–damaged patients, even those with low levels of outright denial, ignore errors and confabulate, argue, and justify them when errors are called to their attention.

Neglect Many right-hemisphere–damaged patients exhibit *left hemispatial neglect,* characterized by diminished responsiveness to stimulation on the left side of the body and diminished awareness of visual or auditory stimuli in left-sided space. When these patients copy drawings or draw figures, objects, or scenes from memory they tend to leave out details on the left side. When they read printed materials aloud they may read only the material on the right side of the page, even as they complain that the material makes no sense. These patients bump into things on the left, and those in wheelchairs sometimes get trapped against the left side of doorways or other obstructions because they fail to perceive their presence and remain unaware of them even when trapped by them. Patients with moderate neglect attend to stimuli in their left hemispace if reminded, but bump into things on the left and may show other signs of inattention such as using only their right-side trousers pockets or the right side of dressers, cupboards, and bureaus. In its mildest form neglect may be detectable only with *simultaneous stimulation,* in which brief stimuli (such as flashes of light, gentle touches, or pinpricks) are presented simultaneously on both sides of the body. Patients with mild neglect (sometimes called *hemispatial inattention*) do not perceive stimuli on the left when both sides are stimulated, but perceive them when only the left side is stimulated.

Neglect seems not to be simply a perceptual problem, but appears to be a result of disrupted mental representations of external space. There are several accounts in the literature of right-hemisphere–damaged adults who, when they are asked to describe familiar spaces or scenes from memory, describe only right-sided space or describe right-sided space in greater detail than left-sided space. For example, a right-hemisphere-damaged adult who is asked to describe his or her home while mentally walking through it from the front to the back provides elaborate description of the rooms on the right and ignores the rooms on the left. When they describe the same living space while mentally walking through it from the back to the front, they describe the rooms on the previously neglected side and ignore those previously described.

Many theories have been proposed to explain why and how neglect happens. *Arousal theories* (Heilman, Schwartz, & Watson, 1978; and others) propose that right-hemisphere-damaged patients' perceptual systems are less sensitive and responsive to stimuli in the neglected space. *Attentional engagement theories* (Arguin & Bub, 1993) propose that patients have difficulty directing attention to the neglected space, and *attentional disengagement theories* (Posner and associates, 1987) propose that patients' attention is captured and held by stimuli in non-neglected space, preventing them from redirecting it to stimuli on the neglected side. As this is written, there is no empirical evidence that clearly favors any one of these theories.

Neglect can be caused by damage in either hemisphere, but usually is more severe and persistent following right-hemisphere damage (Cummings, 1983). It can occur following damage in any cortical region, but is most common and most severe after right parietal lobe damage (Mesulam, 1981; Watson & Heilman, 1979). Patients with left-sided neglect often exhibit left visual field blindness, but visual neglect can happen to patients with no demonstrable visual field blindness (Willanger, Danielsen & Ankerhus; 1981). Neglect sometimes resolves either partially or completely in the first days or weeks after injury.

Constructional Impairment Many brain-injured patients perform poorly when they are asked to draw or copy geometric designs, create designs with colored blocks, reproduce two-dimensional stick figures, or reproduce three-dimensional constructions using wooden blocks. Deficient performance on such tasks, in the absence of visual perceptual or motor impairments that could cause it, is called *constructional impairment* (sometimes erroneously called *constructional apraxia*).* Constructional impairments appear following damage to either hemisphere but are more frequent and more severe following right-hemisphere brain damage, especially when the damage is in the right parietal lobe or right parieto-occipital region. Patients with left-hemisphere brain damage, as well as those with right-hemisphere damage, make errors on constructional tests, and counting the number of errors made does not discriminate between them (Gainotti & Tiacci, 1970). However, patients with right-hemisphere damage and patients with left-hemisphere damage do not make the same kinds of errors. Patients with right-hemisphere damage draw quickly and impulsively. They make mistakes, which they often try to correct by adding more lines. Patients with left-hemisphere damage draw slowly and effortfully, but tend not to make gross mistakes that must be corrected by redrawing or adding lines. Patients with right-hemisphere damage tend to leave out details on the left side of drawings or constructions or omit the left side entirely (see above). When copying drawings they often add extraneous lines, rotate and fragment the drawings, and render three-dimensional drawings in two dimensions. Their drawings look fragmented, disorganized, and crowded, and they often are misplaced to the right on the page. Patients with left-hemisphere damage simplify figures or constructions and produce drawings in which the proportions and dimensionality are accurate, but angles and lines are distorted (Lezak, 1983). Their drawings look incomplete and clumsy, but coherent. Patients with left hemisphere lesions benefit from having a model to copy, while those with right-hemisphere lesions do not (Hecaen & Assal, 1970). Many of these differences are apparent in Figure 7-1, which shows figures copied by a left-hemisphere–damaged patient and the same figures copied by a patient with right-hemisphere damage.

Topographic Impairment Patients with topographic impairments (sometimes called *topologic disorientation*) seem confused about how they relate to the space around them. They have difficulty following familiar routes, reading maps, giving directions, and performing other tasks that depend on internal representations of external space. Myers (1994) has suggested that at least some of right-hemisphere–damaged patients' problems in this domain may arise from failure to recognize familiar landmarks or to learn new ones because they fail to attend to visual cues. Some patients with topographic impairments compensate for them by talking themselves through a sequence of directions. One right-hemisphere–damaged patient found his way back to his room by talking himself through the following sequence.

> *Go to the end of the hall. Look both ways. Find the hall with the window at the end. Go down that hall. The first door past the nurses' station is my room.*

Right-hemisphere–damaged patients' ability to talk themselves through a route sets them apart from patients with generalized disorientation and confusion, who also get lost easily and have no idea where they are or how they got there.

---

* Apraxia is a disorder in which planning and execution of volitional sequential movements are disrupted. Constructional impairments represent visuospatial perceptual and organizational impairments, rather than motor planning impairments

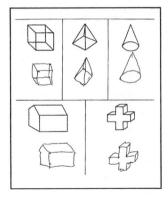 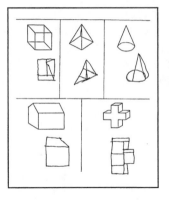

Figure 7-1 ■ Performance on a figure-copying test by a patient with left-hemisphere brain damage (left) and a patient with right-hemisphere brain damage (right).

An unusual disturbance in which the patient believes in the existence of two or more identical persons, places, or things occasionally follows right-hemisphere brain damage. This disturbance is called *reduplicative paramnesia.* One patient with reduplicative paramnesia claimed the existence of two identical hospitals in the same city, another claimed to have two left legs, and a third claimed the existence of two identical husbands, both living in the patient's home. Reduplicative paramnesia apparently is produced by disturbances of spatial perception and visual memory. Most patients who develop it have damage in the right brain hemisphere, but a more precise localization has not been offered.

Geographic Disorientation Geographic disorientation is less common than topographic impairment, but the two often occur together (Tompkins, 1995). Patients with geographic disorientation recognize at least the general nature of their surroundings but are mistaken as to their geographic location. (For example, a patient at Veterans Medical Center in Minneapolis, Minnesota believed that he was in a hospital in South Africa). Geographic disorientation, in its pure sense, is distinct from orientation to time and person. These patients know what day, month, and year it is, and they know who they are and have at least a general sense of who

those around them are.* The reasons for geographic disorientation are unknown, although it may reflect an inference deficit that prevents patients from inferring their location from cues provided by surroundings, or it may be caused by patients' inability to construct a mental representation of geographic locations based on cues available from immediate surroundings. (Tompkins, 1995).

Facial Recognition Deficits (Prosopagnosia) Some patients with right-hemisphere brain damage are unable to recognize otherwise familiar persons by their facial features, and perform poorly on other tasks that depend on perception and integration of facial features, such as identifying famous people from photographs and choosing pictures of people previously shown to them from a group containing previously seen pictures and previously unseen foils. This disorder is called *prosopognosia,* (from the Greek words for *face* and *knowledge*). These patients' facial recognition deficits usually affect perception of cartoons and line-drawn faces as well as actual faces and photographs, and may extend beyond human faces, as indicated by ac-

---

* Many hospitalized adults, non-brain-damaged as well as brain-damaged, lose track of what day it is after several days in the hospital, because there are few reminders of what day it is in most hospitals.

counts of a birdwatcher who no longer recognized different species of birds, and a farmer who no longer recognized his cows, following right-hemisphere strokes (Albert and associates, 1982). Patients who fail to recognize friends and family members by their facial features recognize them when they speak or by their clothing, hair color, hair style, body size, or gait. (Presumably the birdwatcher could still tell different birds by their songs, and perhaps the farmer could tell his cows apart by the sound of their voices, their coloring, or the way they walked.) Some patients with prosopognosia also have difficulty distinguishing between male and female faces, old and young faces, or human and animal faces. Facial recognition deficits are common following posterior right-hemisphere brain damage (Haecan & Angelergues, 1962; Warrington & James, 1967; Whitely & Warrington, 1977), but persisting deficits probably require bilateral damage (Albert and associates, 1982; Cohn, Newman & Wood, 1977; Damasio, 1985; Damasio & Damasio, 1983; Meadows, 1974). Facial recognition deficits seem to be independent of disordered visuospatial perception (McKeever & Dixon, 1981) and recognition of emotion (Cicone, Wapner & Gardner, 1980; Ley & Breyden, 1979). Occasionally, a right-hemisphere–damaged patient with prosopagnosia claims that relatives and friends have been abducted and replaced by imposters—a condition called *Capgras syndrome.*

Visuoperceptual Impairments Right-hemisphere–damaged adults typically have little difficulty identifying real objects or recognizing pictures or drawings of objects when they are portrayed naturalistically, in prototypic views. Their visuoperceptual impairments become apparent when they are asked to recognize objects, pictures, or drawings that are incomplete, distorted, or otherwise changed from their traditional prototypic form (Myers, 1994). They have difficulty identifying line drawings of ob-

jects when one drawing is superimposed on another, they may be unable to identify familiar objects depicted in incomplete or fragmented pictures or drawings, and they may be slow to identify familiar objects depicted in unusual orientations or with unusual size relationships. These visuospatial impairments seem less perceptual than organizational. When visual stimuli are simple, clear, and unambiguous they are perceived normally, but when the stimuli are incomplete, degraded, or distorted, right-hemisphere–damaged patients' recognition and interpretation of them suffers.

Recognition and Expression of Emotion

The experience of emotion is mediated by the limbic system,* but appreciation of others' emotions and expression of personal emotion appear to be mediated in large part by the right hemisphere in right-handed adults. Right-hemisphere–damaged adults' impairments in appreciating emotions generally are attributed to deficiencies in three domains—appreciation of prosodic cues to emotion in others' speech, appreciation of the emotional implications of facial expressions, and appreciation of the emotional tone associated with stereotypic emotional situations (e.g., weddings or funerals).

Many right-hemisphere-damaged adults seem not to appreciate the significance of prosodic indicators of emotion. Whether this deficit actually represents an underlying disturbance of emotional competence is not clear. There is some evidence that right-hemisphere–damaged adults' insensitivity to prosodic indicators of emotion is caused by failure to perceive, dis-

---

* The limbic system includes phylogenetically old portions of the cerebral cortex, subcortical structures, and pathways connecting them to the diencephalon and brain stem. The functions of the limbic system are related to survival of the individual and continuation of the species, including eating behavior, aggression, expression of emotion, and endocrinal aspects of the sexual response.

criminate, and process the acoustic information related to pitch and intonation patterns, rather than failure to attach emotional significance to perceived acoustic information (Robin, Tranel, & Damasio, 1990).

Many investigators have reported that adults with right-hemisphere brain damage fail to correctly interpret facial expressions indicative of emotion (Blonder, Bowers, & Heilman, 1991; Cicone, Wapner, & Gardner, 1980; DeKosky and associates, 1980; and others). Right-hemisphere–damaged adults' interpretation of facial expression typically has been tested by presenting still photographs of people producing static representations of feigned emotions. Because movement cues to the expressions are not available, identification of the emotions portrayed in the photographs depends completely on analysis of visuospatial information (how narrow the eyes are, whether the mouth curves up or down, and so on). Because adults with right-hemisphere brain damage are known to be deficient both in analysis of visuospatial information and in integration of individual features into a composite whole, it may be that what seems to be a problem in interpreting facial expression actually reflects an underlying impairment in the analysis and integration of spatial information (Myers, 1994).

Several studies have reported that adults with right-hemisphere brain damage perform poorly when asked to match the emotional tone of short stories with pictured scenes (Cicone, Wapner, & Gardner, 1980); identify emotions portrayed in pictured scenes (Bloom and associates, 1992; Cancelliene & Kertesz, 1990); or identify emotions portrayed in isolated spoken sentences (Blonder, Bowers, & Heilman, 1991). However, some contradictory evidence has been reported. Tompkins & Flowers (1985) reported that adults with right-hemisphere brain damage performed comparably to adults with left-hemisphere brain damage when they were asked to identify the emotions conveyed by spoken sentences. Myers (1994) has asserted that

determining the emotional tone of situations, sentences, and narratives requires that individuals recognize that emotional tone is present, discriminate cues that signal emotions, and integrate the cues into an overall representation of an emotion—all of which characteristically are problems for adults with right-hemisphere brain damage.

In summary, many adults with right-hemisphere brain damage appear to have diminished appreciation of emotions conveyed by speech prosody, facial expression, narratives, or pictorial representations, at least when they are asked to identify the emotional tone of such materials presented in a test environment. However, it is not clear that their abnormal performance on these tasks actually reflects impaired appreciation of emotions and not impairment of some other cognitive process or processes. Regardless of the underlying reasons, many adults with right-hemisphere damage seem deficient in recognizing and expressing emotion in daily life interactions. They are insensitive to emotional tone conveyed by others' facial expression and tone of voice, and when they do assign emotional significance to spoken materials, facial expressions and body language, or situations, they often assign the wrong emotion.

Attentional Impairments

Attentional impairments are common in brain-damaged adults, and those with right-hemisphere brain damage are no exception. In fact, it is possible that many of the surface manifestations of right-hemisphere brain damage represent, at least in part, disturbances of underlying attentional processes. Many patients with right-hemisphere damage have difficulty focusing, maintaining, and shifting attention. These impairments make them distractible in treatment activities and interfere with many aspects of daily life activities. Attentional impairments make it difficult for these patients to determine the overall meaning of situations and events, separate what is important from what is not, identify relationships among individual elements of information, maintain appropriate patterns of interaction with conversational partners, and maintain coherence in their communications with others. Attentional impairments often make it difficult or impossible for some right-hemisphere–damaged patients to focus on treatment activities.

Attention no doubt represents the interaction of several cognitive processes, and some investigators have divided attentional processes into multiple components that they believe represent different underlying skills. *Sustained attention* denotes an individual's ability to maintain attention on selected stimuli over a period of time, without significant changes in performance. *Selective attention* (sometimes called *focused attention*) denotes an individual's ability to maintain attention on selected stimuli in the presence of competing or distracting stimuli, and to attend to specific stimuli within an array. *Alternating attention* denotes an individual's ability to shift attention from one stimulus to another in response to changing requirements or goals. *Divided attention* denotes an individual's ability to perform more than one activity simultaneously (for example, driving an automobile while carrying on a conversation). Patients with right-hemisphere brain damage may exhibit impairments in any or all of these attentional processes.

Communication Impairments Associated with Right Hemisphere Damage

In addition to perceptual, affective, and attentional impairments, many adults with right-hemisphere damage have communication impairments that compromise their ability to communicate emotions, express themselves coherently and efficiently, comprehend humor, sarcasm, and nonliteral material, and interact appropriately in conversational interactions.

Diminished Speech Prosody Many right-hemisphere–damaged adults lose normal variability in vocal pitch and loudness, making their speech sound monotonous and devoid of emotion. In addition to the monotony and emotional flatness of their speech, many of these patients show reductions in nonverbal movements (head nods, gestures, and so on) that typically accompany speech.

It is not clear which right-hemisphere–damaged patients are most likely to exhibit prosodically flattened speech. Breyden and Ley (1983) and Shapiro and Danley (1985) attributed this phenomenon to damage in the right frontal lobe. Colsher, Cooper, and Graff-Radford (1987) subsequently challenged this conclusion, claiming that adults with anterior right-hemisphere damage have essentially normal variability in vocal pitch. Additionally, Myers (1994) and Tompkins (1995) raise the possibility that right-hemisphere–damaged adults' reduced speech prosody may be caused by muscle weakness (dysarthria) rather than by an underlying affective impairment. Tompkins also notes that diminished speech prosody can occur with brain damage outside the right hemisphere. Finally, some right-hemisphere–damaged adults seem aware that their voice does not communicate their emotional state to listeners, and compensate by communicating their emotional state via propositional speech (e.g., the right-hemisphere–damaged patient who, in the middle of a challenging treatment activity, said to the clinician, *"Since you don't seem to realize it, I guess I have to tell you that I'm tired of this and upset with you."*). That these patients verbally compensate for their prosodic flattening suggests that their prosodic deficiencies are not related to an underlying affective impairment. However, it is true that many of the same patients who fail to communicate emotion via speech prosody also fail to appreciate emotions conveyed by others' speech prosody and facial expression, lending credence to the assumption that they have an underlying emotional impairment.

Anomalous Content and Organization of Connected Speech One of the most striking communication impairments of right-hemisphere-damaged patients is their excessive, confabulatory, and sometimes inappropriate connected speech. These anomalies become apparent when right-hemisphere–damaged adults are placed in narrative production tasks in which they tell (or retell) stories in response to pictures, picture sequences, or stories told to them by another. The speech they produce under these conditions has been described as excessive and rambling (Gardner and associates, 1983); repetitive and irrelevant (Tompkins & Flowers, 1985); and tangential, digressive, and inefficient (Myers, 1994). They use more words but produce less information than either non–brain-damaged adults or adults with left-hemisphere brain damage (Diggs & Basili, 1987; Myers, 1979; Rivers & Love, 1980). Their narratives tend to be fragmented and to lack cohesion and an overall theme or point, because they tend to focus on incidental details, fail to establish relationships among events, insert tangential comments, and permit their personal experiences and opinions to intrude into their narratives. The following description produced by an adult with right-hemisphere brain damage reflects many of these characteristics. (He is describing the "cookie theft" picture shown in Figure 7-2.)

> Well, this is a scene in a house. It looks like a fine spring day. The window is open. I guess it's not Minnesota, or the flies and mosquitoes would be flying in. Outside I see a tree and another window. Looks like the neighbors have their windows closed. There's a woman near the window wearing what appears to be an inexpensive pair of shoes. She's holding something that looks like a plate. On the counter there, there's a hat and two caps that look like they would fit on a child's head. The woman is looking out the window and the water's on, and it's running on the floor. Looks like she needs to call the plumber. (Clinician: Is there anything over here? Points to left side of picture.) Well, I see two people...children...a boy and a girl. The boy is getting cookies from the cupboard and the girl is laughing and waving. There's also a stool. Perhaps the boy is stealing cookies and perhaps the girl...or the stool is going to fall. There's a window beside the cookie jar, but it doesn't have any curtains.

Comments The patient begins by making three inferences. One is correct and relevant *(the scene is in a house),* the other two are potentially correct, but irrelevant *(it looks like a spring day, it must not be Minnesota).* The patient then continues on to enumerate elements on the right side of the drawing, with occasional interjection of irrelevant comments. After misinterpreting the plate and two cups shown on the counter as a hat and two caps (but inferring, from their size, that they must be for children), the patient begins to appreciate the prob-

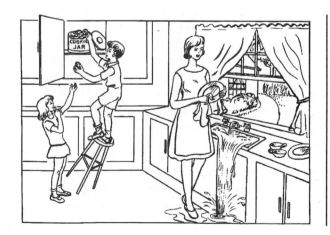

Figure 7-2 ▪ The "Cookie Theft" picture. (From Goodglass H, Kaplan E: *The Boston Diagnostic Aphasia Examination.* Philadelphia, 1983, Lea & Febiger.)

lem with the overflowing sink. When the clinician directs the patient to the left side of the drawing, the patient begins by enumerating pictured elements, then eventually arrives at the appropriate interpretation. He ends by misinterpreting a cupboard door as a window, but correctly perceives that the "window" has no curtains. This patient's narrative contains many right-hemisphere syndrome characteristics. He focuses on the right-hand side of the picture. He begins by enumerating pictured elements and slowly develops intepretations expressing relationships among the elements. He adds irrelevant and tangential comments. He misinterprets visual information. He makes inferences that may be consistent with his interpretation of visual information or underlying relationships, but which are inconsistent with the true sense of what is portrayed.

Impaired Comprehension of Narratives and Conversations Adults with aphasia comprehend discourse better than their performance on tests of single-sentence comprehension suggests that they should, but the converse seems true for most adults with right-hemisphere damage (Brownell, 1988). Right-hemisphere–damaged adults' impairments in discourse comprehension reflect many of the same underlying disabilities that compromise both their production of narratives and their ability to get along in daily life—insensitivity to relationships among events, failure to judge the appropriateness of events or situations, and making premature assumptions based on incomplete analysis of events and situations. Many patients with right-hemisphere brain damage have particular difficulty comprehending implied meanings in narratives and conversations (Brownell and associates, 1986) and are seemingly unable to get beyond literal interpretations of what they hear or read. They interpret idiomatic expressions, figures of speech, and metaphors literally. They fail to identify incongruous, irrelevant, or absurd statements, and offer confabulatory or bizarre reasons for accepting them as true. They are unable to judge the appropriateness of facts, situations, or characterizations in stories or conversations, and cannot extract morals from stories. These deficiencies in discourse comprehension carry over into their comprehension of conversations. Right-hemisphere–damaged patients ". . . often seem to lack a full understanding of the context of an utterance, the presuppositions entailed, the affective tone, or the point of a conversational exchange. They appear to have difficulties in processing abstract sentences, in reasoning logically, and in maintaining a coherent stream of thought." (Gardner and associates, 1983; p. 172).

Right-hemisphere–damaged adults' difficulties with nonliteral material are not always complete. Sometimes patients fail to appreciate nonliteral meanings in one context, but get them in another. For example, some right-hemisphere–damaged adults who cannot select pictures representing the implied meanings of nonliteral statements can explain them orally, some who cannot choose the best punch-lines for printed jokes nevertheless choose endings that are surprising, and some who do not choose the appropriate printed responses to indirect requests such as "Can you open the door?" respond appropriately to their nonliteral meaning in daily life interactions (Tompkins, 1995). Some who misperceive or misinterpret elements of narratives in test situations perceive and interpret similar elements appropriately when narratives occur in daily life situations with more contextual support. Like adults with left-hemisphere damage, those with right-hemisphere damage tend to perform better in naturalistic situations, which provide situational context, than in testing or treatment activities, which limit that context.

Brownell and associates, (1986) have suggested that right-hemisphere–damaged patients can make inferences suggested by discourse, but that their inferences are premature and incorrect. According to Brownell and associates, these patients are trapped by their initial inferences, and are unable to reject or revise them when subsequent material shows their inferences to be incorrect. The problem for these patients seems not to be that they cannot *make* inferences, but that they are too readily led into inappropriate ones. Results reported by Nicholas and Brookshire (1995) support Brownell and associates' suggestion that right-hemisphere-damaged patients can make inferences. Nicholas and Brookshire evaluated the *Discourse Comprehension Test* performance of 20 adults with right-hemisphere damage. Their group of right-hemisphere-damaged adults correctly answered 31 of 40 questions relating to implied information. The right-hemisphere-damaged adults performed as well on questions related to implied information as either aphasic adults with left-hemisphere damage or traumatically brain-injured adults.

Pragmatic Impairments Pragmatic impairments are impairments in the social and interactional aspects of language, such as turn-taking, topic maintenance, social conventions, and eye contact. Pragmatic impairments are common consequences of right-hemisphere brain damage. Many right-hemisphere-damaged adults are poor at maintaining eye contact with conversational partners, talk excessively and without regard for their listener, have difficulty staying on topic, and interject irrelevant, tangential, and inappropriate comments. Many right-hemisphere-damaged adults also are insensitive to rules governing conversational turn-taking, especially those related to "yielding the floor" to conversational partners.

However, not all right-hemisphere-damaged adults exhibit pragmatic impairments. Prutting and Kirchner (1987) evaluated the conversational behavior of 10 right-hemisphere-damaged adults while they engaged in a 15-minute conversation with another adult. They recorded the occurrence of appropriate and inappropriate behaviors in each of 30 pragmatic categories. The right-hemisphere-damaged

adults as a group failed to maintain adequate eye contact, produced speech with diminished emotional tone, were slow in responding to the conversational partner's utterances, deviated from conversational topics, and talked too much. However, not all exhibited this pattern. Of nine right-hemisphere-damaged subjects (data for one subject were not reported), two had violations in only one category (eye contact), whereas one subject had violations in 13 of the 30 categories. Nevertheless, Prutting and Kirchner's results at the group level are consistent with descriptions of right-hemisphere-damaged adults' conversational behavior found in the literature.

Kennedy and associates, (1994) evaluated 12 right-hemisphere-damaged adults' conversational behaviors as they conversed with non-brain-damaged adults. They divided the conversational behaviors into two categories. One category represented *topic-related skills* (introducing, maintaining, elaborating on, and terminating topics). The other represented *turn-taking skills* (making assertions, requesting information or action, communicating emotion, acknowledging the other's contributions, and committing to a future action). The two groups did not differ significantly in topic-related skills, but differed in turn-taking. The right-hemisphere-damaged group made significantly more assertions than the non-brain-damaged group, but significantly fewer requests for information. They also took more conversational turns, but said fewer words in each turn. (Which, as Kennedy and associates commented, may be one reason that they took more turns.) Kennedy and associates commented that several of the right-hemisphere-damaged subjects spent most of their turns talking about themselves and rarely asked their conversational partners for information. However, there was great variability among the right-hemisphere-damaged subjects, with some exhibiting severely impaired conversational skills and others appearing essentially normal, leading

Kennedy and associates to comment that right-hemisphere–damaged patients' premorbid conversational style should be considered when evaluating their postmorbid conversational skills. In combination, Kennedy and associates and Prutting and Kirchner's results show that not all adults with right-hemisphere damage have pragmatic impairments, and they also show that those who do, do not necessarily exhibit the same impairments. Consequently, treatment of right-hemisphere-damaged adults' pragmatic impairments must be based on careful analysis of the performance of individuals.*

■ TESTS FOR ASSESSING PATIENTS WITH RIGHT HEMISPHERE BRAIN INJURY

Objective assessment of right-hemisphere–damaged adults' linguistic, cognitive, and communicative abilities received little attention before the mid 1970s. Consequently, assessment of these patients is considerably less sophisticated than assessment of aphasic adults, who have been studied for over 50 years. At the time this is written, two standardized tests for evaluation of adults with right-hemisphere brain damage and several nonstandardized procedures have been reported in the literature.

Standardized Tests

The *Right Hemisphere Language Battery* (RHLB; Bryan, 1989) is one of the standardized tests. It contains seven subtests.

- The *metaphor picture subtest* assesses comprehension of spoken metaphors such as *under the weather* or *keep it under your hat*.
- The *written metaphor subtest* assesses comprehension of similar metaphors in printed form.
- The *comprehension of inferred meaning* subtest assesses appreciation of implied

meanings expressed by short spoken narratives.
- The *appreciation of humor subtest* assesses the patient's ability to choose the correct humorous punch line for printed jokes.
- The *lexical semantic subtest* is a spoken-word-to-picture-matching subtest in which the patient chooses pictures named by the examiner from among foils representing semantic, phonologic, or visual similarities to the target picture.
- In the *production of emphatic stress subtest* the examiner reads the first clause of a two-clause sentence aloud, and the patient reads the second, which is designed to elicit certain patterns of emphatic stress. (For example: *Clinician:* "He sold the *large* car and . . ." *Patient:* ". . . bought a *small* one.")
- The *discourse analysis rating* permits the examiner to rate a patient's cumulative performance during the test, while in conversation with the examiner, and in a picture description task. Ratings are assigned in 11 categories (such as humor, variety, and turn-taking), using a four-point scale for each rating.

The RHLB manual provides a general description of hemispheric specialization for language, the major behavioral consequences of right-hemisphere brain damage, and a summary of some literature on language processing by the right hemisphere. The manual also provides administration and scoring instructions for RHLB subtests, a summary of studies using the RHLB, a section on test interpretation and applications, and appendices containing a rating scale for discourse and a table for converting RHLB raw scores to T scores.

The RHLB is normed on 30 patients with vascular right-hemisphere damage, 10 patients with nonvascular right-hemisphere damage, 30 patients with vascular left-hemisphere damage, 10 patients with nonvascular left-hemisphere damage, and 30 neurologically normal adults. Means and standard deviations for right-

---

* This can be said for all aspects of communication and related skills for all categories of brain-damaged adults.

hemisphere–damaged, left-hemisphere–damaged, and normal groups on each subtest are provided. Significant and nonsignificant differences among the three groups on each subtest (measured by analysis of variance) are reported. Test-retest reliability (evaluated by *t*-tests and correlation coefficients) is reported for each subtest, and correlations among the subtests of the RHLB are provided. The RHLB provides a reasonably comprehensive look at the major communicative functions likely to be affected by right-hemisphere brain damage. However, as Tompkins (1995) has noted, the RHLB has several fairly serious deficiencies in reliability and validity, and an inadequate normative sample.

The *Mini Inventory of Right Brain Injury* (MIRBI; Pimental & Kingsbury, 1989) is a standardized test that, according to the authors, can be used to identify the presence of right-hemisphere brain injuries, determine the severity of right-hemisphere brain injury, identify the strengths and weaknesses of right-hemisphere-damaged adults, guide treatment, and document progress.

The MIRBI contains 27 test items divided among 10 categories: *visual scanning* (2 items), *integrity of gnosis* (finger identification, tactile perception, two-point tactile discrimination—3 items), *integrity of body image,* including neglect (1 item), *reading and writing* (5 items), *serial 7s* (subtracting 7 from 100, subtracting 7 from the remainder, and so on—1 item), *clock drawing* (1 item), *affective language* (repeating a sentence with happy and sad intonation—2 items), *appreciation of humor, incongruities, absurdities, figurative language* (8 items), *similarities* (8 items), *affect* (observation and rating by examiner—1 item), and *general behavior* (examiner's rating of impulsivity, distractibility, and eye contact—3 items).

The test manual contains sections on administration, scoring, and test interpretation, and a summary of the results of testing 30 adults with right-hemisphere brain damage, 13 patients with left-hemisphere brain damage, and 30 non–brain-damaged adults with the MIRBI. Correlations between MIRBI scores and age, education, and time post-onset are reported. Comparisons of overall MIRBI scores and scores on each item are reported for the three groups. Sections on the reliability and validity of the MIRBI are also included. Because it contains only 27 items spread across 10 categories, the MIRBI seems best-suited as a screening test to identify patients who may have communication impairments that may be further delineated by additional testing.

Nonstandardized Procedures

Gordon and associates, (1984) described an extensive nonstandardized protocol for evaluation of adults with right-hemisphere damage. The protocol provides for assessment of *visual scanning and visual inattention* (neglect and visuospatial abilities), *activities-of-daily-living skills* (arithmetic, reading, copying), *sensorimotor integration* (tactile perception, estimation of body midline, manual dexterity), *visual integration* (face recognition, visual assembly, figure-ground discrimination, and copying geometric forms), *higher cognitive and perceptual functions* (verbal and performance subtests from the *Wechsler Adult Intelligence Scale*), *linguistic and cognitive flexibility* (analogies, auditory comprehension, generative naming, and logical memory), and *affective state* (comprehension of affect, plus depression and mood ratings made by the examiner).

Gordon and associates tested 385 right-hemisphere–damaged patients with their protocol, but the number of patients tested differed across subtests. They provide numerous statistics for each subtest. For many subtests the data are subdivided according to patient variables such as age, education, or presence of visual field deficit. Although not standardized, the protocol describes materials and procedures for numerous tests of linguistic, cognitive, perceptual, and affective functions, and provides a large corpus of data about how adults with right-hemisphere damage perform on those tests. It should prove useful to clinicians who are looking for assessment materials or need information about how adults with right-hemisphere damage perform on tests like those in the protocol. The protocol includes numerous standardized tests as subtests, many of which have been revised since the Gordon and associates report, so the norms provided will not be usable with current versions of the standardized tests (Tompkins, 1995).

The Rehabilitation Institute of Chicago Evaluation of Communicative Problems in Right-Hemisphere Dysfunction (RICE) is a nonstandardized procedure for evaluating deficits associated with right-hemisphere brain injury (Burns, Halper & Mogil, 1985).* The procedure includes an interview with the patient; observation of the patient in interactions with family members and hospital staff; ratings of attention, eye contact, and awareness of illness; orientation to place, time, and person; ratings of facial expression, speech intonation, and topic maintenance in conversation; four tests of visual scanning and tracking; ratings of written expression; a scale for rating pragmatic communication skills; and a metaphoric language test.

Adamovich and Brooks (1981) described a procedure for evaluating the communicative deficits of adults with right-hemisphere brain injury. Their procedure includes tests of auditory comprehension, oral expression, and reading from the *Boston Diagnostic Aphasia Examination* (Goodglass & Kaplan, 1972); the *Revised Token Test* (McNeil & Prescott, 1978); the *Hooper Visual Organization Test* (Hooper, 1983); the *Boston Naming Test* (Kaplan, Goodglass & Weintraub, 1976); the *Word Fluency Task* (Borkowski, Benton & Spreen, 1967); and portions of the verbal absurdities, verbal opposites, and likenesses and differences subtests of

the *Detroit Tests of Learning Aptitude-2* (Hammill, 1965).

The Burns and associates procedures and the Adamovich & Brooks procedures are unstandardized, do not have adequate norms, and do not have documented reliability or validity. However, they may prove useful as a source of materials and ideas for locally constructed protocols for evaluation of patients with right-hemisphere brain injury.

Tests of Pragmatic Abilities

Right-hemisphere–damaged adults' pragmatic abilities typically are assessed with rating scales, not all of which were designed for use with right-hemisphere–damaged adults. The RHLB and the RICE each contain short scales for rating pragmatic behaviors. The RHLB provides a scale for rating discourse that addresses several categories of pragmatic behavior:

- *Supportive routines* (greetings, thanks, and the like).
- *Assertive routines* (complaining, demanding, criticizing, and the like).
- *Formality* (formality of language and behavior).
- *Turn-taking* (taking and yielding the conversational "floor").
- *Meshing* (pace, timing, and pauses).

The RICE scale provides for rating 12 pragmatic behaviors divided among four categories:

- *Nonverbal communication* (intonation, facial expression, eye contact, gestures and movements).
- *Conversational skills* (initiation, turn-taking, verbosity).
- *Use of linguistic context* (topic maintenance, presupposition).
- *Referencing skills* (organization and completeness of a narrative).

The RHLB's coverage of truly pragmatic behaviors is limited. The scale in the RICE has enough detail to make it useful as a screening measure or as a quick assessment of change in pragmatic behaviors in response to treatment.

---

* A revised version of the RICE (RICE-2) was published late in 1996.

The *Pragmatic Protocol* (Prutting & Kirchner, 1987) provides general descriptions of pragmatic behaviors in conversational interactions. Users of the pragmatic protocol score the occurrence of inappropriate pragmatic behaviors while the patient engages in 15 minutes of conversation with a familiar partner. Inappropriate pragmatic behaviors are assigned to one of 30 categories, representing *verbal aspects* (such as speech acts, topic maintenance, turn-taking, and communicative style), *paralinguistic aspects* (such as vocal intensity and quality, prosody, and fluency), and *nonverbal aspects* (such as physical proximity, posture, and eye contact).

The scoring procedures for the *Pragmatic Protocol* overemphasize violations, because any occurrence of inappropriate behavior in a category causes that category to be marked deficient, even though a subject may have had several occurrences of appropriate behavior in the same category. Consequently, subjects are penalized for a single occurrence of inappropriate behavior in a category, but get no credit for appropriate behaviors in the same category, even when the appropriate behaviors outnumber the inappropriate ones.

In its published form, the *Pragmatic Protocol* seems best-suited as a screening instrument to identify problem areas that can then be evaluated in greater detail by counting both appropriate behaviors and inappropriate behaviors in problem categories. Prutting and Kirchner apparently agree, because they suggest that a patient's performance on the *Pragmatic Protocol* should lead to detailed assessment of their pragmatic performance, focusing on the pragmatic behaviors identified as inappropriate by the *Pragmatic Protocol*. They also recommend that clinicians use the results of the detailed assessment to determine the probable impact of the inappropriate behaviors on daily life interactions.

The *Communicative Effectiveness Index* (CETI; Lomas and associates, 1989) is a rating scale designed to assess severely aphasic adults' functional communication, but may be useful for assessing some severely impaired right-hemisphere–damaged adults' functional communication. The CETI is described in Chapter 3.

Communicative Abilities in Daily Living (CADL; Holland, 1980) like the CETI, was designed to assess aphasic adults' functional communication, but could be used to assess the communicative effectiveness of adults with right-hemisphere damage. Because CADL samples communicative behavior in a number of contexts other than conversational interactions, using it together with a conversationally oriented instrument such as the *Pragmatic Protocol* may provide a more comprehensive picture of right-hemisphere–damaged adults' pragmatic strengths and weaknesses than use of either instrument by itself. CADL is described in Chapter 3.

Tests of Visual and Spatial Perception, Attention, and Organization

Patients with right-hemisphere brain damage often have difficulty in tasks requiring perception of complex visual stimuli and appreciation of spatial relationships. These difficulties appear to reflect attentional and integrational impairments, such as inattention to visual stimuli (especially on the side contralateral to the patient's brain injury), diminished ability to perceive or discriminate complex stimuli, and inability to integrate or synthesize individual elements of complex visual stimuli into a meaningful whole. Consequently, tests of visual attention and organization are an important part of the assessment protocol for patients who may have right-hemisphere damage.

Most tests for visual inattention *(neglect)* are paper-and-pencil tests. *Cancellation tests* are the most common. In cancellation tests the patient is asked to mark, circle, or cross out lines, letters, or figures (stars, crosses, and so on) printed at various locations on a printed page.

Patients with neglect tend to miss stimuli on the side of the page contralateral to their brain injury. Albert's (1973) *Test of Visual Neglect* is typical. The patient is given a sheet of paper on which short lines have been drawn in random locations and is asked to cross out each line. A variation on these simple cancellation tests is provided by the *Bells Test* (Gauthier, Dehaut, & Joanette (1989). In the *Bells Test,* the patient is required to circle drawings of bells that are scattered across the page and interspersed with drawings of other objects. Because patients must selectively circle only the drawings of bells, the *Bells Test* is more difficult for most patients than straight cancellation tasks, and it may be a more sensitive test of inattention than straight cancellation tasks (Gauthier and associates, 1989).

Figure 7-3 (left) shows a simple cancellation test in which a patient with left neglect was asked to cross out small squares, and Figure 7-3 (right) shows a more complex cancellation test in which a patient with left neglect was asked to cross out flowers and ignore stars.

Line bisection tests provide another way to test for visual neglect. The patient is given a page on which several horizontal lines of different lengths are printed, and draws a short vertical line on each one to divide it into two equal halves. Patients with neglect tend to divide the lines so that the segment in the neglected visual field is longer than the segment in the intact field (the bisecting line is displaced into the non-neglected half of the visual field (Figure 7-4). Displacement of the patient's dividing mark toward the non-neglected half-field tends to increase as lines move farther into the neglected visual field.

Copying and drawing tests are yet another way to test for visual neglect. In copying tests the patient is given a drawing to copy. (Often the drawing is of a symmetrical object with more-or-less mirror image properties on each side of the drawing's midline; for example, a clock face, a daisy, or a human figure.) Patients with neglect tend to omit detail from the side of the drawing contralateral to their brain injury (Figure 7-5).

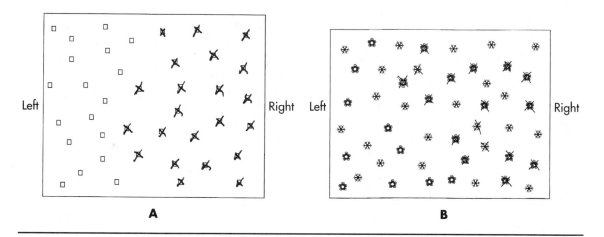

Figure 7-3 ■ (A) A simple cancellation test for neglect and **(B)** a more complex cancellation test completed by a patient with right-hemisphere brain damage. The patient was instructed to cross out all the boxes in **(A)** and to cross out only the flowers in **(B)**. The patient shows evidence of neglect on both tests. The patient also erroneously crossed out several snowflakes in **(B)**.

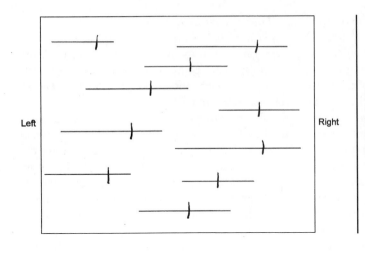

Left   Right

Figure 7-4 ■ A right-hemisphere-damaged patient's performance on a line-bisection test. The patient's line bisection marks are displaced to the right, toward non-neglected space.

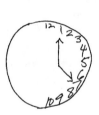

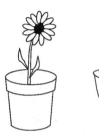

Figure 7-5 ■ A clock face drawn from memory and a flower copied by a patient with right-hemisphere damage and neglect.

In drawing tests the patient is asked to draw familiar objects or simple scenes from memory. Patients with neglect tend to leave out detail on the side of the drawing contralateral to their brain injury (Figure 7-6).

Scanning tests are still another way to test for visual neglect. In scanning tests the patient is given a page on which is printed a horizontal array of numbers, letters, or (less frequently) objects and asked to circle or cross out every occurrence of a target item (e.g., all occurrences of the letter *B* in a line of randomly-arranged alphabet letters). Scanning tests resemble cancellation tests, except that in scanning tests the stimuli are in horizontal linear arrays, rather than random arrays, and in scanning tests there are more distractors (stimuli not to be marked).

The *Behavioural Inattention Test* (BIT; Wil-son, Cockburn, & Halligan, 1987) is a standardized test battery for assessing neglect. It is unique among neglect tests in its inclusion of subtests to assess performance in daily life activities that might be affected by neglect (such as reading maps, dialing telephones, or reading menus and newspaper articles), in addition to traditional paper-and-pencil tests.

Horner and associates, (1989) suggested that it may take more than one test of neglect to identify its presence in many right-hemisphere–damaged adults' test performance. They administered tests of line bisection, drawing from memory, copying simple drawings, reading, and writing to 106 adults with right-hemisphere brain damage, and reported that no single test identified the presence of neglect in all who had neglect. Myers (1994) concurs, and recom-

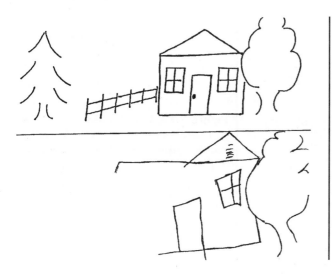

Figure 7-6 ■ A scene drawn by a patient with right-hemisphere damage and neglect. The stimulus drawing is on top and the patient's reproduction is on the bottom. The stimulus is shown to the patient, then removed, and the patient draws the scene from memory.

mends that combinations of neglect tests be administered to ensure that neglect, when present, is detected. She also suggests that a patient's combined score on several tests of neglect may give the best estimate of the overall severity of neglect.

Tests of Component Attentional Processes

Although attentional processes are implicitly tested in many of the tests described above, clinicians sometimes supplement them with tests that assess specific attentional processes in more detail.

Sustained attention can be assessed with cancellation and scanning tests (see above), or with trail-making tasks and mazes. Trail-making tasks and mazes are paper-and-pencil tasks that require sustained attention for successful performance. In trail-making tasks, the patient is given a sheet of paper on which sequences of letters, numerals, or a combination of letters and numerals are printed in a quasi-random array (Figure 7-7). The patient is asked to draw lines connecting the letters or numerals in sequence, according to a rule (such as *A-1-B-2*, and so on). In maze tasks, the patient is asked to draw a continuous line that traces a path

from the beginning to the end of the maze (Figure 7-8). Both tasks require the patient to maintain a mental representation of the appropriate path as he or she draws. Making the paths longer and more complex increases the difficulty of these tasks.

Some *visual sustained-attention tests* can be delivered via a personal computer. Visual stimuli (colored squares, dots, flashes of light, or similar stimuli) appear on the computer monitor screen at unpredictable times and at unpredictable locations. The patient presses a key on the computer keyboard to report the occurrence of each target stimulus. The computer keeps a record of hits, misses, reaction times, and the overall time taken to complete the test. Some *auditory sustained-attention tests* are presented via audiotape recordings and a few can be presented on a personal computer. Both require patients to maintain attention to strings of auditory stimuli and report the occurrence of designated targets (clicks, tones, and the like).

Selective attention customarily is assessed with tasks like those used to test sustained attention, with the addition of competing or distracting stimuli. For example, an auditory sustained attention test in which the patient signals

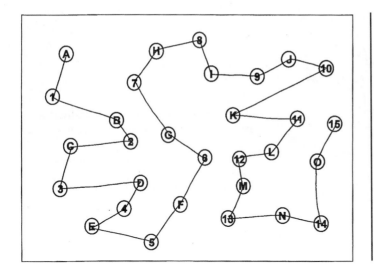

Figure 7-7 ▪ A trail-making test. The test-taker creates a path by alternately connecting letters and numerals.

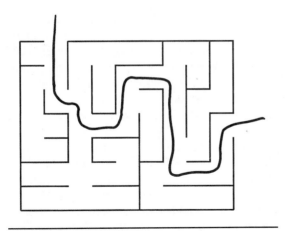

Figure 7-8 ▪ A simple maze.

when he or she hears a designated tone can be made into a selective attention test by presenting competing or distracting sounds along with the designated tones. A sustained attention test in which the patient is expected to report the occurrence of a single target stimulus (such as a chirp or a tone with a given frequency) becomes a selective attention test when the target sounds are embedded in strings of nontarget sounds and the patient is expected to report

only the target sounds. Some paper-and-pencil cancellation tests (described earlier in this chapter) also qualify as selective attention tests, if the patient must identify and mark stimuli meeting a certain criterion and pass over those that do not, or if distracting material is included with or overlaid upon the test stimuli. The *Stroop Test* is a widely used test that is thought to measure selective attention. In the *Stroop Test* the test-taker is shown a set of color names printed in ink colors that conflict with the color names (e.g., the word *red* printed in blue ink). The speed with which the test-taker reads the printed words is compared with the speed at which she or he names the colors in which the words are printed. Typically it takes longer to read words printed in conflicting colors than to identify ink colors. Large differences between the two are considered indicators of impaired selective attention.

The distinction between sustained attention and selective attention is in some respects an artificial one, because even in sustained attention tasks the patient must selectively attend to the visual or auditory stimuli and not on some other aspect of the task such as the label to the computer monitor, the background noise on the auditory stimulus tape, or the pattern on the clinician's neckwear.

Tests of *alternating attention* require the patient to change her or his focus of attention in response to changing task requirements. Most are sustained-attention tests in which response requirements are periodically changed. A patient may be placed in a cancellation task in which he or she is first instructed to cross out all the odd numbers in a random list of numbers. When the patient's performance has stabilized the examiner says *even,* and the patient is expected to begin crossing out only even numbers. The test continues with the examiner periodically changing the target response each time the patient's performance stabilizes. In another, more challenging, alternating attention test, the patient begins a serial calculation task by subtracting 5 from a specified number, subtracting 5 from the remainder, and so on. When the patient's performance stabilizes, the examiner says *add,* and the patient reverses direction and begins adding by 5s. The task continues with the examiner changing from addition to subtraction or vice-versa each time the patient's performance stabilizes.

Divided attention tests come in two formats. One format requires test-takers to monitor two tasks simultaneously and make differential responses to each task. For example, the test-taker may be required to perform a paper-and-pencil cancellation task in which she or he crosses out all occurrences of the letter *b* in randomly arranged letter strings while simultaneously listening to a list of randomly arranged spoken numbers and saying *yes* whenever the number *5* occurs. (This is sometimes called a *dual-task* format.)

Another format requires test-takers to retain several bits of information in immediate memory while performing mental operations on the information. The *digits backward* test is one of the easier tests in this format. In the digits backward test the examiner says a string of randomly arranged single-digit numbers and the patient re-

peats them in reversed order. Some other relatively easy tests in this format are counting, saying the alphabet, days of the week, or months of the year in reverse order, and counting forward by 2s, 3s, 4s, or 5s. More difficult tests include orally spelling words backwards, serial subtractions (beginning with a number provided by the examiner, the test-taker subtracts a specified number, then subtracts the specified number from the remainder, and so on, as in *100-93-86-79*), and saying letters and words alternatively in sequence (*A-1-B-2*). The *Paced Auditory Serial Addition Test* (PASAT; Gronwall, 1977) is a challenging divided-attention test in which strings of single-digit numbers are orally presented at a predetermined rate, and the test-taker is required to add each digit to the immediately preceding one and say the result. (For example, for the string *3-6-5-1-9*, the test-taker should respond with *9-11-6-10.*). Lezak (1995) has commented that the PASAT is a difficult and stressful task even for non–brain-damaged adults, who experience great pressure and a sense of failure even when they are doing well. Consequently, Lezak reserves the PASAT for detection and demonstration of very subtle attentional impairments.

Tests of Visual Organization

Tests of visual organization usually require the patient to identify *incomplete visual stimuli, fragmented visual stimuli* or to discriminate pictured objects from their background *(figure-ground discrimination). Incomplete figure tests,* as the name implies, contain drawings of familiar objects with missing elements. The patient is asked to say or write the name of each test item. Figure 7-9 shows an example of an incomplete figures test item.

In tests of *fragmented visual stimuli* the patient is shown drawings of common objects which have been divided into parts and the parts rearranged to disguise their identity. Tests with fragmented stimuli usually are more sensitive to visual organization impairments than tests with incomplete stimuli (Lezak, 1995). The *Object Assembly* subtest of the *Wechsler Adult Intelligence Scale* (WAIS; Wechsler, 1955, 1981) requires identification of fragmented visual stimuli, as does the *Hooper Visual Organization Test* (Hooper, 1958). In the WAIS *Object Assembly* subtest, the patient is given cut-up pressboard figures of familiar objects (a human figure, a human head in profile, a hand, or an elephant) and is asked to assemble them (Figure 7-10). In the Hooper test, the patient is presented with a series of pictures depicting cut-up line drawings of common objects and is asked to say or write the name of the object portrayed in each picture.

Visual figure-ground tests contain stimuli in which test figures are embedded in more complex figures, as in the *Hidden Figures Test* (Thurstone, 1944), stimuli in which test figures overlap (Poppelreuter, 1917), or stimuli in which lines are drawn over test figures or test figures are partially occluded by masks (Luria, 1965). Figures 7-11, 7-12, and 7-13 give examples of items like those in visual figure-ground tests.

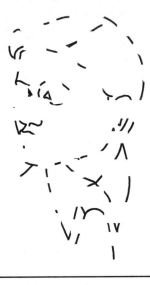

Figure 7-9 ▪ An example of an incomplete-figures test item.

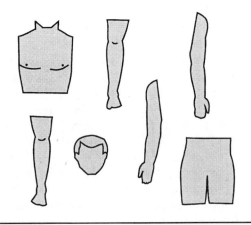

Figure 7-10 ▪ An example an object assembly test item. The components of the figure are made of heavy paperboard or fiberboard. The test-taker assembles them as he or she would assemble a jigsaw puzzle.

▪ TREATMENT OF PATIENTS WITH RIGHT HEMISPHERE BRAIN DAMAGE

We know less about treatment of right-hemisphere–damaged patients than we do about treatment of left-hemisphere–damaged (aphasic) patients, in part because the communication impairments of right-hemisphere-damaged patients were largely unrecognized and untreated until about 15 years ago, and in part because focal right-hemisphere damage seems to produce more diffuse effects on behavior than focal left-hemisphere damage does.

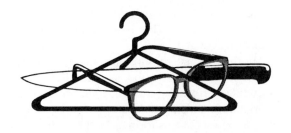

Figure 7-11 ▪ An example of an overlapping-figures test item.

Consequently, identifiable (and treatable) right-hemisphere syndromes are not as well-described as left-hemisphere aphasic syndromes.

Within the last few years a treatment literature on right-hemisphere–damaged patients has begun to develop, although most of it is anecdote and opinion, without much empiric support. Nevertheless, we now know that many right-hemisphere–damaged patients exhibit communicative impairments that can be objectively described, and that treatment can help at least some of these patients overcome or compensate for their impairments. However, there are several major differences between right-hemisphere–damaged patients and left-hemisphere–damaged (aphasic) patients that affect both the nature of treatment and its probable outcome. These differences are largely attributable to the fact that lesions in the left hemisphere tend to produce focal effects on specific linguistic and communicative abilities, whereas lesions in the right hemisphere tend to produce diffuse effects that are not readily reducible to specific communicative abilities.

Communicative impairments of patients with left-hemisphere damage are relatively discrete and can be classified and quantified with reasonable reliability. Their communicative failures are usually relatively obvious and characterized by countable errors (e.g., misnaming pictures, missing the last two parts of a three-part command). The relationships between left-hemisphere-damaged patients' performance on diagnostic tests and their underlying communicative impairments tend to be straightforward—for example, the relationship between errors on tests of confrontation naming and impaired word retrieval. The communicative impairments of patients with right-hemisphere damage are less discrete and tend to be less amenable to simple counts of errors because they represent more diffuse failures, such as treating serious situations as humorous or failing to follow conversational rules. The relationships between right-hemisphere-damaged patients' performance on diagnostic tests and their underlying communicative impairments usually are less straightforward and require more assumptions—for example, the relationship between errors on tests requiring correct interpretations of idioms and metaphors and inability to make inferences.

Treatment of right-hemisphere-damaged adults' communication impairments may target a variety of deficits that affect receptive and expressive aspects of communication—difficulty organizing and synthesizing information; difficulty separating what is important from what is not; inability to use contextual cues to ascertain

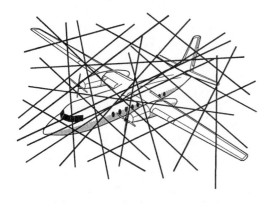

Figure 7-12 ■ **An example of a figure-ground test item in which lines have been drawn over a drawing of an object which the test-taker is asked to identify.**

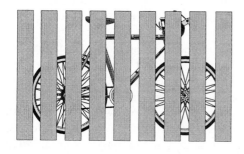

Figure 7-13 ■ **An example of a figure-ground test item in which the test stimulus is partially occluded by a mask.**

meanings; interpreting figurative language literally; overpersonalization; reduced sensitivity to pragmatic or extralinguistic aspects of communication; and tangentiality and excessive detail in speech. Right-hemisphere–damaged adults' communicative impairments can be exacerbated by cognitive and behavioral abnormalities, including denial of illness, indifference and denial of impairments, distractibility, problems maintaining attention, impulsivity, and impaired reasoning and problem-solving.

Cognitive and Behavioral Abnormalities

Denial and Indifference Right-hemisphere–damaged patients' indifference to or denial of errors can be a major impediment to treatment of their communicative impairments. Denial and indifference usually are greatest in the first days and weeks post-onset, and usually diminish with neurologic recovery. However, some patients remain indifferent to or deny impairments for months and years. Not much has been written about treating denial and indifference, perhaps in part because treatment often is not completely successful in reducing them to a point at which they are no longer a significant problem for the patient, family members, and friends.

Most right-hemisphere–damaged patients are compliant and willingly participate in treatment programs, although their participation is more likely to be passive than active. If asked to participate in making decisions about the content and focus of treatment, they may talk a good game, but fail in its execution. They tend not to do more than is specifically required, and may resist, either overtly or covertly, even doing what is specifically required. They often fail to carry out assignments unless they are closely supervised. Homework assignments are likely to be neglected unless someone in the patient's living environment provides supervision and direction. When confronted about their failure to carry out assignments, they may confabulate or offer implausible reasons for their failure.

According to Tompkins (1995) patients who remain uncritical of their poor performance and unconcerned about their impairments are poor treatment candidates, and she recommends that treatment be deferred until denial and indifference resolve. While the clinician waits for resolution, Tompkins suggests that he or she establish baselines, identify impairments, and select potential treatment approaches. For patients who are neurologically recovered, but still exhibit indifference and denial, Tompkins recommends simplifying treatment goals, modifying the patient's living environment to limit the negative effects of indifference and denial, and teaching compensatory strategies to family members and associates. Clinicians can also compensate for the effects of indifference and denial by making treatment activities highly structured, defining a clear set of treatment goals, and communicating the treatment goals to the patient and family. Indifference and denial can sometimes be treated indirectly, in the context of activities directed toward other goals, by giving the patient immediate feedback after erroneous or inappropriate responses, by confronting the patient when he or she denies errors, and by improving the patient's self-monitoring, first in highly structured activities and later in less structured ones.

Indifference and denial also can be worked on more directly by having the patient (or the patient and family) collaborate with the clinician in making a list of the patient's strengths and weaknesses. Entries in the list can then be singled out for attention in treatment activities. Sometimes videotaping treatment activities and reviewing them with the patient can improve patients' awareness of errors or inappropriate responses. For patients with extreme denial, one might begin by reviewing, with the patient, videotapes of interactions involving others, or staged interactions in which one participant makes errors or inappropriate responses that resemble those made by the patient. (Many right-hemisphere–damaged patients who deny their own errors are quick to spot errors when others make them.) When the patient becomes adept at identifying errors and inappropriate responses in the behavior of others, videotapes in which the patient is a participant can gradually be introduced. It is vital that family members and other caregivers be involved in the treatment program to ensure that the patient and family understand the relationship between treatment activities and treatment goals, to ensure that homework assignments are completed, and to facilitate transfer of treatment gains from the clinic to the patient's daily life.

Finally, a few words of caution. Many right-hemisphere–damaged patients can, with help, make lists describing their own pattern of errors and inappropriate responses, talk constructively about the lists, and even identify their own errors and inappropriate responses in structured treatment activities, but fail to anticipate them or do much about them either in treatment activities or daily life. The transition from identifying and talking about these behaviors to doing something about them can be an arduous one, requiring carefully programmed generalization procedures and the active participation of the patient's family members and daily life associates.

Attentional Impairments, Distractibility
Treatment of attentional impairments takes many forms, ranging from paper-and-pencil or computer-presented attention drills to activities that require the patient to focus and maintain attention in natural contexts. A sampling of these activities follows.

Sustained Attention Drills to improve sustained attention range from paper-and-pencil tasks such as letter cancellation and solving mazes, to vigilance drills that require the patient to monitor a visual display or strings of auditory stimuli and press a key when a target stimulus occurs. The easiest visual and auditory sustained attention tasks are those in which a single target stimulus appears against a constant background. Increasing the time between stimuli,

making the intervals between stimuli less predictable, and increasing the overall duration of the task all make sustained attention tasks more difficult. Patients with attentional impairments often do well as sustained attention tasks begin, but have increasing difficulty as the task progresses and the load on sustained-attention increases. The *starry night* task (Rizzo & Robin, 1990) is a computerized visual sustained-attention task that permits manipulation of task difficulty across a wide range. A pattern of dots (which resembles a starry night sky) is displayed on the monitor screen, and dots appear and disappear at unpredictable times and locations. The patient presses a key when he or she sees a dot appear or disappear. The computer keeps a record of the patient's "hits," "misses," and reaction times. The density of the dots, the rate at which they appear or disappear, and the duration of the task can be adjusted to manipulate task difficulty.

Paper-and-pencil sustained-attention tasks usually are less challenging than computer-based tasks, because paper-and-pencil tasks do not require a constant level of sustained attention across the task. Patients can slow down or stop when their attention flags and resume when their level of attention increases, thereby minimizing errors, although the time it takes them to finish the task increases (Tompkins, 1995).

Selective Attention Treatment of selective attention usually involves drills in which the patient performs sustained attention tasks in the presence of competing or distracting stimuli. A common way to treat impairments in selective attention is to place the patient in a sustained attention task and play a tape containing distracting sounds (such as conversations, radio programs, or popular music) in the background. Choosing distractions that the patient is likely to encounter in daily life helps to prepare the patient for resisting distraction, in daily life and helps to ensure that improvements in selective attention obtained in treatment activities carry over to the patient's daily life.

Alternating Attention Almost any sustained-attention task can be modified to create an alternating attention task by periodically changing stimulus characteristics or response requirements during the task. For example, a patient might practice shifting attention from one conversational partner to another in conversational interactions. Alternating-attention tasks also can be created by combining two different tasks and alternately switching between them. For example, a patient might practice alternating between doing a paper-and-pencil sustained-attention task and participating in a conversational interaction.

Divided Attention Treatment to improve right-hemisphere–damaged patients' ability to attend to two or more aspects of a task may involve drills in tasks that are similar to those used to test divided attention, described above. Tompkins (1995) commented that one objective of divided-attention treatment for patients with right-hemisphere damage might be to give them training in volitional allocation of mental resources. According to Tompkins this is necessary because some patients can no longer perceive which aspects of a task are most important and should receive the most attention. Tompkins recommends training these patients to systematically analyze tasks and situations to decide which aspects are most important, followed by practice in volitional allocation of attention.

Attention tasks no doubt fall along a continuum. At one end are simple cancellation or vigilance tasks, which demand considerable attentional stamina but do not put much strain on the patient's ability to ignore distracting or competing stimuli. At the other end are the most challenging sustained attention tasks, which demand both attentional stamina and the ability to ignore distracting or competing stimuli.

There is no strong empirical evidence showing that right-hemisphere–damaged adults' improved performance on attention drills generalizes to natural contexts, although anecdotal reports suggest that such generalization occurs, at least for some patients. Clinicians sometimes attempt to ensure generalization to daily life contexts by working on attention in contexts that resemble those the patient will encounter in daily life. Patients may be placed in conversational interactions in which they must maintain eye contact, stay on topic, respond appropriately to changes in topic, and get and retain a reasonable amount of specific information. For patients who can handle such interactions in quiet and nondistracting environments, noise, movement, or interruptions may be gradually introduced to increase the patient's resistance to distracting conditions. (See Chapter 8 for more on treating attentional impairments.)

Impulsivity Impulsivity can have major effects on many right-hemisphere–damaged patients' performance in treatment and in daily life. In treatment they may respond before the clinician has finished delivering task instructions or stimuli, interrupt treatment activities with tangential and irrelevant comments, begin tasks before they understand what is expected, and terminate tasks before finishing them. In daily life they may respond to their first impressions of messages, events, or situations, creating mistakes, misinterpretations, and social blunders. Clinicians can sometimes manage right-hemisphere–damaged patients' impulsiveness by incorporating distinctive stimuli as *stop* and *go* signals for patient responses. For example, patients might be taught to monitor a clinician-controlled signal light as an indicator of when they are permitted to respond. If the light is off, the patient cannot respond, but must wait until it comes on. As the patient's impulsive responses diminish under the control of the light, the light may gradually be replaced by verbal or gestural cues from the clinician (*wait* or *a 'stop' hand gesture*). The clinician's cues may then gradually be reduced and control transferred to patient self-cueing.

Impaired Reasoning and Problem-Solving Right-hemisphere–damaged patients' impaired reasoning and problem-solving can have important effects on the conduct of treatment as well as on its outcome. Right-hemisphere–damaged patients tend to get lost in the details of treatment activities and lose track of general goals and objectives. They are not very good at anticipating when a treatment task is likely to give them trouble, and when they do get into trouble, their responses are likely to be impulsive, inappropriate, and unreasoned. Their impaired reasoning and problem-solving makes them of little help to the clinician in deciding treatment objectives and the way in which the objectives are to be reached. Treatment of right-hemisphere–damaged patients' reasoning and problem-solving impairments requires structured practice in a variety of tasks that require reasoning, foresight, and problem-solving; for example role-playing situations in which problem-solving skills are needed (such as getting a refund for defective merchandise); proposing solutions to problems posed by the clinician; and planning activities such as vacations, field trips, and picnics. A formal, prescriptive, and highly structured approach to problem-solving should help most right-hemisphere–damaged patients get started:

- Identify the problem.
- Think of several possible solutions.
- Evaluate the feasibility and potential consequences of each solution.
- Choose the best solution.
- Apply it.
- Evaluate the results.

With extensive practice, some right-hemisphere–damaged patients can move away from a highly structured and prescriptive problem-solving strategy toward a less formal and less laborious one. Few, however, progress to the point at which problem-solving becomes automatic and instinctive.

Communicative Impairments

Reading Impairments Right-hemisphere–damaged patients' visual neglect is a common target of treatment because neglect has impor-

tant effects on their ability to read and comprehend printed materials. Numerous procedures for treating neglect have been described in the literature, but little is known of their effectiveness or generalizability.

Diller and Weinberg (1977) described a comprehensive treatment program for treating visual neglect. The program teaches patients to scan both sides of visual space, with emphasis on left-side space. Patients in Diller and Weinberg's program receive systematic practice in visual tasks such as visual tracking of a moving target across visual fields, detection of flashing lights in various locations in both visual fields, letter cancellation, or reading printed paragraphs projected on a wall so that they encompass both visual fields. The primary objectives of Diller and Weinberg's program are to make patients aware of their neglect, to force patients to view visual stimuli systematically, and to make newly acquired skills automatic by means of massed repetition.

Several techniques for getting patients with left neglect to attend to the left side of printed texts have been reported in the literature. Typically, salient markers (such as colored vertical lines, colored dots, or rulers) are placed at the left margin of printed material. The patient is instructed to scan leftward until she or he sees the marker whenever beginning a new line of text. Sometimes the patient is instructed to keep one finger on the marker and to scan back to it when beginning each new line. The patient's dependence on the markers is gradually reduced by making the markers less salient and by eventually replacing them with the patient's internal monitoring of whether or not the material makes sense.

Stanton, and associates (1981) described a comprehensive approach to treating neglect in reading. Their treatment program includes several tasks designed to enhance patients' awareness of, and attention to, the neglected side. In one task, patients match printed letters, numbers, and words from a column in the right visual field with numbers, letters, and words printed in a column in the left visual field. In another task they read aloud printed sentences, beginning with large-print sentences and large blank spaces separated by and progressing to single-spaced small-print sentences. In another task they read printed paragraphs aloud, progressing from paragraphs printed in large letters and with double spacing between lines to standard books, magazines, and newspapers, some in double-column format. Stanton and associates use verbal cues to remind patients to attend to the left side of the materials. They begin with the clinician instructing the patient to, *"Tell yourself out loud, Look to the left."* at the end of each line, and progress to self-initiated verbal cues by the patient, who vocalizes (or subvocalizes) *Look to the left* at the end of each line. As the patient progresses, overt verbal cues are gradually eliminated and replaced by covert ones. Stanton and associates recommend that clinicians take advantage of right-hemisphere–damaged patients' good verbal skills by having them ask themselves *"Does that make sense?"* at the end of each sentence or periodically while they read.

Myers (1994) suggests that the most effective techniques for treating neglect are those in which patients internalize the need to look to the left, rather than depending on external cues or self-cueing. One such procedure was described by Myers and Mackisack (1990). The procedure is built around two techniques, called *edgeness* and *bookness.* The edgeness technique requires the use of a work space with a raised border (a rectangular board or grid). First the patient familiarizes himself or herself with the spatial boundaries for a task by tracing the perimeter of the work space with one finger. Then the clinician places colored cubes at various locations on the work space. The patient is told how many cubes are on the work space, and that he or she is to find and remove all of them. The clinician does not tell the patient where to look, but simply encourages him

or her to continue looking until he or she finds all the cubes. The difficulty of the task is determined by the number of cubes (more cubes = greater difficulty), their placement (more cubes in neglected space = greater difficulty), and the presence of foils (cubes may be in two colors, only one of which the patient is to find and remove). To extend improved scanning from this task to other tasks, Myers and Mackisack suggest that patients be encouraged to extend the edgeness technique to other tasks by tracing the boundaries of other appropriate surfaces (such as writing tablets and books).

The bookness technique resembles the edgeness technique and is specific to reading. Patients first orally describe a closed book placed in front of them at their visual midline, then trace its perimeter with a finger. Then they open the book and trace its perimeter, again describing what they see. Reading tasks printed in the book are then administered, beginning with matching tasks that require the patient to match stimuli on the left and right sides of the book. Patients trace the perimeter of the book before each trial. The reading tasks then increase in difficulty by manipulation of number of stimuli, presence of foils, and so on. As the patient's attention to the left side of the book improves, the requirement that she or he trace the perimeter of the book is gradually eliminated. Myers (1994) sees two advantages to the edgeness and bookness techniques. First, they teach the patient to search to the left without the need for external cues, which increases the likelihood of generalization to other tasks. Second, they help to maximize the patient's overall level of attention, which may then transfer to other treatment tasks.

Treating right-hemisphere-damaged adults' attentional impairments is thought by many investigators and clinicians to have positive effects on their neglect. Myers (1994) suggests that treatment for neglect might include tasks to increase right-hemisphere–damaged patients' overall level of arousal, their capacity to sustain attention, and their capacity to selectively attend to certain stimuli while ignoring others. Because many models of neglect attribute a prominent role to attentional abnormalities, indirect treatment of neglect by direct treatment of attention seems intuitively reasonable, although verification of the relationship between attentional skills and neglect awaits empiric results.

Pragmatic Impairments Treating right-hemisphere–damaged patients' pragmatic impairments can capitalize on their preserved verbal skills. This approach alternates clinician coaching and clinician-patient strategizing with structured practice. The approach emphasizes the use of videotapes to provide feedback to patients regarding their pragmatic behaviors in conversational interactions. The videotapes also serve as a record of patients' progress (or lack thereof) in improving their pragmatic appropriateness. The approach proceeds roughly as follows.

At the beginning of treatment, one or more 10- to 20-minute conversations between the patient and another person (the clinician or someone chosen by the clinician and patient) are recorded on videotape. These videotapes provide baseline measures of the patient's conversational behaviors. After the baseline videotapes are made, the clinician leads the patient through a short general discussion of language pragmatics. When the patient has a good sense of what language pragmatics are and how pragmatic behaviors function to maintain and regulate communication, the clinician and patient jointly view several videotapes of conversations not involving the patient (e.g., television talk shows, excerpts from movies, or videotapes made specifically for this purpose) and evaluate the occurrence and appropriateness of pragmatic behaviors, with special attention to violations of pragmatic rules and conventions (interruptions, tangentiality, monopolizing the conversation, and so on). When the patient has demonstrated some facility at identifying violations of pragmatic and conversational rules in interactions involving others, the clinician and

patient jointly view the baseline videotape(s) and identify instances in which the patient engages in appropriate and inappropriate pragmatic behaviors. The clinician and patient use the results of their evaluation of the patient's performance to select pragmatic behaviors to be targeted in treatment. They formulate immediate and long-term goals and set up a plan for reaching the goals. The plan usually includes structured conversational interactions between the patient and clinician in which the patient practices the agreed-upon strategies for improving a targeted behavior, alternating with videotaped conversational interactions in which the patient employs the strategies either with the clinician or with others. These videotapes provide the patient with documentation of progress made and provide the clinician and patient with indications of pragmatic behaviors that should be attended to in the next phase of treatment. The process is repeated for successive pragmatic behaviors until all behaviors selected for treatment have been addressed.

Eye contact, turn-taking, and *topic maintenance* are frequent targets for treatment because they often are a problem for patients with right-hemisphere damage and because improving them can have striking effects on a right-hemisphere–damaged patient's conversational appropriateness. Increasing a patient's eye contact may require only that the clinician say *look at me* at appropriate times in treatment interactions. When the patient responds consistently to the clinician's cues, they can be gradually faded and eventually replaced by self-cueing by the patient. Giving the patient specific points at which to make eye contact may be helpful if the patient has difficulty making the transition from clinician cues to self-cues. Teaching the patient to make eye contact when he or she begins and ends each utterance, and then extending eye contact to the beginning and end of the conversational partner's utterances may provide a structured way for patients to maintain appropriate eye contact in conversations.

Teaching right-hemisphere–damaged patients to follow conversational turn-taking rules is approached systematically and in stepwise fashion. The clinician's explanation of turn-taking rules and how conversational participants know when to take or yield conversational turns leads into structured practice in which the patient can concentrate on turn-taking without having to concentrate on other aspects of communication such as message formulation or inferential reasoning. The structured practice may include (1) watching videotapes of conversational interactions (such as television talk shows) and discussing how the participants knew when to talk and when to let the other person talk; (2) preparing a script for a conversational interaction with appropriate conversational turns, videotaping it, then critiquing it; (3) videotaping a free conversation, viewing it, and identifying appropriate and inappropriate turn-taking behavior. When the patient begins to exhibit reasonably good appreciation of normal turn-taking, turn-taking can be incorporated into other treatment activities and into free conversation with the clinician.

Teaching right-hemisphere–damaged patients to maintain conversational topics usually requires some instruction and much structured practice. The instruction involves pointing out to the patient that conversations usually have a central theme or topic that lasts through several conversational turns, and convincing the patient that he or she often strays from the topic during conversations. Structured practice may involve activities such as (1) identifying topics in printed materials such as newspaper or magazine articles; (2) watching videotapes of conversational interactions and identifying topics, identifying when the topic changes, and discussing how the topic change was brought about by the participants; and (3) engaging in structured conversations with the clinician while maintaining a specified topic for a given length of time or a given number of conversational turns.

Some of what appear to be pragmatic impairments, such as appreciating a speaker's implied intent and responding appropriately to figurative language, may actually represent problems in making inferences. These impairments can be more effectively and efficiently treated, at least in the initial stages of treatment, by treating the underlying impairment in making inferences than by working on conversational interactions. In later stages of treatment, work on making inferences in conversational interactions may be appropriate.

Inference Failure and Communication Impairments Myers (1990) has asserted that most of right-hemisphere–damaged patients' communication impairments can be accounted for by a central impairment in making inferences. She called this impairment "inference failure." According to Myers, inference "requires an interaction between two types of recognition—the recognition of key elements and the recognition of their relationship to one another and to other contextual cues" (p. 4). Myers considers right-hemisphere–damaged patients' tendency to interpret metaphor, humor, idioms, and indirect requests literally, their pragmatic deficits in conversations, their impaired expression of emotion, their impulsivity and denial of illness, their facial recognition deficits, their verbose, tangential, and inefficient speech, and their failure to produce integrated stories and descriptions to be the result of a general failure to go beyond the superficial meaning of events or situations to their deeper (implied) meanings. If Myers is correct, treatment of right-hemisphere–damaged patients' communicative impairments would be most efficient and effective if it focused on teaching them to make inferences. As their ability to make inferences improves, the surface impairments that depend on making inferences should improve. Myers's hypothesis has yet to be tested, but it suggests a promising alternative to current treatment-by-symptom approaches to remediation of right-hemisphere–damaged patients' communicative impairments.*

The following short list of tasks contains examples of activities that would be appropriate for treatment that focuses on teaching patients to make inferences.

Appreciation of Humor The patient is given a printed joke, minus its punch line, and chooses the humorous punch line from a set containing a humorous punch line and nonhumorous foils. The patient is given a cartoon minus its caption, and then chooses the humorous caption from a set containing a humorous caption and nonhumorous foils.

Appreciation of the Implied Meanings of Metaphors and Idioms The patient hears (or reads) a common metaphor or idiomatic expression, then chooses the correct interpretation from a group containing the correct interpretation and foils that include a literal interpretation of the metaphor or idiom.

Identification of Verbal and Pictorial Absurdities The patient listens to a short spoken narrative in which there are absurd or inconsistent statements, identifies the absurd or inconsistent statements, and explains why they are absurd or inconsistent. The patient is shown pictures containing absurd or unlikely relationships (for example, a rabbit chasing a dog), identifies the absurd or unlikely relationships, and explains why they are absurd or unlikely.

Comprehension of Implied Information in Discourse The patient listens to spoken discourse, answers questions testing implied information, and tells the main point or moral for the discourse. The patient reads printed discourse and does the same things.

Retelling Stories The patient listens to a story, then retells it, paraphrasing and interpreting it, rather than repeating it verbatim.

Perceiving Relationships The patient categorizes items according to similarities and differences or class membership; for example, telling why a scissors and a saw are alike, listing things that one might find at a picnic, naming ferocious animals, and so forth. The patient analyzes familial relationships (e.g., *"How is your son's uncle related to you?"*). The patient generates lists of divergent functions (Chapey, 1994); for example, telling the clinician all the ways in which one could use a brick. (Divergent tasks may exacerbate some patients' tendency toward tangentiality. If carefully controlled, divergent tasks may provide ways of working on tangentiality. If not carefully controlled, they may reinforce it.)

The Potential Role of Attention in Right-Hemisphere-Damaged Adults' Communication Impairments Tompkins (1995) comments that attentional impairments may cause or exacerbate communication impairments following right-hemisphere brain damage. She notes that sustained attention is crucial for comprehension and production of discourse, and that selective attention is important for maintaining coherent interpretations of printed and spoken materials, establishing referential relationships, and making inferences. According to Tompkins, control of attention is important in keeping track of plots in movies and television shows, revising interpretations, and resisting distractions (and no doubt in other daily life communicative activities). She suggests that working on attentional capacity and control may provide a greater clinical payoff than working on their surface manifestations.

---

* As noted, earlier, Brownell and associates (1986) have reported that right-hemisphere-damaged adults make inferences, but make the wrong ones, based on their initial surface interpretations, and fail to revise their initial inferences based on subsequent information. The transcript of a right-hemisphere-damaged adults' picture description earlier in this chapter is striking not so much because the patient failed to make inferences, but because he made incorrect ones. These findings somewhat weaken Myers's arguments for inference failure as a general explanation for right-hemisphere-damaged adults' impairments.

Generalization

Generalization of improved performance from level to level within treatment tasks, from one treatment task to another, and from treatment tasks to the patient's daily life often poses substantial problems for right-hemisphere–damaged patients and their clinicians. As a group, right-hemisphere–damaged adults tend not to spontaneously generalize responses or strategies from one context to another. Their progress through successive levels of treatment tasks may be slowed by failure to apply skills and strategies learned at one level to the next level. Transitions between treatment tasks may be compromised by failure on the part of the patient to extend what is learned in one task to other related tasks. Finally (and perhaps most importantly), extension of gains made in the clinic to the patient's daily life may be compromised by the patient's failure to apply what is learned in the clinic to daily life interactions. Consequently, successful treatment of right-hemisphere–damaged adults requires that clinicians give careful attention to procedures for enhancing generalization, both within treatment activities and from treatment activities to daily life.

Generalization Across Treatment Tasks

The generalization procedures described in Chapter 5 provide some methods by which clinicians can build generalization into their treatment of right-hemisphere–damaged patients. These procedures may be modified or elaborated on as needed to account for the behavioral and cognitive impairments exhibited by right-hemisphere–damaged patients (impaired attention, impaired inferencing, impulsiveness, indifference, and so on). Because of these impairments, generalization procedures for right-hemisphere–damaged patients tend to be more prescriptive and more carefully structured than generalization procedures for patients with left-hemisphere damage.

One way of dealing with right-hemisphere–damaged patients' stimulus boundedness and impaired inferencing abilities is to make the steps between treatment levels small. Making the steps small helps right-hemisphere–damaged patients by diminishing the need for making inferences and by minimizing changes in stimulus processing and response sets between levels. Yorkston's (1981) description of a program to teach a right-hemisphere–damaged patient to transfer from his wheelchair to his bed dramatically underscores the need for small-step transitions for some patients with right-hemisphere brain damage. Yorkston began with a seven-step procedure, which proved completely beyond the patient's capacity. She then expanded it to 17 steps, then 27 steps, and eventually added the self-cue *"Have you finished this step?"* at the end of each step before the patient eventually learned to transfer. Yorkston cautioned that clinicians should never assume that a right-hemisphere–damaged patient will make logical transitions from one step to another, and commented that, "Rarely, if ever, does one err in the direction of breaking a task into too many steps" (p. 283).

Generalization from task to task within treatment activities can be enhanced by making the source task (the one in which the patient has learned a set of responses or a strategy) resemble the target task (the one to which generalization is intended). Similarity between tasks can be manipulated by adjusting the task stimuli, the responses required in the task, or the context in which the task is presented (e.g., paper-and-pencil versus computer presentation). Requiring new responses to new stimuli in a new context maximizes between-task differences and works against generalization, whereas maintaining consistency of stimuli, responses, and context minimizes between-task differences and increases the probability that learning will generalize. (For related information, see *programming common stimuli,* Chapter 5.)

Loose training (see Chapter 5) is another way in which clinicians can enhance right-hemisphere–damaged patients' generalization across tasks. By allowing stimulus conditions, response requirements, and reinforcement contingencies to vary within a controlled range, the clinician prevents the patient's performance from becoming too tightly bound to a restricted set of conditions, and thereby increases the probability that learned responses and strategies will transfer across treatment tasks. (Many clinicians routinely begin treatment in a task under tightly controlled conditions, and when the new learning has stabilized, gradually loosen the training conditions.)

Generalization From the Clinic to Outside Environments

Right-hemisphere–damaged patients' tendency not to generalize from task to task or from level to level within tasks in the clinic is mirrored in their tendency not to generalize what they acquire in the clinic to outside environments. However, clinicians are not powerless. Tompkins (1995) identifies several ways in which clinicians can ensure or enhance generalization across settings.

Provide enough training trials to consolidate and stabilize responses so that patients can produce them in novel or stressful contexts.

Poorly consolidated and incompletely learned responses or strategies tend not to spontaneously generalize from the context in which they are acquired to other contexts, although some disciplined and motivated patients may, with careful coaching by the clinician, volitionally make such generalizations. However, few patients with right-hemisphere damage have the discipline and motivation to volitionally generalize from one context to another, because of indifference and difficulty sustaining effort and focus. It usually is necessary to bring these patients' responses to an overlearned, automatic level to ensure that they generalize what they learn in the clinic to the outside.

Train a variety of related responses (for example, eye contact, turn-taking and relevance in conversations), rather than single responses.

This resembles loose training. The idea behind this principle is that training several related responses both provides the patient with alternatives when the primary response is not available, and creates a network of associations that raises the overall probability of appropriate responses in the target contexts.

Train responses and strategies in a variety of tasks and present the tasks in a variety of contexts (for example, role-playing, simulated natural environments, and natural environments).

This principle incorporates elements of *programming common stimuli* and *sequential modification* (see Chapter 5). Training responses or strategies in a variety of tasks helps to stabilize and consolidate them and diminishes their dependence on the exact conditions under which they are acquired. Presenting treatment tasks in a variety of contexts increases the patient's tolerance for changes in context and thereby increases the probability that the treated responses or strategies will generalize from the treatment setting to other settings. By incorporating stimuli from other settings (topics, situations, people) into treatment tasks, the clinician can enhance generalization from the treatment setting to the other settings.

Incorporate aspects of the target environment into treatment activities (topics, stimuli, contingencies, people, situations).

This principle is related to the preceding one, and speaks more directly to how clinicians go about ensuring generalization from clinic activities to the patient's daily life environment. Topics, situations, response contingencies, and sometimes people can be transplanted from the patient's daily life environment to the clinic, where they are incorporated into treatment activities. Their presence in treatment activities imbues them with power to elicit, maintain, and control the patient's strategies and behaviors in daily life enviroments.

Train self-instruction and verbal mediation.

Self-instruction and verbal mediation can be important adjuncts to other generalization procedures for patients with right-hemisphere brain damage. Clinicians can exploit these patients' well-preserved verbal skills by teaching them self-instructional or self-cueing strategies that are (overtly or covertly) verbally mediated. (For example, a patient with neglect might be taught to compensate while reading by covertly saying to him or herself, *"Find the left-hand side of the page,"* at the beginning of every line of text.)

Enlist the help of others (family members, friends, caregivers).

Family, friends, and caregivers can be a powerful force for generalization of learned responses and strategies from the clinic to the patient's home environment. In many respects these individuals can function as surrogate clinicians by manipulating stimuli, arranging situations and experiences, and administering response contingencies under the direction of the speech-language pathologist. Family, friends, and caregivers can also monitor the patient's daily-life performance and provide the clinician with information about how much generalization actually is taking place.

Generalization is one of the most challenging components of treatment for clinicians who work with right-hemisphere–damaged adults. Unless generalization is specifically targeted and systematically trained, what the right-hemisphere–damaged patient learns in the clinic is likely to stay there. Fortunately, procedures to enhance and ensure generalization are available, and their systematic application can help to ensure that improvements in right-hemisphere–damaged adults' communication transfer to their daily life.

■ KEY CONCEPTS

- Adults with right-hemisphere brain damage typically exhibit a variety of nonlinguistic impairments related to underlying impairments of perceptual and attentional processes. These nonlinguistic impairments include denial of illness, neglect, constructional impairment, topographic impairment, geographic disorientation, and visuoperceptual impairments.

- Adults with right-hemisphere brain damage also typically exhibit communication impairments, including diminished speech prosody, excessive, confabulatory, and tangential connected speech, failure to appreciate nonliteral or abstract material in conversations and narratives, and failure to observe pragmatic conventions such as turn-taking, topic maintenance, and eye contact.

- Treatment of right-hemisphere-damaged adults' communication impairments requires attention to several impairments that either directly or indirectly affect the individual's communicative effectiveness and efficiency—difficulty organizing and synthesizing information, difficulty separating what is important from what is not, inability to use context to ascertain meanings, interpreting figurative language literally, and overpersonalization.

- Generalization of improved performance from level to level within treatment tasks, from treatment task to treatment task, and from the clinic to the patient's daily life is a major concern of treatment for right-hemisphere-damaged adults, who tend not to spontaneously generalize responses or strategies from one context to another.

Traumatic Brain Injury

Traumatic brain injuries are a consequence of abrupt external forces acting on the head. These forces are generated when a moving object (such as a bullet, a club, or a baseball) strikes the head, or when the moving head strikes a stationary object (such as an automobile windshield, a tree, or a sidewalk). If the skull is fractured or perforated and the meninges torn or lacerated, the injury is called a *penetrating head injury* or *open-head injury*. If the skull and meninges remain intact, the injury is called a *nonpenetrating head injury* or, more frequently, a *closed-head injury*. Penetrating injuries often are caused by missile wounds or blows to the head by sharp objects. Closed-head injuries often are caused by motor vehicle accidents and falls.

■ INCIDENCE AND PREVALENCE OF TRAUMATIC INJURIES

About 7 million United States residents incur traumatic brain injuries each year (Rosenthal and associates, 1990). Most (about two-thirds) are caused by motor vehicle accidents, with falls and assaults accounting for most of the rest. Males are more likely than females to re-ceive traumatic brain injuries (Figure 8-1). Over-all there are about two male traumatic brain injuries for every female injury, but the differ-ence is larger for young adults. For young adults between 15 and 25 years old 3 to 5 males are traumatically brain injured for every female, and for 20-year-olds, the ratio is approximately 4:1 male/female (Annegers and associates, 1980).

Toddlers and older adults are less likely to incur traumatic brain injuries than 15- to 25-year-olds, but more likely to incur them than the general population (Finlayson & Garner, 1994). Falls account for most of the traumatic brain injuries in toddlers and the very old, whereas motor vehicle accidents account for most traumatic brain injuries in young adults (Finlayson & Garner, 1994; Van Houten and associates, 1994). Traumatic brain injury is the leading cause of neurologic disability in per-sons under the age of 50 (Finlayson & Garner, 1994).

■ RISK FACTORS

Several variables other than age and sex affect the probability of traumatic brain injury. One of

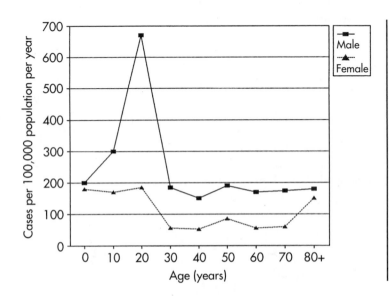

Figure 8-1 ■ The frequency of traumatic brain injuries in males and females according to age. (Modified from Annegers JF and asso-ciates: The incidence, causes, and secular trends of head trauma in Olm-sted County, Minnesota, *Neurology* 30: 912-919, 1980.)

the most conspicuous is *alcohol and drug use and abuse.* From 40% to 60% of patients admitted to hospitals with traumatic brain injuries are intoxicated at the time of admission (Rutherford, 1977; Brismar, Engstrom, & Rydberg, 1983). Motor vehicle accidents, falls, and assaults, in that order, cause most of the traumatic brain injuries sustained by intoxicated adults. Many assault-related injuries also are related to the use of alcohol and/or drugs by the aggressor, the victim, or both (Giles & Clark-Wilson, 1993). Hillbom and Holm (1986) estimate that the incidence of brain injury in alcoholic adults is two to four times greater than the incidence in the general population.

School adjustment and social history seems to be related to the probability of traumatic brain injury. Haas, Cope, and Hall (1987) reported that 50 percent of a large group of severely brain-injured patients had a history of poor academic performance (failure in two or more subjects, diagnosed learning disability, or school dropout). Giles and Clark-Wilson (1993) comment that poor academic performance may be related to underlying neurologic impairments that can in turn lead to distractibility, attentional impairments, lowered frustration tolerance, impulsivity, rebelliousness, egocentrism, sociopathic behavior, and substance abuse, all of which increase the probability of head injuries from motor vehicle accidents, assaults, and falls.

Socioeconomic status also affects the probability of traumatic brain injury. Individuals with low income, especially those who live in areas with high population density (central cities) have a higher probability of traumatic brain injury (primarily from assaults and falls) than individuals with higher income who live in areas of low population density (Macniven, 1994).

The influence of *personality type* on the probability that an individual will sustain a traumatic brain injury has received a fair amount of attention. The general conclusion is that *type A* personalities (characterized by competitiveness, impulsivity, belligerence, and hostility) are more likely to sustain traumatic brain injuries than *type B* personalities (characterized by cooperativeness, deliberateness, and helpfulness) (Evans, Palsane, & Carrere, 1987).

A *history of traumatic brain injury* is associated with increased probability of additional traumatic brain injury. The probability of a second traumatic brain injury is three times higher in individuals who have sustained a previous traumatic brain injury than the probability for the general population. The probability of a third traumatic brain injury for an individual who has had two traumatic brain injuries is eight times higher than the probability of traumatic brain injury for an individual with no previous brain injury (Annegers and associates, 1980).

Participation in sporting activity increases the risk of traumatic brain injury. Professional and amateur boxers have a particularly high rate of diffuse brain injury, which gradually increases in severity throughout the boxer's career, presumably because of repeated mild brain trauma. Motorcycling, bicycling, snowmobiling, and rock climbing are associated with increased risk of traumatic brain injury, although wearing appropriate safety helmets significantly diminishes the risk of head injury. Bicycle riders wearing helmets have an 88% reduction in risk of traumatic brain injury (Thompson, Rivara, & Thompson, 1989), and comparable reductions in injury are no doubt associated with use of helmets in other sporting activities.

Although each of the foregoing variables affects the probability of traumatic brain injury, it seems certain that many interactions among variables exist, making it difficult or impossible to isolate the effects of any single variable. For example, alcohol and drug abuse are likely to be related to socioeconomic status, school adjustment, educational achievement, and personality variables, and each of the latter variables is likely to interact with one or more of the others. (Most young head-injured adults are unmarried, unemployed individuals of low socioeconomic status—Barber & Webster, 1974.) Consequently, it is impossible to estimate the amount by which the presence of any single variable increases the probability of traumatic brain injury. However, it seems clear that the presence of several risk factors increases that probability more than the presence of only one or two.

■ PATHOPHYSIOLOGY OF TRAUMATIC BRAIN INJURY
Penetrating Brain Injuries

As noted above, most penetrating brain injuries are caused by high-velocity missiles (bullets or other projectiles). High-velocity penetrating injuries perforate or fracture the skull and penetrate the brain substance. The projectile creates a pressure wave that has an explosive impact on the skull and brain, destroying tissue on both sides of the projectile's track. Hair, skin, and bone fragments are carried into the brain by the projectile, where they become sites for potential bacterial infections. Low-velocity impacts (for example, blows to the head received in altercations or automobile accidents) may cause penetrating injuries if the force of the impact is concentrated in a small area. Low-velocity penetrating injuries fracture rather than perforate the skull. If the fracture is severe, bone fragments are carried into the brain, and there is substantial destruction of brain tissue at the impact site.

Mortality is high following penetrating injuries to the brain. Penetrating injuries to the brainstem usually are fatal, because of damage to structures that regulate respiratory, cardiac, and other vital functions. If the patient survives the first day after a penetrating brain injury, infection, bleeding, and increased intracranial pressure, either from swelling of the brain or from hydrocephalus, become important threats to the patient's survival. Adults who survive penetrating head injuries and their sequelae often make surprisingly good recoveries, although they are almost invariably left with physical,

cognitive, or linguistic deficits. These deficits usually are focal, rather than diffuse, and reflect loss of functions served by the regions of the brain destroyed by the injury.

Nonpenetrating Brain Injuries

In nonpenetrating brain injuries (closed-head injuries) the meninges remain intact and foreign substances do not enter the brain. Nonpenetrating injuries can be divided into two general categories—*acceleration injuries* and *nonacceleration injuries.*

Acceleration injuries (sometimes called *moving-head injuries*) are produced when the unrestrained head is struck by a moving object or the moving head strikes a stationary object.* Nonacceleration injuries (sometimes called *fixed-head injuries*) are produced when the restrained head is struck by a moving object (the patient is lying on a hard surface or sitting with his or her head against an unyielding surface when the head is struck).

Nonacceleration Injuries Nonacceleration injuries are much less likely to produce severe traumatic brain injury than acceleration injuries. Blows to a moveable head are estimated to be 20 times more devastating than blows to a fixed head (Pang, 1989). The primary consequences of nonacceleration injuries are related to deformation of the skull by the impact of the moving object. Because the skull is rigid, but slightly elastic, the blow deforms the skull at the point of impact and drives it against the brain surface. This causes localized damage to the meninges and brain cortex at the point of impact—damage called *impression trauma* (Figure 8-2). It is not clear whether impression trauma is caused by the impact of the depressed skull against the brain or by negative pressure that develops when the skull snaps back to its original shape.

---

* Acceleration injuries can also occur when the rapidly-moving head abruptly changes direction without striking a surface (shaken-baby syndrome).

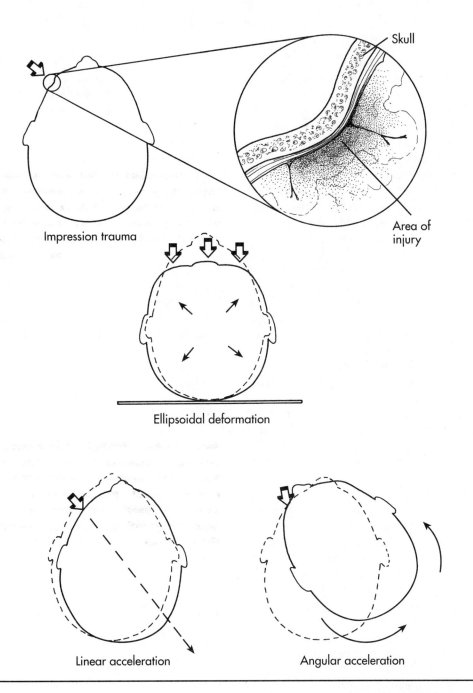

Figure 8-2 ■ Physical consequences of blows to the head. Impression trauma is caused by blunt force applied to a small area of the skull. The skull is depressed at the point of impact with consequent injury to meninges and brain tissue beneath the point of impact. Ellipsoidal deformation is caused by blunt force applied to a large area on the restrained head. The skull is forced from its usual ellipsoidal shape to a more nearly circular shape. Linear acceleration of the skull and its contents is caused by blunt force applied on a line through the central axis of the unrestrained head. Angular acceleration of the skull and its contents is caused by blunt force applied at an angle to the central axis of the unrestrained head, causing the head to rotate away from the point of impact.

If a nonacceleration injury is caused by a slow-moving object with a large surface area, *ellipsoidal deformation* of the skull may occur (Figure 8-2). When the skull is forced from its customary oval shape to a more circular one, its volume increases. This creates a pressure gradient that causes general expansion of brain tissue outward from the center, which in turn generates stretching and shearing forces that are concentrated around central structures (the ventricular walls, corpus callosum, and basal ganglia).

Some nonacceleration brain injuries are accompanied by skull fractures. Fractures at the base of the skull are more serious than ones higher up, because basal skull fractures may damage cranial nerves or the carotid arteries. Regardless of its site, any skull fracture is dangerous if the meninges beneath the fracture are torn, because of bleeding from damaged meningeal blood vessels and the potential for infection by bacteria penetrating the damaged meninges. At one time the severity of closed head injuries was measured by whether or not the skull was fractured. However, it is now clear that the presence (or absence) of skull fracture does not predict the severity of brain damage.

Acceleration Injuries When traumatic brain injury is caused by acceleration, the brain and brainstem sustain considerable indirect damage, most of it caused by their movement inside the skull. This movement is the result of inertial forces generated either when the head is rapidly moving through space and comes to a sudden stop (as when it strikes the floor after a fall) or when the head is at rest and is suddenly accelerated (as when it is struck by a blunt object). Acceleration injuries can in turn be subdivided into two categories—*linear acceleration injuries* and *angular acceleration injuries.*

Linear acceleration injuries happen when the head is suddenly accelerated by an outside force, which is applied on a linear path that passes through the center axis of the head (Figure 8-2).* Because resting bodies tend to stay at rest, the head and its contents resist acceleration, but within a few milliseconds the skull begins to move in line with the direction of the outside force. However, the brain has its own resting inertia, which keeps it at rest for a few milliseconds after the skull begins to move. As a result the brain is compressed against the inner surface of the skull at the point at which the accelerating force is applied. This compression may cause bruises and abrasions on the surface of the brain where it strikes the skull. Such injuries are sometimes called *coup injuries* (*coup* is a French word, pronounced *coo,* that means *blow* or *impact*). Within a few milliseconds the brain accelerates to the rate at which the skull is moving. Then the movement of the skull is abruptly stopped, either by the tethering action of the vertebrae and neck muscles, or by striking a surface or object. Because moving bodies tend to keep moving, the head and its contents resist deceleration, so it takes a few milliseconds for the skull to decelerate and a few milliseconds more for the brain to decelerate. The mismatch in deceleration rates causes the brain to be compressed against the inner surface of the skull at the point at which the decelerating force is applied.[†] This compression causes localized injury to the surface of the brain on the opposite side from the blow that first started the head moving. These injuries are called *contre-*

---

* The same physical processes operate when the head is moving in a linear path and is suddenly stopped. In this case the force opposes movement, rather than initiating it, but the consequences for the skull and brain are equivalent to those generated by sudden acceleration of the head. To keep things simple, I will limit my description to what happens when the head is accelerated, and trust the reader to keep in mind the equivalence of acceleration and deceleration processes.

† Technically the skull is pressed into the brain at the beginning of the movement, and the brain is pressed into the skull at the end. However, it is the brain that suffers the consequences in both cases. Consequently, visualizing the process from the brain's point of view seems appropriate.

coup (pronounced *contra-coo*) injuries. Coup and contrecoup injuries cause focal damage to the meninges, brain cortex, and immediately subcortical brain regions where the brain is compressed against the skull. Coup and contrecoup injuries are sometimes called *translational trauma* (Teasdale & Mendelow, 1984) and only occur with linear acceleration and deceleration of the head. Translational trauma is more likely following blows to the front or back of the head than to the side of the head. This is because the space between the brain and the skull (the epidural space) is greater at the front and back than at the sides. Consequently the potential for linear brain movement within the skull is greater when the head moves front-to-back than when it moves side-to-side.

Blows that strike the head off-center propel it at an angle from the direction of the blow and rotate it away from the blow (Figure 8-2). This causes what is called *angular acceleration* of the skull and its contents. Inertial forces are generated by angular acceleration, but the forces are rotational rather than linear. Within a few milliseconds of impact the skull begins to rotate and move at an angle away from the point of impact. The brain's inertia causes it to remain at rest for a few milliseconds after the skull begins to move, generating twisting and shearing forces which are concentrated in axial structures (the midbrain, basal ganglia, brainstem, and cerebellum). Then the brain begins to move away from the point of impact and to rotate in the same direction as the skull. Within a few milliseconds the tethering action of the vertebrae and neck muscles abruptly stop the movement of the head and cause it to rebound in the opposite direction, but the brain's inertia causes it to continue rotating in its original direction for a few milliseconds, causing a second episode of twisting and shearing forces concentrated in axial structures. Shearing forces tend to be greatest at the boundaries between gray matter (supportive tissue) and white matter

(fiber tracts). For this reason, bleeding and swelling tend to be more severe around major white fiber tracts, especially the internal capsule, the corpus callosum, and the brainstem. Angular acceleration of the head and rotation of cranial contents within the skull usually produces more severe brain injuries than linear acceleration of the head, wherein cranial contents are not subjected to twisting forces (Ommaya, Grubb & Naumann, 1971).

The twisting and shearing forces created within the brain by angular acceleration, and the stretching and tearing forces created by linear acceleration cause damage to nerve-cell axons diffusely scattered throughout the brain substance—a condition called *diffuse axonal injury.* Diffuse axonal injury is a common consequence of traumatic brain injury and is assumed to be responsible for many of the diffuse cognitive and behavioral impairments that follow. Some diffuse axonal injury probably occurs whenever consciousness is lost following head injury (Giles & Clark-Wilson, 1993), and widespread diffuse axonal injury is considered to be a common cause of *persistent vegetative state,* in which the patient has sleep-wake cycles, but makes no purposeful movements, does not talk, cannot follow instructions, and does not track visual stimuli. Persistent vegetative state is the result of severe diffuse damage to cortical and subcortical regions with relative preservation of the brainstem—damage that can also be caused by conditions other than diffuse axonal injury, such as cerebral anoxia or bacterial or viral infections.

Rapid acceleration and deceleration of the head also causes abrasions and lacerations of cortical tissues. These injuries are a consequence of movement of the brain within the cranial vault. As the brain moves inside the skull, it scrapes against bony ridges and projections on the floor of the cranial vault. Because the floor of the cranial vault is uneven and irregular and the walls and roof are relatively smooth

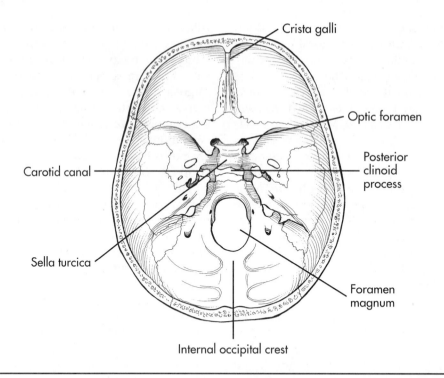

Crista galli

Optic foramen

Posterior
clinoid
process

Carotid canal

Sella turcica

Foramen
magnum

Internal occipital crest

Figure 8-3 ▪ The floor of the skull. The crista galli, the clinoid process, and the sella turcica are ridges in the skull floor. These and other prominences on the skull floor contribute to contusions and abrasions on the bottom surface of the brain in acceleration injuries.

and featureless (Figure 8-3), abrasions and lacerations tend to concentrate on the bottom surfaces of the frontal lobes and the anterior temporal lobes. Abrasions and lacerations in the parietal lobes, occipital lobes, and the convexities of the frontal lobes are uncommon, because the walls and roof of the cranial vault are smooth and featureless (Figure 8-4).

The foregoing consequences of traumatic brain injury are the result of the forces exerted on the brain at the time of injury. They are accounted for by the mechanical effects of compression, stretching, shearing, abrasion, and laceration of the brain and meninges. For this reason they are sometimes called *primary consequences.* The primary consequences usually generate several *secondary consequences,* which represent the brain's responses to trauma

or to the failure of other somatic functions (such as cardiac output or pulmonary function). These secondary consequences often are more devastating than the primary consequences. Although no statistics are available, it is probably true that more patients with traumatic brain injuries die from the secondary consequences of their injuries than from the physical damage to the brain sustained at the time of the accident. (Death rates from traumatic brain injuries are highest in the first three days, with 50% to 75% percent of deaths occurring within 72 hours.)

Secondary Consequences of Traumatic Brain Injury

Traumatic Hemorrhage Hemorrhages lead to accumulations of blood called *hematomas.* There are four major categories of traumatic

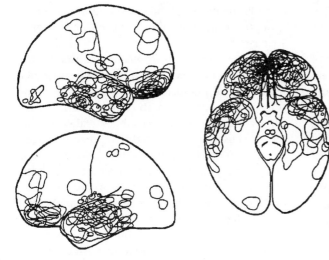

Figure 8-4 ▪ **The location of brain contusions in a series of 40 traumatically brain-injured adults. The most frequent location for contusions is the bottom surface of the frontal lobes, followed by the bottom surface of the anterior temporal lobes.** (From Courville CB: *Pathology of the central nervous system,* Mountain View, Calif, 1937, Pacific.)

hematomas, depending on where the blood accumulates—*epidural hematoma, subdural hematoma, subarachnoid hematoma,* and *intracerebral hematoma.*

Epidural hematomas, as the label suggests, are accumulations of blood between the dura mater and the skull. They are caused by lacerations of the middle meningeal artery, middle meningeal vein, or a dural venous sinus. Automobile accidents are their most common cause, but trivial events, such as falls and sports injuries also may cause them. Ninety percent of epidural hematomas are associated with skull fracture (Teasdale & Mendelow, 1984). About 20% to 30% of patients who have epidural hematomas die as a consequence of their head injuries. Mortality from epidural hematoma is strongly related to whether the bleeding is from an artery (death in about 85% of cases) or a vein (death in about 15% of cases). Arterial bleeding usually is marked by massive hemorrhage, with symptoms progressing rapidly, often culminating in death within a few hours. Venous bleeding usually follows a less dramatic course, with slow progression of symptoms. Small venous hemorrhages may ooze blood so slowly that they produce no overt symptoms, and the bleeding may be detected only with imaging scans of the head during routine evaluation of the patient.

The magnitude of the symptoms caused by epidural hemorrhages depends to some extent on the location of the hemorrhage. Bleeding into the posterior inferior epidural space can cause compression of the brainstem, with respiratory depression, decreased heart rate, and increased blood pressure. Bleeding into the frontal and superior epidural space is likely to be less serious, because centers for vital functions are far away, and because there is more epidural space to accommodate the hematoma before it begins to displace brain structures. The most common treatment for epidural hematomas is surgical removal, which usually is relatively easy to do because of the hematoma's accessibility, just beneath the skull.

Subdural hematomas, as the name suggests, are accumulations of blood between the dura and the arachnoid. Subdural hematomas are twice as common as epidural hematomas, and twice as deadly, with 60% (or greater) overall mortality. Motor vehicle accidents are their most common cause, and about half are associated with skull fractures. The source of most subdural hematomas is laceration of cortical blood vessels caused by abrasions and contusions on the brain surface. Acute subdural hematomas usually develop within a few hours, and almost always within a week of the injury. The combination of increasing pressure and displacement of brain tissue by the expanding hematoma, if not controlled, usually leads to coma and death within a few hours. Surgical removal of the hematoma is the most common treatment for acute subdural hematomas. In some cases surgical removal of swollen brain tissue caused by contusions also is necessary to control increased intracranial pressure, if medication to manage brain swelling is unsuccessful.

Chronic subdural hematomas are most common in older patients and in patients with long-term alcoholism, "who usually have some degree of brain atrophy with a resultant increase in the size of the subdural space" (Friedman, 1983, p. 10). In many, if not most, cases the injury that precipitates the hematoma is relatively trivial (usually a fall, with a bump on the head). The hemorrhage gradually fills the subdural space, and within a few weeks a membrane forms around it. Eventually the hematoma may reach a size at which it produces symptoms, which often wax and wane. Headache and tenderness in the affected area are the most common symptoms, although progressive dementia and decreasing levels of consciousness may develop. Surgical evacuation of the hematoma was for many years the treatment of choice, but mortality rates were distressingly high. In the last decade or so a more conservative procedure has been successful. In this procedure a catheter is inserted into the hematoma through a burr hole in the skull. The fluid is then continuously drained into a container below the level of the head.

Subarachnoid hematomas, caused by rupture of pial vessels within the subarachnoid space, are a less common consequence of traumatic brain injury than epidural or subdural hematomas, although they often are associated with subdural hemorrhages. Little is known about the long-range consequences of slowly ac-cumulating blood in the subarachnoid space, although it is known to contribute to cerebral vasospasm.*

Intracerebral hematomas are caused by rupture of blood vessels within the brain substance. Intracerebral hemorrhages are most commonly seen in combination with diffuse axonal injury. They are most frequent in subcortical white matter, the basal ganglia, and the brainstem, and are a common consequence of translational trauma. Occasionally a large intracerebral hematoma bleeds into the ventricular system, creating a secondary subarachnoid hematoma, usually with devastating effects on the patient. A pattern of multiple small intracerebral hemorrhages is sometimes seen in combination with diffuse axonal injury—a combination that often leads to coma and death of the patient (Adams, Graham, & Scott, 1980).

Cerebral Edema Accumulation of fluid is the brain's generic response to a wide variety of insults, such as trauma, anoxia, infection, and inflammation. The fluid may accumulate between the brain and skull, within the ventricles, or within brain tissues. Cerebral edema almost always surrounds the primary site of brain injury, but can occur throughout the brain, especially following diffuse injuries such as those caused by translational trauma. Cerebral edema is an important contributor to increased intracranial pressure. It usually becomes significant within 4 to 6 hours post-injury and peaks in 24 to 36 hours.

Traumatic Hydrocephalus Swelling of brain tissues (especially in midbrain regions) sometimes compresses the passages through which cerebrospinal fluid moves between the ventricles and from the ventricles to the subarachnoid space. As a result, the cerebrospinal fluid pressure within the ventricles increases,

---

* Rapid accumulation of blood following massive subarachnoid hemorrhage is associated with massive headache and rapid neurologic deterioration, often ending in death.

causing expansion of the ventricles, compression of brain structures, and elevation of intracranial pressure

Increased Intracranial Pressure Perhaps the most dramatic (and deadly) consequence of brain injury is increased pressure inside the cranial vault. The pressure is generated by accumulations of fluid (blood, cerebrospinal fluid, or water) within the skull. The resulting pressure build-up compresses and displaces brain tissues, with increasing neurologic impairment as the pressure increases. Increased intracranial pressure is the most frequent cause of death from traumatic brain injury, and one of the primary concerns in medical management of traumatically brain-injured patients is monitoring and controlling intracranial pressure.

Generalized pressure on brain tissue can, by itself, cause neurologic impairments, but only if the pressure becomes very high. The brain seems reasonably tolerant of modest increases in pressure, provided the pressure is distributed equally throughout the cranial vault. Unfortunately, traumatic injuries produce pressure gradients in which pressure is greatest at and around the site of injury and decreases with increasing distance from the injury. These pressure gradients displace brain tissues away from areas of high pressure into areas of low pressure. The tissues are compressed, distorted, stretched, forced against the skull, and forced against projections and partitions within the skull, usually with ominous consequences, for the brain is as intolerant of displacement and distortion as it is tolerant of moderate increments in generalized intracranial pressure. Damaged cell walls leak fluid into extracellular space. Damaged blood vessels leak into brain tissue or into adjacent spaces. The already swelled brain swells further, increasing the forces that displace and distort it. If uncontrolled, this sequence of events quickly leads to coma and brain death.

The most dangerous consequence of regional increases in intracranial pressure is *herniation,* in which cerebral structures are pushed around rigid partitions in the cranial vault, or extruded through cranial orifices. See Chapter 1 for a description of what happens in herniation.

Prolonged high levels of intracranial pressure inevitably cause irreversible brain damage, with coma and death the frequent outcome. Fortunately, intracranial pressure can be monitored and controlled. To monitor intracranial pressure a pressure transducer is inserted into the cerebrospinal fluid through a hole in the skull. If intracranial pressure becomes dangerously high, the patient may be hyperventilated. (Increased blood oxygen causes constriction of cerebral arteries, decreases cerebral blood volume, and provides at least temporary reductions in intracranial pressure.) Steroids (antiinflammatory medications) may be administered to reduce cerebral edema. Diuretics (medications that increase the body's excretion of fluids) may be administered. If these treatments are unsuccessful, the patient may be put into a barbiturate coma to decrease cerebral metabolism and constrict cerebral blood vessels.

Ischemic Brain Damage In addition to the impairments caused by the effects of tissue destruction, swelling, and tissue displacement, most traumatically brain-injured patients sustain at least some ischemic brain damage. Graham, Adams, and Doyle (1978) reported ischemic damage in 91% of patients who had died of head injuries. Ischemic brain damage can occur for several reasons. Injury to cardiovascular and pulmonary systems may compromise respiratory and cardiac output, leading in turn to diminished blood oxygenation and reduced blood supply to the brain. Elevated intracranial pressure and pressure on blood vessels may reduce the volume of blood reaching the brain. Cerebral vasospasm (see below) may decrease the carrying capacity of the cerebral vessels, especially when cardiac output is reduced. The distribution of damage from these ischemic processes varies, but damage is most common in the basal ganglia and surrounding structures, and the watershed cortical areas adjacent to the distributions of the three major cerebral arteries.

Cerebral Vasospasm Cerebral vasospasm (contraction of the muscular layer surrounding blood vessels) occurs in 15% to 20% of head injuries. Cortical arteries that are inflamed by the presence of blood from a subarachnoid hemorrhage are most frequently affected by vasospasm, although any artery can be affected, especially if it is in or near the site of primary injury. Other causes of cerebral vasospasm include stimulation of cerebral blood vessels by chemical or metabolic disruptions or injury to control centers that regulate dilation and constriction of cerebral arteries. Cerebral vasospasm, by itself, rarely is responsible for major neurologic complications. However, when it is inflicted on a system already compromised by other consequences of brain injury, it may be responsible for significant worsening of the patient's condition.

The primary and secondary physical consequences of traumatic brain injury are important determinants of traumatically brain-injured patients' eventual level of recovery, but not the only ones. Patient variables such as age, gender, and personal history also can affect recovery, although their influence is not as strong as that of physical consequences. In the following section we will consider how some of these variables relate to recovery from traumatic brain injury and to each other.

Prognostic Indicators in Traumatic Brain Injury

Nature and Severity of Brain Injury Not surprisingly, patients who have severe brain injuries recover less than patients with milder injuries. This relationship has been recognized and accepted for over 100 years, and during that time investigators have worked not so much to confirm the relationship as to discover reliable indicators of the severity of brain injury that do not require taking the brain out and inspecting it. One of the most reliable indirect indicators of the severity of brain injury is the magnitude and duration of alterations in consciousness (Macniven, 1994). Deeper and longer-lasting unconsciousness (coma) is associated with poorer eventual recovery (Carlsson, Svärdsudd, & Welin, 1987; Gilchrist & Wilkinson, 1979; Jennett, Teasdale, & Galbraith, 1977; Ruesch, 1944; and others). Katz and Alexander (1994) reported outcomes based on length of coma for 119 traumatic brain-injury patients with diffuse axonal injury. Outcomes were progressively worse as length of coma increased (Figure 8-5).

Until the 1970s, specification of the relationship between severity of brain injury and outcome was compromised because different investigators measured the level and duration of unconsciousness in different ways and used different measures of outcome, which prevented comparisons across studies. Then, in the early 1970s, investigators began to develop standardized measures of consciousness and outcome.

Teasdale and Jennett (1974) helped bring uniformity to how levels of consciousness were measured with the *Glasgow Coma Scale,* which provided a consistent way of rating a patient's level of consciousness based on eye opening, verbal responses, and motor responses observed during the immediate post-injury period (Table 8-1). To arrive at a GCS score, the examiner determines the patient's highest level of eye-opening, motor, and verbal responses, and sums the scores for the three levels. GCS total scores can range from 3 to 15, and *coma* is operationally defined as a GCS total score of 8 or less (Eisenberg & Weiner, 1987). Practitioners routinely divide patients into three levels of severity based on GCS score. Scores of 3 to 8 denote *severe head injury,* scores of 9 to 12 denote *moderate head injury,* and scores of 13 to 15 denote *mild head injury.*

Initial GCS scores have been shown to be strong predictors of traumatically brain-injured patients' eventual recovery, if the patient is assessed during the early stages of recovery, but

Duration of coma

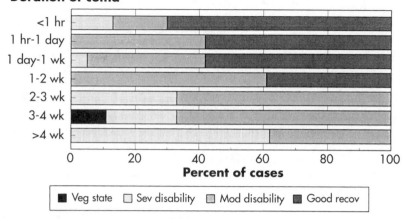

Figure 8-5 ▪ The relationship between the duration of coma following severe traumatic brain injury and eventual recovery. Longer durations of coma are associated with poorer eventual recovery. (From Katz DI, Alexander MP: Traumatic brain injury. In Good DC, Couch JR, eds: *Handbook of neurorehabilitation,* New York, 1994, Dekker.

TABLE 8-1

The *Glasgow Coma Scale*

Category of behavior	Description	Value
Eye Opening	Opens eyes spontaneously.	4
	Opens eyes to verbal command.	3
	Opens eyes in response to pain.	2
	No response.	1
Motor Responses	Obeys verbal commands.	6
	Attempts to pull examiner's hand away during painful stimulation.	5
	Moves limb away from painful stimulus.	4
	Flexes body in response to pain.	3
	Extends limbs, becomes rigid in response to pain.	2
	No response.	1
Verbal Responses	Converses and is oriented.	5
	Converses but is disoriented.	4
	Utters intelligible words, but does not make sense.	3
	Produces unintelligible sounds.	2
	No response.	1

Data from Teasdale and Jennett, 1974.

T A B L E   8 - 2

The *General Responsiveness* and *Best Communicative Effort* scales from the *Comprehensive Level of Consciousness Scale*

Scale 7: general responsiveness

8   The patient is fully aroused and alert or, if asleep, arouses and attends to the examiner following only mild or moderate stimulation. The arousal outlasts the duration of the stimulus.

7   The patient is aroused by mild or moderate stimulation, but upon cessation of stimulation returns to his/her former state, or the patient displays marked psychomotor agitation shortly after stimulus onset.

6   The patient is aroused only by noxious stimulation.

5   In response to noxious stimulation, the patient displays a purposeful withdrawal or a typical facial grimace. There is no arousal.

4   In response to noxious stimulation, the patient displays gross, disorganized withdrawal. There is no facial grimace or arousal.

3   In response to noxious stimulation, the patient displays only a feeble, disorganized withdrawal or flexion. There is no arousal or facial grimace.

2   Any decorticate rigidity.

1   Any decerebrate rigidity.

0   Total absence of discernible motor activity, even in response to noxious stimulation.

Scale 8: best communicative effort

7   Normal communication is possible through speech, writing, gesturing, and so on.

6   Profuse spontaneous or elicited verbalizations (signs, gestures). The communication is intelligible, but may be bizarre, jargonistic, and/or perseverative.

5   The patient responds to verbal, written, or signaled instructions with spontaneous but unintelligible or poorly articulated verbalizations (signs, gestures) or in a coded manner such as eye blinking, finger tapping, or hand squeezing. If intubated, the patient responds appropriately to commands.

4   The patient spontaneously vocalizes, verbalizes, makes signs or gestures, but gives no indication that he/she comprehends any form of receptive language.

3   The patient visually tracks an object passed through his/her visual field and/or turns his/her head toward the examiner as if wishing to communicate, or the patient generates spontaneous moaning or muttering coupled with reliable eye contact or searching behaviors.

2   Spontaneous, random muttering or moaning only.

1   Muttering or moaning in response to noxious stimulation.

0   No elicited or spontaneous vocalizations, searching behaviors, or eye contact.

Data from Stanczak and associates, 1984. **Decorticate rigidity:** Upper limbs are flexed at the elbows, wrists, and fingers, and are adducted (drawn toward the midline) at the shoulders. The lower limbs are extended and rotated inward and the feet are flexed downward. (Appears with damage in subcortical white matter, thalamus, and internal capsules bilaterally.) **Decerebrate rigidity:** Upper limbs are extended, drawn toward the midline, and rotated inwardly. The lower limbs are extended and rotated inward and the feet are flexed downward. The head and heels are bent backward and the body is bowed forward. The patient's jaw may be clenched. (Appears with temporal lobe herniation and midbrain compression.)

long enough after injury that noncranial contributors to the patient's impairments (such as alcohol intoxication) have dissipated (Bowers & Marshall, 1980; Jennett and associates, 1976; Langfitt, 1978; and others). Most studies of the relationship between GCS scores and outcome have used the GCS score at 6 hours post-accident as the reference value for predicting outcome.

The *Glasgow Coma Scale* has been shown to be highly reliable (Teasdale & Jennett, 1976), but is relatively insensitive, because wide ranges of behavior must be reduced to a small number of possible scores. Because no exceptions are made for untestable categories of behavior, the GCS may overestimate the severity of impairment for some patients, such as intubated patients who are verbally competent but cannot talk because of intubation, patients with facial injuries whose eyes are swollen shut, or patients with paralyzed or immobilized limbs for whom motor responses are difficult or impossible. The timing of assessment can also affect the predictive reliability of the GCS. Some patients with traumatic brain injuries are alert and clear-headed in the first few hours post-injury and then deteriorate, so GCS scores obtained at the standard 6 hours post-injury may give an unduly optimistic estimate of recovery for these patients.

The *Comprehensive Level of Consciousness Scale* (*CLOCS;* Stanczak and associates, 1984) was designed to compensate for some of the deficiencies of the Glasgow Coma Scale by assessing a broader range of responses. The CLOCS provides for measurement of posture, resting eye position, spontaneous eye opening, ocular movements, pupillary reflexes, motor functioning, responsiveness, and communicative effort. Behaviors in these eight categories are subjectively rated using 5-point to 9-point scales. Table 8-2 shows the rating scales for two behavioral categories—*general responsiveness* and *communicative effort.* Similar scales are used to rate behaviors in the other six behavioral categories. The CLOCS is more sensitive to subtle changes

in patients' responsiveness than the GCS. Stanczak and associates (1984) have shown that the CLOCS reliably predicts the recovery of traumatically brain-injured patients at discharge from the hospital. Nevertheless, the quick and easy-to-administer GCS remains the most widely used measure for assessing traumatically brain-injured patients' level of consciousness in the immediate post-injury period.

The *Glasgow Coma Scale* and the *Comprehensive Level of Consciousness Scale* are designed to measure patients' responsiveness in the immediate post-injury period. In the 1970s and 1980s, several procedures designed for measuring brain-injured patients' eventual level of recovery (outcome) were published.

Jennett and Bond (1975) proposed a standardized procedure for characterizing recovery in traumatic brain injury, called the *Glasgow Outcome Scale* (*GOS,* Table 8-3). The GOS was a substantial improvement over the poorly defined measures of outcome previously used, but is insensitive to less dramatic but still meaningful differences in outcome than the five levels specified by the GOS. Livingstone and Livingstone (1985) described a more sensitive procedure for measuring outcome—the *Glasgow Assessment Schedule* (*GAS,* Table 8-4), which permits users to rate outcome in six domains (physical condition, subjective complaints, personality change, cognitive functioning, occupational functioning, and proficiency in activities of daily living). However, the majority of clinicians and investigators continue to opt for the simpler and easier-to-use Glasgow Coma Scale.

The duration of posttraumatic amnesia (the time following coma during which the patient is unable to store new information and experiences in memory) has also received attention as an indirect indicator of the severity of brain injury and predictor of outcome. Several studies have shown the duration of posttraumatic amnesia to be inversely related to eventual level of recovery from traumatic brain injury (Bond, 1976; Levin and associates, 1979; Katz, 1992;

T A B L E   8 - 3

The Glasgow Outcome Scale

Rating	Definition
1	**Death.** Includes death clearly attributable to indirect or secondary effects of brain injury, such as pneumonia.
2	**Persistent Vegetative State.** The patient displays sleep-wake cycles, but makes no organized responses to stimulation during periods of wakefulness.
3	**Severe Disability (conscious but disabled).** The patient is dependent on others for daily care by reason of mental or physical disabilities, or a combination of both.
4	**Moderate Disability (disabled but independent).** The patient can travel by public transportation and work in a sheltered workshop. The patient may have motor impairment, language impairment, intellectual and/or memory impairment, and personality disruption.
5	**Good Recovery.** The patient resumes normal life, but may have minor neurological and psychological impairments. Return to work is not a prerequisite for this rating.

Data from Jennett and Bond, 1975.

and others). Katz (1992) reported Glasgow outcome scores for 114 consecutive patients with diffuse axonal injury. Posttraumatic amnesia lasting less than two weeks was associated with good recovery in 80% of cases, whereas no patient with posttraumatic amnesia lasting longer than 12 weeks made a good recovery.

In the late 1970s investigators began to question the reliability of the retrospective estimates of posttraumatic amnesia that were being used in studies that related posttraumatic amnesia to recovery. Consequently, efforts were made to replace subjective estimates of posttraumatic amnesia with standardized procedures to permit more detailed and more reliable assessment.

The *Galveston Orientation and Amnesia Test* (*GOAT;* Levin, O'Donnell, & Grossman, 1979) was designed to track recovery of orientation and memory in traumatically brain-injured patients who are emerging from coma (Table 8-5). The GOAT is made up of 10 questions that assess the patient's ability to remember and produce biographic information (orientation to person), the patient's orientation to place and time,

and the patient's memory for events immediately preceding his or her injury.

The patient begins the GOAT with 100 points and points are subtracted for each failed test item. Scores from 80 to 100 are considered average, scores from 66 to 79 are considered borderline, and scores from 0 to 65 are considered impaired. Scores on the GOAT have been found to correlate with the severity of brain injury as indicated by CT scans and GCS scores, and also have been found to correlate with traumatically brain-injured patients' eventual level of recovery (Levin, O'Donnell, & Grossman, 1979).

The GOAT can be a useful screening test for getting a general idea of a patient's level of cognitive functioning and responsiveness, although orientation is weighted more heavily than amnesia and memory. Because it requires spoken responses, it may overestimate the severity of impairment for patients with focal language–dominant-hemisphere pathology in addition to the diffuse damage typical of traumatic brain injury.

The *Rancho Los Amigos Scale of Cognitive Levels* (*RLAS;* Hagen & Malkamus, 1979) pro-

T A B L E 8 - 4				
The *Glasgow Assessment Schedule*				

Patient characteristic	Scoring	Patient characteristic	Scoring
Personality Change		**Cognitive Functioning**	
Emotional lability	a	Immediate recall	a
Irritability	a	Two-minute recall	a
Aggressiveness	a	Attention, concentration	a
Other behavioral change	a	Orientation	a
		Current intelligence	a
Subjective Complaints			
Sleep disturbance	a	**Physical Examination**	
Incontinence	a	Dysphasia	a
Family stress	a	Dysarthria	a
Financial problems	a	Abnormal tone: R leg	a
Sexuality problems	a	Abnormal tone: L leg	a
Alcohol: excess, poor tolerance	a	Abnormal tone: upper limbs	a
Reduced leisure, sporting activities	a	Walking	a
Headache	a	Cranial nerves	a
Dizziness, loss of balance	a	Seizures	a
Paresthesia	a		
Reduced sense of smell	a	**Activities of Daily Living**	
Reduced hearing	a	Cooking	b
Reduced vision	a	Other domestic tasks	b
		Shopping	b
Occupational Functioning		Traveling	b
Working: same job	0	Personal hygiene	b
Working: similar job	0	Feeding	b
Working: less skilled job	1	Dressing	b
Not working: employable	2	Mobility	b
Not working: not employable	3		

Data from Livingstone and Livingstone, 1985. **Scoring a:** normal (0), moderate (1), severe (2). **b:** on own (0), with help (1), unable to do (2).

vides a standard set of categories with which clinicians can describe a patient's cognitive and behavioral recovery following traumatic brain injury (Table 8-6). Rancho Los Amigos levels are commonly used by clinicians to identify a traumatically brain-injured patient's level of cognitive and behavioral recovery, and many clinicians assume that individual patients' recovery follows RLAS levels. (Many do, although the length of time spent at each level differs across patients.) There is some evidence that the length of time spent at the lower levels is related to eventual outcome (Hagen & Malkamus, 1979). The longer the patient remains at levels 1 through 4, the poorer the prognosis for recovery, but the relationship is not perfect, and sizeable errors in prediction can occur. The three highest RLAS levels are more sensitive to language impairments than the five lowest levels. Consequently, higher-level pa-

T A B L E 8 - 5	

Galveston Orientation and Amnesia Test (GOAT)

Question	Point value
What is your name?	2
When were you born?	4
Where do you live?	4
Where are you now? (City)	5
Where are you now? (Hospital)	5
On what date were you admitted to this hospital?	5
How did you get here?	5
What is the first event you can remember *after* the injury?	5
Can you describe in detail (e.g., date, time, companions) the first event you can recall *after* injury?	5
Can you describe the last event you recall *before* the accident?	5
Can you describe in detail (e.g., date, time, companions) the first event you can recall *before* the injury?	5
What time is it now?	(A)
What day of the week is it?	(B)
What day of the month is it?	(C)
What is the month?	(D)
What is the year?	(E)

(A) 1 for each ½ hour removed from correct time to maximum of 5

(B) 1 for each day removed from correct one

(C) 1 for each day removed from correct date to maximum of 5

(D) 5 for each month removed from correct one to maximum of 15

(E) 10 for each year removed from correct one to maximum of 30

tients with focal damage in the language-dominant hemisphere tend to be rated somewhat lower on the RLAS than patients with diffuse but symmetric damage or patients with foci of damage in the non–language-dominant hemisphere.

Sbordone (1991) developed a scale with fewer levels, but which covers a greater range of recovery than the Rancho Los Amigos Scale (Table 8-7). However, the Rancho Los Amigos Scale continues to be more widely used.

The Nature of the Patient's Traumatic Brain Injury Although the severity of traumatic injury plays the most prominent role in determining patients' eventual recovery, the nature of the injury also plays a part. Focal injuries

usually have a better prognosis than diffuse injuries. Neurologic recovery following focal injuries proceeds faster and plateaus earlier (but usually at a higher level) than recovery from diffuse injuries (Katz & Alexander, 1994). However, when focal injuries are superimposed on diffuse injuries the prognosis for recovery suffers (Filley and associates, 1987). The presence of diffuse axonal injury customarily is associated with poor outcome (Uzzell and associates, 1987), as is the presence of secondary brain damage caused by increased intracranial pressure, cerebral edema, anoxia or hypoxia (Andrews and associates, 1990; Miller and associates, 1978). Patients with diffuse hypoxic injury have a particularly ominous prognosis. Patients with

The *Rancho Los Amigos Scale of Cognitive Levels*

Level	Definition
1. No response	No response to pain, touch, sound, or sight.
2. Generalized response	Inconsistent, nonpurposeful, nonspecific responses to intense stimuli. Responds to pain, but response may be delayed.
3. Localized response	Blinks to strong light, turns toward/away from sound, responds to physical discomfort. Inconsistent responses to some commands.
4. Confused-agitated	Alert, very active, with aggressive and/or bizarre behaviors. Attention span is short. Behavior is nonpurposeful, and patient is disoriented and unaware of present events.
5. Confused-nonagitated	Exhibits gross attention to environment. Is highly distractible, requires continual redirection to keep on task. Is alert and responds to simple commands. Performs previously learned tasks but has great difficulty learning new ones. Becomes agitated by too much stimulation. Can engage in social conversation, but with inappropriate verbalizations.
6. Confused-appropriate	Behavior is goal-directed, with assistance. Inconsistent orientation to time and place. Retention span and recent memory are impaired. Consistently follows simple directions.
7. Automatic-appropriate	Performs daily routine in highly familiar environment without confusion, but in an automatic robot-like manner. Is oriented to setting, but insight, judgment, and problem-solving are poor.
8. Purposeful-appropriate	Responds appropriately in most situations. Can generalize new learning across situations. Does not require daily supervision. May have poor tolerance for stress and may exhibit some abstract reasoning disabilities.

Data from Hagen and Malkamus, 1979.

diffuse hypoxic injury who remain comatose for one week or more are virtually certain to remain severely disabled for the rest of their lives (Katz, 1992).

Patient-Related Variables Of several patient-related variables, *age* is the most important predictor of outcome following traumatic brain injury. Older patients are more likely to sustain hemorrhages than younger patients, and the hemorrhages are likely to be larger (Katz & Alexander, 1994). Older patients with traumatic brain injuries have higher mortality than younger patients—the mortality of traumatically brain-injured patients age 60 and up is approximately twice that of patients age 20 or below

(Wilson and associates, 1987). Older traumatically brain-injured patients recover less rapidly and are more likely to exhibit persistent confusion, attentional impairments, and memory impairments than younger patients (Jennett & Teasdale, 1981). Consequently older patients are more likely to remain dependent on caregivers than younger patients.

Abuse of alcohol or drugs also has negative effects on outcome following traumatic brain injury. Alcoholic traumatically brain-injured patients have longer periods of coma, lower levels of consciousness after emerging from coma, longer hospitalizations, and greater impairments of memory and verbal learning than

Cognitive and behavioral stages of recovery from traumatic brain injury

Stages of recovery	Characteristics
Stage 1	In coma
Stage 2	Opens eyes
	Severe agitation-restlessness or vegetative state
	Severe confusion
	Disoriented to place and time
Stage 3	Oriented to place but not time
	Moderate confusion
	Denial of cognitive deficits
	May complain of somatic problems
	Fatigues very easily
	Poor judgment
	Marked to severe attention deficits
	Severe memory deficits
	Severe social difficulties
	Severe problem-solving difficulties
Stage 4	Oriented to place and time
	Becoming aware of cognitive deficits
	Mild confusion
	Mild to moderate attention difficulties
	Marked problem-solving difficulties
	Moderate to marked memory deficits
	Early onset of depression-nervousness
	Unsuccessful attempts to return to work or school
	Poor endurance
	May appear relatively normal
	Moderate to marked social difficulties
Stage 5	Significant depression-nervousness
	Mild to moderate memory deficits
	Mild to moderate problem-solving difficulties
	Frequent comparison to premorbid self
	Given little hope of additional recovery
	Has returned to work or school
	Mild to moderate social difficulties
Stage 6	Mild memory impairment
	Mild problem-solving difficulties
	Acceptance of residual deficits
	Improving social relationships
	Return of most premorbid responsibilities
	Generally positive self-image

From Sbordone RJ: Overcoming obstacles in cognitive rehabilitation of persons with severe traumatic injury. In Kreutzer JS, Wehman PH, editors: *Cognitive rehabilitation for persons with traumatic brain injury: a functional approach*, Baltimore, 1991, Brookes, pp. 112-113.

non-alcoholic patients (Alfano, 1994). These relationships may be explained, at least in part, by the physiologic consequences of alcohol intoxication at the time of brain injury. Patients who are alcohol-intoxicated at time of injury are more likely to experience cerebral hypoxia, hemorrhage, or cerebral edema than their non-intoxicated counterparts (Alfano, 1994). The effects of abuse of substances other than alcohol on recovery from traumatic brain injury have received little empiric study, although presumably chronic drug abuse would have similar negative effects on recovery.

Several other patient-related variables have been shown to have minor effects on recovery from traumatic brain injury. *Intelligence* and *socioeconomic status* apparently have some effect on outcome. More intelligent individuals and those with higher socioeconomic status seem to recover better than those characterized by low levels of these variables. *Premorbid personality* and *emotional disturbances* also may have negative effects on the amount of anticipated recovery. Patients with maladaptive personality characteristics and premorbid emotional instability have a somewhat poorer prognosis than those without such disturbances (Rutter, 1981; Humphrey & Oddy, 1981).

The effects of individual patient-related variables on outcome are weak and easily overwhelmed by other more potent variables such as the severity and nature of brain injury. Additionally, many patient-related variables are correlated and tend to occur in combination (e.g., low intelligence, low socioeconomic status, and substance abuse), making determination of the effects of individual variables difficult, if not impossible. Finally, even the most dependable prognostic variables are best at predicting average outcomes for groups of patients and are less reliable when applied to individual patients. Experienced clinicians give the greatest prognostic weight to the most robust indicators (severity and nature of brain injury), but recognize that outcome for individual patients may not replicate group findings, even for the most robust indicators.

Behavioral and Cognitive Recovery Following Traumatic Brain Injury

The general course of recovery following traumatic brain injury is one of improvement, but the pattern of improvement usually differs from that seen following vascular accidents. Recovery from vascular accidents usually progresses predictably and regularly, with relatively rapid recovery in the early post-onset period and gradually slowing recovery thereafter. Recovery from traumatic brain injuries may progress in stepwise fashion, with periods of little or no change interspersed with periods of sometimes rapid improvement. The relationship between the severity of the patient's impairments in the first few weeks post-onset and the patient's permanent level of impairment is much stronger for vascular accidents than it is for traumatic brain injury. Consequently, it is more difficult to predict traumatically brain-injured patients' permanent level of impairment in the first weeks post-onset than to do the same for vascular patients.

Traumatically brain-injured patients typically progress through a fairly predictable sequence of stages during recovery. Most patients lose consciousness immediately after the accident. The unconsciousness can last from a few seconds to weeks or, rarely, months. Return to consciousness begins a period of undifferentiated activity, in which the patient is awake but responds indiscriminately and purposelessly to events. The patient does not maintain focused attention for more than a few seconds and his or her overall level of arousal fluctuates unpredictably from moment to moment. During this period the patient is hyperresponsive to stimulation and is agitated and irritable. Repetitive stereotypic movements (rocking, thrashing) are common, as are striking out, shouting, biting, and emotional lability. As recovery continues the patient becomes more lucid, and behavior becomes more purposeful; however, restlessness, agitation, and irritability persist, although at lower levels.

As recovery continues, the patient becomes oriented to time and place and begins to respond appropriately to simple requests, although the patient's attention span is short and distractibility is high. With the passage of time the patient begins to manage his or her daily routine with careful supervision and direction, but judgment, memory, and abstract reasoning remain impaired. Eventually the patient may function independently in familiar situations, but almost all continue to have problems with memory and abstract reasoning. A few patients eventually resume premorbid activities, but almost always with subtle but important deficiencies in memory, abstract reasoning, and tolerance for noise and distractions.

▪ REHABILITATION OF TRAUMATICALLY BRAIN-INJURED ADULTS: AN OVERVIEW

Rehabilitation of traumatically brain-injured patients requires the collaboration of many professionals, including physicians, nurses, speech-language pathologists, occupational therapists, physical therapists, neuropsychologists, clinical psychologists, social workers, and vocational counselors. Interdisciplinary collaboration is especially important in the early stages of the patient's recovery, when medical, physical, and behavioral impairments are most severe. The physical, cognitive, and behavioral impairments exhibited by traumatically brain-injured patients cross professional boundaries, and require a unified, integrated program of treatment that extends from the clinic to the patient's daily environment. According to Kay and Silver (1989),

> . . . rehabilitation [of traumatically brain-injured patients] must be interdisciplinary in the truest sense of the word. There must be ongoing communication among team members (not just with a central leader), care planning that cuts across disciplines, and coordination by a professional who is

an expert in the cognitive and behavioral problems of head injured persons (p. 147).

The first programs for treatment of traumatically brain-injured adults did not arise out of any particular theoretic rationale and were not based on sophisticated analyses of traumatically brain-injured adults' performance. The practitioners who designed and carried out these programs generally were operating under the assumption that stimulation of mental processes is the key to improving traumatically brain-injured adults' performance. Consequently, the early treatment programs immersed patients in drill activities that were designed to stimulate and restore mental processes. These programs usually used a *teach-to-the-test* approach, in which tests of generic skills (reading, reasoning, problem-solving) were administered, deficient performance in specific skills was identified, and treatment consisted of drills to stimulate the patient with activities that targeted the deficient skills. The treatment activities often resembled the tests that were used to identify the patient's deficient skills, and treatment frequently relied on workbooks and computer-based programs designed for remedial education in the schools. Sohlberg and Mateer (1989) call this treatment approach the *general stimulation* approach. General stimulation approaches to rehabilitation of traumatically brain-injured adults have largely been abandoned in favor of theory-driven or model-driven approaches.

One early reason for clinicians' disenchantment with stimulation approaches to traumatic brain injury rehabilitation was their recognition that stimulation treatment had little effect on traumatically brain-injured adults' daily life. Immersing patients in a program of general stimulation sometimes produced favorable changes in their test scores, but rarely led to improvements in their ability to get along in daily life. This realization led some clinicians to abandon stimulation treatment in favor of a *functionally oriented* approach to treatment. Functionally oriented treatment programs focused on improving patients' daily life competency by training them to perform specific daily life tasks in situations that paralleled daily life situations. (For example, a patient might be trained to plan a meal, make a shopping list, go to a market, and purchase the items on the list, either in a real market or in a mock-up in the rehabilitation facility.)

Functionally oriented treatment is based on the assumption that traumatically brain-injured adults' rehabilitation is most efficient and effective when treatment is carried out in contexts that replicate the daily life contexts to which improved performance is to generalize. Treatment activities typically consist of structured experience in mock-ups of real-life settings and situations, in which patients are coached in the skills and behaviors needed for successful performance. Functionally oriented treatment proved to be a quick way to train traumatically brain-injured adults to operate with maximum success in specific activities of daily life, producing "individuals who can perform particular activities under the conditions in which they were taught" (Sohlberg & Mateer, 1989, p. 20). A major drawback of most functionally oriented treatment is that generalization across tasks and situations often is limited or absent, which means that patients must be trained in a very large number of daily life tasks to function independently in an everyday environment.

Cognitive rehabilitation approaches to treatment of traumatically brain-injured adults seek to promote patients' capacity for independent function in daily life by focusing on remediation of specific cognitive processes such as attention, memory, and language. Cognitive rehabilitation treatment typically consists of hierarchically-organized drills. The choice of cognitive processes and the hierarchic arrangement of drills are based on a theoretic rationale that is either explicitly or implicitly defined. Improvements in a cognitive process are assumed to create improved performance in a broad range of activities that depend on that process. (For example, improving a patient's sustained attention should improve the patient's performance in all tasks that require sustained attention.) Cognitive rehabilitation is sometimes called *component training,* because it focuses treatment on specific components of a patient's overall pattern of impairment.

Behavior therapy represents yet another approach to rehabilitation of traumatically brain-injured adults. Behavior therapy focuses on direct modification of abnormal behaviors with procedures based on learning principles. Behavior therapy emphasizes direct, objective measurement of target behaviors and the use of stimulus control, reinforcement, and punishment to modify the frequency and/or the form of target behaviors. Behavior therapy is not necessarily (or usually) a stand-alone treatment. It is a part of many functionally oriented treatment programs, and often is a central focus of residential treatment and transitional living programs for traumatically brain-injured adults.

Most contemporary treatment programs for traumatically brain-injured adults include a mix of functionally oriented treatment, cognitive rehabilitation, and behavior therapy. Behavior therapy usually plays a prominent role in the immediate post-coma phase of treatment when control and modification of aberrant behaviors are major concerns. Cognitive rehabilitation usually plays a prominent role in the middle stages of treatment when restoration of cognitive abilities is the primary focus. Functionally oriented treatment becomes more prominent as traumatically brain-injured patients move into the later stages of recovery, when preparation for life after the rehabilitation facility and reintegration into society become primary concerns.

■ ASSESSMENT AND TREATMENT OF TRAUMATICALLY BRAIN-INJURED ADULTS

Assessment and treatment of traumatically brain-injured adults is an evolutionary process. As a patient's physical, cognitive, and behavioral characteristics change with recovery, what happens in testing and treatment also changes. Tests that are appropriate for patients in the immediate post-injury period, when confusion and agitation are prominent, may be irrelevant for patients in later stages of recovery, when subtle cognitive impairments are the primary concern.

Not all traumatically brain-injured adults spend time at each stage of recovery. Some with mild brain injuries skip the early stages or pass through them so quickly that intervention during those stages is not an issue. Some with severe brain injuries do not make it to the later stages. The rate at which individuals pass through each stage varies. Some linger at a given stage longer than others, and some pass through stages very rapidly or skip stages entirely. The reader should keep in mind that these stages are as much an index of the severity of brain injury as a timetable for recovery. That is, a severely injured patient may still be at Sbordone Stage 2 at 3 weeks post-injury, whereas a patient with a less severe brain injury may be at Sbordone Stage 5 at the same time post-injury.

■ GENERAL CHARACTERISTICS OF PATIENTS AT VARIOUS STAGES OF RECOVERY
Comatose and Semi-Comatose*

Stage 1 patients are bedbound, usually in an intensive-care unit. Most are comatose or minimally responsive. Many have tubes in place to maintain an open airway, assist breathing, and provide for removal of secretions. Most have intravenous lines and urinary catheters in place. Some are attached to sensors used to monitor intracranial pressure, heartbeat, and respiration. Some have nasogastric tubes in place for administration of liquid nutrition, and a few have gastrostomies (openings into the stomach through which liquid diets are administered). Low-level Stage 1 patients are unresponsive or minimally responsive to all external stimulation. High-level

---

* See Table 8-7 for descriptions of the Sbordone stages.

Stage 1 patients may respond intermittently and inconsistently, but nonpurposefully, to intense stimulation.

Responsive and Agitated

Patients at Stage 2 are awake and responsive, but their responses are inconsistent, nonpurposeful, inappropriate, and sometimes bizarre. These patients invariably are agitated, restless, impulsive, and highly distractible, and they inevitably exhibit massive impairments in attention, memory, reasoning, and problem-solving. Their interaction with others is primitive and socially inappropriate. They are not sensitive to environmental or social cues that normally regulate behavior. The most severely impaired are not oriented to person, place, or time, whereas those with less severe impairments usually are oriented to person, but not place or time.* Stage 2 patients have little tolerance for stress or frustration, which can lead to explosive emotional outbursts, including physical aggression. They do not monitor their own behavior, do not notice mistakes, and may deny the existence of impairments.

Restless and Distractible

Patients at Stage 3 are restless, distractible, and impulsive, but not agitated. Most are oriented to place but not to time. Most are aware that they have been injured but are unaware of the nature of their impairments and do not notice errors and inappropriate responses. These patients customarily exhibit profound impairments in attention, memory, reasoning, judgment, and problem-solving. Patients at this stage of recovery do not tolerate long or challenging tests or treatment tasks. They fatigue easily and have short attention spans, which prevents them from participating meaningfully in tasks that require sustained attention and ef-

---

* The usual progression in recovery of orientation is person-place-time. Orientation to time often proves to be especially impervious to the effects of recovery or rehabilitation.

fort. Their interactions with others are at a less primitive level than is true for patients at earlier stages of recovery, although their impulsivity and impaired judgment may contribute to frequent episodes of inappropriate behavior. They are inconsistently responsive to social cues and observe basic social conventions with occasional lapses. They can perform familiar tasks, but have great difficulty learning new ones. Stressful or challenging situations often provoke these patients into emotional outbursts that are striking in their intensity and equally striking in how quickly and completely they dissipate. Patients at Stage 3 remain highly controlled by their immediate environment and exhibit little capacity for independent thought or behavior.

Oriented, Purposeful

Patients at Stage 4 are not strikingly restless, distractible, or impulsive. Most are oriented to person, place, and time, although time sense may remain impaired for some. Most know that they have been injured, but do not have good understanding of the specifics of their injuries. Patients at Stage 4 usually have a general sense of their impairments and recognize most errors, although they may not be able to correct them. They behave appropriately in most interpersonal interactions, although the content of what they say may be inappropriate. Many exhibit subtle impairments in word retrieval and verbal fluency, and most exhibit more obvious problems in the pragmatic aspects of communication. These patients' performance on structured tasks may be within normal limits, but their performance breaks down in unstructured settings, or when they are faced with challenging or stressful situations. Stage 4 patients invariably have pronounced difficulty dealing with abstraction, implication, and inference. They tend not to get beyond surface interpretations of nonliteral material, situations, and events. They have moderate ability to control their immediate environment, and limited ability to work independently if given highly structured assignments and substantial coaching.

Dependent

Patients at Stage 5 typically have mild to moderate attentional, memory, and problem-solving impairments and subtle communication impairments (occasional word-retrieval failures, excessive repetition and filler, false starts and circumlocutions, and mild deficits in conversational turn-taking and topic maintenance). The self-monitoring skills of patients at Stage 5 are better than those of patients at lower levels, but occasional lapses occur. Patients at Stage 5 perform well in structured tasks in which instructions and response requirements are clear and unambiguous, and are capable of generalizing what they learn in one context to other similar contexts. However, their performance may deteriorate when they encounter unanticipated challenging or stressful situations. Patients at Stage 5 continue to have moderate problems with abstractions, implications, and inferences. They often get lost in details and fail to grasp the overall meaning of events, situations, or communications. Depression and anger often become prominent for patients in Stage 5 as it becomes obvious that complete recovery of premorbid abilities is unlikely or impossible.

Semi-Independent

Patients at Stage 6 function independently in structured and familiar situations, but most need supervision and direction in unfamiliar and unstructured ones. Almost all exhibit subtle cognitive impairments, although communication and interpersonal skills usually are within normal limits. Many of these patients can invoke compensatory strategies to help them cope with new or unusual situations. However, when they become fatigued or find themselves in stressful situations, their performance deteriorates. Many patients at Stage 6 have returned to school, work, or resumed other pre-injury responsibilities, although usually at a reduced level.

■ ASSESSMENT OF TRAUMATICALLY BRAIN-INJURED ADULTS
Assessing Level of Consciousness and Responsiveness to Stimulation

The speech-language pathologist's primary concerns with comatose and semicomatose (Stage 1) patients are to determine their level of consciousness, to get a sense of the nature and severity of their injuries, and to learn something about the progression of their physical, behavioral, and cognitive state since the time of injury. Most of this information comes from the patient's medical record and from discussion with other professionals involved in the patient's care, and some comes from direct observation of the patient.

Assessment of comatose and semicomatose patients focuses on establishing their arousability, wakefulness, and responsiveness to stimulation. Standard rating scales such as the *Glasgow Coma Scale* or the *Glasgow Assessment Schedule* provide a general subjective estimate of these characteristics, but the speech-language pathologist often supplements the impressions provided by rating scales with objective measurement of the patient's arousability, wakefulness, and responsiveness to stimulation. The first step is to determine the nature of the patient's sleep-wake cycles, either by direct observation or by consulting the patient's medical chart, family members, or patient-care personnel. The speech-language pathologist ascertains how much of the day the patient spends sleeping, what parts of the day the patient typically is awake, and the times of day during which the patient is most alert and responsive.

The next step is to determine how easily the patient is aroused from sleep. The most easily aroused patients awaken to environmental sounds or verbal commands. More difficult to arouse patients may require light touch, shak-ing, or even painful stimulation (squeezing, pinching) to awaken them.*

Finally, the patient's responsiveness to stimulation is evaluated, at a time at which the patient is at her or his highest level of arousal and alertness. The patient's responsiveness to environmental stimuli (such as a television or radio playing, people entering and leaving the patient's room, being talked to, touched, and moved by nursing personnel) is observed and recorded. Then the patient is systematically stimulated and the frequency and nature of the patient's responses are recorded.

The patient's *comprehension of speech* may be assessed by means of one-step commands requesting responses that are known to be within the patient's physical capability (such as *open your eyes, look at the ceiling*).

The patient's responsiveness to *visual stimulation* may be assessed by introducing lights or brightly colored objects into the patient's field of vision and noting whether the patient orients toward them, then moving the light or object through the patient's visual field and noting whether the patient visually tracks them. For patients who do not orient to or track moving objects, the speech-language pathologist may rapidly move a hand or some other object toward the patient's eyes and note whether a protective eyeblink response occurs.

The patient's responsiveness to *tactile stimulation* is assessed by lightly touching and stroking the patient's limbs. For patients who do not respond to light touch and stroking, the speech-language pathologist may assess their response to pressure (pinching, squeezing), hot and cold, or rough and smooth tactile stimulation. Assessment of the patient's responsiveness to *olfactory stimuli* may include pleasant ones such as cologne, vanilla extract, or almond ex-

---

* Comatose and semicomatose patients who do not respond to neutral or pleasant stimuli often respond to unpleasant or noxious stimuli, usually by some sort of avoidance response (withdrawing a limb, averting the head, closing the eyes).

tract and unpleasant ones such as ammonia or rubbing alcohol. Finally, the speech-language pathologist may assess the patient's responsiveness to pleasant *taste sensations,* such as fruit juice or honey, and unpleasant ones, such as lemon juice or vinegar.*

During the assessment the speech-language pathologist watches the patient for subtle responses to stimulation, such as acceleration or slowing of respiration, changes in muscle tone, subtle movements or changes in facial expression, eyeblinks, or brief vocalizations contingent on stimulation. The speech-language pathologist records the nature and magnitude of the patient's responses to each stimulus, as well as their consistency.

In this way the speech-language pathologist documents the nature and consistency of the patient's responses to several categories of stimuli. The information from the assessment serves as a baseline against which the rate and magnitude of the patient's subsequent recovery may be evaluated. During the days which follow, the speech-language pathologist periodically samples the patient's responsiveness and documents the results, providing the treatment team with important information regarding the patient's progression through the early stages of recovery.

Assessing Orientation

As traumatically brain-injured patients return to consciousness and begin responding to environmental stimuli, they enter a state of profound disorientation, confusion, and agitation (Stage 2). When this happens, the clinician becomes concerned with getting baseline measures of orientation and memory. However, because of these patients' behavioral and cognitive impairments, administering long or difficult tests of cognition, language, or communication is out of

the question. Objective assessment of these patients usually is limited to brief tests that provide a limited sample of performance representing basic levels of communication and cognition. Screening tests of orientation, memory, and amnesia such as the *Mini Mental Status Examination* (Folstein, Folstein, & McHugh, 1975), or the *Galveston Memory and Orientation Test* (Levin, O'Donnell, & Grossman, 1975), often suffice to track patients' progress during this stage of recovery. Performance data obtained with such tests can be supplemented with subjective ratings, using any of several rating scales designed for use with traumatically brain-injured adults. The simplest rating scales (such as the *Glasgow Coma Scale*), which are intended for frequent ratings (daily or more often) are too insensitive to be of much value for tracking traumatically brain-injured adults' performance at this stage of recovery. Consequently, the speech-language pathologist usually chooses a more detailed rating scale, such as the *Glasgow Assessment Schedule* (Livingstone & Livingstone, 1985) or subsections of the *Comprehensive Level of Consciousness Scale* (Stanczak & associates, 1984) to track these patients' recovery.

Orientation (awareness of self and appreciation of how one relates to others or to the environment) is a major problem in the post-coma phase of recovery. Orientation customarily is divided into orientation for *person* (who one is and who others in one's environment are), *place* (where one is), and *time* (what year, month, day, and hour it is, plus a sense of the passage of time). A few standardized procedures for assessing orientation have been reported in the literature, but most clinicians rely on the orientation items from screening examinations of mental status such as the *Mini-Mental Status Examination* (Folstein, Folstein, & McHugh, 1975) or the *Galveston Orientation and Amnesia Test* (Levin, O'Donnell, & Grossman, 1975), plus questions asked during the patient interview.

---

* Taste and smell are phylogenetically more primitive senses and may elicit responses from brain-damaged patients when visual and auditory stimuli do not.

Most mental status screening examinations contain items that test basic orientation to time, place, and personal information such as the patient's name, age, and marital status. The clinician can gather supplementary information about a patient's orientation to place by asking questions to assess the patient's concepts of direction and distance during an interview. For example, the clinician might ask the patient to indicate the direction of various locations (including the patient's home) from the place of the interview and to estimate distances between the place of the interview and those locations. To assess the patient's sense of time beyond the standard questions relating to day, hour, month, year, and season, the clinician can ask questions about what time of the day certain events happen (such as meals, group meetings, visits by family). The clinician can test the patient's sense of elapsed time by asking questions such as, *"How long have you been in this medical center?"* or *"How long has it been since your family last came to visit?"*.

Assessing Cognitive and Communicative Abilities

Patients at Stages 3 and above tolerate testing, although those at Stage 3 may not tolerate long or challenging tests. By the time patients reach these stages, their agitation and confusion have substantially resolved and underlying cognitive and communication impairments become more prominent. Cognitive and communication impairments become a major focus of assessment with Stages 3 and 4 patients, and it is at these stages that patients first receive detailed assessment of alertness, attention, visual perceptual abilities, memory, language and communication, and reasoning and problem-solving. Patients at Stages 5 and 6 tolerate challenging tests and do not have the profound and sweeping cognitive impairments typical of traumatically brain-injured patients at lower stages. Their cognitive performance in some domains may be within normal limits, although islands of substantial impairment may remain. For many it

may be apparent that restitution of remaining cognitive impairments is not in the cards, leading to a shift in clinical focus away from retraining cognitive abilities and toward providing the patient with strategies to compensate for cognitive impairments that cannot be repaired.

The scope and pattern of testing depends, of course, on each patient's tolerance for testing and her or his particular pattern of impairments. However, most clinicians attempt to at least sample each patient's test performance in the cognitive domains mentioned above, with follow-up testing to explore in more detail impairments identified in the initial tests.

Alertness Van Zomeren, Brouwer and Deelman (1984) divide alertness into *tonic alertness* and *phasic alertness. Tonic alertness* refers to an individual's ongoing, continuing receptivity to stimulation. Tonic alertness changes slowly and reflects the individual's overall state of arousal. Diurnal rhythms, increasing drowsiness in monotonous tasks, and the "mid-afternoon slump" are examples of changes in tonic alertness. Most traumatically brain-injured patients appear to have lower-than-normal resting levels of tonic alertness, but the magnitude of their cyclical changes in tonic alertness does not seem greater than normal. Traumatically brain-injured patients who drift off or fall asleep during testing or treatment do so because of lowered tonic alertness.

Phasic alertness refers to momentary, rapidly occurring changes in receptivity to stimulation. Changes in phasic alertness occur within milliseconds. Phasic alertness is strongly affected by the individual's intentions and interests. Increased alertness in response to warning signals or important events are examples of changes in phasic alertness.

Lowered tonic alertness is an inconvenience for the patient, and may slow the patient's progress in treatment, but diminished phasic alertness usually is more disruptive, both in treatment activities and in daily life. In treatment activities patients with diminished phasic alertness tend to make errors on initial stimulus items, and their performance deteriorates when treatment tasks change. They may fail to perceive short-duration stimuli unless given a warning signal, and they may fail to perceive subtle changes in instructions or treatment stimuli. In daily life they may miss key elements in others' spoken messages, and they may respond slowly or erroneously to rapidly occurring events or stimuli, such as traffic signals.

Attention Attentional impairments are a universal consequence of traumatic brain injury, and assessment and treatment of traumatically brain-injured patients' attentional impairments is a primary concern of most treatment programs. Most traumatically brain-injured patients have impaired *selective attention,* which means that they are distractible and have difficulty maintaining attention in the face of competing stimuli. In figure-ground tasks (both visual and auditory) these patients have difficulty discriminating figures from backgrounds, and may be distracted by irrelevant aspects of stimuli, such as the border around a picture or irrelevant details in stories or events. Traumatically brain-injured patients typically perform poorly on visual figure-ground tests (embedded figures, overlapping figures, masked or occluded figures), and they may have difficulty separating what is important from what is not in spoken and printed materials.

Impairments in *sustained attention* are not clearly separable from impairments in alertness and selective attention, because diminished alertness and impaired selective attention are certain to disrupt performance on tasks that require sustained attention. However, there are traumatically brain-injured patients who perform well on tasks requiring momentary alertness and have few problems discriminating figure from ground who nevertheless perform poorly on tests requiring sustained attention. These patients' performance deteriorates as the interval during which attention must be sustained increases, and as the complexity of the task increases. They do poorly on tests such as digits backward, backward spelling, oral arithmetic, and challenging vigilance tasks. Tests for evaluating selective attention and sustained attention are described in Chapter 7. Most traumatically brain-injured patients have difficulty in quickly shifting attentional focus from one stimulus to another or from one aspect of a task or situation to another *(alternating attention).* They perform poorly in tasks, in which response requirements change, or in which they are required to transfer attentional focus from one characteristic of task stimuli to another.

Divided attention tasks create major problems for most traumatically brain-injured patients, who cannot maintain attentional focus on two aspects of a task. Traumatically brain-injured patients usually have great difficulty with dual-task divided attention tasks such as those described in Chapter 7.

Visual Processing Visual processing impairments are most common in traumatically brain-injured patients who are in the early stages of recovery, although some patients in later stages of recovery (especially those with posterior brain damage) continue to have significant problems processing visual information into the middle and late stages of recovery. These patients perform poorly on tests that require identification of incomplete or fragmented visual stimuli, partially occluded stimuli, and on visual figure-ground tests such as those described in Chapter 7.

Memory Impaired memory is an important early consequence of traumatic brain injury, and memory disturbances plague most traumatically brain-injured patients throughout the course of their recovery and thereafter. Memory has been divided up in many ways by different writers. One useful way is to divide it into *retrospective memory* and *prospective memory.*

Retrospective memory is memory for past events and experiences, and for information acquired in the past. Most traumatically brain-injured patients have problems with retrospective memory—they fail to remember conversations, events, people, or situations from minute to minute or (more often) from hour to hour or day to day. Most standardized memory tests are designed to assess retrospective memory.

Prospective memory is the ability to remember to do things at specific points in time—keep an appointment, prepare dinner, or feed the cat. Impairments in prospective memory are considered by some (such as Lezak, 1995) not to be impairments of the memory system itself, but inability to use contextual cues to facilitate recall *(remembering to remember).*

Retrospective memory can be divided into *declarative memory* and *procedural memory* (Tulving, 1983). Declarative memory can be loosely characterized as *what we know about things,* and procedural memory as *what we know about how to do things.* Knowledge of who we are, our parent's names and birthdates, the capital city of Poland, how many eggs make a dozen, the composition of a protein molecule, the names of the cranial nerves, and other such material is stored in declarative memory. Information in declarative memory can be brought to conscious awareness and verbally reported. Declarative memory almost always is compromised by traumatic brain injury.

Remembering how to perform previously-learned behavioral routines (driving an automobile, making a tuna salad sandwich, repairing a television set, diagnosing diabetes mellitus) calls upon information in procedural memory. Information in procedural memory cannot be brought to conscious awareness, but must be accessed via performance of the activity to which the information relates.* Procedural

memory has been described as "a collection of habits which can be applied automatically without having to think about new response strategies" (Garner & Valadka, 1994; p. 95). Procedural memory apparently is less affected by traumatic brain injury than declarative memory, and there are reports that traumatically brain-injured patients can learn and use new procedural routines, even though they are not aware of learning them and cannot verbally describe them (Ewert and associates, 1989; Parkin, 1982; Verfaelli, Bauer, & Bowers, 1991).

But we are not finished chopping memory into smaller pieces, because declarative memory can in turn be divided into *episodic memory* and *semantic memory* (Tulving, 1972). Episodic memory can loosely be characterized as memory for personally experienced events. Experiences stored in episodic memory are time- and place-specific. Our knowledge of who we were with and what we were doing at certain points in time comes from episodic memory, as well as our sense of relationships between events that took place at different points in time. In many respects our sense of who we are comes largely from information in episodic memory.

Semantic memory contains our organized knowledge of the world, including most of what we learned in school or other educational settings (facts, dates, names, places, and so on). Semantic memory contains information that permits us to report that John Quincy Adams was the sixth President of the United States, that there are 12 eggs in a dozen, that gasoline stations usually are found on busy highways, or that some barking dogs do indeed bite.*

One more chop, and our cutting up of memory will be complete. Impairments of retrospec-

---

* One's memory of having performed a procedure can be brought into consciousness and the steps in the procedure verbally reported. However, one's knowledge of the exact sequence, timing, amplitude, and other characteristics of the behaviors in the procedure can only be accessed by performing the procedure. (Every good mechanic can tighten a nut on a bolt tightly enough so that it will not loosen, but not so tightly that it breaks the bolt or the nut, but none can tell a novice how to do it, and a novice can only learn how by doing it many times.)

---

* However, one's knowledge that some barking dogs bite may be based on one incident stored in episodic memory, which illustrates the interactions and overlap between episodic memory and semantic memory. It also shows that much of what we "remember" is *constructed,* rather than *remembered,* but that is another (too long) story.

tive memory in adults with traumatic brain injuries have been divided into two categories—*pretraumatic memory loss* and *posttraumatic memory loss.*

The concepts of pretraumatic and posttraumatic memory loss were developed by Russell and associates (Russell, 1971; Russell & Espir, 1961; Russell & Nathan, 1946), based on their studies of traumatically brain-injured British armed forces personnel during and after World War II. Russell and his contemporaries called pretraumatic memory loss *retrograde amnesia* and posttraumatic memory loss *anterograde amnesia.* Over the years these difficult-to-keep-straight labels have been gradually replaced by the more descriptive and easier-to-remember labels *pretraumatic memory loss* and *posttraumatic memory loss.* However, some contemporary writers still use the original labels.

Both labels refer to a period of time for which a traumatically brain-injured patient has no subsequent recollection of experiences that happened during the period—hence the terms *amnesia* and *memory loss.* As the labels suggest, *pretraumatic memory loss* is loss of memory for experiences that happened before the patient's brain injury and *posttraumatic memory loss* is loss of memory for experiences that happened after the injury (Figure 8-6).

Pretraumatic memory loss may have two components. Loss of memory for the seconds to minutes immediately preceding the patient's injury apparently is caused by disruption of the neurochemical processes responsible for embedding information in long-term memory. Loss of memory for hours (or days) preceding the injury apparently is caused by disrupted access to material in long-term memory. Pretraumatic memory loss usually shrinks as the patient recovers, and most patients eventually recover memory for all but the last few minutes before their brain injury. (Presumably because experiences in the last few minutes never made it into long-term memory.)

Corkin and associates (1987) reported the duration of pretraumatic memory loss in 121 cases of penetrating or nonpenetrating traumatic brain injury from the Korean conflict. About one third of the patients experienced no pretraumatic memory loss, and for most that did, the interval of memory loss lasted less than one hour (Figure 8-7). The duration of pretraumatic memory loss was not significantly related to whether the injuries were penetrating or nonpenetrating. These results are consistent with results reported by Russell and Nathan (1946) who studied the duration of pretraumatic memory loss in 973 traumatically brain-

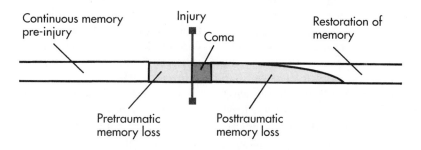

Figure 8-6 ▪ A schematic representation of memory loss associated with traumatic brain injury. Pretraumatic memory loss is loss of memory for experiences preceding the injury and posttraumatic memory loss is loss of memory for experiences following the injury. Postraumatic memory loss almost always covers a longer time interval than pretraumatic memory loss.

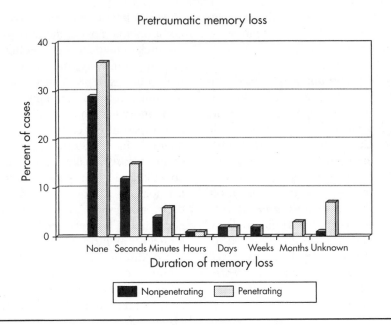

Figure 8-7 ▪ The duration of pretraumatic memory loss in 121 cases of penetrating or nonpenetrating traumatic brain injuries from the Korean conflict. (From Corkin and associates: Consequences of penetrating and nonpenetrating head injury: posttraumatic amnesia, and lasting effects on cognition. In Levin HS, Grafman J, Eisenberg HM, eds: *Neurobehavioral recovery from head injury,* New York, 1987, Oxford University Press.)

injured survivors of World War II. Eighty-six percent of Russell and Nathan's subjects experienced pretraumatic memory loss, but only 14 percent experienced loss that lasted more than 30 minutes.

Posttraumatic memory loss is "inability to retain new information in the minutes, hours, days, or weeks following the injury" (Corkin and associates, 1987, p. 318). It usually begins at the time of injury, but some patients may have brief intervals of memory for events that happened immediately after their injury, with loss of memory for later-occurring events. Russell's original definition of posttraumatic memory loss included both the period of coma and the period following it in which the patient fails to remember experiences. Contemporary writers exclude the period of coma, and most assume that posttraumatic memory loss coincides roughly with the period of confusion and dis-

orientation following the patient's emergence from coma (Baddelly and associates, 1987). Posttraumatic memory loss almost always lasts longer than pretraumatic memory loss. Figure 8-8 summarizes results reported by Corkin and associates (1987) for Korean conflict survivors. Whereas pretraumatic memory loss rarely lasted more than seconds to minutes, posttraumatic memory loss often lasted for days or weeks. Russell (1971) and Jennette (1976) have reported similar results.

As mentioned earlier, the problem in posttraumatic memory loss is getting information into long-term memory. Patients with posttraumatic memory loss may participate in conversations, take tests, and carry out activities of daily living, but have no subsequent recollection of those experiences. They do not remember meetings, conversations, or people from hour to hour or from morning to afternoon. Posttraumatic

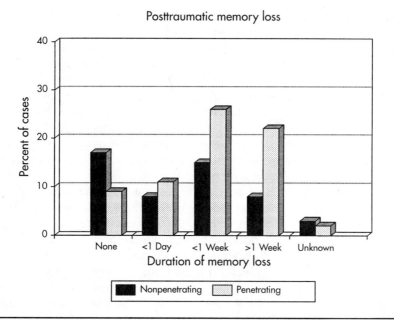

Figure 8-8 ■ **The duration of posttraumatic memory loss in 121 cases of penetrating or nonpenetrating traumatic brain injuries from the Korean conflict.** (From Corkin and associates: Consequences of penetrating and nonpenetrating head injury: posttraumatic amnesia, and lasting effects on cognition. In Levin HS, Grafman J, Eisenberg HM, eds: *Neurobehavioral recovery from head injury,* New York, 1987, Oxford University Press.)

memory loss has far more serious consequences for the patient than pretraumatic memory loss and causes greater disruption in the patient's daily life.*

The duration of posttraumatic memory loss is moderately related to the duration of coma, and may be a better predictor of eventual recovery than duration of coma (Levin, Benton, & Grossman, 1982), with longer posttraumatic memory loss suggesting greater residual deficits. Patients with posttraumatic memory loss of 1 month or more are likely to have permanent memory deficits, and if posttraumatic memory loss lasts 3 months or more, the patient is likely to have permanent and substantial impairments of cog-

nition, learning, and memory (Brooks, 1989; Katz & Alexander, 1994).

Most measures of the duration of pretraumatic and posttraumatic memory loss are actually retrospective estimates based on patients' accounts of when they first began remembering things after their accidents, and there are no standard procedures for obtaining these estimates. Consequently, it seems likely that considerable unaccounted-for variability exists in the measures. (For example, it is difficult, and perhaps impossible, to separate what a patient actually remembers from the time immediately following her or his accident from what family members, staff, or others have told the patient about that period.) Even so, there is sufficient consistency of results across studies of pretraumatic and posttraumatic memory loss to give us reasonable confidence about the relative duration and time-course of these two memory impairments.

---

* According to Lezak (1983) traumatically brain-injured patients are most troubled by posttraumatic memory loss, while their lawyers are most troubled by pretraumatic memory loss.

Assessment of Memory For patients who can tolerate the testing, clinicians are likely to administer a comprehensive retrospective/declarative memory assessment battery that includes tests of immediate retention span, short-term retention, retention of new information, retrieval of information from remote memory, and visual memory.

The most common way of testing *immediate retention span* is *digit span* testing, in which the examiner reads lists of single-digit numbers aloud and the patient says each list back when the examiner finishes reading it. These tests usually begin with two- or three-digit lists, and the number of digits in successive lists increases until the patient can no longer repeat them without error. Digit span tests are found in several test batteries for assessing memory, as well as most general intelligence tests such as the *Wechsler Adult Intelligence Scale—Revised* (Wechsler, 1981) and the *Stanford-Binet Intelligence Test* (Terman & Merrill, 1973). Similar tests, in which the examiner reads lists of randomly arranged letters or lists of unrelated words, are less commonly used to measure immediate retention span. Normal spans for digits, letters, and words are similar, and range from 5 to 7 items.

Digit span, letter span, and word span tests are auditory-verbal tests, in that the patient must comprehend and retain strings of spoken words long enough to repeat them. A few span tests in which the stimuli are visual and nonverbal have been described in the literature. The most common are *block-tapping* tests, in which a set of blocks is placed before the patient and the examiner taps some of them in prearranged order. The patient then is asked to tap the blocks in the same order as the examiner. As in digit span tests, the number of blocks in the sequence increases until the patient can no longer duplicate the examiner's tapping patterns without error. The *Knox Cube Test* (Arthur, 1947) is the best-known block-tapping test. However, the cubes in the *Knox Cube Test* are arranged in a row, permitting test-takers to mentally number them, thus incorporating a verbal strategy into the test. The *Corsi Block-tapping Test* (Milner, 1971) eliminates this possibility by arranging the blocks in a random array.

Clinicians customarily test *short-term retention* by administering retention-span tests with a delay imposed between the examiner's presentation of test items and the patient's opportunity to respond. The delay interval usually lasts for only a few seconds, and rarely exceeds one minute.

Short-term retention with interference tests are like short-term retention tests, except that the patient must perform an activity (such as counting or saying the alphabet) to prevent rehearsal of stimulus sequences during the delay interval.

Retention of new information tests come in two forms, both of which resemble word span tests. In the *subspan format* the examiner repeats a 3- or 4-word list until the patient can repeat them back. Then the examiner goes on with other activities, and after five minutes or so asks the patient to recall the list. In some variants, the examiner prompts the patient for unremembered words at the time of recall testing by giving a related word or category, and sometimes follows with recognition trials for items the patient fails to remember after the prompts. In recognition trials the examiner provides several words, one or more of which are words the patient has failed to remember, and the patient is asked if any of the words were those that were to be remembered.

In the *supraspan format* the examiner reads a list of words that exceeds the patient's immediate retention span. (Lists usually contain 15 or more words.) After the first reading the examiner asks the patient to repeat as many of the words as he or she can remember. The examiner writes down the words produced by the patient and the order in which they were produced. Then the examiner repeats the list and again asks the patient to say as many as he or she can remember. This procedure continues until the patient has learned the entire list, or for a predetermined number of trials (usually four or five). In some tests, a recognition trial is provided after the final recall trial for patients who have not learned the list in the prescribed number of trials. The *Auditory-Verbal Learning Test* (Rey, 1964), and the *California Verbal Learning Test* (Delis and associates, 1987) are frequently administered supraspan tests.

When testing *retrieval of information from remote memory,* the examiner asks the patient questions related to biographical information, such as the place and time of the patient's school attendance, the nature of the patient's first employment, and so on. It is not always necessary to administer a separate test of remote memory, because some items in most screening tests of mental status test remote memory. Biographic information also may be obtained during the patient interview, or as part of routines for gathering patient information when filling out test forms.

In typical tests of *visual (nonverbal) memory* the examiner shows the patient cards on which are printed geometric designs (such as the one shown in Figure 8-9) and asks the patient to draw them from memory. Many such

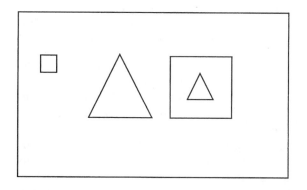

Figure 8-9 ▪ A plate from the *Revised Visual Retention Test*. The inclusion of smaller figures in the periphery make these designs sensitive to visual inattention. (From Benton AL: *The Revised Visual Retention Test,* ed 4, San Antonio, TX, 1974, The Psychological Corporation.)

tests are available, but the *Memory for Designs* subtests from the *Stanford-Binet Intelligence Scale* (Terman & Merrill, 1973), the *Memory for Designs Test* (Graham & Kendall, 1960), the *Visual Reproduction Test* (Wechsler, 1987), the *Rey Complex Figure Test* (Rey, 1941), and the *Benton Visual Retention Test* (Benton, 1974) are among the most popular with clinicians who work with traumatically brain-injured adults. The Benton test differs from the others in that its designs are designed to be sensitive to the presence of hemispatial neglect (Figure 8-9).

If a patient fails a drawing-from-memory test, the clinician may administer a visual memory test in which the patient is asked to recognize, rather than draw, previously presented visual stimuli. Some of these tests resemble visual reproduction tests, in that the stimuli are geometric designs (e.g., the *Recurring Figures Test;* Kimura, 1963 and the *Visual Retention Test;* Warrington & James, 1967). In others the stimuli are drawings of real objects, as in the *Continuous Recognition Memory Test* (Hannay, Levin, & Grossman, 1979), in which the stimuli are plants, sea creatures, and animals. In a third kind of recognition memory test the patient is shown a series of cards, each containing a different drawing or picture. Then a second set of cards, which contains the previously seen items plus additional foils, is shown to the patient, and the patient indicates which ones he or she has previously seen.

Language and Communication Most traumatically brain-injured adults produce speech that is phonologically, syntactically, and semantically within normal limits. The primary exceptions are those with brainstem, cerebellar, or peripheral nervous system damage who are dysarthric. Assessment of these patients follows the same pattern as assessment of patients with dysarthria from other causes (see Chapter 10).

Traumatically brain-injured patients often make errors on tests of confrontation naming, but most errors reflect visual misperceptions or the patient's inability to inhibit competing responses, rather than word-retrieval impairments *per se*. Although word-retrieval failures in spontaneous speech sometimes occur, they do not constitute a serious impairment for most patients. Not so for relevance and efficiency. Most traumatically brain-injured adults, except for those with mild head injuries, produce speech that is intermittently (at least) irrelevant, confabulatory, circumlocutory, tangential, fragmented, and noncohesive, but (usually) linguistically acceptable. Add to this their faulty appreciation and observance of pragmatic rules and conventions, and the stereotypic picture of the traumatically brain-injured speaker emerges. On the comprehension side, most traumatically brain-injured adults do well if the material to be comprehended is structured and literal, but their comprehension deteriorates when they are confronted with unstructured material, or when appreciation of the meaning of the material depends on appreciation of indirect meanings such as metaphor, humor, or sarcasm.*

Few traumatically brain-injured adults exhibit patterns of language impairment that justify calling them aphasic, although many exhibit mild word-retrieval problems, diminished auditory and reading comprehension for complex materials, and occasional literal or verbal paraphasias. The communication impairments seen following traumatic brain injuries usually are secondary consequences of underlying impairments in attention, memory, reasoning, and problem-solving. Consequently, standard aphasia tests are not suitable for assessing the language and communication impairments of traumatically brain-injured adults. Standard aphasia tests highlight skills such as word retrieval, syntactic pro-

cessing, and comprehension of literal material (skills that usually are preserved following traumatic brain injury) and downplay or ignore skills such as organization and integration of complex information and appreciation of nonliteral and implied meanings (skills that are most likely to be compromised by traumatic brain injury). As a result, performance on an aphasia test usually overestimates traumatically brain-injured adults' actual communicative competence. Ylvisaker and Urbanczyk (1994) describe the reasons why:

> To the extent that communication is negatively affected by attentional, perceptual, organizational, and executive system dysfunction, language testing by its very nature may compensate for the underlying weakness. For example, the controlled testing environment reduces attentional challenges; clear instructions and well defined tasks help to ensure orientation to task and reduce the effects of cognitive inflexibility; test items that include only relatively small amounts of language compensate for organizational weakness; the deliberate rate at which information is presented compensates for difficulties with speeded performance; the supportive and encouraging manner of the examiner may compensate for an inability to cope with interpersonal stress; and commonly used tests fail to measure the individual's ability to learn new information and skills and to generalize new skills from one setting or task to another.

This does not mean, however, that tests used to evaluate aphasic adults have no place in the evaluation of adults with traumatic brain injuries. Selective testing of reading, writing, speaking, and listening that focuses on perceptual and processing impairments likely to be affected by traumatic brain injury may be useful in quantifying traumatically brain-injured patients' language and communication abilities. Depending on the severity of the patient's brain injury and the pattern of the patient's impairments, some or all of the following tests may be appropriate. The tests are described in Chapter 5.

• A receptive vocabulary test such as the *Peabody Picture Vocabulary Test* (Dunn &

---

* The speech and comprehension performance of traumatically brain-injured adults has much in common with that of patients with right-hemisphere brain damage. One reason for this commonality may be the large proportions of patients with frontal-lobe damage in groups of right-hemisphere-damaged adults and the high probability that traumatically brain-injured adults will have frontal lobe damage (McDonald, 1993).

Dunn, 1981) to estimate usable listening vocabulary.

- A confrontation naming test such as the *Boston Naming Test* (Kaplan, Goodglass, & Weintraub, 1983) to assess the patient's ability to retrieve and produce words on demand.
- A test of generative naming such as the *Word Fluency Measure* (Borkowski, Benton, & Spreen, 1967) to assess the patient's ability to produce conceptually related words under time pressure.
- A test of sentence comprehension such as the *Token Test* (DeRenzi & Vignolo, 1962) to assess the patient's short-term auditory retention span and comprehension of short spoken messages.
- A sample of connected speech production elicited by picture description or story narration to assess the content, organization, and efficiency of the patient's connected speech.
- A test of spoken discourse comprehension to assess the patient's comprehension of stated and implied main ideas and details from spoken narratives.
- A sample of conversation in which the presence and appropriateness of pragmatic aspects of the patient's communication are rated.*

Depending on the patient's pattern of communication impairments, other tests of speech, language, and communication may be appropriate. Comprehensive testing of spelling and reading comprehension may be important for high-level patients concerned with return to school or work. Extended evaluation of pragmatic skills may be important for patients who are contemplating return to work that requires interactions with others. Comprehensive evaluation of verbal planning and problem-solving may

---

* The sample should represent a true conversation and not an interview (sometimes called "semi-structured conversation") in which the examiner asks questions and the patient answers them. Such "conversations" do not discriminate traumatically brain-injured adults from adults without brain injuries (Snow, Douglas, & Ponsford, 1995).

be important for patients who intend to return to jobs in which those skills are required.

Abstract Thinking Impaired abstract thinking is almost a universal consequence of brain damage. Lezak (1995) describes it as " . . . inability to think in useful generalizations, at the level of ideas, or about persons, situations, events not immediately present (past, future, or out of sight)" (p. 602) and comments that tests of other cognitive processes such as planning, organizing, problem-solving, and reasoning also supply information about abstract thinking.

Adults with severe traumatic brain injuries do poorly on tests of abstract thinking regardless of the modality in which test items are presented or the nature of the responses required. Those with less severe injuries may perform well on some tests and poorly on others, depending on the complexity of the test and whether the test addresses an impaired stimulus or response modality (Lezak, 1995).

Commonly administered verbal tests to assess abstract thinking include *proverb interpretation tests,* in which the patient tells the meaning of common proverbs such as *Don't put the cart before the horse* (Delis, Kramer, & Kaplan, 1988; Gorham, 1956); and *similarities and differences tests,* in which the patient tells how two words are similar *(orange/banana)* or different *(bird/dog)* (Terman & Merrill, 1973; Tow, 1955; Wechsler, 1981).

Commonly administered nonverbal (visual) tests to assess abstract thinking include the *Progressive Matrices* (Raven, 1960, 1965) and *categorization and sorting tests.*

Raven's *Standard Progressive Matrices* (Raven, 1960), and *Coloured Progressive Matrices* (Raven, 1965) are tests of intelligence and reasoning ability with low verbal loadings. They are useful in estimating the intellectual and reasoning abilities of patients with language impairments. Both matrices tests are multiple-choice tests in which the patient is shown visual patterns in which a part is missing. The patient is asked to choose from a set of six or eight choices the one that completes the stimulus (Figure 8-10). The *Standard Progressive Matrices* consists of 60 items divided into five sets of 12 items each. The *Coloured Progressive Matrices* consists of 36 items, is easier, and is for testing children and for testing adults 65 years old and up. The *Standard Progressive Matrices* has numerous difficult items that may require verbal reasoning for their solution. For most brain-injured patients, the *Coloured Progressive Matrices* are appropriate. However, for patients with mild brain injuries, the standard (more difficult) version may be appropriate.

In *categorization and sorting tests,* the patient must determine the rules for assigning stim-

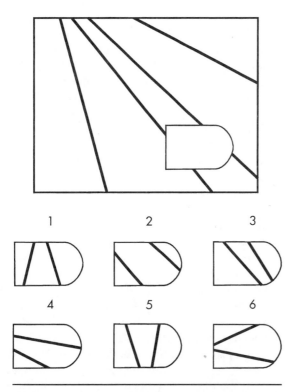

1   2   3

4   5   6

Figure 8-10 ■ An example of a *Progressive Matrices* task. The person taking the test chooses the pattern segment at the bottom that best completes the overall pattern at the top.

uli to categories by means of a trial-and-error process in which the examiner tells the patient only *right* or *wrong* following correct or incorrect assignments (Mahurin & Pirozzolo, 1986; Reitan & Wolfson, 1993). The *Wisconsin Card Sorting Test (WCST;* Grant & Berg, 1948) is a widely used categorization and sorting test. In the WCST the test-taker is given a deck of cards, each of which contains one of four symbols *(triangle, cross, star, circle).* The symbols on each card are printed in one of four colors *(red, green, yellow, blue).* The test-taker is instructed to sort the cards into four stacks according to the examiner's feedback. The test-taker begins sorting the cards and the examiner says *right* or *wrong* after each placement. When the test begins, color is the principle governing the sort, and the examiner says *right* whenever the patient sorts a card by its color. When the subject has deduced the color sorting principle (10 consecutive correct placements), the principle for sorting changes to form. (The only sign of the change to the test-taker is a change in the feedback provided for sorting responses.) When the test-taker has deduced the form sorting principle, the principle changes to number, and so on, for two cycles of color-form-number. Performance on the WCST can be scored in several ways, but most users score the number of runs of 10 consecutive correct sorts, plus the number of perseverative errors (failure to change sorting responses to match changes in the sorting principle).

Reasoning According to Lezak (1995), tests of reasoning assess an individual's capacity for logical thinking, appreciation of relationships, and practical judgment. Reasoning tests can be divided into three categories: *verbal reasoning tests, arithmetic and numerical reasoning tests,* and *visual/spatial reasoning tests.*
Verbal reasoning tests include:

- *Tests of reasoning and judgment* such as items in the *Wechsler Intelligence Scale* (Wechsler, 1981) in which the patient is asked to respond to questions such as

What would you do if you find a letter on the street?

- *Verbal absurdities tests* such as items in the *Stanford-Binet Intelligence Scale* (Terman & Merrill, 1973) in which the patient is asked to identify the logical inconsistencies in items such as *Bill Jones's feet are so big that he has to pull his trousers on over his head*.
- *Logical relationship tests* such as *Verbal Reasoning* in which the patient must arrive at a conclusion based on analysis of logical relationships presented in a short narrative *(Fred is taller than Bill but shorter than Oliver. Helen is taller than Oliver and shorter than Bill . . .)*.

Arithmetic and numerical reasoning tests include:

- *Arithmetic story problems* (Fasotti, 1992; Walsh, 1985; Wechsler, 1981), in which the patient is asked to solve story problems such as *Bill has 8 pencils. Frank has 4 times as many pencils as Bill. How many pencils do they have together?*
- *Block-counting tests* (McFie & Zangwill, 1960; Newcombe, 1969; Terman & Merrill, 1973) require the patient to count how many blocks are depicted in drawings of three-dimensional stacks of blocks (Figure 8-11). The difficulty of items in these

tests depends on the number of blocks depicted and the number of blocks in the stack that are hidden from view.

Visual/spatial reasoning tests include:

- *Picture completion tests* such as those in the *Wechsler Intelligence Scale* (Wechsler, 1981) in which the patient tells what is missing from drawings of common objects, human figures, or animal figures drawn with missing parts (Figure 8-12).
- *Picture arrangement tests* (Wechsler, 1981) in which the patient arranges scrambled pictures to portray a story-like sequence of events (Figure 8-13).
- *Pictured absurdities tests* (Terman & Merrill, 1973) in which the patient tells what is wrong with pictures depicting bizarre or impossible relationships or situations (Figure 8-14).

Planning and Problem-solving Planning and problem-solving call into play several abilities, including the ability to think ahead, the ability to conceptualize future consequences of present actions, the ability to consider alternatives, and the ability to make choices. Deficiencies in any of these abilities can disrupt or devastate planning and problem-solving. There are

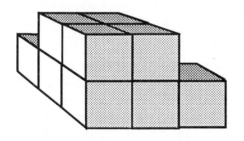

Figure 8-11 ▪ **An example of a block counting test stimulus. The difficulty of a block counting test item depends on the number of blocks and the number of blocks hidden from view.**

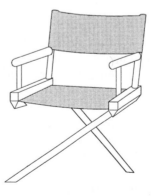

Figure 8-12 ▪ **An example of a picture completion test stimulus. The person taking the test tells what is missing from the test stimulus.**

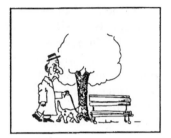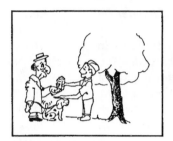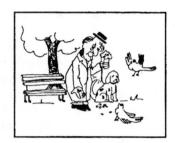

Figure 8-13 ■ **An example of a picture arrangement test stimulus. The person taking the test rearranges the pictures to tell a story. The pictures in Figure 8-13 are shown in story order. The examiner gives them to the person taking the test in scrambled order.**

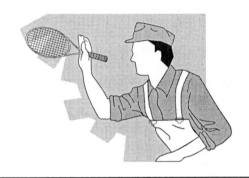

Figure 8-14 ■ **A picture absurdities test item. The person taking the test tells what is wrong with the picture.**

few standardized tests designed exclusively to measure planning and problem-solving ability, although most construction tests involve some degree of planning, and maze tests (see Chapter 7) require both planning and problem-solving. Two less well-known tests that require planning and problem-solving for successful performance are the *tower tests* (Shallice, 1982; Glosser & Goodglass, 1990; Saint Cyr & Taylor, 1992) and the *Tinkertoy test* (Lezak, 1995). In the *tower tests* the test-taker must rearrange colored rings, beads, or blocks on upright dowels to end with a specified arrangement (Figure 8-15). Performance is scored as the number of moves re-

quired to get from the starting position to the specified final arrangement.

In the *Tinkertoy test*, 50 pieces of a standard Tinkertoy set* are placed in front of the patient, who is told *make whatever you want with these*. The patient is then given 5 minutes to plan and execute the construction, after which the examiner asks, *What is it?* and writes down the patient's response. The final construction is scored with a 7-category system that takes into account the number of elements in the construction, whether it has moving parts, whether it is freestanding and three-dimensional, the appropriateness of the name given by the patient, and errors (misfits, incomplete fits, failed fits). According to Lezak, the *Tinkertoy test* allows patients to initiate, plan, and structure a potentially complex activity and carry it out independently.

■ TEST BATTERIES USEFUL IN EVALUATION OF TRAUMATICALLY BRAIN-INJURED ADULTS

Several test batteries for assessment of traumatically brain-injured adults' cognition and lan-

---

* Tinkertoys are collections of small dowels of various lengths and colors, plus connectors, wheels, and other parts that can be assembled into constructions of considerable complexity, complete with moving parts.

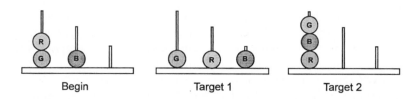

Begin   Target 1   Target 2

Figure 8-15 ▪ A tower test. The test-taker starts with the blocks arranged in a pattern by the examiner. (*Begin* in Figure 8-15.) Then he or she is given a drawing that shows the blocks rearranged in a new pattern, and is asked to move the blocks to create the new pattern with the smallest number of moves possible. The number of moves the test-taker makes to create the new pattern is recorded. *Target 1* in Figure 8-15 can be accomplished in two moves. *Target 2* cannot be accomplished in less than five moves. (From Shallice, 1992.)

guage have been published, but most have weaknesses in coverage, norms, reliability, or standardization that compromise their value as a stand-alone assessment for traumatically brain-injured adults. However, some may be useful as screening instruments to identify gross impairments that can then be evaluated in more detail with follow-up tests that focused on those impairments. Brief descriptions of some of the major test batteries follow. Because there is considerable variability in their psychometric properties, potential users should examine a test's validity, reliability, norms, and coverage before adopting it for routine clinical use.

The *Brief Test of Head Injury* (*BTHI;* Helm-Estabrooks & Hotz, 1991) is a screening test for evaluating adults with severe impairments following traumatic brain injury. The BTHI contains 31 items in seven sections: *orientation/attention, following commands, linguistic organization, reading comprehension, naming (pictures, objects), memory (immediate, recent, remote),* and *visual-spatial skills.* Section scores and BTHI total score can be converted into percentile ranks and standard scores for comparison with the norm group. Clinicians may find the BTHI a useful supplement to (or replacement for) rating scales such as the *Rancho Los Amigos Scale of Cognitive Levels* (Hagen & Malkamus, 1979) for establishing baseline per-

formance and tracking recovery of severely impaired traumatically brain-injured patients.

The *Ross Information Processing Assessment* (*RIPA;* Ross, 1986) contains 10 subtests to assess *immediate memory, recent memory* (2 subtests), *remote memory, spatial orientation, orientation to the environment, recall of information, problem solving/reasoning, organization of information,* and *auditory comprehension and retention.* The RIPA test manual provides normative information for a group of traumatically brain-injured adults and adults with right-hemisphere brain injuries, but does not report normative information separately for each group. Tompkins (1995) has noted that the RIPA has serious deficiencies in validity and reliability.

The *Scales of Cognitive Ability for Traumatic Brain Injury* (*SCATBI;* Adamovich & Henderson, 1992) contains 41 subtests divided among five sections: *perception and discrimination, orientation, organization* (categorization, association, sequencing), *recall,* and *reasoning.* The total score for each section can be converted to a percentile rank and a standard score, and the overall score on the SCATBI can be converted to a severity rating. These converted scores are based on the performance of a norm group that included 244 traumatically brain-injured adults and 78 non–brain-injured adults. The SCATBI has a greater range of item difficulty than most tests for traumatically brain-injured adults. (It contains some items that non–brain-damaged adults are likely to find difficult.) Because of its length (it takes approximately 2 hours to administer the entire SCATBI) and the range of difficulty of test items, clinicians are unlikely to administer the entire test on any single test occasion. It is practical for clinicians to administer individual sections because normative information is provided for individual sections. The SCATBI appears to be a reasonable general-purpose test battery for higher-level traumatically brain-injured adults, although clinicians may wish to supplement information provided by the SCATBI with the results of other tests that provide more detailed information about areas of impairment identified with the SCATBI.

Although not normed on traumatically brain-injured adults, the *Woodcock-Johnson Psycho-educational Battery—Revised* (*WJR;* Woodcock & Johnson, 1989) includes several tests that are appropriate for assessing specific cognitive abilities of higher-level patients with traumatic brain injuries. The WJR has two components—the *Woodcock-Johnson Tests of Cognitive Ability—Revised* (WJR-COG) and the *Woodcock-Johnson Tests of Achievement* (WJR-ACH). The range for most of the subtests in the WJR is from age 2 to 90. The design and standardization of the WJR permit use of most subtests in isolation. For these reasons, the WJR-COG can provide a valuable set of tests for assessing a broad range of abilities across a wide range of ability levels, and performance of traumatically brain-injured patients can reliably be compared with that of non–brain-damaged individuals of equivalent age.

The Woodcock-Johnson Tests of Cognitive Abilities are divided into two sections (batteries). The *standard battery* contains seven subtests. In the *memory for names* subtest, the patient must remember nonsense names (such as *jawl, kiptron*) for cartoon figures, with a name added on each trial until the patient is responsi-

ble for remembering 9 names. In the *sentence recall* subtest, the patient must repeat words and sentences, beginning with a single one-syllable word and progressing to a 33-syllable sentence. In the *visual matching* subtest, the patient must search an array of numbers for a designated target. In the easiest item the patient searches for a single-number target (such as the number *9* in the sequence *8 5 9 2 9 7*). In the hardest item the patient searches for a 3-number combination in a string of 3-digit numbers all of which contain the numbers in the target, but in different order (e.g., the target *493* in the sequence *943 439 493 394 349 943*). In the *incomplete words* subtest, the patient is asked to give a complete word in response to spoken words with missing sounds (for example *koo—ie* for *cookie* or *—anz—or—a—eeuhn* for *transportation*). In the *visual closure* subtest, the patient says the names of common objects represented by incomplete drawings of common objects and photographs of common objects taken from unusual angles. In the *picture vocabulary* subtest, the patient is asked to say the name of pictured items, ranging from familiar high-frequency names *(ball)* to unfamiliar low-frequency names *(fluke)*. In the *analysis-synthesis* subtest, the subject is asked to solve puzzle-like problems by applying symbolically-represented rules.

The *supplemental battery* of the WJR-COG contains 14 supplemental subtests that relate to the subtests in the standard battery in specified ways. In the *visual-auditory learning* subtest, the patient must learn real-word names for non-representational symbols, then "read" sentences made up of the symbols. In the *memory for words* subtest, the patient must learn and recall word lists ranging from one word to eight words. The *cross-out* subtest is a cancellation task in which the patient crosses out target symbols in a linear array of targets and foils. The complexity of the symbols increases across the subtest. In the *sound blending* subtest, the patient is asked to identify fragmented spoken words (such as *p—I—k—n—I—k* for *picnic*).

In the *picture recognition* subtest, the patient is shown drawings of one or more objects (fish, flowers, houses, dogs, and the like) and then is asked to choose them from an array containing the previously shown items plus foils. In the *oral vocabulary* subtest, the patient is asked to provide synonyms and antonyms for familiar words (such as *big*) and unfamiliar words (such as *munificent*). In the *concept formation* test, the patient must learn rules that determine the placement of large and small colored forms. The *delayed recall-names* subtest is a delayed-recall trial (2 to 4 days later) of the *memory for names* subtest in the standard WJR-COG battery. The *delayed recall-visual/auditory learning* subtest is a similarly delayed version of the *visual-auditory learning* subtest in the supplemental battery. In the *sound patterns* subtest, the patient must tell whether pairs of nonsense words are "same" or "different." The "words" range in length from one to eight syllables. In the *spatial relations* subtest, the patient is asked to choose jigsaw-puzzle-like forms that would combine to form a more complex figure. In the *listening comprehension* subtest, the patient is asked to provide a missing word to complete a sentence. The easiest items are single sentences with familiar vocabulary (*Candy tastes —.*) and the most difficult items are sentences in short paragraphs with unfamiliar vocabulary (*Observation of behavior when errors are made can lead to hypotheses regarding learning characteristics. Some people become so frustrated that their emotions cause them to quit. The rigid persist with a strategy that has —.*). In the *verbal analogies* subtest, the patient completes two-word analogies ranging from simple (*bird—flies, fish—*) to complex (*wine is to vat, as water is to —*).

Achievement test batteries provide another important resource for clinicians who wish to evaluate the performance of higher-level traumatically brain-injured patients in tasks that provide an indication of potential success in school or other activities that depend on mathematics, reading, writing, spelling, and vocabulary skills.

The *Woodcock-Johnson Tests of Achievement—Revised* (*WJR-ACH;* Woodcock & Johnson, 1989) are divided into two sections. The *standard battery* contains 12 tests to assess reading, mathematics, and written language. The *supplemental battery* contains two reading subtests and two writing subtests. The *Peabody Individual Achievement Test—Revised* (*PIAT-R;* Markwardt, 1989) contains five subtests. The *mathematics* subtest includes multiple-choice problems ranging from number and symbol recognition to complex algebra and geometry problems. The *reading recognition* subtest includes single-letter and word recognition items, plus items in which the patient reads aloud printed words ranging from familiar *(run)* to unfamiliar *(apophthegm).* Each item in the *reading comprehension* subtest requires the patient to choose from a set of four pictures the one that is described by a printed sentence. Sentence length and vocabulary difficulty increase across the test. The *spelling* subtest is a multiple-choice test in which the patient identifies printed letters and words and chooses correctly spelled words from sets containing a correctly spelled word and three incorrect spellings. The *written expression* subtest requires the patient to write a short narrative related to a picture stimulus. The *general information* subtest is a question-answer test of information gained in daily life, reading, or school. The questions range from easy *(What do you hear with?)* to difficult *(What is a quasar?).*

The PIAT-R manual provides norms for each subtest, so the PIAT-R subtests, like the WJR subtests, can be administered and interpreted individually. Subtest scores can be converted into percentile ranks for ages from 5 to 18, and into grade equivalents and age equivalents.

■ TREATMENT OF TRAUMATICALLY BRAIN-INJURED ADULTS

Treatment of traumatically brain-injured adults is an evolutionary process. Treatment goals and procedures change as traumatically brain-injured patients progress from coma or semi-coma to progressively higher levels of responsiveness and goal-directed behavior. Treatment of comatose or semi-comatose (Stage 1) patients consists primarily of sensory stimulation, and the purposes of treatment are to increase the patient's responsiveness to his or her environment and to accelerate the patient's return to consciousness.

Treatment of confused and agitated (Stage 2) patients usually combines (1) environmental control to reduce the patient's confusion and disorientation and control maladaptive behavior, (2) response contingencies to directly manage and modify inappropriate or maladaptive behavior, and (sometimes) (3) pharmacologic management to reduce the patient's agitation and facilitate new learning or relearning. The overall treatment objectives for patients at this stage of recovery are to stimulate basic motor and sensory functions, reestablish basic self-care skills (feeding, dressing, toileting, grooming), facilitate basic cognitive skills (orientation, attention, memory), facilitate organized thinking and use of knowledge, and reestablish functional communication skills.

Treatment of restless and distractible (Stage 3) patients focuses on increasing the patient's control over his or her immediate environment, stimulating the patient's basic cognitive skills, and increasing the patient's appropriateness in interactions with others.

Treatment of Stage 4 (oriented, purposeful) patients usually is more strongly oriented toward cognitive skills. As patients reach Stage 5 (dependent), it usually becomes apparent that some cognitive impairments will not yield to direct treatment, and the emphasis of treatment shifts to providing the patient with compensatory strategies for dealing with their chronic cognitive impairments. For patients in the late phases of recovery (Stage 6 and beyond), the emphasis shifts toward facilitating the patient's re-entry into family, community, school, and work environments.

Sensory Stimulation

Treatment of comatose and semi-comatose patients depends primarily on *sensory stimula-*

tion, in which the patient is repeatedly stimulated in auditory, visual, tactile, olfactory, and taste modalities. Comatose patients often receive several short (10- to 15-minute) intervals of stimulation every day, together with passive range of motion activities to prevent muscle deterioration. The purposes of sensory stimulation are ". . . to increase the patient's alertness/ arousal and responsiveness to the environment and to prevent sensory deprivation . . . to facilitate changes in responsiveness such as increased consistency and specificity of response and/or decreased latency of response" (Cherney, Halper, & Miller, 1991, p. 59). Many practitioners believe that sensory stimulation hastens traumatically brain-injured patients' emergence from coma, but there is no empirical evidence supporting this belief.[*] Nevertheless, the idea makes intuitive sense, and as Kay and Silver (1989) point out, "It would seem to make sense on rational grounds that it is better to provide regular, gentle sensory input to comatose patients than to let them lie unattended and unstimulated (physically and sensorially) for long periods of time" (p. 149).

Sensory stimulation is an uncomplicated procedure and most adults of average intelligence can learn it within two or three training sessions. Consequently, many speech-language pathologists train family members or caregivers to provide the stimulation and keep a record of the patient's responses. After they are trained, the family members or caregivers provide the stimulation. The speech-language pathologist periodically reviews the response records to de-

---

[*] There is some indirect evidence from studies of animals. Some studies have shown that animals with experimenter-induced brain damage who are then placed in a stimulating environment recover their ability to learn new behaviors to a greater degree than animals with equivalent brain damage kept in a nonstimulating environment. Other studies have shown that animals raised under conditions of sensory deprivation are less active and learn less well than animals raised under normal conditions. (The relevance of the latter research to traumatically brain-injured adults depends on the assumption that their comatose or semi-comatose state causes sensory deprivation.)

termine if changes in the patient's responsiveness are taking place, and also periodically (usually weekly) personally assesses the patient's responsiveness to the stimuli used in the stimulation program.

The nature of sensory stimulation depends on the patient's general level of arousal. Stuporous and lethargic patients may be stimulated with intense stimuli to increase their level of arousal. Excitable and restless patients may receive gentle, rhythmic stimulation to calm them. Some practitioners stimulate phylogenetically older senses (touch, movement, olfaction) first, and stimulate phylogenetically younger senses (vision, audition) later. Most change the form and modality of stimuli frequently to avoid habituation on the part of the patient. Many practitioners believe that familiar voices, touches, and activity are intrinsically more effective than unfamiliar ones, but there is no evidence to confirm this belief.

Environmental Control

Environmental control refers to procedures by which confused and agitated patients' confusion and agitation are controlled and lessened by controlling how the patient's environment is arranged and what happens in it. The objective of environmental control is to alter the patient's daily life environment to create highly stable and predictable surroundings to minimize the patient's confusion and agitation and to maximize successful performance. Significant events (such as therapy appointments, meals, or visits from family members) are organized into a consistent routine, so that they happen at the same time, in the same place, and with the same people each day.

As the patient's agitation and confusion diminish, the controls over the patient's environment are gradually loosened and the salience of cues and reminders within the environment is gradually modulated. These changes permit the patient gradually to assume responsibility for some daily routines while keeping challenges and stresses manageable.

Manipulation of Response Contingencies

Behavior management complements environmental modification by directly targeting certain behaviors to increase the frequency of adaptive behaviors and diminish the frequency of maladaptive ones. Environmental modification controls and shapes behavior and facilitates successful performance by reducing or eliminating stimuli that produce agitation and confusion and replacing them with stimuli that help the patient cope with the environment in spite of cognitive limitations and alterations in emotions and personality. These manipulations of the environment control what behaviorists call *antecedent stimuli* (stimuli that function to elicit or maintain certain behaviors). Another, more direct, way of managing traumatically brain-injured patients' behavior is by manipulation of *response contingencies.*

In Chapter 5, two main categories of what was called *feedback* were identified. *Incentive feedback* denotes a class of stimuli that can maintain (or eliminate) behaviors whose only function is to elicit (or avoid) the feedback stimuli. *Information feedback* denotes a class of stimuli that provides information about the appropriateness, correctness, or accuracy of the responses that elicit the feedback. Traumatically brain-injured patients who are in the early stages of recovery usually are not affected by intangible consequences (information feedback) such as verbal praise or reproof.* Tangible, primary consequences (incentive feedback) are needed. Tangible consequences include positive consequences such as sweets, music, touching, massaging, or other pleasurable stimuli, and negative consequences such as noise, bright light, or painful stimuli.

---

* These patients do not meet the conditions set forth in Chapter 5 under which intangible consequences (information feedback) are effective. They are not internally motivated to get better. Much of their behavior is primitive and unmodulated by cortical control mechanisms. Consequences that depend on interpretation by the cerebral cortex and appreciation of others' intentions and desires are unlikely to affect these patients' behavior.

Four procedures for directly managing behavior by manipulation of response contingencies are available to clinicians. In *positive reinforcement* pleasurable stimuli are delivered contingent on desired responses. In *negative reinforcement,* aversive stimuli are removed contingent on desired responses. In *punishment,* aversive stimuli are delivered contingent on undesired responses. In *extinction,* selected responses elicit neither pleasurable or aversive stimuli.

When response contingencies are used to modify or maintain the behavior of confused and agitated traumatically brain-injured patients, the stimuli used as response contingencies must have incentive value, and they must be delivered consistently following each occurrence of the target behavior(s). Positive reinforcement can increase the frequency of some target behaviors, provided that the behaviors do not require great effort and do not lead to conditions that the patient finds aversive (such as the clinician asking the patient to repeat or elaborate on the behavior).

Negative reinforcement can sometimes be a surprisingly powerful tool for modifying the behavior of severely agitated and confused patients, who prefer being left alone to being harassed by the clinician to make effortful responses that have no immediate payoff. The negative reinforcement procedure proceeds as follows. Initially the clinician makes termination of the session contingent on the patient performing one or two simple responses. As treatment continues, the criterion gradually shifts upward, so that more responses, or more effortful responses, are required to terminate the session. Eventually, as the patient's agitation and confusion lessen and she or he becomes more responsive to pleasurable stimuli the focus shifts from negative to positive reinforcement. (For most patients, the valence associated with the clinician and treatment tasks changes from negative to positive within several treatment sessions, thus nullifying termination of the session as a negative reinforcer.)

Punishment has a limited role in managing the behavior of confused and agitated patients. Physical punishment (slapping, pinching, and so on) is morally and legally impermissible. Milder forms of punishment, such as the sound of a buzzer or loud verbal reproof may sometimes help suppress a confused and agitated patient's inappropriate behavior. However, the suppressive effects of punishment usually are temporary—the behavior usually reappears as soon as the punishment is discontinued. More durable changes in behavior usually can be obtained by other forms of reinforcement and by controlling the patient's environment to minimize undesirable behavior.

Sometimes caregivers unintentionally provide positive reinforcement for undesirable behaviors by paying attention when the patient behaves unacceptably and ignoring him or her at other times. Extinction (removing positive consequences contingent on a behavior) may help eliminate such unacceptable behaviors, especially if extinction is combined with positive reinforcement of alternative behaviors. Extinction may not be very effective at modifying confused and agitated patients' behavior because, as noted above, these patients may consider being ignored by the clinician a positive consequence rather than a negative one.

The response contingencies employed and the schedule on which they are delivered change as the patient recovers. When patients are confused and agitated, only a few important behaviors are treated, response-contingent stimuli have incentive value, and consequences follow every occurrence of the targeted behavior. Negative reinforcement may be an important treatment procedure. As the patient recovers, the number and complexity of behaviors targeted for treatment increase, the emphasis shifts from negative reinforcement to positive reinforcement, and partial reinforcement schedules, in which not every occurrence of the target behavior receives consequences, replace continuous schedules of reinforcement.

Pharmacologic management

Sedatives or antipsychotic drugs are prescribed to reduce some traumatically brain-injured patients' agitation and assaultiveness. The positive result of such medication is that the patients become calmer and less assaultive. The negative result is that many become lethargic and sleepy. Finding the dosage at which a patient's agitated behavior is controlled without making him or her too lethargic and sleepy to benefit from treatment requires careful tuning of the patient's dosage and medication schedule.

Stimulant drugs sometimes are prescribed to improve a traumatically brain-injured patient's alertness and attention, thereby increasing the potential benefits of treatment. (Some stimulants also have antidepressive effects.) Although some studies apparently have shown acceleration of recovery by administration of stimulant drugs, others have shown no meaningful effects. At this time there is no conclusive evidence for their efficacy in facilitating traumatically brain-injured adults' recovery of cognitive abilities.

Some traumatically brain-injured patients become clinically depressed in the later stages of recovery, perhaps in part as a consequence of their experiences with social and vocational dislocation, compromised physical and mental state, financial hardship, isolation, and inactivity, and in part as a consequence of neurochemical imbalances. Antidepressant medications may be prescribed for these patients. However, some antidepressant medications have potential side effects that can compromise memory and motor performance. If possible, they should be avoided, as well as those that are fatal in overdose, if a patient has suicidal tendencies.

A few traumatically brain-injured patients develop psychotic conditions (paranoia, delusional states, schizophrenic-like disorders) several years after their injuries. Antipsychotic medications may be prescribed for these patients. However, most of these medications have extrapyramidal side effects They may cause dyskinesia, suppress volitional movement, or cause Parkinson's-disease–like symptoms. They usually are administered at minimum effective dosage, and patients are carefully monitored for potential side effects.

Anticonvulsant medications are routinely prescribed for patients in the acute stages of recovery from traumatic brain injuries, whether or not the patient actually has had a seizure. These medications have several potential side effects, including sedation, depression, motor impairments, and memory impairments. Consequently, anticonvulsants should not be prescribed indiscriminantly or continued unnecessarily.

Orientation Training

In some respects, procedures to enhance traumatically brain-injured patients' orientation resemble procedures used in environmental control, and orientation training often is the next stage of treatment for patients who are progressing beyond the confused and agitated stage of recovery. Orientation training typically relies on a combination of environmental prompts in the patient's living space, and systematic stimulation, training, and behavior management by patient-care staff and family members.

Environmental prompts come in a variety of forms. Signs, notes, appointment calendars, and appointment books help the patient anticipate upcoming events and assume responsibility for daily routines. Prominently-displayed calendars, clocks, and schedules help orient the patient to time. Signs, labels, and maps showing city, state, and facility names and locations, and signs, posters, and pictures identifying significant locations within the treatment facility (such as the patient's room, lounges, and dining areas) help the patient orient to place. The patient's room may be identified by signs displaying the patient's name and photograph, and by the presence of significant personal possessions. Orientation to person is facilitated by pictures of home and family members displayed in the patient's room and by name tags worn by staff. These passive reminders of time, place, and person are augmented by overt reminders provided by patient-care staff and family members. Patient-care staff and family members include references to time, place, and person in routine interactions with the patient, and may carry out orientation drills to stimulate the patient to acquire and retain a sense of time, place, and person.

Orientation drills come in two basic forms (Cherney, Halper, Miller, 1991). *Passive orientation drills* are best suited for patients in the immediate post-coma phase of recovery, when confusion, agitation, and profound attentional and memory impairments make their active participation in structured treatment activities unlikely. In passive orientation, the clinician provides didactic instruction, demonstration, prompts, and cues to help the patients understand who they are, what has happened to them, where they are, and what hour, day, month, and year it is. Passive orientation sometimes is carried out in group settings. Patients usually are asked to repeat orientation information after the clinician, but are not expected to produce it without prompts or cues. When patients can repeat orientation information after the clinician, the focus of training moves on to training them to verbalize accurate information about person, place, and time. However, the ability to verbalize this information does not mean that the patient has internalized the concepts well enough to incorporate the concepts into daily life activities. That often requires active orientation training.

Active orientation training helps patients incorporate their imperfectly developed sense of person, place, and time into daily life activities. In active orientation training the patient is given responsibility for carrying out daily life activities that depend on internalized concepts of person, place, and time. Passive orientation training usually precedes active orientation training. For example, patients are taught how to tell time (passive orientation) before they are expected to monitor the passage of time or follow appointment schedules (active orientation), and they are taught where they are (passive orientation) before they are expected to find their way around their environment (active orientation).

Component Training

As traumatically brain-injured patients become less disoriented and their confusion dissipates, the focus of treatment shifts toward remediation of impaired cognitive and linguistic processes. Individual processes (attention, memory, language and communication, and so on) are treated individually and in a sequence governed either by a theoretical rationale or the clinician's intuitions and preferences—an approach called *component training*. The objective of component training is to facilitate cognitive and linguistic processes by means of drill activities. The drill activities often have little surface similarity to natural contexts. Specific cognitive or linguistic impairments are sequentially targeted for treatment, and treatment usually consists of repetitive drill, to facilitate and repair the targeted processes, often with paper and pencil or computer-based materials. The expectation is that as the cognitive and linguistic processes improve, general skills that depend on the underlying processes also will improve. In this respect, component training has much in common with the *treat underlying processes* approach to aphasia treatment described in Chapter 6. Component training is most often the mode of treatment for patients at Stage 4, although some patients at late Stage 3 and early Stage 5 may be candidates.

Training Attention Treatment of attentional impairments occupies a prominent place in component training—in part because most traumatically brain-injured adults have attentional impairments, and in part because attention is so important for other cognitive processes. Component training of attention typically addresses *focused attention, selective attention, sustained attention, alternating attention,* and *divided attention* in that order, apparently in the belief that the order represents a hierarchy and that focused, selective, and sustained attention are prerequisites for alternating and divided attention.

Sohlberg and Mateer (1989) described an organized program of treatment for attentional impairments called *Attention Process Training (APT).* APT is based on Sohlberg and Mateer's 5-component model of attentional processes *(focused attention, sustained attention, selective attention, alternating attention,* and *divided attention)* and provides treatment activities to target each of the last four, in the belief that attentional impairments are best treated by targeting specific attentional processes.*

Sustained attention is treated in APT with a series of tasks. In APT *visual cancellation tasks* the patient scans visual arrays that differ in size and spacing and crosses out specified targets. In APT *auditory vigilance tasks* the patient pushes a button to sound a buzzer whenever he or she hears specified targets. The auditory vigilance tasks range from simple *(Push the buzzer every time you hear the number 6)* to complex *(Push the buzzer every time you hear two months in a row, such that the second month comes just before the first one on the calendar).* In APT *serial numbers activities* patients perform tasks such as backward counting, adding 4 and subtracting 2 from successive numbers, and so on.

APT treats *visual selective attention* with materials such as those used in visual sustained attention activities, but in which overlays with distracting designs are placed over the stimuli. *Auditory selective attention* is treated with audiotapes containing the same stimuli as the APT auditory sustained attention tasks, but with targets presented against a background of distract-

ing noise (conversations, news broadcasts, and so on).

APT treats alternating attention with several response-switching activities. In *alternating cancellation tasks* the patient begins crossing out a specified target, such as all the even numbers in an array of numbers. Then, when the examiner says *change,* the patient crosses out all the odd numbers. This continues for several changes in target. In *add-subtract cancellation* the patient begins by adding numbers presented in pairs until the examiner says *change,* at which time the patient begins subtracting, and so on, for several changes in direction. In *Stroop-like activities* the words *high, mid,* and *low* are printed in high, middle, and low positions on a line. The patient is directed to alternate between reading the words and saying their position on the line. Likewise, when the words *big* and *little* are printed in large and small letters.

Divided attention is treated with tasks requiring simultaneous attention to two aspects of a single task, or simultaneous attention to two different tasks. An example of the former is the *card sort task,* in which the patient sorts playing cards by suit, but cards whose name contains a designated target letter must be turned face-down. For example, if the target letter is *e,* all *1s, 3s, 5s, 7s, 8s, 9s,* and *queens* must be turned face down. An example of the latter is requiring the patient to do a letter-cancellation task while simultaneously saying *yes* each time the examiner says the number *5* in a string of randomly arranged spoken numbers.

Sohlberg and Mateer present some preliminary evidence supporting the efficacy of APT in improving four traumatically brain-injured patients' attentional abilities, but conclusive evidence of APT's efficacy awaits additional empirical investigation. Nevertheless, APT represents an innovative, model-driven approach to attention training, and provides a worthwhile source of procedures for systematic treatment of attentional processes. (See also Chapter 7 for more on treating attentional impairments.)

---

* According to Sohlberg and Mateer, focused attention usually is disrupted only in the early stages of emergence from coma. Consequently, it is not a concern for most patients who can participate in structured treatment activities.

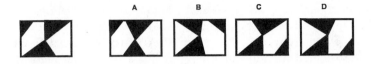

Figure 8-16 ▪ A visual rotation test item. The test-taker chooses from patterns A through D the one that represents a rotated version of the pattern on the left.

Training Visual Processing Treatment of traumatically brain-injured patients' visual perceptual impairments has received less attention than treatment of their attention, memory, and language impairments, and for speech-language pathologists, treatment of visual impairments may seem to lie somewhat outside their usual clinical territory. However, as Sohlberg and Mateer (1989) have noted, visual and visuospatial processing are crucial for carrying out activities of daily living, for adequate job performance, and for performing academic and clerical tasks. Consequently, speech-language pathologists may find that treatment of visual processing impairments is an important part of the overall plan of care for a traumatically brain-injured patient, especially if the visual processing impairments compromise the adequacy or effectiveness of the patient's communication. Some treatment programs for visual processing impairments focus on *discrimination and recognition* of visual stimuli, and others focus on *visuospatial processes.* Work on discrimination and recognition usually precedes work on visuospatial processes, the rationale being that discrimination and recognition are prerequisites to more complex visuospatial processing.

Visual discrimination and recognition treatment activities include visual scanning drills in which the patient scans an array of symbols, designs, or pictures to find those that match a target; visual closure tasks in which the patient must identify familiar objects or scenes based on partial information; and visual figure-ground discrimination tasks in which the patient must identify familiar objects or scenes

presented on an interfering or distracting background.* Sometimes these tasks are presented with a time limit, to increase the speed and efficiency of the patient's visual processing. (See Chapter 7 for examples of some of these tasks.)

Treatment of visuospatial processing impairments usually incorporates drills that emphasize analysis of spatial relationships. Tasks that require the patient to copy or draw simple or complex geometric figures from memory or to construct duplicates of a model constructed by the clinician with sticks or blocks are commonly used in treating visuospatial impairments. These tasks usually are arranged from simple to complex. For example, paper-and-pencil tasks might begin with copying two-dimensional figures, then progress to drawing two-dimensional figures from memory, copying three-dimensional figures, and drawing three-dimensional figures from memory. Tasks that require the patient to mentally rotate printed visual stimuli (Figure 8-16) may also be used to treat visuospatial impairments.

Other tasks require manipulation of stimuli. For example, a patient may arrange blocks in a row to replicate a model constructed by the clinician, then move on to arranging blocks in several rows with different numbers in each row based on the clinician's model, and then move on to duplicating complex three-dimensional constructions (Figure 8-17). More naturalistic stimuli that require visuospatial processing such as

---

* Treatment of attention often precedes treatment of visual perception and discrimination, and sometimes accompanies it.

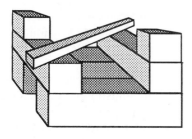

Figure 8-17 ■ A complex block construction test item. The test-taker constructs from a set of blocks a duplicate of a model constructed by the examiner.

maps, floor plans, and flow charts also can be incorporated into treatment of visuospatial impairments.

Training Memory Memory impairments are a common and stubborn consequence of traumatic brain injury, often persisting for years in spite of intensive treatment. The pervasiveness of memory impairments following traumatic brain injury and their resistance to treatment have challenged patients, clinicians, and scientists for several decades. In response to that challenge, clinicians and scientists have developed numerous programs for improving traumatically brain-injured adults' memory.

Most of the early programs attempted to *restore* memory by means of what Sohlberg and Mateer (1989) called the *muscle building* approach to memory rehabilitation—repetitive drills intended to strengthen and revitalize memory. These drills typically required patients to memorize and recall lists of numbers or words, or to read printed texts or listen to spoken narratives and later retell them or answer questions about them. As personal computers became more common and less expensive, computer-based memory retraining programs were marketed to clinics and individuals. These programs resembled their noncomputerized ancestors in that they focused on drills in which patients practiced remembering letters, num-

bers, words, pictures, shapes, and stories. They differed from their predecessors in that they controlled stimulus presentation rate and exposure time with great consistency and accuracy, they kept precise records not only of correct and error responses, but also how long it took a patient to respond to each stimulus, and they did not require the presence of a clinician throughout the treatment session. These advantages contributed to a proliferation of computerized memory rehabilitation programs and their incorporation into the activities of clinics throughout the United States and many other countries.

It gradually became apparent that the payoff of these computerized programs was considerably less than their promise. Articles began to appear in the literature asserting that stimulation approaches to memory rehabilitation in general, and computerized stimulation programs in particular, are of little value for creating meaningful changes in traumatically brain-injured adults' daily life memory performance (Brooks, 1984; Godfrey & Knight, 1985; Gloag, 1985; Hart & Hayden, 1986; Kreutzer & Wehman, 1991; Prigitano and associates, 1984; Robertson, 1990; Schacter, Rich, & Stampp, 1985; and others). As a consequence, stimulation treatment of traumatically brain-injured adults' memory impairments has largely been abandoned in favor of compensatory approaches. However, there are indications that treating attentional impairments may indirectly facilitate memory (Sohlberg & Mateer, 1989).

Training Language and Communication As noted earlier, except for dysarthria, most traumatically brain-injured patients' language and communication impairments are attributable to underlying impairments in basic cognitive processes such as attention, memory, reasoning, abstract thinking, and problem-solving. Attentional impairments can contribute to:

- Poor comprehension of spoken and written verbal materials, especially when they are long or complex.

- Missing details in spoken and written material.
- Fragmented, disjointed, noncoherent spoken discourse.
- Failure to observe turn-taking rules and conventions, and weak or inappropriate topic maintenance.
- Failure to appreciate and respond appropriately to social cues in conversational interactions.

Memory impairments can contribute to:

- Tangentiality, irrelevance, and failure to stay on topic in conversations and writing.
- Excessive repetition and redundancy in spoken and written language.
- Inability to keep goals, objectives, and strategies for improving communication in mind.

Impairments in reasoning and abstract thinking can contribute to:

- Concrete language and inability to appreciate inferences and indirectly stated material.
- Inability to appreciate relationships in spoken or written discourse.
- Egocentrism in social interactions, and inability to appreciate others' points of view.

Impairments in problem-solving can contribute to:

- Failure to implement prescribed strategies to enhance communicative effectiveness.
- Inappropriate conversational content and maladaptive interpersonal behaviors.

These secondary effects of cognitive impairments are most effectively and efficiently treated by treating the underlying cognitive impairments. However, many patients can benefit from direct treatment of communication impairments concurrently with work on the underlying impairments. Direct treatment of communication impairments most often targets the social and interpersonal (pragmatic) aspects of communication. The general objective is to increase the appropriateness, relevance, and efficiency of the traumatically brain-injured patient's par-

ticipation in conversational interactions, and to enhance the patient's ability to follow shifts in topic and appreciate nonliteral aspects of communication.

Traumatically brain-injured patients and patients with right-hemisphere brain damage often exhibit similar impairments in communicative interactions. Both tend to be impulsive and egocentric in interpersonal interactions, to miss nonliteral and implied meanings, to make faulty assumptions based on first impressions, and to be tangential, verbose, circumlocutory, and inappropriate in what they say. Consequently, treatment for traumatically brain-injured patients' impairments in communicative interactions often resembles that for patients with right-hemisphere brain damage (see Chapter 7).

Training Reasoning and Problem-Solving
Reasoning and problem-solving are involved in almost any treatment activity that a clinician might carry out with traumatically brain-injured adults. Nevertheless, clinicians often focus treatment specifically on reasoning and problem-solving, either with paper-and-pencil workbook-like exercises or with on-line coaching and training in simulated or (less often) actual daily life problem-solving situations.

Many workbooks and paper-and-pencil programs for treating reasoning and problem-solving have been published. There is no strong evidence that doing such paper-and-pencil activities has any significant effects on patients' ability to reason and solve problems in daily life. Nevertheless, many clinicians incorporate them into their treatment, usually as homework. Because such exercises may do at least some patients some good, and are unlikely to cause harm, their use in treatment programs seems appropriate, provided clinicians ensure that improved performance on the paper-and-pencil exercises also leads to improved reasoning and problem-solving in daily life activities, and provided that the paper-and-pencil exercises do not take the place of other activities with documented effectiveness.

Training in daily life problem-solving typically entails practice, coaching, and role-playing in simulated daily life situations. Patients with substantial impairments practice reasoning and problem-solving in simple, highly-structured activities such as planning a meal, planning a trip to a shopping center on public transportation, or balancing a checking account. Patients with less severe impairments practice with less structured and more complex activities such as planning a vacation trip, role-playing the return of a defective item to a store for a refund, or role-playing an employment interview. (see also Chapter 7 for more on treatment of reasoning and problem-solving).

Compensatory Training

When component treatment leaves a patient with residual impairments that interfere with daily life activities, the focus of treatment shifts to teaching the patient compensatory strategies by which she or he can circumvent the impairments. These compensatory strategies are deliberate, volitional (and sometimes unconventional) behaviors that allow a patient to carry on activities that would otherwise be impossible. For example, a traumatically brain-injured college student who cannot take notes fast enough to keep up with lectures may be trained to tape-record the lectures, write down only major points while the lecture is going on, and later use the tape recording to fill in the details.

Ylvisaker and Holland (1985) cite four principles of compensatory training:

- Select strategies that fit the patient's strengths and weaknesses.
- Train the patient in the use of efficient and effective strategies.
- Help the patient control or eliminate inefficient, maladaptive, or escapist strategies.
- Guide the patient through practice with the strategies until they become automatic, thereby limiting demands on attention, memory, and other cognitive processes.

Not every traumatically brain-injured patient can learn compensatory strategies, and many that can learn them cannot apply them outside the environment in which they were learned. According to Ylvisaker and Holland, the success of compensatory strategy training depends partly on the patient and partly on the strategy. The patient must recognize the existence of impairments that cannot be alleviated by restitution of underlying processes, must be capable of recognizing problems as they occur or better yet anticipate problems before they occur, and must be capable of invoking a strategy based on recognition of a present or potential problem situation. The strategy must be fitted to the patient's needs, personality, and abilities. It must fulfill an obvious and apparent need that is personally felt by the patient. (Teaching a patient a strategy for remembering information from printed texts will be of little use for a patient who is uninterested in reading.) It must fit the personal inclinations and attitudes of the patient. (Teaching a shy and reclusive patient strategies that require assertiveness and social poise is unlikely to lead to the patient's use of the strategy in daily life.) It must be easy enough that the patient can eventually invoke it automatically and effortlessly. (Strategies that require substantial mental effort from the patient are unlikely to be used outside the environment in which they are learned.)

Barco and associates (1991) addressed the problem of matching compensatory strategies to the ability of the patient by dividing compensatory strategies into four categories, each of which is appropriate for patients at a given level of ability.

External compensations are appropriate for patients who are oriented and responsive but unaware of their impairments and do not recognize when their impairments cause problems. External compensations are changes in the environment initiated by an agent other than the patient. External compensation appears to be synonymous with *environmental control,* discussed earlier.

Situational compensations are appropriate for patients who are aware of their impairments but do not recognize problems as they occur. These patients are taught compensatory strategies to be used habitually in all situations in which they might be appropriate. The patient invokes the strategy when she or he enters the situation and continues it throughout the situation whether or not problems targeted by the strategy occur. For example, a patient who occasionally misses some of the steps in a daily life procedure may routinely use a checklist whenever performing that procedure.

Recognition compensations are appropriate for patients who can recognize problems when they occur but cannot anticipate them. These patients are trained to invoke a strategy when they perceive that a problem of a given nature is occurring. For example, patients may be trained to begin writing down key points whenever they find themselves becoming confused when reading printed materials. Situational and recognition compensations may be identical in content. The difference is that situational compensations are routinely invoked within a specified context, whereas recognition compensations are invoked only when the patient perceives that she or he is having a problem.

Anticipatory compensations are appropriate for patients who can anticipate problems before they occur. These patients are taught to invoke a strategy at the first sign of an impending problem, thereby avoiding the problem. Anticipatory compensations are the most flexible and most effective, but require relatively high levels of awareness and problem-solving ability. Consequently they are beyond the reach of many traumatically brain-injured patients.

The following short list gives examples of some compensatory strategies that may be useful for traumatically brain-injured patients, if the strategies are appropriately matched to the patients.

- A daily log or journal in which the patient (and/or those around the patient) record daily-life happenings, to help orientation.
- Photographs of people who are significant participants in the patient's daily-life activities, with printed names attached, to help the patient's orientation to person.
- Printed maps or diagrams showing routes to and from familiar destinations, to help patients who get lost easily.
- Checklists that show the steps of commonly-performed daily-life activities and procedures.
- Symbols or printed reminders posted in prominent places as cues to perform certain activities.
- Writing down important information and covertly or overtly rehearsing it, to facilitate memory.
- Developing and using standard routines for organizing thinking and problem-solving. (For example, ordering elements from first to last, from most important to least important, or best-known to least-known.)
- Mentally rehearsing problem situations. Using visual imagery and written plans to organize responses to problem situations.
- Organizing the workspace and materials, with tools and materials that are used together, grouped together, and arranged in the order in which they are used.
- Eliminating distractions from the workspace.
- Asking for repetition or clarification when confused or uncertain about others' instructions, plans, or wishes.
- Asking others to write down important information and instructions.
- Asking others to speak slowly or to repeat key points.
- Requesting extra time for performing tasks or taking tests.

Compensatory Approaches to Treatment of Memory Impairments Helping traumatically brain-injured patients compensate for memory impairments is a major focus of treatment for most patients. Compensatory strategies with which traumatically brain-injured adults can circumvent problems generated by impaired memory can be divided into two general categories—those entailing the use of *internal strategies* and those entailing the use of *external aids* (Sohlberg & Mateer, 1989).

Approaches that teach patients to make use of *internal strategies* depend primarily on mnemonic devices or imagery, and are best-suited for facilitating *retrospective memory*. Most mnemonic devices are verbal. In *verbal chaining strategies* patients are taught to arrange lists of to-be-remembered items into sentences or short stories to facilitate subsequent recall of the items. For example, a patient who has to remember the words *dog, book, rain,* and *bus* might put them into a sentence such as *The dog chewed up the book and ran under the bus to get out of the rain.* In *first-letter mnemonic strategies* patients are taught to associate the first letters of words to be remembered with words that can be arranged into easy-to-remember sayings, phrases, or rhymes. (The mnemonic for remembering the names of the cranial nerves is an example of a first-letter mnemonic strategy.)

Sometimes patients may be trained to create a mental image that organizes the words in a to-be-remembered list into a visual scene; for example, a dog lying beside a bus in the rain chewing on a book, or to place to-be-remembered items in a certain location within an imagined scene. When it comes time to retrieve the item from memory, the patient mentally "looks" for it in the imagined scene.

Giles and Clark-Wilson (1993) described a method for helping traumatically brain-injured adults encode, store, and retrieve information from printed materials. They called the method the *PQRST* method (for *preview, question, read, state, test*). First the patient skims the material to learn its general content (*preview*). Then the patient asks himself or herself questions about the central features of the material (*question*). Then the patient actively reads the material with emphasis on answering the questions asked in the previous step (*read*). Then the patient repeats and rehearses the information from the printed material (*state*). Finally,

the patient uses the information to answer the previously-posed questions (*test*).

Some studies have shown that training traumatically brain-injured adults to use such internal strategies improves their performance on tests of recall (Cermak, 1975; Wilson, 1981; 1982; and others), but many more have shown that the beneficial effects of training decay rapidly over time and do not generalize to natural situations (Glisky & Schacter, 1986; Lewinsohn, Danaher, & Kikel, 1977; Schacter & Glisky, 1986; and others). Sohlberg and Mateer (1989) point out that most traumatically brain-injured patients do not have sufficient cognitive resources to carry out such internal strategies successfully:

> The utility of internal memory aids for this population should be suspect. These techniques place heavy demands on patients' already deficient cognitive systems; they are thus ineffectual for many persons with significantly compromised intellectual functions (p. 153).

Parente and DiCesare (1991) also have pointed out that the practical application of internal mnemonic strategies is likely to be limited by traumatically brain-injured patients' general cognitive impairments in attention, planning, and encoding, all of which are necessary for successful use of mnemonic strategies. However, step-by-step strategies such as *PQRST* can be used successfully by some traumatically brain-injured adults if they write down the results of each step in the strategy before moving on to the next step.

External memory aids usually prove more practical for brain-damaged adults than internal strategies. External memory aids are devices that provide cues and reminders to allow traumatically brain-injured patients to compensate for their problems in remembering. They are well-suited for aiding *prospective memory*—remembering to do things at some point in time. They span a range of sophistication from hand-written notes, calendars, and checklists to computers that permit the patient to organize, store, and retrieve complex information. They also include modifications to a patient's environment to facilitate prospective memory.

The simplest, cheapest, and easiest-to-use prospective memory devices are calendars, schedules, checklists, and memory notebooks. Carrying a pocket calendar or printed schedule in which appointments and important events are listed may be sufficient for some high-level traumatically brain-injured patients who can remember to carry the calendar or schedule and periodically check it. However, many traumatically brain-injured patients cannot remember to check the calendar or schedule often enough to prevent missing appointments or other important events. Checklists are helpful for patients who cannot keep track of which tasks they have attended to and which remain undone, but checklists, like calendars, are of little value if the patient cannot remember to check the checklist. The solution for many of these patients is a signaling device (such as an alarm watch) that can be set to sound an alarm at pre-set times to remind them to check their calendar, schedule, or checklist.

Another solution for patients who cannot manage portable memory devices is *environmental modification,* in which memory props are posted in conspicuous locations in the patient's living environment. For these patients, reminder notes can be posted on mirrors and other conspicuous places, and large-print schedules of appointments and activities and check-off sheets to permit the patient to keep track of completed and pending tasks can be posted in strategic locations. Cupboards, shelves, and drawers can be labeled according to their contents, and closets and cupboards can be arranged systematically (for example, items that are used together may be placed adjacent to each other, or items may be arranged alphabetically or by color).

Electronic memory devices may be appropriate for some higher-level traumatically brain-injured adults. Electronic organizers (pocket-sized devices for storing and retrieving informa-

tion electronically) and computer-based personal information managers are more expensive and not as easy to use as calendars, schedules, and checklists, but provide more power and greater flexibility in storing names, addresses, phone numbers, appointments, and other personal information, and are more versatile in sounding alarms and displaying reminders at times programmed into the device. Some of these devices also permit users to print a paper copy of appointment lists or calendars, which can be kept in a notebook. Programming these devices requires sustained attention, reasoning ability, and problem-solving skills, which means that programming will not be in the cards for many traumatically brain-injured patients. However, many who cannot program the devices can still use them successfully in daily life, provided someone in the patient's life is available to do the programming for him or her.

Environmental Compensation

Another way to help traumatically brain-injured adults compensate for residual impairments is to restructure the patient's daily life environment to minimize the effects of the impairments on the patient, family members, and associates. This may require physical modifications to the patient's home, school, or work environment to facilitate access and ease of movement. (For example installation of ramps and modifications of living spaces to accommodate a patient in a wheelchair.) Such physical modifications usually are the province of physical and occupational therapists.

Environmental modifications can also include educating family members, teachers, supervisors, and others who associate with the patient to promote constructive attitudes and to minimize unrealistic expectations. Such education is especially important for families and associates of traumatically brain-injured patients who have residual cognitive impairments but few or no major physical impairments, and who talk and behave much as they did before their injury. Because these patients appear so normal, family members, friends, teachers, and supervisors often expect patients to perform as they did before their injury. When the patient does not meet their expectations, these individuals may become irritated or angry and conclude that the patient is uncooperative, unmotivated, stubborn, or acting out covert hostility and anger. In such situations, environmental modification may entail education of family members about why the patient behaves as she or he does, teaching family members appropriate strategies for interacting with the patient, and helping the patient and family organize the patient's daily life environment to maximize successful interactions and minimize unsuccessful ones.

Environmental modifications might include:

- Establishing consistent routines and regular schedules for daily life activities.
- Instructing family members, friends, and associates in how best to facilitate the patient's success in daily life activities.
- Limiting or eliminating distractions by keeping radios and televisions turned down, and by closing doors and windows to reduce noise from outside or from other rooms.
- Keeping the patient's possessions in designated places, and putting them away when they are not being used.
- Organizing the patient's workspace and scheduling work at difficult tasks for times at which the patient is rested and alert.
- Setting time limits (using alarms, timers) for working at difficult tasks to avoid fatigue and minimize mistakes.

Environmental compensation for higher level traumatically brain-injured patients resembles *environmental control* for confused and agitated patients. The primary difference is one of intent. The intent of environmental control, as the label implies, is to bring the patient's agitated, confused, and maladaptive behaviors under control. The patient does not plan, initiate, or use environmental control procedures in a purposeful way—the patient's behavior is controlled by the environment, rather than the other way around. The intent of environmental compensation is to provide the patient with strategies, prompts, or cues to enhance performance in certain contexts or in certain cognitive or linguistic domains. The patient typically participates in planning the compensations, is actively trained in their use, and employs them in a purposeful and goal-directed way.

■ GROUP TREATMENT

Group treatment usually is an integral part of the overall treatment plan for patients with traumatic brain injuries, especially those at Stages 4, 5, and 6. Group treatment provides a number of benefits, not all of which are related to improvements in cognitive and behavioral adequacy. Some of these auxiliary benefits include helping patients overcome feelings of isolation and loneliness, increasing patients' self-confidence and sense of self esteem, and helping patients express and deal with negative feelings such as anger and hostility.

Groups for traumatically brain-injured patients can serve several purposes, either separately or in combination. The most common purposes are *support, self-assessment, communication, cognitive rehabilitation, generalization,* and *education.* Less common ones are *sensory stimulation* and *orientation.*

Sensory Stimulation Sensory stimulation of groups of patients with traumatic brain injuries is controversial, owing in large part to the questionable efficacy of sensory stimulation for individual patients. Sensory stimulation groups usually are made up of high-level Stage 1 patients and sometimes some low-level Stage 2 patients. Group sessions typically are short (30 minutes or less), and include a mix of orientation activities and sensory stimulation. Orientation activities may include a round of greetings in which the group leader and support staff greet each patient by name and announce to the group each patient's name and an item of interest or two about each patient; announce the date, day of week, and time of day, often supported by visual aids such as a large clock and calendar; announce the name of the treatment facility, its location, and purpose; describe what the weather is like outside the facility and describe the predicted weather for the rest of the day. Stimulation may be provided to the group with recorded music, recordings of radio or television programs or sporting events, movies, slide shows, or other auditory or visual materials. Group stimulation activities sometimes are supplemented with tactile, taste, or movement stimulation of individual patients.

Orientation Group orientation activities may be carried out with Stage 3 and high-level Stage 2 patients. Group orientation activities are similar to those for patients in sensory stimulation groups, except that patients actively participate by acknowledging and repeating the information provided by the group leader and support staff. Some basic interactional skills, such as acknowledging and taking turns, may also receive attention.

Support Group support activities are most appropriate for patients at Stage 4 and higher. Participation in support activities with other traumatically brain-injured patients can help individual patients dispel feelings of isolation, loneliness, and having been unfairly singled out by fate. Observing other group members who are coping with their impairments and progressing may help motivate individual patients and provide hope for the future. Support from other group members may help individual patients deal with failure and overcome disappointments, and by providing a forum for expression of feelings, group activities can help individual patients express and deal with feelings of anger, rage, hostility, and frustration.

Self-assessment Group self-assessment activities are most appropriate for patients at Stages 4 and 5, although some high-level Stage 3 patients may profitably participate. Participation in self-assessment activities can help traumati-

cally brain-injured patients toward a more objective sense of their own abilities and disabilities. Group experiences can serve this function both for patients who minimize or deny their impairments and have unrealistic expectations, and for patients who exaggerate their impairments and minimize or ignore their remaining strengths. (One-on-one treatment, with its highly structured format and the presence of a supportive and helpful clinician, sometimes gives patients an unduly optimistic impression of their potential success in daily life interactions.) Group experiences can also provide opportunities for individual patients to observe and evaluate others' successful and unsuccessful performance as a prelude to evaluating their own performance. (As mentioned earlier, traumatically brain-injured patients usually are better at evaluating others' behavior than their own.)

Communication Group communication activities are most appropriate for patients at Stages 4, 5, and 6. Group communication activities can provide traumatically brain-injured patients with a sheltered but realistic context in which to work on interpersonal interactions. Group members can practice conversational and pragmatic skills such as turn-taking, topic maintenance, requesting, asserting, and clarifying, repairing conversational breakdowns, and monitoring and responding to others' verbal and nonverbal communication. Feedback concerning appropriate and inappropriate behavior can come from group leaders or, more importantly, from other group members. Videotaped role-playing activities, in which participants act out and discuss daily life problem situations, are a common vehicle for providing participants with practice in developing communication and interactional skills. Group review and discussion of the videotapes provide the opportunity for group members to exchange opinions and ideas regarding appropriate and inappropriate behavior in communicative interactions.

Erlich and Sipes (1985) described a communication group format for traumatically brain-injured adults in which group activities center around videotaped role-plays. Target behaviors are specified by group leaders in advance of each role-play. Group leaders make the first videotape, in which they act out a common problem situation to illustrate appropriate and inappropriate behaviors. Then the interactions are replicated by group members in a second videotaped role-play. The videotaped role-plays are reviewed and commented on by the group, with emphasis on behaviors that contribute to or interfere with communicative success. Group members are assigned personal goals in each interaction, and members' successes and failures relative to their goals are discussed by the group. Erlich and Sipes's group format addresses *nonverbal communication* (voice inflection, facial expression, eye contact, posture, and gesture), *communication in context* (topic initiation, topic maintenance, and responsiveness to social context), *message repair* (awareness of communication failure, appreciation of listener needs, and clarification strategies), and *cohesiveness* (organization and sequencing of information, temporal and spatial integrity).

Sohlberg and Mateer (1989) describe several group activities for working on traumatically brain-injured patients' communication skills, including a collaborative drawing task in which group members are divided into pairs. One participant in each pair draws, out of sight of the other, three simple geometric shapes in two colors. Then that participant instructs the other in how to reproduce the drawings without seeing them. When the second participant has finished, they compare drawings and discuss communication successes and failures. In another activity, participants wear hats labeled with phrases such as *ignore me* or *talk down to me.* (Group members cannot see what is printed on the hat they are wearing.) The group members discuss a topic and respond to each participant according to what is printed on her or his hat. After the discussion each member tries to guess

what is printed on their hat, and the group talks about what happened and how they felt.

Cognitive Rehabilitation Group cognitive rehabilitation activities may address attention, memory, reasoning, problem solving, and visual processing, either individually or in combination. Activities may resemble those employed in one-to-one treatment activities, but group members may be divided into teams which compete with one another, collaborate on solving problems posed by the group leader, or take turns in game-like activities that call upon the cognitive processes that are the focus of the day. Competition among teams to finish a task first or to finish a task with the highest accuracy often has a prominent place in cognitive rehabilitation group activities, both to motivate group members to participate, and to keep levels of interest and attention high.

Generalization Generalization of skills, attitudes, strategies, and behaviors acquired in one-to-one treatment to less structured and more natural contexts is an objective of most group activities. Generalization is targeted by means of group activities in which members can practice strategies newly acquired in controlled, structured, and supportive group situations that resemble daily life.

Education Instruction about the physical, cognitive, emotional, psychosocial, and vocational effects of brain injury sometimes is incorporated into group activities. Some instruction may be didactic, with group leaders providing group members with instruction and handouts. Videotapes or films about the effects of traumatic brain injury may be viewed and discussed by the group. Group exercises in which group members make lists of changes in their own lives caused by their brain injury, present the lists to the group, and discuss them with the group also may serve an educational purpose. Guest speakers, such as physicians, social, workers, vocational counselors, or survivors of traumatic brain injury may talk to the group and lead subsequent group discussions.

Efficacy of Group Activities for Traumatically Brain-Injured Adults

Just as there is no convincing empiric evidence for the efficacy of group treatment of aphasic or right-hemisphere damaged adults, there is no convincing empirical evidence for the efficacy of group treatment of adults with traumatic brain injuries, although numerous non–data-based anecdotal reports have appeared in the literature. Deaton (1991) concludes her discussion of group interventions for traumatically brain-injured adults as follows:

> At present, the most glaring gaps in the use of group interventions have to do not with the availability of various models and formats, but rather with the documentation of group effectiveness in improving cognitive skills in particular, as these skills generalize to other social environments. This remains the most significant issue needing to be addressed in future work in this area (p. 199).

By far the most controversial purpose of group treatment is that of sensory stimulation. The appropriateness of sensory stimulation for groups of traumatically brain-injured patients is questionable because, as noted earlier, there is no evidence that sensory stimulation of individual patients hastens their return to consciousness or accelerates their recovery of orientation to person, place, and time. Group experiences for Stage 1 and Stage 2 patients seem unlikely to provide unique benefits, because these patients are at best only dimly aware of the other group members and are unlikely to contribute to or benefit from a group experience. Proponents might argue that group stimulation, like individual patient stimulation, is unlikely to do harm and should be administered because it may do some good. Proponents might also argue that stimulation groups represent a cost saving over individual-patient stimulation. Whether the possible good merits the time and expense of professionals to provide the stimulation remains an important question, and one might argue that providing an ineffective treatment more cheaply is no bargain.

Although there is no convincing evidence for the efficacy of purely orientation groups, the fact that participants are actively responding to the group leaders and to other group members suggests that the group experience may enhance participants' orientation and help them get started on the road toward interpersonal adequacy. However, it is unlikely that patients who qualify for purely orientation groups receive much benefit from the group experience itself. Consequently, the primary advantage of putting them into a group for orientation may be cost savings. Whether orientation groups require professionals as leaders, however, seems questionable.

The widespread use of group activities to provide support, facilitate self-assessment, improve communication, enhance cognitive processing, promote generalization, and educate higher-level patients about the effects of brain injury, and the presence of numerous anecdotal reports of the positive effects of such group activities on traumatically brain-injured patients' performance provide some nonempirical support for their efficacy. At present, there seems to be no compelling reason to reject group activities for traumatically brain-injured adults, provided group members are appropriately selected (they must have adequate comprehension, expressive abilities, and intellectual function to participate, and they must be able to control disruptive behavior), there is at least some degree of homogeneity among group members, and activities and objectives are appropriately selected and matched to the group. However, as Deaton has noted, there is an immediate and pressing need for objective verification of the effectiveness of group treatment for traumatically brain-injured adults.

■ COMMUNITY REENTRY

The final stage of rehabilitation for many traumatic-brain-injury patients is reentry into family, vocational, and community settings. Preparation for community reentry can take several months, and usually takes place in residential facilities *(transitional living facilities)*, wherein a group of traumatically brain-injured patients lives around the clock. Patients in transitional living facilities spend their daytime hours in activities to prepare them for reentry into the community. Less often, preparation for community reentry is carried out in day treatment centers, wherein patients spend their daytime hours, returning home at the end of each workday.

Treatment objectives in reentry facilities differ across facilities and, of course, differ for different patients. However, most facilities offer programs directed toward the following objectives.

- Provide patients with a supportive context in which to practice and perfect strategies and procedures for increasing their daily-life competence.
- Prepare patients for carrying out routine self-care activities (personal hygiene, eating, sleeping, grooming, and so on) in daily life.
- Develop patients' interest in domestic, vocational, leisure, and social activities, and develop the patient's ability to perform them.
- Establish routines for commonly-occurring daily life domestic, vocational, leisure, and social activities, and train patients to perform them.
- Train patients to allocate appropriate amounts of time for daily activities and to use time constructively.
- Evaluate patients' competence for vocational, school, and leisure-time activities.
- Place patients in appropriate work, school, and leisure activities and work with employers, teachers, family, and others to ensure success.

These objectives are approached by means of one-to-one training sessions, group activities, and structured experiences in real-life situations. Patients typically spend part of the day working on specific behavioral goals and strategies for increasing daily-life competence, and

part of the day in group activities wherein they practice daily-living skills, discuss problems and their potential solutions, and provide each other with social and emotional support. Sometimes patients spend time in real-life or simulated vocational, school, or social settings in which they can practice strategies that may be needed for success in work, school, or social endeavors. Family members, employers, and other individuals who may play important parts in a patient's daily life also may participate.

Treatment activities within reentry facilities are carried out by teams made up of occupational therapists, recreational therapists, speech-language pathologists, vocational counselors, neuropsychologists, social workers, and other professionals. As the patient progresses, the team gradually withdraws structured treatment, training, and support, and expects increasing independence on the part of the patient. Discharge from the facility and return to home, family, work, and/or school mark the end of formal rehabilitation for most patients, although periodic counseling visits may continue for some.

■ WORKING WITH THE FAMILY

Providing support, reassurance, information, and direction to family members is an important part of the clinical management of patients with traumatic brain injuries. The family's need for support, reassurance, and information is greatest in the acute post-injury interval, and their need for direction is greatest in the middle and later stages of recovery. Polinko (1985) has divided the time following traumatic brain injury into three stages: *injury to stabilization, return to consciousness,* and *rehabilitation.*

For the family, the first stage (injury to stabilization), when the patient remains unconscious, is a period of apprehensive waiting. The patient is in the care of strangers and is surrounded by an alarming array of monitors and support systems. The family may have been told that the patient may not recover. They anxiously watch for the first signs of consciousness, and often misinterpret the patient's purposeless activity as purposeful behavior. According to Polinko, this is a time of shock and denial, with occasional breakthroughs of panic, and family members need extensive support and reassurance. During this time, family members also need objective information about what has happened and what the outcome is likely to be, but they may have difficulty assimilating it because of their emotional upset. Consequently, information may have to be reiterated a number of times. As time goes on, denial may be replaced by bargaining, in which family members attempt to strike a deal with a deity or with fate by promising acceptance of the patient's condition, acts of contrition, changes in attitudes, or changes in behavior, if only the patient survives.

The second stage (return to consciousness) usually brings feelings of relief that the patient will live, together with apprehension about the extent to which he or she will recover. Family members continue to watch anxiously for hopeful signs, and may continue to interpret incidental patient behaviors as signs of recovery. Because the patient's emergence from coma often occurs rapidly, family members may be led into overly optimistic predictions about the patient's eventual recovery. Educating family members about the usual course of recovery from traumatic brain injury and helping them separate true prognostic indicators from fallacious ones is an important part of the clinician's responsibility during this stage.

By the time the third stage (rehabilitation) is reached, most families have accommodated to the accident and its aftermath, and have moved past the stage of denial to reasonably realistic expectations about the future. The beginning of structured treatment activities usually is a time of increased hope and optimism for family members, often leading to rosy expectations of what will be accomplished in treatment. This time of hope and optimism often gives way to anxiety, confusion, and eventually anger with the patient and with professional staff, as the patient's recovery fails to meet their optimistic expecta-

tions. The unpredictable nature of recovery from traumatic brain injury adds to the family's confusion, and sometimes to their anger. When periods of rapid recovery alternate with periods of little change, family members may accuse the patient of slacking off, or clinicians of not doing their job. When it becomes apparent that the patient will not recover to premorbid levels, the family will need help in planning how they will cope with a future that includes an impaired family member.

As time goes on, families usually return to a semblance of normal functioning. Family members who once stayed with the patient during major parts of the day return to work, and the patient no longer is the central focus of family life. Responsibility for the patient may be divided among family members. One family member may assume primary responsibility for visiting the patient and interacting with caregivers, and another may take responsibility for dealing with financial and logistical adjustments. During this time the family may need the help of psychologists, social workers, rehabilitation therapists, speech-language pathologists, and community service agencies in setting up a long-term plan for incorporating the brain-injured patient into family life in a way that is maximally beneficial for the patient and the family. Throughout the course of the patient's recovery the family will need continuing and conscientious assistance from all members of the patient-care team in order to survive the mental, emotional, and physical consequences of the patient's injury.

■ KEY CONCEPTS

• Traumatic brain injuries can be divided into those caused by high-velocity missiles, in which the skull and meninges are penetrated *(penetrating brain injuries),* and those caused by the head striking a stationary object or by a low-velocity object striking the head, but leaving the skull and meninges intact *(nonpenetrating brain injuries).* Nonpenetrating injuries are more common, except in armed conflicts.

- Traumatic brain injuries have both *primary consequences* (damage caused by forces acting on the brain at the time of injury) and *secondary consequences* (the body's physiologic responses to the primary consequences). Secondary consequences often are more devastating than primary consequences.

- Recovery from traumatic brain injury depends primarily on the amount of tissue damage caused by the injury. Length of coma is one of the most dependable indirect indicators of the amount of tissue damage sustained by a traumatically brain-injured patient. Patient-related variables such as age, chemical abuse, and socioeconomic status have less strong effects on recovery.

- Assessment of traumatically brain-injured patients' communicative/cognitive status requires materials and procedures that are appropriate for patients spanning a range of impairment from comatose to minimally impaired. For severely-impaired patients, assessing level of consciousness and responsiveness to stimulation are primary concerns. For moderately impaired patients, assessment tends to focus on orientation, attention, memory, and problem-solving. For mildly impaired patients, assessment tends

to focus on abstract thinking, reasoning, planning, and problem-solving.

- Treatment of traumatically brain-injured patients, like their assessment, requires materials, procedures, and treatment goals that are appropriate for patients spanning a range of impairment from comatose to minimally impaired. For severely impaired patients, sensory stimulation, environmental control, behavior modification, and pharmacologic management are important treatment procedures. For moderately impaired patients, component training of attention, visual processing, memory, language and communication, reasoning, and problem-solving may be appropriate. For mildly impaired patients, treatment often focuses on compensatory training and environmental compensation.

- Group treatment plays an important part in most comprehensive treatment programs for traumatically brain-injured adults. Treatment groups may serve any of several functions, individually or in combination, including stimulation, orientation, support, self-assessment, communication, cognitive retraining, generalization, and education.

- The final stage of treatment for most traumatically brain-injured patients is *community reentry,* in which the patient is prepared for reentry into family, vocational, recreational, and community settings.

Dementia

Dementia is a condition in which the affected individual exhibits diffuse impairment of intellect and cognition. The intellectual and cognitive impairments usually are accompanied by behavioral and personality changes, and sometimes by physical impairments such as movement disorders or sensory disturbances. The most widely used definition of dementia is from the *Diagnostic and Statistical Manual of Mental Disorders–Revised* (*DSMIII-R*; American Psychiatric Association,

1987). The *DSMIII-R* definition requires that a patient have impaired short-term and long-term memory, plus impairment in at least one of the following: *abstract thinking, personality, judgment, language, praxis, constructional abilities,* or *visual recognition.* The patient's impairments must be severe enough to interfere with work, social activities, and relationships with others.

Cummings and Benson (1992) provide a slightly different definition of dementia. They define dementia as "an acquired persistent impairment of intellectual function with compromise in at least three of the following spheres of mental activity: language, memory, visuospatial skills, emotion or personality, and cognition (abstraction, calculation, judgment and executive function, and so forth)" (Cummings & Benson, 1992, pp. 1-2). Cummings and Benson's definition requires that the condition is acquired, distinguishing it from congenital conditions such as mental retardation; that it is persistent, distinguishing it from transitory states such as acute confusional states; and that the deficits cross several areas of mental function, distinguishing it from more focal impairments such as aphasia or psychiatric disturbances.

Dementia almost always begins late in life and its incidence increases rapidly with age. The presence of dementia doubles with every 5-year increment in age after age 65 (Jorm, Korten, & Henderson, 1987). Dementia is the most common single diagnosis in nursing-home occupants. Estimates of its prevalence vary greatly, because of differences in where samples were obtained, variable definitions of dementia, and differences in the ages of the patients studied. Estimates of the prevalence of dementia in the over-65 population range from 6% to about 30%, with the highest rates in the oldest age groups. Because of declining birth rates and longer life expectancy, the proportion of elderly persons in the world population is increasing, and with it the incidence of age-related illnesses, including dementia.

Three major categories of dementia have been identified, based on the neuroanatomic location of the causative central nervous system pathology. *Cortical dementias* are caused by pathology that affects the cerebral cortex. *Subcortical dementias* are caused by pathology that primarily affects the basal ganglia, thalamus, and brainstem. *Mixed dementias* are caused by pathology that affects both cortical and subcor-

tical structures. The most common causes of cortical dementia are *Alzheimer's disease* and *Pick's disease.* The most common causes of subcortical dementia are *Parkinson's disease* and *lacunar state.*

Dementia often occurs as the primary (or only) symptom of neurologic impairment, as in Alzheimer's disease and Pick's disease. Vascular disease sometimes causes dementia, and dementia often appears in the late stages of extrapyramidal diseases such as Huntington's or Parkinson's disease. Depression, metabolic disorders, nutritional deficiencies, drug overdoses or drug side-effects, infections (encephalitis, meningitis), and poisoning with toxic substances (mercury, lead, arsenic) may also lead to dementia. Some dementias (such as those caused by metabolic and nutritional disorders, drugs, infections, or toxins) are reversible, but most are irreversible and progressive. The most frequent single cause of dementia is Alzheimer's disease.

■ CORTICAL DEMENTIAS
Alzheimer's Disease

Alzheimer's disease is the fastest-growing and most expensive clinical population in the United States (Bayles, Kazniak, & Tomoeda 1987). It accounts for 25% to 30% of all dementias, and comprises up to 50% of all progressive dementias (Cummings, 1990). Alzheimer's disease is two to three times more common in women than in men (Cummings & Benson, 1983). The cause of Alzheimer's disease is not known, and a massive research effort currently is underway to determine its causes and to develop preventive and palliative medical treatments.

Neuropathology of Alzheimer's Disease
Alzheimer's disease is characterized by microscopic changes in the neurons of the brain, particularly in the cerebral cortex. These changes are detectable only by direct examination of brain tissue. They are not visible on CT scans or MRI scans. Definitive diagnosis of Alzheimer's

disease depends on the presence of *neurofibrillary tangles, senile plaques,* and *granulovacuolar degeneration.* *

Neurofibrillary Tangles Neurofibrils are "filamentous structures seen with the light microscope in the nerve cell's body, dendrites, axon, and sometimes synaptic endings" (Stedman's Medical Dictionary, 1990). In Alzheimer's disease, the neurofibrils become twisted, tangled, and contorted. These changes are easily seen using standard microscopic techniques. Neurofibrillary tangles are not unique to Alzheimer's disease. They sometimes are present in the brains of patients with Parkinson's disease, patients with hereditary cerebellar ataxia, and occasionally in the brains of elderly patients with no obvious neurologic disease. Neurofibrillary tangles may be the neuron's nonspecific reaction to central nervous system damage (Cummings & Benson, 1983; Bayles & associates, 1987).

Neuritic Plaques Neuritic plaques (sometimes called *senile plaques*) are "minute areas of tissue degeneration consisting of granular deposits and remnants of neuronal processes" (Cummings & Benson, 1992, p. 67). Neuritic plaques tend to concentrate in the cortex and subcortical regions of the brain. Neuronal synapses are markedly reduced by neuritic plaques; consequently synaptic transmission is adversely affected. In addition to Alzheimer's disease, neuritic plaques are seen in Down syndrome, Creutzfeldt-Jakob disease (a rare disease characterized by progressive degeneration of corticospinal nerve fibers), and in the brains of some normal elderly adults.

Granulovacuolar Degeneration Granulovacuolar degeneration refers to a condition in which small fluid-filled cavities containing granular debris appear within nerve cells. The pyramidal neurons in the hippocampus (a deep brain structure that seems to be important in memory) are most frequently affected. Granulovacuolar degeneration also is seen in other diseases, and occasionally appears in the brains of normal elderly persons. However, Tomlinson and Henderson (1976) report that if 10% or more of hippocampal neurons are affected, dementia is always present.

Neuropathologic changes in Alzheimer's disease are not diffuse and equally distributed throughout the brain. Neurofibrillary tangles and senile plaques are most frequent in the temporoparietal-occipital junctions and the inferior temporal lobes (Figure 9-1). The frontal lobes, the motor and sensory cortex, and the occipital lobes usually are spared.

The cause of Alzheimer's disease is unknown, although several causes have been proposed, including aluminum poisoning, disturbed immune function, infection with a slow virus, and genetically transmitted disturbance of neuronal function. There is no cure for Alzheimer's disease, and no specific medical treatment other than management of the patient's symptoms. Tranquilizers may be administered to control combativeness and aggression, or if the patient is depressed, antidepressants may be administered. The patient's diet and fluid intake can be monitored and managed to prevent dehydration and maintain adequate nutrition. The patient's environment can be managed to stimulate the patient, maintain orientation and cognitive abilities, and prevent social isolation. Counseling and other support services can be provided to the patient and the patient's family.

The Course of Alzheimer's Disease The course of Alzheimer's disease is one of gradual deterioration. The first symptoms are subtle, and include lapses of memory (usually the first symptoms reported), impairments in reasoning, periods of poor judgment, disorientation except in highly familiar environments, and alter-

---

* In the late stages of Alzheimer's disease the brain shrinks, the ventricles become larger, and sulci become wider. These changes are visible on CT or MRI scans.

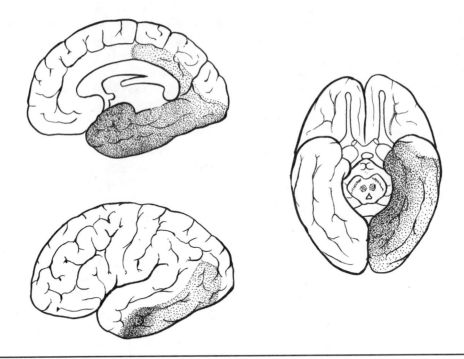

Figure 9-1 ■ Cortical brain regions most often affected by Alzheimer's disease. The darker shading represents the cortical regions most frequently affected.

ations of mood (depression, apathy, irritability, suspiciousness). Personality and interpersonal behaviors remain relatively intact during the early stages of the disease, although the patient may withdraw from social contact. As the disease progresses the patient's mental impairments become more obvious and general. Intellect and cognition become increasingly impaired, and disturbances of language and communication appear. The patient becomes restless and agitated, gets lost even in familiar environments, and wanders off when not supervised. Episodes of incontinence appear. These symptoms gradually worsen, and in the final stages leave the patient with profound motor problems (rigidity or spasticity), complete incontinence, and loss of almost all intellectual and cognitive abilities. The patient usually dies of aspiration pneumonia or infection.

Language and Communication in Alzheimer's Disease Language usually is less affected than cognition and intellect in the early stages of Alzheimer's disease, although mild word-retrieval problems, verbal paraphasias, and subtle comprehension impairments may appear early. Phonology, syntax, articulation, and voice quality are well-preserved until the late stages. Highly practiced responses (counting, reciting the alphabet, reciting the days of the week, and so on) are spared until the late stages of the disease, but responses calling for sustained attention and mental flexibility (describing pictures or objects, explaining proverbs, comprehending abstract material) are compromised early. As the patient's dementia progresses into the middle stages, perseverative responses and literal paraphasias appear, and the content of the patient's speech becomes empty,

T A B L E   9 - 1

Effects of dementing illnesses on communication

Early stages

Sounds:	Used correctly.
Words:	May omit a meaningful word, usually a noun, when talking in sentences. May report trouble thinking of the right word. Vocabulary is shrinking.
Grammar:	Generally correct.
Content:	May drift from the topic. Reduced ability to generate series of meaningful sentences. Difficulty comprehending new information. Vague.
Use:	Knows when to talk, although may talk too long on a subject. May be apathetic, failing to initiate a conversation when it would be appropriate to do so. May have difficulty understanding humor, verbal analogies, sarcasm, and indirect and nonliteral statements.

Middle stages

Sounds:	Used correctly.
Words:	Difficulty thinking of words in a category. Anomia in conversation. Difficulty naming objects. Reliance on automatisms. Vocabulary noticeably diminished.
Grammar:	Sentence fragments and deviations common. May have difficulty understanding grammatically complex sentences.
Content:	Frequently repeats ideas. Forgets topic. Talks about events of past or trivia. Fewer ideas.
Use:	Knows when to talk. Recognizes questions. May fail to greet. Loss of sensitivity to conversational partners. Rarely corrects mistakes.

Late stages

Sounds:	Generally used correctly, but errors are not uncommon.
Words:	Marked anomia. Poor vocabulary. Lack of word comprehension. May make up words and produce jargon.
Grammar:	Some grammar is preserved but sentence fragments and deviations are common. Lack of comprehension of many grammatic forms.
Content:	Generally unable to produce a sequence of related ideas. Content may be meaningless and bizarre. Subject of most meaningful utterances is the retelling of a past event. Marked repetition of words and phrases.
Use:	Generally unaware of surroundings and context. Insensitive to others. Little meaningful use of language. Some patients are mute; some are echolalic.

From Bayles KA: Management of communication disorders associated with dementia. In Chapey R, editor: *Language intervention strategies in adult aphasia.* Baltimore, 1994, Williams & Wilkins, p. 542.

circumlocutory, and littered with jargon. As the patient's dementia progresses into the late stages, the patient's speech becomes rapid and incoherent *(flight of ideas),* and echolalia (automatic and uncontrollable repetition of what others say) or pallilalia (uncontrollable repetition of what the patient has previously said) may appear. Table 9-1 summarizes the progression of communication impairment as Alzheimer's disease progresses.

Although aphasic adults and those with Alzheimer's disease may both perseverate and circumlocute, the nature of the perseveration and circumlocution differ. The perseverative responses of patients with Alzheimer's disease represent intrusion of unrelated thoughts rather than persistence of response sets, as is true for perseverative responses of aphasic persons. An aphasic patient might say, *That's a comb* to *comb,* and *That's a comb* to *fork* on the next trial, whereas a patient with Alzheimer's disease might say, *That's a comb—I lost my comb when I was four* to *comb* on one trial, and *It was a pretty red comb* to *fork* on the next trial. (The *thought* is stuck in the mind of the patient with Alzheimer's disease; the *word* is stuck in the mind of the patient with aphasia.) The patient with Alzheimer's disease circumlocutes because he or she has forgotten the topic or lost her or his train of thought, whereas the aphasic patient circumlocutes because of word-retrieval failure. The aphasic patient's circumlocution is strategic and directed either toward retrieving the missing word or replacing the missing word with other words. Patients with Alzheimer's disease circumlocute because they cannot maintain a consistent train of thought, do not comprehend what their conversational partner is saying, or do not grasp the overall sense of the interaction.

Language pragmatics usually are affected early and progressively deteriorate as Alzheimer's disease progresses. In the early stages the patient observes conversational turn-taking rules but talks too long, strays from the topic, and repeats himself or herself without awareness. The patient has difficulty grasping implicit meanings such those involved in humor, sarcasm, or nonliteral statements. As the disease progresses the patient stops initiating conversations and ignores social conventions such as greetings and farewells. In the terminal stages the patient loses all orientation to self and surroundings and does not use language in any meaningful way.

Pick's Disease

Pick's disease, like Alzheimer's disease, is a degenerative disease affecting neurons in the cerebral cortex. Its etiology is unknown. It is characterized by two neuronal abnormalities—the presence of *Pick bodies* within neurons and a proliferation of *enlarged neurons.* Pick bodies are dense globular formations within the neuron cytoplasm. They are about the same size as the cell nucleus and contain numerous neurofibrils. The progression of Pick's disease is marked by gradual reduction in brain mass (particularly in the frontal lobes and anterior temporal lobes) and neuron loss throughout the cortex. There is no cure for Pick's disease, and its treatment, like that of Alzheimer's disease, is symptomatic, consisting of medications to control changes in mood and temperament and behavioral intervention to maintain orientation and manage the patient's daily life behavior.

The Course of Pick's Disease The progression of symptoms in Pick's disease differs from that of Alzheimer's disease. Whereas intellect is compromised early in Alzheimer's disease and personality is spared, in Pick's disease personality disturbances usually are the first symptoms observed. The initial stages of Pick's disease are dominated by alterations in personality and emotion. Social behavior deteriorates early, with general disinhibition of behavior. The patient exhibits inappropriate jocularity, inappropriate comments and behavior (often sexual), and "loss of personal propriety" (Cummings & Benson, 1992). Judgment and insight are soon compromised, and stereotypic repetitive sequences of behavior often develop (such as folding napkins and putting them away, taking them out, refolding them, and putting them away again and again). Increased eating and weight gain are common in the early stages of Pick's disease.

Language and Communication in Pick's Disease As Pick's disease progresses, the patient's intellectual functions begin to deteriorate. The pattern of deterioration differs from that of Alzheimer's disease. In Alzheimer's disease, memory and orientation to place are compromised early, but language remains relatively intact. In Pick's disease, memory and orientation usually are well preserved until the late stages of the disease, but language breakdown appears early and remains prominent in the middle and late stages of the disease. Word-retrieval failures, impaired confrontation naming, circumlocution, and empty speech (use of generic words such as *thing* for specific words) are common expressive abnormalities. Echolalia and verbal stereotypes *(mama-mama-mama, me-me-me)* may be present. The patient may repeat the same story over and over. Comprehension impairments for both spoken and printed materials become prominent by the middle stages of Pick's disease and become progressively more profound as the disease progresses. In the final stages patients with Pick's disease become completely mute and profoundly demented, with severely impaired memory, orientation, and cognition. Like patients with Alzheimer's disease, those with Pick's disease usually succumb to aspiration pneumonia or infection.

▪ SUBCORTICAL DEMENTIAS

Alzheimer's and Pick's disease primarily involve cortical neurons. Consequently, impairments of cortical functions (memory, intellect, language) are seen early, and motor impairments are seen late in the course of the disease. Dementia also appears in the late stages of more than a dozen subcortical degenerative diseases. Although there are differences in symptoms and in the manner in which they appear, all dementias associated with subcortical pathology are characterized by early motor impairments and relative preservation of mental abilities until late in the course of the disease.

Parkinson's Disease

Parkinson's disease is a degenerative disease affecting nuclei in the midbrain and brainstem. The primary symptoms are motoric and include muscle rigidity, tremor, and slowness or abolition of movement. Parkinson's disease usually becomes evident between the ages

of 50 and 65 years and is more likely to affect men than women. The usual first symptom of Parkinson's disease is tremor, but sometimes immobility and "poverty of movement" (Adams & Victor, 1981) are noticed by family members before tremor appears. As the disease progresses, memory, problem-solving, abstract reasoning, and other mental functions requiring sustained mental effort become increasingly compromised. Affect becomes progressively flattened, and many patients become depressed. Treatment with L-dopa or similar medications suppresses dyskinesia and slows mental deterioration for about two thirds of patients with Parkinson's disease. Many patients eventually reach the point at which their disease progresses in spite of medications, at which time their mental functions also deteriorate.

Huntington's Disease

Huntington's disease is a hereditary degenerative neurologic disorder characterized by increasingly severe chorea and dementia. The first symptoms usually are the appearance of involuntary movements (chorea). At first the movements are slight and the patient may simply appear restless and fidgety. Personality changes develop as the involuntary movements become more obvious. "Patients begin to find fault and complain about everything and to nag other members of the family; they may be suspicious, irritable, impulsive, eccentric, or excessively religious, or may exhibit a false sense of superiority" (Adams & Victor, 1981, p. 804). Irritability is common, and emotional outbursts frequently occur. Mental deterioration usually follows, sometimes becoming obvious several years after the first signs of chorea. Memory usually is affected first, followed by general mental slowing and attentional impairments. Language usually remains relatively intact until the late stages of the disease, except for language tasks requiring sustained attention, memory, and judgment. Dysarthria frequently accompanies the development of the patient's movement disorder. In the final stages of the disease patients with Huntington's disease are mute, incontinent, and profoundly demented. Death usually occurs within 10 to 20 years of the onset of symptoms.

Progressive Supranuclear Palsy

Progressive supranuclear palsy (PSP) is a rare progressive disorder that usually begins during the sixth or seventh decade of life. Death usually occurs 5 to 10 years after the onset of symptoms. The first symptoms are motor abnormalities: paresis of gaze (downward gaze first, then upward gaze), rigidity of the neck and trunk (axial rigidity) which gradually extends to the limbs, and pseudobulbar palsy (exaggerated palatal and laryngeal reflexes, drooling, swallowing disturbances, and heightened emotionality). Slowly progressive dementia may eventually appear but usually remains mild. Language usually remains well-preserved, but the patient's speech is dysarthric, slow, and deficient in loudness, sometimes with stuttering-like repetitions (Albert, Feldman, & Willis, 1974). In the late stages of PSP, speech may be completely unintelligible, and mutism is not uncommon.

Human Immunodeficiency Virus Encephalopathy (Aids Dementia Complex)

Active HIV infections often lead to pathologic changes in the subcortical white matter and basal ganglia, which eventually extend to the cortex (Navia, Jordan, & Price, 1986). Consequently, the early symptoms usually are extrapyramidal (weakness, slowness, rigidity, dyskinesia), with later appearance of cortical involvement (impaired perception, memory, intellect, and language). In the early stages, AIDS patients' spontaneous speech is slow, labored, sparse, and dysarthric, but their language is well-preserved. As the disease progresses, memory disturbances become more prominent and impairments in visuospatial abilities, abstract thinking, and reasoning appear. In the terminal stages of the disease patients become incontinent, mute, and immobile. Death usually occurs within 6 months after the onset of central nervous system pathology.*

■ CEREBROVASCULAR DEMENTIA (MULTI-INFARCT DEMENTIA)

Vascular disease is second to Alzheimer's disease as a cause of dementia (Cummings & Benson, 1992). Three etiologic subgroups of cerebrovascular dementia have been described in the literature.

Multiple cortical infarcts are the result of thrombotic or embolic occlusions of cortical arteries. The occlusions cause focal neurologic symptoms, and repeated occlusions yield an increasingly diffuse pattern of impairment, eventually culminating in dementia. The patient's symptoms depend on the cortical areas involved in each incident and include those commonly associated with cortical damage (aphasia, apraxia, neglect, and so on). Hemiparesis and hemiplegia are commonly associated with cortical infarcts, but dysarthria and swallowing impairments are not.

Lacunar state results from multiple small infarcts in the lenticulostriate arteries supplying the basal ganglia, thalamus, midbrain, and brainstem. The first symptoms include dysarthria, swallowing disturbances, pseudobulbar palsy, weakness, and sometimes tremor, because of involvement of extrapyramidal and brainstem structures. Intellect and language are preserved until late in the course of the disease. Dementia is the end-state for 70% to 80% of patients with lacunar state (Celesia & Wanamaker, 1972).

Binswanger's disease is a rare disease caused by multiple infarcts in subcortical white matter, usually in patients with severe hypertension. It is caused by thrombotic or embolic occlusion of long penetrating arteries from the cortex that

---

* However, at the time this is written, new combinations of drugs appear to have promise for slowing the progression of AIDS and extending AIDS patients' life span.

supply subcortical white matter tracts. The first symptoms of Binswanger's disease usually are focal, but repeated infarcts yield more pervasive mental and physical impairments, eventually culminating in dementia. Clinically, the symptoms of Binswanger's disease resemble lacunar state, but combinations of cortical and subcortical neurologic signs are common, and motor impairments appear somewhat later in Binswanger's disease than in lacunar state.

Most patients with multi-infarct dementia have a history of hypertension, heart disease, or both, and a history of multiple strokes is a common finding. The first symptoms typically are abrupt in onset and generate focal neurologic signs (perceptual, motor, or sensory impairments) which represent the localized effects of the first infarct. Subsequent infarcts produce a stepwise progression of symptom development, as additional focal impairments are added with each new infarct. The slow accumulation of neurologic events eventually produces diffuse cerebral involvement and dementia. The patient's personality and intellect usually are preserved until the late stages of the disease, although depression, irritability, and emotional lability may appear early.

■ DIAGNOSIS AND ASSESSMENT OF DEMENTIA

Scales for Rating Dementia Rating scales occupy a prominent place in the diagnosis of dementia. Most can be completed after observing the patient and interviewing family members and caregivers, and most require little or no specialized training to complete. Rating scales provide a quick but usually insensitive estimate of a patient's intellectual abilities. Most can identify the presence of moderate to severe dementia but are insensitive to subtle intellectual decline. Detecting the subtle signs of early dementia requires standardized, sensitive, and reliable tests of cognitive and linguistic performance administered by a specialist trained in their administration and interpretation.

Well over a dozen scales for rating dementia severity have been published, of which six or eight are in fairly general use. Two that have gained relatively wide acceptance are the *Blessed Dementia Scale* (*BDS;* Hachinsky, Illiff, Zihlka, & associates, 1975) and the *Global Deterioration Scale* (*GDS;* Reisberg, Ferris, DeLeon, & Crook, 1982). The *Blessed Dementia Scale* uses information obtained from family members, caregivers, and the patient's medical record to estimate the patient's ability to get along in daily life activities. The BDS has two sections (Table 9-2). In one section the patient's performance of eight general daily life activities is rated. In the other section the patient's performance in 14 specific activities is rated. For some items the severity of the patient's impairments, as well as their presence, is rated. Increasing scores on the BDS represent increasing severity of impairment. The maximum possible score is 28. Patients scoring below 4 are considered unimpaired; scores of 4 to 9 represent mild impairment; and scores of 10 and higher represent moderate to severe impairment (Eastwood, Lautenschlaeger, & Corbin, 1983).

The *Global Deterioration Scale* provides a scale by which patients can be assigned to one of six levels representing increasing severity of intellectual impairment (Table 9-3). The GDS is completed by a clinician after interviewing the patient, family members, and caregivers. Ratings are based on general descriptions of behavior provided in the GDS and, raters must use some judgment and intuition to arrive at a rating because few patients are likely to precisely match the descriptions provided. The GDS provides for relatively coarse estimates of intellectual level. However, it covers a wide range of levels of impairment and ratings are easy to make and fairly reliable. Consequently, it occupies a place in rating dementia similar to the place occupied by the *Rancho Los Amigos Scale of Cognitive Levels* (Hagen & Malkamus, 1979) for rating cognitive functioning following traumatic brain injury.

T A B L E   9 - 2

The Blessed Dementia Scale

Feature	Score
Changes in Performance of Everyday Activities	
1. Inability to perform household tasks	1
2. Inability to cope with small sums of money	1
3. Inability to remember short lists of items, e.g., in shopping	1
4. Inability to find way about indoors	1
5. Inability to find way about familiar streets	1
6. Inability to interpret surroundings	1
7. Inability to recall recent events	1
8. Tendency to dwell in the past	1
Changes in Habits	
9. Eating	
Messily with spoon only	1
Simple solids, e.g., biscuits	2
Has to be fed	3
10. Dressing	
Occasionally misplaces buttons, etc.	1
Wrong sequence, commonly forgetting items	2
Unable to dress	3
11. Sphincter control	
Occasional wet beds	1
Frequent wet beds	2
Doubly incontinent	3
12. Increased rigidity	1
13. Increased egocentricity	1
14. Impairment of regard for feelings of others	1
15. Coarsening of affect	1
16. Impairment of emotional control	1
17. Hilarity in inappropriate situations	1
18. Diminished emotional responsiveness	1
19. Sexual misdemeanor (appearing *de novo* in old age)	1
20. Hobbies relinquished	1
21. Diminished initiative or growing apathy	1
22. Purposeless hyperactivity	1

Diagnosis

Diagnosing Subcortical Dementia Most subcortical dementias are delayed consequences of extrapyramidal system disease, and are preceded by characteristic impairments of volitional movements (for example, the rigidity, tremor, and slowness of movement of Parkinson's disease, the choreiform movements of Huntington's disease, or the eye muscle and axial muscle paralysis of progressive supranuclear palsy). For these patients diagnosis of subcortical dementia is a relatively straightforward mat-

TABLE 9 - 3

**Stages of the *Global Deterioration Scale* and clinical characteristics
of patients at each stage**

GDS stage	Clinical phase	Clinical characteristics
1. No cognitive decline	Normal	No complaints of memory impairment, no evidence of memory impairments in the clinical interview.
2. Very mild cognitive decline	Forgetfulness	Subjective complaints of memory impairment, such as decline, forgetting where one has placed familiar objects, or forgetting formerly well-known names. No objective evidence of memory impairment in the clinical interview. No objective impairment in work or social situations. Patient is appropriately concerned with regard to symptoms.
3. Mild cognitive decline	Early confusional	The patient exhibits the first obvious impairments. Exhibits more than one of the following: (1) The patient gets lost when traveling to an unfamiliar location. (2) Co-workers are aware of patient's impairments. (3) Family or caregivers note word-retrieval and naming impairments. (4) The patient does not remember material from recently read printed material. (5) The patient has unusual difficulty in remembering names upon introduction to new people. (6) The patient loses or misplaces items of value. (7) Attentional impairments are obvious in clinical testing. Objective evidence of the patient's memory impairment is observable only with an intensive interview conducted by a trained professional. The patient exhibits impaired performance in demanding work and social situations. The patient begins to deny impairments and exhibits mild to moderate anxiety.
4. Moderate cognitive decline	Late confusional	The patient exhibits obvious impairments in a careful clinical interview. Impairments consist of: (1) Diminished knowledge of current and recent events. (2) Mild impairment of personal history. (3) Attentional impairments on difficult tasks. (4) Impaired ability to travel, handle personal finances, and so on. The patient usually has minimal or no impairments in: (1) Orientation to time and person. (2) Recognition of familiar persons and faces. (3) Ability to travel to familiar locations.
5. Moderately severe cognitive decline	Early dementia	The patient can no longer survive without assistance from others. In a clinical interview patients cannot provide major, relevant, current information (such as address or telephone number, the names of close members of their family, the name of the high school or college from which they graduated). The patient frequently exhibits some disorientation to time (date, day, season) or place. The patient knows his own name and usually knows the names of spouse and children. He or she eats and toilets him or herself unassisted but may need assistance in choosing what to wear.

Continued.

Stages of the *Global Deterioration Scale* and clinical characteristics of patients at each stage—cont'd

GDS stage	Clinical phase	Clinical characteristics
6. Severe cognitive decline	Middle dementia	The patient may occasionally forget the name of his or her spouse or primary caregiver. The patient is largely unaware of recent events and experiences, but retains sketchy knowledge of his or her past life. The patient is generally disoriented to time and place. The patient usually requires assistance with activities of daily living, and may be incontinent. The patient may retain the ability to travel to familiar locations, but cannot travel to unfamiliar locations without assistance. The patient remembers his or her own name and recognizes familiar persons. Personality and emotional changes become obvious, and may include: (1) Delusional behavior. They may accuse their spouse of being an imposter, talk to imaginary persons, or to their own image in the mirror. (2) Obsessive behavior, such as continual repetition of a simple cleaning activity. (3) Anxiety, agitation, and occasional violent behavior. (4) Loss of willpower because the patient cannot maintain thought long enough to determine a purposeful course of action.
7. Very severe cognitive decline	Late dementia	The patient loses all verbal ability. Speech may consist only of grunting. The patient is incontinent of urine and requires assistance with eating and toileting. The patient loses the ability to walk. Generalized neurologic signs and symptoms are obvious.

Data from Reisberg and associates: The global deterioration scale for assessment of primary degenerative dementia. *Am J Psychiatry* 139:1136-1139, 1982.

ter, because the diagnosis of the original disease precedes and leads to the diagnosis of dementia. When the first signs of mental decline appear the clinician can reasonably assume that the signs portend onset of dementia, because the clinician knows that dementia often appears in the late stages of these diseases. However, a few patients with subcortical disease exhibit signs of mental decline before detectable motor impairments appear. For these patients there is no pre-existing disease that points to a diagnosis of dementia, and the clinician must base the diagnosis on the pattern and progression of the patient's mental impairments. The diagnostic routine for these patients is essentially the same as the routine for patients with cortical dementia.

Diagnosing Cortical Dementia Diagnosing early-stage cortical dementia is a challenging assignment. Patients in the early stages of cortical dementia rarely exhibit overt signs that point unequivocally to a diagnosis of dementia. They usually arrive at the medical facility with vague complaints of forgetfulness, mental slowing, apathy, depression, fatigue, and similar non-definitive symptoms. The reports of family members often are not helpful in diagnosing dementia because they tend to focus on the most disruptive alterations in the patient's behavior and overlook subtle signs of general cognitive decline that signal the beginning of dementia.

Diagnosis of early cortical dementia usually requires comprehensive testing to detect subtle disturbances of intellect and cognition. The most sensitive tests for detecting early dementia are mentally challenging tests that require abstraction, analysis and integration of information, reasoning, and problem-solving. Highly practiced and automatic activities (counting, reciting the days of the week, reciting the alphabet), or structured tasks with highly constrained responses (confrontation naming, phrase and sentence repetition, copying) are too easy to be of much use in detecting early dementia. The most sensitive tests of language and communication are likely to be those that call for mental flexibility and creativity, such as generative naming, story telling or retelling, or comprehension of abstract or implied spoken or printed material.

Diagnosis of middle- and late-stage cortical dementia usually poses no great clinical challenge to experienced practitioners. Patients in the middle and late stages of dementia exhibit such striking impairments of intellect, orientation, and behavior that a patient interview, the reports of family members and caregivers, and brief assessment of orientation, memory, and intellect usually are sufficient to confirm the diagnosis.

One diagnostic question that occasionally confronts speech-language pathologists is whether a patient has cortical dementia or is aphasic.* Patients who have cortical dementia

are most likely to be confused with patients who have Wernicke's aphasia (and sometimes vice-versa), because both produce vague, empty, paraphasic, and circumlocutory speech, and both have significant comprehension impairments. The key to differential diagnosis of these syndromes is administering nonverbal tests of intelligence and problem-solving. Patients with aphasia do better on nonverbal tests than on verbal ones, whereas patients with dementia perform poorly on both. Additional diagnostic help may come from knowledge of the onset and progression of symptoms. Dementia usually has insidious onset and develops slowly, with gradual worsening from subtle impairments of memory, reasoning, and problem-solving to gross impairments of intellect, personality, and behavior. Aphasia usually has abrupt onset and symptoms develop rapidly, peaking within a few minutes to a few hours, followed by slow improvement over weeks to years.*

Measuring the Patient's Impairments and Plotting Their Course

Speech-language pathologists make perhaps their most important contribution to management of dementia by administering standardized and reliable tests to identify the patient's communicative strengths and weaknesses and to provide dependable baseline measures against which the effects of interventions can be assessed. Tests of language and communication supplement tests of verbal and nonverbal intelligence, immediate and remote memory, and attention and perception to provide a compre-

---

* Physicians and other health-care personnel sometimes use the label *aphasia* in a broad sense to refer to any language impairment caused by brain damage, whether or not it is the patient's primary impairment. Speech-language pathologists use the label in a narrow sense to refer to specific patterns of language impairment disproportionate to any other cognitive or behavioral impairments the patient may have.

* Several cases of slowly progressive aphasia have been reported in the literature (Duffy, 1987; Heath, Kennedy, & Kapur, 1983; Kirshner, Tanridag, Thurman, & Whetsell, 1987; Mesulam, 1982). Slowly progressive aphasia is a poorly understood phenomenon, and some patients who initially exhibit slowly progressive aphasia eventually become demented. Nevertheless, the potential existence of slowly progressive aphasia makes the rate of symptom onset a slightly less dependable sign for differentiating dementia from aphasia.

hensive description of the patient's impairments. Evaluation of the patient's speech, language, and communicative abilities may include a comprehensive aphasia test such as the *Boston Diagnostic Aphasia Examination* (Goodglass & Kaplan, 1983), the *Western Aphasia Battery* (Kertesz, 1982), or a test of functional communication such as *Communicative Abilities in Daily Living* (Holland, 1980).* Separate tests of auditory and reading comprehension, spelling, arithmetic, vocabulary, and confrontation naming may also be appropriate, depending on the patient's level of impairment.

The *Arizona Battery for Communication Disorders of Dementia (ABCD;* Bayles & Tomoeda, 1991) is a clinical assessment instrument for identifying and quantifying communicative deficits of persons with dementia (specifically that caused by Alzheimer's disease). The ABCD contains four screening subtests to evaluate *speech discrimination, visual perception and literacy, visual fields,* and *visual agnosia,* plus 14 subtests to evaluate *mental status, linguistic expression, verbal memory, linguistic comprehension,* and *visuospatial construction.* The subtests in the ABCD are based on the authors' research on the language performance of 175 normal older adults and 300 adults with dementia-producing illnesses. The ABCD is standardized on 50 adults with Alzheimer's disease and 50 age-matched normal adults. Reliability and validity information as well as cut-off scores for normal performance are provided in the test manual. The ABCD appears to be an efficient and informative instrument for assessing communicative disabilities of persons with either suspected or confirmed dementia, and the au-

thors report that the ABCD correlates with several other measures of dementia severity.

■ MANAGEMENT OF DEMENTIA

When dementia is progressive (most is), the objectives of treatment are to slow the progression of the dementia, facilitate constructive interactions between the patient and his or her environment, ensure the patient's safety, keep the patient healthy, and provide support and direction for the patient and caregivers. Achieving these objectives requires the coordinated efforts of medicine, nursing, speech-language pathology, neuropsychology, clinical psychology, occupational, recreational, and physical therapy, social work, dietetics, and others.

Helping the Patient Cope with Dementia

Memory impairments, disorientation, and confusion are particularly distressing to patients in the early and middle stages of dementia (and their families). Managing these impairments is an important part of the overall plan of care for patients in the early and middle stages of dementia.

Memory Impairments Memory impairments usually are the most salient concern of patients in the initial stages of dementia, and helping the patient cope with them can enhance both the patient's mental health and his or her competence in daily life. There are no effective procedures for improving demented patients' memory, so the goal of treatment is to help the patient find and use compensatory strategies. Many of the compensatory memory strategies for traumatically brain-injured adults described in the last chapter of this book also work well for patients with dementia. The following strategies are likely to be particularly useful for patients with dementia-related memory impairments.

- Establish a routine schedule of activities that remains constant from day to day, to minimize demands on memory. Keep a written

---

* The *Western Aphasia Battery* and *Communicative Abilities in Daily Living* have been used to evaluate communicative abilities of persons with dementia, and some normative information has been published (Appell, Kertesz, & Fishman, 1982; Fromm & Holland, 1989; Murray, Marquardt, Richardson, & Nalty, 1984).

schedule of things to be done each day, and cross out or check off entries as they are completed.

- Set an alarm clock to go off when specific things are to be done. Put a note by the clock telling what is to be done when the alarm goes off.
- Keep a list of important phone numbers near the telephone, with emergency numbers listed first and the others listed in order of frequency of use.
- Make up a checklist of things to be done when leaving the house (turn off lights, turn off the stove, get keys to house, and so on). Put the list by the exit customarily used by the patient.
- Keep personal possessions in a consistent location.
- Keep things used at the same time or in the same activity together (for example, keep coffee pot, filters, coffee, and coffee measure on the same shelf).
- Carry a card listing the home address and telephone numbers of at least two caregivers.
- Wear an identification bracelet containing the same information.

Disorientation and Confusion Episodes of disorientation and confusion often occur during the early stages of dementia and increase in frequency and magnitude as the patient's dementia progresses. The first episodes often cause the patient emotional upset and anxiety disproportionate to their actual effects on the patient's life. Helping the patient deal with disorientation and confusion in a constructive way, and reassuring the patient that occasional episodes of disorientation and confusion are manageable, are important aspects of patient care in the early stages of dementia. The following list gives examples of strategies and compensations that may help early stage dementia patients minimize disorientation and manage confusion.

- Keep a large calendar in a highly visible place. Cross off the current day before going to bed at night. (Caregivers may have to do this, if the patient can't remember to.)
- Wear a digital calendar watch that shows time (preferably with AM and PM indicated) and date in a legible size. Some have built-in alarms that can be set to signal repetitive events, although most are too faint to be heard by patients with diminished hearing.
- Have someone draw maps showing how to walk to nearby stores, shops, and businesses. The maps can be illustrated with pictorial representations of landmarks that can be used for orientation by the patient.
- Put cards showing the contents of cabinets, dressers, and bureaus on doors and drawer fronts.

For more on managing disorientation and confusion, see the discussion of orientation procedures for traumatically brain-injured patients in the preceding chapter.

Language and Communication Speech-language pathologists play an important part in facilitating communication between the demented patient and her or his caregivers, and in helping the patient maintain communicative competence. This requires attention to both the patient and her or his caregivers. During the early stages, when the patient's dementia is mild, the patient can be an active participant in efforts to maintain and enhance communication. As the patient becomes less able to comprehend instructions, remember communicative strategies, and carry them out, caregivers assume more of the responsibility for maintaining communication with the patient.

Patients in the early stages of dementia usually have sufficient language comprehension and speech to manage routine daily life situations. However, subtle attention and memory impairments compromise the patient's retention of spoken or printed materials, comprehension deteriorates in noisy and distracting environments or when several people are talking, and intermittent word-retrieval failures create annoying gaps in the patient's output, although they do not seriously interfere with communication. Patients in the early stages of dementia (and their families and caregivers) need help in identifying how communication is affected by the patient's impairments, assistance in identifying the most important targets for management, help with devising strategies for working around the patient's communication impairments, and direction in putting the strategies into practice.

By working with the patient the speech-language pathologist can identify impairments that compromise the patient's communicative functioning and help the patient develop strategies for working around compromised communicative functions and emphasizing intact ones. A patient who cannot remember spoken instructions but who can read and write might compensate by writing down the instructions and reading them when needed. A patient who cannot get the gist of reading material might compensate by underlining or highlighting the main point of each paragraph and making marginal notes about the current topic of the material.

The speech-language pathologist also can help the patient differentiate communication impairments that actually interfere with communication from those that are primarily annoyances. Word-retrieval failures in which the patient comes up with synonyms may be annoying but usually do not cause communication breakdown, whereas failing to provide listeners with accurate referents for pronouns has more serious consequences. As the patient's communication impairments worsen, the speech-language pathologist provides emotional support and helps the patient change his or her communicative strategies to compensate for changes in the severity and nature of the communication impairments.

As the patient's competence diminishes, the responsibility for maintaining communication shifts to family members and caregivers, and they become the primary focus of intervention. The speech-language pathologist instructs caregivers about how the patient's impairments affect communication and how caregivers can modify communicative interactions to capitalize on the patient's strengths and circumvent his or her weaknesses. The family may be taught to keep messages short, simple, and concrete, to increase message redundancy by repetition and paraphrase, to slow speech rate to provide more time for the patient to process what he or she hears, and to confirm that the patient understands by having her or him repeat back what the family member or caregiver says. As the patient's communicative abilities continue to decline, the speech-language pathologist helps caregivers make the adjustments needed to maintain and maximize communication with the patient.

■ THE LONG HAUL: THE FAMILY AND THE DEMENTIA PATIENT

The speech-language pathologist, as a part of the professional team, works closely with the dementia patient's family, providing support and reassurance together with information, guidance, and instruction. Understanding what the family experiences as the patient's dementia progresses is crucial if the speech-language pathologist's contributions to care and management are to be appropriate and effective. The magnitude and the nature of the problems, stresses, and issues faced by the family inexorably increase as the patient's intellectual and behavioral dysfunction progress from annoying to enervating.

The Early Stages: Onset of Symptoms to Diagnosis

The first symptoms of dementia usually are subtle and may be overlooked by the family. The patient becomes forgetful, irritable, and inattentive, but remains oriented and socially appropriate. These initial symptoms often are interpreted by family members as depression, stubbornness, or normal aging. As the patient's gradual decline continues, family members may remain unaware that something ominous is happening, until seizures or dyskinesia appear, or until a change in routine (such as going on vacation) leaves the patient disoriented, confused, and frightened.

As the family's concern deepens, they seek professional help in finding out what is wrong. The diagnosis of dementia almost always begins a period of intense stress for the patient and family members, during which counseling and support for the patient and family are crucial. The patient needs help in dealing with feelings of grief and anger about what is happening, help with diffuse anxiety about the future, and a plan for coping with the future. The family needs information about what is happening to the patient and information about what the course of the patient's illness is likely to be. The family, like the patient, needs help in dealing with the grief, anger, and anxiety that almost invariably follow the diagnosis.

During the very early stages of dementia, most of the patient's symptoms are inconveniences, and families often spontaneously adapt to them. They no longer permit the patient to run errands unaccompanied, because they discover that she or he tends to get lost. They take away the patient's car keys because they sense that impaired judgment and slow reactions place the patient and other drivers in danger. They gradually assume the patient's responsibilities for shopping, paying bills, and housecleaning, and they take over the patient's legal and financial affairs. They shape family routines around the patient's eccentricities. If the patient lives alone, the family keeps track of the patient with frequent telephone calls and visits, but gradually the family is forced to assume more and more responsibility for the patient, until the family decides that the patient must move in with a family member. This decision often is precipitated by a dramatic incident (the patient may start a fire by leaving a stove or iron unattended, may get lost and be picked up by the police, or may enter neighbors' houses uninvited and at inopportune times).

As the patient's dementia progresses it becomes apparent that something more ominous than normal aging is taking place. The patient's lapses of memory increase in frequency and duration, until they constitute a profound impairment in storing and retrieving new information. The patient begins to neglect self-care and has to be reminded, cajoled, or nagged to bathe, keep clothing clean, and maintain oral hygiene. Progressive impairments in judgment, attention, and memory put the patient and others at risk when the patient uses gas stoves, ovens, power tools, ladders, or other appliances, tools, or machinery. As the patient's confusion and disorientation progress, he or she becomes progressively more anxious, depressed, and irritable and withdraws from interactions with family members and others. Periodic violent emotional outbursts may occur. The patient takes frequent naps during the day and wakes up and wanders about during the night. For some patients the wake-sleep cycle is reversed, and the patient sleeps all day and is awake all night. Some patients become indifferent to food and fail to maintain adequate caloric and fluid intake without supervision. Others become gluttonous, eating continuously and indiscriminantly unless they are supervised.

The Middle Stages: Caring for the Demented Patient in the Home

Most demented patients are cared for by family members at home until the burden becomes intolerable, at which time the patient is placed in a nursing home. The period of at-home care can range from 1 or 2 years to 10 or 15, depending on how rapidly the patient's dementia progresses, and on the family's tolerance for the disruptions caused by the patient's dementia. During the middle stages of dementia the patient and family members must cope with the patient's increasingly severe mental impairments and the disruptive effects of the impairments on family relationships and routines. Most patients go through a period of frustration and anger about what they have lost, combined with worry and anxiety about the future. As time goes on, many become depressed and apathetic and withdraw from family and friends, with intervals of self-imposed social isolation punctuated by angry outbursts over trivial incidents.

Family members are distressed by the patient's increasing mental impairments and her or his unpredictable changes in mood. They may be angry and resentful about the burden that has been imposed on them, although they are unlikely openly to express or acknowledge their anger and resentment and may feel guilty about it. Family relationships and routines are disrupted as caregivers become increasingly responsible for the patient and are forced to neglect other family activities and responsibilities. As the patient's deterioration progresses and his or her appreciation of reality declines, depression and apathy may be replaced by hyperactivity, wandering, and stereotypic repetitive behaviors. The patient can no longer be left alone and requires continuous supervision. Family members have to take responsibility for bathing the patient and supervising her or his oral hygiene. When incontinence develops, the burden of caring for the patient escalates. Additional deterioration often brings verbal abusiveness, aggressiveness, and episodes of physical violence, further disrupting family relationships and increasing family members' anger, resentment, and guilt.

This phase of the patient's illness requires continuing education, support, and therapy for the family. Family members need education about why the patient behaves as she or he does, and about how disruptive behaviors can be controlled or eliminated by manipulating the patient's environment or by medications. Family members need help in setting up a safe, predictable, and stable environment for the patient. They may need help in dividing caregiving responsibilities among family members, and they may need encouragement and direction in taking advantage of respite-care and day-care services and support groups. As the burden of caring for the patient escalates, family members need help in planning for and accomplishing nursing home placement. Throughout this phase of the patient's illness family members need help in dealing with their feelings of resentment, anger, apprehension, and guilt, the latter becoming especially prominent as the family begins to contemplate the patient's placement in a nursing home.

The Late Stages: The Patient in a Nursing Home

Most demented patients spend their last years in a nursing home. Although the physical burden of caring for the patient has been removed by nursing home placement, the emotional burden carried by family members continues, often augmented by feelings of guilt over abandoning the patient to the care of strangers and by feelings of loss that accompany the patient's departure from home. As the patient's physical condition becomes more fragile, family members are faced with decisions about whether or not heroic measures should be employed to sustain the patient's life. During this time family members need continuing help in resolving their often conflicting feelings about their own needs and their obligations to the patient, and in making decisions about when and how to terminate procedures for prolonging the patient's life.

The patient's demise does not end the family's need for advice, support, and reassurance. The period of mourning following the death of the demented family member usually is brief, perhaps because the family has been mentally preparing for the patient's demise for months or years. Although the mourning period may be short, the grief felt by family members may be intense, owing perhaps to the release of emotional tensions that have built up over years of the patient's illness. Professional counseling and support during this period may help family members acknowledge and understand their feelings and reactions to what they have been through and may help them reconstruct and repair family relationships that have been damaged or distorted by the pressures of caring for the demented patient.

Helping Caregivers Cope with Dementia

Caregivers for demented patients face numerous problems related to the patient's declining intellect, mood swings, and changes in behavior. Although the decline in the patient's abilities cannot be arrested or reversed, the effects of the patient's intellectual impairments can be minimized, the patient's mood swings can be diminished, and distressing behaviors often can be controlled or eliminated by environmental manipulation and behavior management techniques similar to those used with traumatically brain-injured adults.

Rabins, Mace, and Lucas (1982) surveyed the families of 55 patients with irreversible dementia to determine what they considered the major problems in caring for their demented family member. Their results are summarized in Table 9-4. The five most frequently reported behaviors were *memory disturbance, catastrophic reactions, demanding and critical behavior, night waking,* and *hiding things.* The five behaviors most frequently reported *as problems* were *physical violence, memory disturbance, catastrophic reactions, incontinence,* and *delusions.* Every respondent reported the presence of memory problems and almost all (88%) considered it a problem. On the other hand, fewer than half of the respondents (47%) reported the presence of physical violence, but almost all (94%) who reported it considered it a problem. Only 11% reported unsafe or excessive smoking, but two thirds of those reporting it considered it a problem. Clearly, the perceived importance of a behavior problem is not determined by its frequency of occurrence alone, but reflects the amount of emotional stress or inconvenience the problem causes for family members.

Hostility, Verbal Abuse, and Physical Violence Combative, aggressive, and accusatory behaviors rank high on the list of problem behaviors, both in Rabin and associates' report and in the general literature on management of patients with dementia. Caregivers need to understand that emotional outbursts, combativeness, and physical attacks often are predictable, based on previous incidents, that they frequently are preceded by warning signs, and that they often represent the patient's response to being pushed beyond his or her ability to deal with a situation or event. Many times such outbursts can be eliminated by removing their precipitating stimuli.

> A man with dementia became violently angry when he saw his wife paying the monthly bills, perhaps because he felt that she was usurping his role as head of the household. The wife realized what precipitated her husband's outbursts and began paying the bills while her husband took his usual morning nap. This eliminated the outbursts.

Many outbursts are preceding by warning signs that, if heeded, can prevent the patient's emotional state from escalating out of control. Warning signs can be diverse and tend to be idiosyncratic. They range from subtle signs such as increased body rigidity, aversion of gaze, or increased respiration rate to more obvious behaviors such as crying and arguing. Teaching caregivers to recognize such warning signs and respond to them by slowing the pace of the activity, doing something else, or diverting the patient's attention can reduce the frequency of such outbursts.

If caregivers understand that the demented patient's outbursts may be an involuntary response to demanding or too-difficult situations, their responses to the outbursts are likely to change in constructive ways. They are less likely to regard the patient as stubborn and uncooperative and less likely to see the patient's

T A B L E 9 - 4			

Percentage of families reporting the occurrence of behaviors and the percentage considering the behavior to be a problem

Behavior	Mention behavior (%)	Behavior	Considered a problem (%)
Memory disturbance	100	Physical violence	94
Catastrophic reactions	87	Memory disturbance	93
Demanding, critical behavior	71	Catastrophic reactions	89
Night waking	69	Incontinence	86
Hiding things	69	Delusions	83
Communication difficulties	68	Making accusations	82
Suspiciousness	63	Hitting	81
Making accusations	60	Suspiciousness	79
Uncooperative at meals	60	Uncooperative at bathing	74
Daytime wandering	59	Communication difficulties	74
Uncooperative at bathing	53	Demanding, critical behavior	73
Hallucinations	49	Unsafe driving	73
Delusions	47	Hiding things	71
Physical violence	47	Daytime wandering	70
Incontinence	40	Unsafe or excessive smoking	67
Unsafe cooking	33	Night waking	59
Hitting	32	Uncooperative at meals	55
Unsafe driving	20	Unsafe cooking	44
Unsafe or excessive smoking	11	Hallucinations	42
Inappropriate sexual behavior	2	Inappropriate sexual behavior	0

Data from Rabins, Mace, and Lucas, 1982.

emotional outbursts as a personal affront. They are more likely to look for what pushed the patient out of control and to eliminate or control the precipitating stimuli. Understanding that accusations and suspicion may be the patient's attempts to reconcile misplaced possessions, forgotten appointments, and unexpected changes in routine may lead caregivers to increase the predictability and orderliness of the patient's environment rather than arguing with the patient about the accuracy of their suspicions.

Finally, caregivers should understand that hostile and aggressive behavior can be caused by physical pain or illness and that patients who exhibit sudden increases in aggressive behavior may need medical evaluation. Because some medications can cause increased aggressiveness, changes in mood or tolerance for frustration that occur when medications are begun or dosages changed should be evaluated by a physician. Sometimes medication may be prescribed to control a patient's violent behavior, but because of their depressive effects on alertness and general mental functioning, they should be prescribed only when behavioral methods fail to provide sufficient control.

Memory Impairments Caregivers can help the patient cope with her or his memory impairments by maximizing the orderliness and predictability of the patient's living environment. Keeping schedules and activities consistent from day to day lessens the amount that the patient has to remember in order to manage daily life activities. Keeping the patient's possessions in a consistent place and putting them away when they are not in use lessens the patient's need to remember where they are and increases the likelihood that she or he will find them when they are needed. Providing a checklist of the day's activities and the patient's responsibilities for the day helps the patient keep track of what has been done and what needs to be done. Order, consistency, and predictability in the patient's daily life environment together with systematic use of schedules, lists, and check-offs may help patients compensate for their memory impairments. As mentioned earlier, many of the compensatory techniques for traumatically brain-injured patients described in the last chapter of this book also are appropriate for patients with dementia.

Sleep Disturbances Most people sleep less as they get older and, as mentioned earlier, disrupted sleep patterns are particularly common in dementia. Helping the patient get adequate sleep helps him or her begin each day well-rested and makes it easier for the patient to deal with challenges and frustrations. Sleep medications are commonly prescribed to normalize dementia patients' disrupted sleep-wake cycles, probably more often than necessary. Adjusting the patient's daily schedule and sleep environment may normalize his or her sleep pattern, and should be tried before medications are prescribed. Even when medications are prescribed, changes in daily schedules and the patient's sleep environment can lower the dosage needed. The following adjustments help some patients (as well as some of the rest of us) sleep through the night.

- Cut back on the number of naps the patient takes during the day. Do not let the patient nap later than midafternoon.
- Have the patient go to bed at the same time every night.
- Make sure the patient gets 20 to 30 minutes of mild exercise in the early evening. A brisk walk is ideal.

- Give the patient a light snack (carbohydrates and milk are good) about an hour before going to bed.
- Provide the patient with comfortable sleeping attire that does not constrict, twist, or bind.
- Keep the patient's bedroom door and windows closed to cut down on extraneous noise.
- Keep the patient's room dimly illuminated with a night light to avoid confusion and anxiety when the patient awakens in the night.

Health Maintenance The mental impairments associated with dementing illness usually disrupt the patient's normal eating and drinking habits and judgment regarding adequate nutrition and fluid intake. Consequently, maintaining adequate nutrition and fluid intake is an important part of the patient's general health care. Ensuring that the patient has properly fitting dentures and maintaining oral hygiene are additional important, but sometimes overlooked, aspects of patient care. Some patients in the later stages of a dementing illness develop swallowing problems, in which case compensatory swallowing techniques may be prescribed, diet may be adjusted, or alternatives to oral feeding may be recommended.

Other illnesses sometimes accompany dementia. Diabetes, heart disease, pulmonary disease, kidney failure, or other diseases of internal organs may require medical care. Metabolic or chemical imbalances are common in both the normal and demented elderly. Demented patients are particularly susceptible to bacterial and viral infections; therefore prevention and treatment of infections is an important part of the general program of health care. Providing hearing aids for the hard-of-hearing patient and properly fitting eyeglasses for those with impaired vision prevent sensory deprivation and contribute to the patient's constructive interaction with her or his environment. Canes, walkers, crutches, or wheelchairs provide physically impaired patients with the mobility needed to get around in their environment.

■ KEY CONCEPTS

- Three major categories of dementia have been identified, depending on the location of the nervous system pathology responsible for the dementia. *Cortical dementias* are caused by pathology affecting the cerebral cortex. *Subcortical dementias* are caused by pathology affecting the basal ganglia, thalamus, and brainstem. *Mixed dementias* are caused by pathology affecting both cortical and subcortical structures.
- Alzheimer's disease causes cortical dementia and is the most frequent single cause of dementia. Its usual course is one of gradual intellectual deterioration followed by increasingly severe motor impairments and death.
- Pick's disease, like Alzheimer's disease, is a progressive disease affecting cortical neurons. Its usual course is one of progressive deterioration of personality and emotion, followed by intellectual deterioration, motor impairments, and death.
- Parkinson's disease is the most common cause of subcortical dementia. It is a progressive disease in which the initial symptoms are muscle rigidity, tremor, and slowness of movement. As Parkinson's disease progresses, intellectual functions usually are increasingly compromised.

- Multi-infarct dementia is a generic label for dementias caused by several disease processes, including *multiple cortical infarcts, lacunar state,* and *Binswanger's disease.* Multi-infarct dementia usually has a stepwise progression congruent with the occurrence of consecutive small infarcts.
- Diagnosis of middle- and late-stage dementia usually is relatively straightforward for experienced practitioners because disturbances of intellect, orientation, and behavior are obvious and distinctive. Diagnosis of early-stage dementia usually is more difficult, because the symptoms of early-stage dementia often resemble symptoms of nondementing conditions such as aphasia.
- Speech-language pathologists contribute to assessment of patients with dementia by measuring their communication impairments with sensitive and reliable tests to provide baseline measures against which the progression of dementia or the effects of intervention can be assessed.
- Speech-language pathologists work with patients and families to identify impairments that compromise the patient's communicative functioning and to devise and implement strategies and make environmental modifications to maximize the patient's daily life communicative success.

Dysarthria

ysarthria is a generic label for a group of speech disorders caused by weakness, paralysis, slowness, incoordination, or sensory loss in the muscle groups responsible for speech. Darley, Aronson, and Brown (1975) define dysarthria as follows:

> Dysarthria is a collective name for a group of speech disorders resulting from disturbances in muscular control over the speech mechanism due to damage of the central or peripheral nervous system. It designates problems in oral communication due to paralysis, weakness, or incoordination of the speech musculature. It differentiates such problems from disorders of higher centers related to the faulty programming of movements and sequences of movements (apraxia of speech) and to the inefficient processing of linguistic units (aphasia) (p. 246).

■ NEUROPATHOLOGY OF DYSARTHRIA

The most common cause of dysarthria is weakness or paralysis of muscles required for speech. The most common cause of muscle weakness or paralysis is damage to motor nerves. Less common causes are diseases affecting nerve-muscle junctions, diseases affecting the muscles themselves, damage in nerve fiber tracts connecting motor nerves to higher centers, compression or irritation of motor nerves, and psychosomatic conditions. The nature and time-course of dysarthria depend mainly on what causes it. Dysarthrias caused by progressive neurologic diseases are likewise progressive. Dysarthrias caused by destruction of motor nerves are irreversible, although patients may learn compensatory techniques to lessen their effects on communication. Dysarthrias caused by compression or inflammation of motor nerves are reversible if the compression and inflammation are successfully treated.

Upper Motor Neuron Damage

Unilateral lesions in the primary motor cortex or the pyramidal tract (upper motor neurons) sometimes produce what Duffy (1995) calls *uni-lateral upper motor neuron dysarthria.* As Duffy notes, unilateral upper motor neuron dysarthia has received little attention in the literature, perhaps because most writers consider it a temporary phenomenon. Darley, Aronson, and Brown (1975) asserted that unilateral lesions in upper motor neurons produce only transitory speech disturbances, which usually resolve within the first month post-onset. However, Duffy (1995) asserts that unilateral upper motor neuron pathology can sometimes cause significant dysarthria that persists after spontaneous neuorologic recovery is complete.

The muscles of the pharynx, larynx, and jaw receive input from both cerebral hemispheres. Consequently, unilateral lesions in upper motor neurons usually have only transitory effects on their function. The external muscles of the lower face receive input primarily from the contralateral hemisphere. Consequently, lesions in their upper motor neurons usually cause weakness or paralysis. The muscles of the tongue receive most of their input from the contralateral hemisphere, but have sufficient input from the ipsilateral hemisphere that unilateral damage in their upper motor neurons causes some mild weakness contralateral to the side of the lesion (Duffy, 1995). For these reasons, unilateral pyramidal tract damage does not usually cause lasting paralysis of most of the muscles responsible for speech, which no doubt is why unilateral upper motor neuron dysarthria tends to be mild and transitory.

Patients with *bilateral* upper motor neuron pathology in nerve fiber tracts serving the speech muscles usually exhibit significant dysarthria that does not spontaneously resolve. These patients' dysarthria is part of a syndrome called *pseudo-bulbar state,* in which the patient exhibits dysarthria, dysphagia (swallowing impairment), and poorly controlled laughing or crying.

Lower Motor Neuron Damage

Dysarthria often follows damage in the pons and medulla, where the cranial nerve nuclei for nerves supplying the facial, oropharyngeal, and laryngeal muscles are located. Damage to the cranial nerves proper invariably creates dysarthria if the damaged nerves supply muscles involved in producing speech. Damage to cranial nerves or their nuclei causes flaccid paralysis of muscles served by the nerve on the side of the lesion, fasciculations (twitching) in the affected muscles, and eventual atrophy of the muscles. The symptoms depend on whether the lesion affects the cranial nerve or the cranial nerve nucleus. If only the cranial nerve is damaged, the muscles served by the nerve are paralyzed and there is no hemiplegia or hemiparesis of either arm or leg. If the cranial nerve nucleus is damaged, spastic hemiparesis or hemiplegia of the contralateral arm and leg often follows. This happens because corticospinal fiber tracts serving the arm and leg pass through the brainstem near the cranial nerve nuclei. Consequently, lesions that destroy cranial nerve nuclei often destroy corticospinal fibers serving the arm and leg (Figure 10-1). Because the corticospinal fibers decussate below the level of the cranial nerve nuclei, lesions affecting cranial nerve nuclei on the left side of the brainstem create right-sided hemiplegia, and vice-versa.

Symptoms of Cranial Nerve Damage If the motor branch of the *facial nerve (7)* is damaged, weakness or flaccid paralysis of the ipsilateral eyelid muscles and muscles of facial expression follows. Disruption of the sensory branch of the facial nerve leads to loss of taste in the anterior two thirds of the tongue. *Bell's*

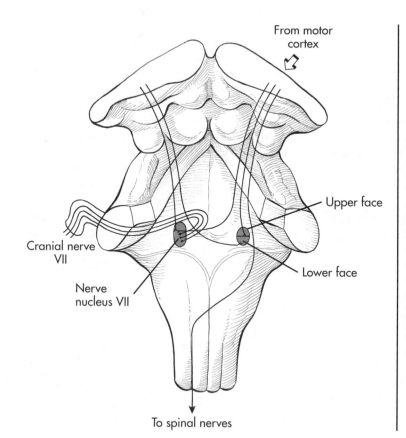

Figure 10-1 ▪ Diagram of cranial nerves and their nuclei. A lesion that destroys a cranial nerve nucleus often destroys corticospinal tract fibers that descend alongside the nucleus. Muscles that depend on the destroyed cranial nerve nucleus are paralyzed on the side of the lesion. Because the corticospinal tract decussates below the level of the cranial nerve nuclei, a lesion that destroys a cranial nerve nucleus and adjacent corticospinal fibers causes contralateral paralysis of muscles that are innervated by spinal nerves (such as the muscles of the arm and leg).

palsy is a relatively frequent (and in most cases reversible) facial nerve syndrome in which one-sided facial paralysis occurs. It usually is caused by inflammation of the facial nerve within the narrow channel through which it exits from the skull. The inflamed nerve swells and is compressed. Paralysis and sensory loss in the ipsilateral face follow. Bell's palsy usually resolves spontaneously within a few weeks. Sometimes the palsy does not resolve, the facial muscles atrophy and droop, and the eye on the affected side may have to be covered because of irritation caused by loss of the automatic eye blink.

Damage to the *glossopharyngeal nerve (9)* causes loss of the gag reflex. The muscles that elevate the palate and larynx and those that constrict the pharynx are weakened or paralyzed on the side of the lesion. Tactile sensation to the posterior wall of the pharynx and back of the tongue on the side of the lesion may be diminished or abolished. Hypernasality and swallowing problems (dysphagia) are likely.

Damage to the *vagus nerve (10)* causes ipsilateral paralysis of the soft palate. If the recurrent laryngeal branch of the vagus nerve is affected, unilateral vocal fold paralysis follows. If the sensory branch of the vagus nerve is damaged, pharyngeal sensation is impaired, with consequent disruption of the mechanics of swallowing.

Damage to the *spinal accessory nerve (11)* usually has no direct effects on speech, because the spinal accessory nerve innervates muscles in the neck and shoulders rather than muscles directly involved in speech. Occasionally accessory nerve damage can have indirect effects on speech, if muscle weakness causes shoulder and head droop that in turn compromises respiration and phonation.

Damage to the *hypoglossal nerve (12)* causes ipsilateral (usually mild) weakness of the tongue. Patients with hypoglossal nerve damage have difficulty protruding the tongue (it devi-

ates to the weak side) and moving the tongue laterally toward the side of the lesion.* Hypoglossal nerve damage can contribute to swallowing impairment if the patient has difficulty controlling the movement of food during chewing and positioning the food preparatory to swallowing it.

Anterior Horn Cell Disease

Several neurologic diseases are characterized by degeneration of anterior horn cells in the spinal cord. Most also cause degeneration of motor neurons in the motor nuclei of the lower cranial nerves, and some extend to the corticospinal and corticobulbar tracts. Degeneration of anterior horn cells causes symptoms typical of lower motor neuron disease, namely flaccid paralysis and fasciculations of muscles served by the damaged nerves. Anterior horn cell disease by itself has only indirect effects on speech. Weakness of respiratory muscles or muscles of the shoulders and rib cage may compromise breath support for speech, leading to diminished vocal intensity and short breath groups. When the disease also affects cranial nerves or corticospinal or corticobulbar tracts, speech movements are compromised, with consequent direct effects on articulation, speech rate, speech prosody, and vocal quality, depending on which nerves or tracts are affected. Anterior horn cell diseases are almost always progressive (except for poliomyelitis). Consequently, many patients require augmentative or alternative communication systems during the final stages of their disease.

Spinal Nerve Disease

Spinal nerves may be the focus of inflammatory or destructive disease. Inflammatory spinal

---

* It deviates to the weak side because the muscles on the strong side pull the tongue out, and the paralyzed side lags behind.

nerve diseases (such as Guillain-Barré disease)* usually are general rather then focal. They typically affect the longest nerve fibers first, and motor fibers before sensory fibers. Muscles in the limbs often are affected before the muscles in the torso, and distal muscles of the limbs are affected before proximal limb muscles. Spinal nerve diseases produce symptoms typical of lower motor neuron disease—weakness, hypotonia, and diminished reflexes, with variable sensory impairment. As is true for anterior horn cell disease, spinal nerve disease usually affects speech indirectly by compromising respiration. However, if the disease extends into the brainstem, corticobulbar tracts, or corticospinal tracts, speech movements may be directly affected.

Diseases of the Neuromuscular Junction

Diseases of the neuromuscular junction are characterized by abnormalities in the neurotransmitters responsible for transmission of nerve impulses across synapses. The abnormalities may be a deficiency or excess of the neurotransmitters themselves, or alterations in the sensitivity of receptor cells to neurotransmitters. *Myasthenia gravis* is the most common of the neuromuscular junction diseases. Myasthenia gravis is caused by autoimmune-mediated damage to the acetylcholine receptors on muscle cells, which interferes with neuromuscular transmission. Symptoms of myasthenia gravis include generalized and fluctuating muscle weakness (with a predilection for the extraocular, bulbar, and proximal limb muscles), rapid fatigability of muscles, and quick recovery of strength when the muscles are rested. Myasthenia gravis often causes a unique dysarthria syndrome, in which the patient's speech intelligibility deteriorates as

the patient talks for extended periods of time and recovers following periods of time during which the patient does not talk.

Primary Diseases of Muscle (Myopathy)

Some diseases affect the muscle fibers themselves and produce atrophy of muscle tissue. Myotonic dystrophy is a relatively common inherited myopathy that may affect muscles responsible for speech. Myositis, an acquired inflammatory muscle disease, usually does not affect speech, but may affect respiratory muscles and produce swallowing problems.

Cerebellar Damage

Damage to the *cerebellum* causes disruption of motor coordination and rhythm, usually with loss of muscle tone. Rapid alternating movements are slow and awkward. The range and force of movements are distorted (*dysmetria*), and movements become jerky and segmented (*decomposition of movement*). Intentional movements are accompanied by tremor, which disappears when the muscles are at rest.

Extrapyramidal System Damage

Damage in the *extrapyramidal system* compromises volitional movements and creates abnormal movements. Depending on the location of the damage, volitional movements may be abnormally slow (*hypokinetic*), or abnormally quick and overactive (*hyperkinetic*). Involuntary movements (*dyskinesia*) such as tremor, choreiform movements, athetosis, and dystonia are common symptoms of extrapyramidal system disease.

Sensory Loss

Damage to sensory branches of the cranial nerves or to the sensory cortex may impair sensation in the face, mouth, and neck. Such sensory disruptions sometimes cause transient and mild speech disturbances, usually lasting no more than a few weeks. Persisting dysarthria

---

* Guillian-Barré disease is a progressive but self-limiting neurologic disease characterized by progressive muscle weakness. Recovery usually begins sponaneously within 4 weeks of onset. Its cause is unknown, but it sometimes develops following inoculations or surgical procedures.

from sensory disturbance alone is rare. However, when sensory disturbances are superimposed upon coexisting motor impairments, the resulting dysarthria may be more severe than if the sensory problem were not present. A normal motor system usually has enough resilience to compensate for sensory disturbances, but an impaired one often does not.

■ EFFECTS OF NEUROLOGIC IMPAIRMENTS ON SPEECH PROCESSES

Bilateral Upper Motor Neuron Disease

As noted earlier, unilateral upper motor neuron disease usually causes mild and often transitory dysarthria. Patients with unilateral upper motor neuron dysarthria often are hemiplegic on the side contralateral to the brain lesion, have weakness in the lower face on the side contralateral to the lesion, and sometimes have weakness in the tongue muscles on the side contralateral to the brain lesion. Deviant speech characteristics for these patients include imprecise articulation, slow speech rate, harsh voice quality, reduced loudness, and (sometimes) hypernasality (Duffy, 1995).

Bilateral upper motor neuron disease may cause what Darley, Aronson, and Brown (1975) called *spastic dysarthria,* in which phonation, articulation, resonation, and prosody are affected. Spasticity of laryngeal muscles contributes to *strained-strangled-harsh* voice quality (Darley, Aronson, & Brown, 1975). Spasticity of articulatory muscles leads to imprecise consonant articulation, especially for complex and rapid movements. Spasticity of velopharyngeal muscles may prevent the velum from occluding the velopharyngeal port, contributing to hypernasality. The vocal pitch of patients with spastic dysarthria tends to be low, and variations in pitch and loudness diminish, contributing to monotonous vocal quality.

Lower Motor Neuron Disease

Problems in respiratory support for speech are common in lower motor neuron disease, disease of the neuromuscular junction, or disease of the muscle fibers themselves. The patient's weak and flaccid respiratory muscles do not fully inflate the lungs, and fail to provide adequate breath pressure at the vocal folds. The patient's respiratory insufficiency may be further complicated by weak and flaccid laryngeal muscles, which fail to fully adduct the vocal folds for phonation, wasting the already insufficient air supply. Consequently, patients with lower motor neuron disease usually speak in short utterances, with frequent pauses for breath. Their vocal intensity is weak and their voice quality breathy, particularly at the end of utterances. Their vocal pitch tends to be low and monotonous.

Extrapyramidal Disease

In *Parkinson's disease,* muscle rigidity leads to shallow respiration, and the patient speaks in short utterances, with abnormally long pauses between utterances. The patient's voice quality is strained and breathy, because rigid laryngeal muscles fail to fully adduct the vocal folds. The loudness of the patient's voice is reduced, sometimes to inaudibility. Articulation is markedly imprecise and indistinct, as rigid articulatory muscles fail to reach full excursion. The patient's connected speech is characterized by frequent rushes of rapid and indistinct speech in which most consonant articulation disappears. Speech rate usually is highly variable, with periods of normal rate interspersed with rushes of rapid and indistinct speech, punctuated by inappropriately placed pauses.

In *dyskinesia,* respiration may be disrupted periodically by involuntary movements that cause involuntary changes in breath pressure at the glottis, leading to abrupt changes in vocal intensity. Articulatory accuracy often falls victim to the dyskinesic movements, with periods of normal articulation alternating with intervals of articulatory inaccuracy coincident with the dyskinesic movements. Dyskinesic patients' speech rate is slow, variations in loudness and pitch are exaggerated by dyskinesic movements of respiratory muscles, and inappropriately placed pauses and periodic explosive articulation interrupt the flow of speech.

Cerebellar Disease

The speech of patients with cerebellar disease is characterized by anomalies of force, timing, and amplitude of movements in the muscles responsible for speech. Uncontrollable changes in breath pressure at the glottis produce irregular, sometimes explosive changes in pitch and loudness. Ataxic articulatory muscles create similar irregular disruptions of articulation. The patient's speech may be alternately normal in nasality and hypernasal.

■ EVALUATION OF DYSARTHRIA

Dysarthric patients are referred to speech-language pathologists because their speech sounds abnormal to physicians, nurses, family members, or to the patients themselves. The speech-language pathologist's assessment of a dysarthric patient usually has five purposes:

- To determine whether the patient's speech is abnormal.
- To evaluate the nature and severity of the abnormalities.
- To determine the cause(s) of the abnormalities.
- To determine if treatment is appropriate.
- To identify potential directions for treatment.

Because dysarthria is a problem with talking, it seems logical that one should look to the mouth for its source. The mouth is the appropriate place to start, but the search must also extend to the throat, chest and abdomen, and up into the pharynx and nasal cavities. To talk we have to breathe, so assessment of dysarthria includes assessment of respiration. To talk we have to produce voice, so assessment of dysarthria includes assessment of vocal fold function. To talk normally, we have to nasalize and denasalize sounds, so assessment of dysarthria includes as-

sessment of the muscles of the posterior pharynx and the soft palate. To talk intelligibly, we have to shape the breath stream into consonants and vowels, so assessment of dysarthria includes assessment of how well the tongue, lips, and jaw move, and how accurately they reach their targets. Comprehensive assessment of dysarthria entails assessment of *respiration, phonation, resonation,* and *articulation.* However, one cannot consider these four processes piece by piece, because they interact. Assessment of dysarthria is as much a search for interactions among processes underlying speech as it is a diagnosis of abnormalities within speech itself.

Evaluation of Breath Support for Speech

Characteristics of Normal Respiration

In neurologically normal adults, respiration for biologic purposes and respiration for speech differ in subtle but important ways. In normal passive breathing, the diaphragm provides most of the respiratory drive by contracting during inhalation. This contraction compresses the abdominal contents downward, increases the volume of the chest cavity, and generates negative pressure in the lungs. Muscles in the chest wall and shoulder girdle contribute by elevating the shoulders and rib cage, further increasing the volume of the chest cavity and adding to the negative pressure in the lungs. Outside atmospheric pressure then forces air into the lungs.

Expiratory force for exhalation is generated by a combination of torque generated by the expanded rib cage as it seeks to return to its resting position, and upward pressure on the bottom of the diaphragm as the compressed abdominal contents seek to regain their normal volume. During normal passive breathing most expiratory force is provided by the elasticity of the rib cage and by upward pressure generated by compressed abdominal organs. During speech, active contraction of abdominal muscles to increase upward pressure on the diaphragm is necessary, because the elasticity of the rib cage and the pressure exerted by compressed abdominal contents, by themselves, do not generate enough breath pressure for speech (Hixon, 1987).

During passive breathing, normal adults inflate their lungs to about 20% of total capacity, but when they speak they increase the amount of air in their lungs to from 35% to 60% of total capacity (Hixon, 1987). The usual respiratory pattern during speech consists of quick inhalation to about 60% of lung capacity, followed by slow exhalation until the lungs reach about 30% of total capacity, when the speaker takes another breath. The normal ratio of inhalation to exhalation is about 1:6. That is, the expiratory phase lasts about six times as long as the inspiratory phase (Yorkston, Beukelman, & Bell, 1988).

Observation of Passive Respiration Visual evaluation of the patient's posture and general appearance often provide important information about potential sources of respiratory insufficiency. If the patient is slouched and bent over, and her or his head droops forward, the patient's chest cavity is likely to be compressed and respiration for speech compromised.

Observation of the rate and depth of the patient's resting respiration can also provide information about potential respiratory problems. Normal resting respiration rates range from 12 to 20 cycles per minute, although there is substantial variability in the normal adult population. Normal respiration is not accompanied by overt movement of the shoulders or head. Fast, shallow breathing in the absence of exertion or elevated emotions may be a sign of weakness in the muscles of respiration, and suggests that the patient may have difficulty speaking with normal loudness and phrase length. Irregularities in resting breathing rate may be caused by cerebellar or extrapyramidal system pathology. Irregular breathing patterns may produce comparable aberrations in phonation.

Assessment of Respiration for Speech
The clinician's first objective in evaluating respiration for speech is to determine if comprehensive evaluation of respiratory function is necessary. This usually is accomplished by asking the patient to produce sustained phonation and repeat syllables. If the patient can sustain effortless phonation of an open vowel *(ah)* with normal loudness for 4 to 5 seconds and can say at least three consonant-vowel syllables on a single breath with normal loudness, respiration is likely to be adequate for speech, and direct work on respiration may not be needed.*

If the patient fails sustained phonation tests, one cannot immediately conclude that the problem is with respiratory support, because sustained phonation requires not only that the patient impound an adequate supply of air but also that she or he has enough strength in the respiratory muscles to generate subglottic air pressure and enough laryngeal muscle movement and strength to keep the vocal folds adducted against the pressure of the breath stream. Problems with vocal fold adduction usually are obvious during phonation. If the vocal folds are not closing, the patient's voice sounds weak and breathy. If the vocal folds are hypertonic, the patient's voice sounds harsh and strangled.

Measuring Respiratory Pressure and Flow Sophisticated (and expensive) instruments are available for measuring respiratory pressure and flow. They are not commonly available clinically. However, two inexpensive and relatively simple instruments for measuring intraoral breath pressure and flow can be constructed.

Netsell and Hixon (1978) described a U-tube manometer suitable for measuring intraoral breath pressure (Figure 10-2). The manometer is a U-shaped glass tube fastened to a board. The U-tube is approximately half-filled with col-

---

* Patients with 4- to 5-second maximum phonation times will be able to say only short phrases (three to six words) on a single breath. For these patients, respiration may be worked on indirectly, by increasing the numbr of words the patient can say on a single breath.

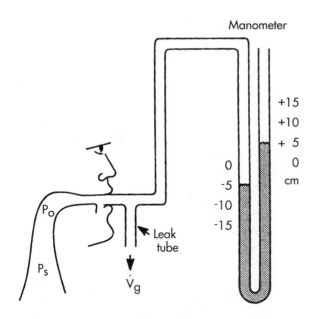

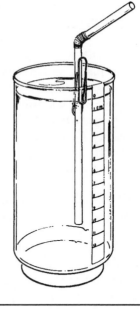

Figure 10-2 ■ A U-tube manometer. The patient blows into the mouthpiece. A leak tube permits a constant amount of air to escape. The height of the liquid in the U-tube is determined by the amount of breath pressure the patient can sustain. (From Netsell R, Hixon TJ: A noninvasive method for clinically estimating subglottal air pressure. *J Speech Hear Disord,* 43:326-330, 1978.)

Figure 10-3 ■ A water glass manometer. The deeper the straw is in the water, the more breath pressure is needed to sustain a string of bubbles at the deep end of the straw. (From Hixon TJ, Hawley JT, Wilson KJ: An around-the-house device for the clinical determination of respiratory driving pressure. *J Speech Hear Disord,* 47:413-415, 1982.)

ored water and calibrated in centimeters (see Netsell & Hixon for specifications). A flexible tube is attached to one end of the U-tube. A rigid T-shaped tube serves as a mouthpiece and bleed tube. The patient blows into the mouthpiece, and breath pressure displaces the column of water. The leak tube provides a constant escape for the airstream so that the person being tested must maintain continuous air flow to sustain displacement of the water. According to Netsell and Hixon, an individual who can maintain a 5 cm displacement of the water column for 5 seconds has sufficient breath pressure for basic speech requirements (the *5 for 5 rule*).

Hixon, Hawley, and Wilson (1982) suggested a similar but simpler device. A tall drinking glass (12 cm or more) is filled with water. The glass is calibrated in centimeters (Figure 10-3). A drinking straw is affixed to the glass so that it reaches a given depth (for example, 5 cm). An individual blowing into the straw must maintain breath pressure equal to the depth to which the straw is inserted in the water to generate a stream of bubbles at the end of the straw. By inserting the straw to 5 cm, one can evaluate whether a patient meets the *5 for 5 rule*.

Assessment of Phonation

Phonation Time and Voice Quality The typical first step in evaluating phonation is to ask the patient to sustain an open vowel *(ah)* for as long as he or she can, while the clinician times the duration of the patient's phonation. As the patient phonates, the clinician also evaluates the loudness, pitch, and quality of the patient's voice. Phonation times below 12 to 15 seconds are considered abnormally low, and suggest problems either with glottal valving or with breath support for speech.

Damage to cranial nerves, especially the laryngeal branches of the vagus nerve, can cause weakness or paralysis of laryngeal muscles. The weakened muscles cannot fully adduct the vocal folds, and the patient's voice is breathy, weak, and abnormally low in pitch.

Bilateral damage to upper motor neurons causes strained, strangled, harsh voice quality (Darley, Aronson, & Brown, 1975). Spastic laryngeal muscles constrict the glottal opening, increasing its resistance to airflow and reducing maximum phonation time. However, most patients with bilateral upper motor neuron pathology should have sufficient respiratory drive to produce 5 to 10 seconds of sustained phonation, although with strained, strangled, harsh voice quality.

Cerebellar damage often generates abrupt perturbations in vocal pitch and loudness caused by ataxic laryngeal muscles. However, most patients with cerebellar pathology can produce 5 to 10 seconds of sustained phonation, although voice quality is likely to be abnormal, and both loudness and quality may fluctuate abruptly. Anomalies in coordination of respiration and vocal fold adduction often causes aspiration of voiced sounds or strained, strangled voice quality at the onset of phonation.

Extrapyramidal diseases may affect vocal fold adduction, shortening phonation time and affecting voice quality. Patients with *Parkinson's disease* typically have breathy, hoarse voices and their maximum phonation time is reduced by rigidity of laryngeal muscles. Patients with Parkinson's disease often begin phonation nor-

mally, but as phonation continues their voice deteriorates, either into a voiceless whisper or a strained squeak. Patients with *dyskinesias* often produce alterations in vocal pitch, loudness, and quality that coincide with episodes of dyskinesia. The alterations may be slow or rapid, continuous or intermittent, depending on the nature of the patient's movement disorder. Patients with *tremor* usually produce regular, cyclic perturbations of pitch and loudness. Patients with *chorea* produce irregular prolonged distortions of vocal pitch and loudness that occur during episodes of choreiform movement. Maximum phonation times for patients with extrapyramidal disease range from substantially reduced (3 to 4 seconds) to normal, depending on the efficiency of glottal valving and the degree to which respiratory muscles are affected.

Vocal Flexibility and Coordination Assessing phonation time and voice quality provide important information about the efficiency of laryngeal valving and respiratory support for speech. However, since continuous phonation requires only that the vocal folds be adducted and maintained in a constant state of tension, the results of such tests do not provide much information about how well the laryngeal muscles can accomplish the more intricate movements of connected speech. That information is obtained by asking the patient to change vocal pitch and loudness in prescribed ways. The patient may be asked to:

- Count aloud from one to ten, beginning with a whisper and ending in a shout, and vice-versa.
- Sing up and down a musical scale.
- Count aloud, beginning with the lowest pitch that the patient can produce and gradually increasing pitch until the patient can go no higher.
- Say short sequences of numbers aloud, alternating loud and soft voice or high and low pitch.
- Repeat sentences at a whisper, normal loudness, and a shout.

- Read a paragraph or story aloud with exaggerated emphatic stress patterns.

The changes in pitch and loudness achieved by the patient in these tasks may be compared with what the patient does in less structured speech tasks (such as conversational speech). Many dysarthric patients sound more nearly normal in structured tasks when their attention is on controlling the pitch and loudness of their speech than in unstructured tasks in which they must attend to other things (such as formulating ideas or taking turns) in addition to monitoring pitch and loudness.

The patient's ability to coordinate respiration and speech may be evaluated by asking the patient to:

- Produce a series of short vowels (*uh-uh-uh—*, *ee-ee-ee—*).
- Alternate aspirate-vowel and voiced continuant-consonant pairs *(huh-muh–huh-muh)*.
- Alternate voiced and voiceless consonant-vowel pairs *(puh-buh–puh-buh)*.

If nervous system pathology is sufficient to produce significant dysarthria, vocal flexibility is almost always reduced. Constricted pitch and loudness range can be caused by upper motor neuron, lower motor neuron, extrapyramidal, or cerebellar pathology. Problems with coordination of respiration and voice onset are most often caused by extrapyramidal or cerebellar pathology.

Evaluation of Velopharyngeal Function

Velopharyngeal structures serve to isolate the pharyngeal and oral cavities from the nasal cavity during swallowing and during production of denasalized speech sounds. Although the exact means by which velopharyngeal closure is achieved differs somewhat across individuals (Yorkston, Beukelman, & Bell, 1988), closure is achieved primarily by movement of the velum (soft palate) up and back to meet the posterior pharyngeal wall, and movement of the lateral pharyngeal walls toward the midline to meet

the sides of the velum. Occasionally the posterior pharyngeal wall may move forward toward the velum (Croft, Shprintzen, & Rakoff, 1981). When normal speakers produce denasalized sounds, velopharyngeal muscles contract to close the nasopharyngeal port and prevent the passage of air from the oral cavity through the nasal cavity. When the speaker produces nasal sounds, the velopharyngeal muscles relax, opening the nasopharyngeal port and allowing part of the air stream to pass through the nasal cavity, adding nasal resonance to the sounds.

The clinician first estimates the adequacy of velopharyngeal function as the patient sustains phonation and repeats syllables, listening for hypernasality, nasal escape of air, and distorted consonants during production of denasal sounds. Judging hypernasality is one of the clinician's most difficult tasks. Such judgments often are unreliable, in part because they are affected by other speech characteristics (Moll, 1968). The more severe a patient's articulatory deviations are, the more likely it is that the patient will be judged hypernasal. Furthermore, patients who speak loudly tend to be judged more hypernasal than those who speak softly (Yorkston, Beukelman, & Bell, 1988). However, no satisfactory substitute for subjective judgments of hypernasality exists.

One of the easiest tests for hypernasality is to alternately pinch and release the patient's nostrils as the patient produces a sustained vowel. If the patient is hypernasal, the sound of the vowel changes as the nostrils are occluded and opened. However, this test does not always predict hypernasality in connected speech. Some patients can successfully occlude the velopharyngeal port during sustained phonation but cannot do so during the more complex movement patterns of connected speech. One can, of course, pinch and release the patient's nostrils as she or he produces connected speech. If the hypernasality is dramatic, changes in vocal resonance will be apparent. Moderate hypernasality may not be apparent, and mild hypernasality will not be. Fortunately, moderate hypernasality, either by itself or in combination with mild articulatory imprecision, usually does not make speech grossly unintelligible. Direct treatment of hypernasality usually is reserved for those patients in whom velopharyngeal incompetence is so severe that it significantly compromises their speech intelligibility.

The primary means of assessing nasal escape of air also is perceptual. The clinician listens for sounds of air escaping through the nose as the patient sustains phonation or repeats syllables, phrases, or sentences containing stop consonants. Other techniques have been used (feathers or small pieces of tissue on a card held under the nose, a cold mirror held under the nose), but they usually yield positive results only when the patient has severe velopharyngeal incompetence. Instrumentation that measures nasal emission is available, but it is expensive and not available in most clinics. Consequently, the clinician's ears (and sometimes, eyes) remain the most common instrument for measuring nasal escape.

Velopharyngeal incompetence often causes distortion of consonants, especially those requiring interruption or constriction of the air stream (stop consonants such as /p/ and /b/ and continuants such as /s/ and /sh/). Stop consonants and continuants are weak and accompanied by nasal emission of air and voiced consonants (such as /b/ or /d/) are weak and hypernasal. When articulation of consonants requiring increased oral breath pressure (stops and continuants) seems markedly poorer than articulation of open consonants (such as /h/, /l/, /r/), velopharyngeal incompetence is likely.

Evaluation of Articulation

Syllable and phrase repetition are the primary vehicles for assessing dysarthric patients' articulatory accuracy. The syllables and phrases are chosen to highlight the contribution of the various articulatory structures to the overall speech product. Lip closure is evaluated by asking the patient to repeat bilabial consonant-vowel com-

binations *(pa-pa-pa—, ba-ba-ba—)*. Tongue tip elevation is evaluated by asking the patient to repeat tongue-tip alveolar-ridge combinations *(ta-ta-ta—, da-da-da—)*. Elevation of the back of the tongue is evaluated by asking the patient to repeat high-back-consonant combinations *(ka-ka-ka—, ga-ga-ga—)*. Articulatory flexibility and coordination is evaluated by asking the patient to repeat strings of syllables in which articulation points change *(pa-ta-ka, da-ba-ga)*. Articulatory accuracy in longer segments of speech is estimated by asking the patient to repeat multisyllabic words *(gingerbread-gingerbread-gingerbread, artillery-artillery-artillery)* phrases *(the national Republican convention),* and sentences *(Nelson Rockefeller drives a Lincoln Continental).*

Standard articulation inventories such as those used to evaluate children rarely are administered to dysarthric patients. Articulatory problems in dysarthria usually are part of a constellation of respiratory, phonatory, and resonance disturbances. Consequently, clinicians are not interested so much in what sounds are in error, as in what impaired speech processes account for the *pattern* of articulatory impairment. Second, the goal of most treatment for dysarthric patients is intelligibility rather than articulatory accuracy. Because articulatory accuracy has only a general relationship to intelligibility, measuring intelligibility usually provides more therapeutically valuable information than measuring articulatory accuracy.

Yorkston, Beukelman, and Bell (1988) offer several objections to the use of traditional articulation inventories with dysarthric speakers. They make three assertions:

- A judge's perceptions of articulatory accuracy may not reflect the adequacy of the patient's articulatory movements.
- Articulation inventories fail to discriminate between sounds that are accurate and sounds that are distorted but still within phoneme boundaries.
- When judges know the target words, as in traditional articulation inventories, they

are likely to overestimate a patient's articulatory accuracy.

Yorkston, Dowden, Beukelman, and Traynor (1986) advocate use of the *phoneme identification task* to eliminate some of these problems. In the phoneme identification task, the speaker is tape-recorded as she or he produces a list of single words and sentences. The list is designed to elicit 57 target phonemes. A judge (not the examiner) then listens to the tape recording and identifies the target phonemes using the following procedure. A word or sentence is played. The judge looks at a printed word with the target phoneme missing (for example, ma_), and identifies the missing phoneme. Then the judge rates the patient's production of the perceived phoneme using a four-point scale, ranging from *no basis for a guess,* to *correct, undistorted.*

Evaluation of Intelligibility Yorkston and Beukelman (1981) published an assessment tool called *Assessment of Intelligibility of Dysarthric Speech.* The test has two sections. One measures single-word intelligibility; the other assesses sentence intelligibility and speaking rate. In the *single-word task,* a patient's oral reading of 50 single words is tape recorded. Each word is selected by the examiner (before the test) from a pool of 12 similar-sounding words. One or more judges (not the examiner) then listen to the tape and either write down each spoken word or choose each spoken word from a set of 12 words that are similar in sound to the target word. In the *sentence task* the patient reads aloud 22 sentences, ranging in length from 5 to 15 words (2 sentences at each length). One or more judges (not the examiner) then listen to the recording and write down the sentences. Judges' transcriptions are then scored by the examiner to yield several measures:

- *Percent intelligibility*
- *Speech rate for sentences* (words per minute)
- *Intelligible words per minute*

- *Unintelligible words per minute*
- *Communicative efficiency ratio* (intelligible words per minute divided by normal speech rate, which is 190 words per minute)

Assessment of Intelligibility of Dysarthric Speech appears to be a sensitive and reliable estimator of speech intelligibility if administered and scored according to instructions. The measures obtained are useful for predicting a speaker's intelligibility in daily life, for measuring changes in intelligibility over time, and in planning treatment to improve a speaker's intelligibility. Patients who are both aphasic and dysarthric may have difficulty with the sentence production part of the test because of reading problems, problems in auditory comprehension and retention, or paraphasic errors in oral reading. Consequently, the test may not be practical for patients who are both dysarthric and more than mildly aphasic.

■ TREATMENT OF DYSARTHRIA

Dysarthria is caused by various neurologic disturbances that cause weakness, slowness, clumsiness, incoordination, diminished range of movement, or sensory loss in speech structures. Some patients do not have the muscle strength or range of movement needed for normal speech. Others may have the muscle strength but not the coordination. Still others may lack the respiratory support necessary for normal speech. Consequently, there is no single treatment for dysarthria.

Treatment of dysarthria must take into account both the causes of a patient's dysarthria and the nature of the speech disturbances. Some treatment procedures may be concerned with causative mechanisms, while others may focus on the speech disturbances themselves. The goal of dysarthria treatment is to maximize the dysarthric patient's communication effectiveness and efficiency. This goal can be achieved in various ways—for example, by improving the physiologic support for speech, by direct work on speech, by environmental control, education, and counseling, by providing compensatory techniques or alternatives to speech for communication, by providing prosthetic facilitation of speech, or (occasionally) by medical or surgical intervention.

Treatment of dysarthric patients may rely on indirect approaches, whereby speech is improved by improving sensory and motor functions that are involved in speech, rather than directly, by working on speech itself. Indirect treatment procedures include sensory stimulation, muscle strengthening, modifying muscle tone, and modifying respiration. Direct procedures include modifying phonation, resonation, articulation, and prosody. For most dysarthric patients, treatment is a combination of direct and indirect procedures. If a patient is severely dysarthric and can produce little or no volitional speech, treatment is likely to be directed toward enhancing physiologic support for speech. If a patient can produce some voice, approximate a few vowel sounds, and produce a few articulatory movements, treatment is likely to focus on production of speech. Nonspeech exercises to strengthen muscles and increase their agility and range of movement may also be appropriate for these latter patients, but primarily as an adjunct to direct work on speech. The more severe the patient's dysarthria, the more likely it is that the clinician will work to strengthen muscles and improve sensory function outside the context of speech. Patients with mild or moderate dys-arthria may get stronger muscles and improved sensory function from treatment, but almost always this is better accomplished by controlled experiences with speaking rather than by stimulation of oral structures or by movement exercises in isolation.

Indirect Treatment Procedures

Sensory Stimulation The intent of sensory stimulation is to increase the dysarthric patient's motor control by increasing the amount and fidelity of sensory feedback from oral structures. Stimulation may include brushing, stroking, vibrating, or applying ice to the patient's lips, tongue, pharyngeal walls, or soft palate. There is little empiric evidence that sensory stimulation improves motor performance in dysarthria, and its use remains controversial, except perhaps for stimulation of the soft palate. Rosenbek and LaPointe (1985) suggest that massaging and lifting the soft palate concurrent with the patient's attempts to raise it may improve velopharyngeal competence. Johns (1985) reports that movement of the lateral pharyngeal walls toward the midline sometimes increases following installation of palatal prostheses. He attributes this to increased sensory feedback generated by contact of the pharyngeal walls with the prosthesis. However, Dworkin and Johns (1980), after reviewing various approaches to managing velopharyngeal insufficiency, assert that neither stimulation nor muscle strengthening are likely to be effective if the insufficiency is caused by neurologic impairment. It may be that clinicians' willingness to use stimulation to remediate velopharyngeal incompetence comes as much from the paucity of other methods for remediation as from the clinician's belief that stimulation actually works. Nevertheless, stimulation of the soft palates and pharyngeal walls of dysarthric patients with gross velopharyngeal incompetence is likely to continue, at least until something better comes along.

Muscle Strengthening Muscle strengthening exercises are intended to improve the dysarthric patient's respiration, phonation, articulation, and resonance by enhancing movement of weakened muscles. There is no conclusive evidence confirming the efficacy of muscle strengthening in treating dysarthria, but it appears to have positive effects for at least some patients (Powers & Starr, 1974; Yules & Chase, 1969; Massengill, Quinn, Pickrell, & Levinson, 1968). Rosenbek and LaPointe (1978) suggest that muscle strengthening is most appropriate for patients whose dysarthria is severe and whose physiologic support for speech is substantially compromised. They recommend muscle strengthening when adjustment of posture, muscle tone, and respiration, and direct treatment of articulation, phonation, and prosody leave the patient unintelligible, but only if the patient will remain in treatment for several weeks and can carry out assignments outside the clinic. In practice, muscle strengthening usually is reserved for severely dysarthric patients who can produce little intelligible speech or can produce it only in fragments and under ideal conditions.

It is important that clinicians not exaggerate the importance of muscle strength for adequate speech movements. Intelligible speech rarely requires forceful muscle activity. In fact, forceful articulatory movements, such as those seen in ataxia, dystonia, and chorea, may actually diminish intelligibility. Agility and range of movement are more important contributors to intelligible speech than strength. Consequently, muscle strengthening exercises that include movement (*isotonic* exercise) are likely to be more effective than those requiring exertion against stationary resistance (*isometric* exercise). As a general rule, clinicians move from isometric to isotonic movements as soon as the patient can accomplish short sequences of simple movements. Muscle strengthening activities lead into agility and range of motion exercises as soon as the muscles have enough strength to carry out the exercises at low levels of speed and efficiency.

Muscle strengthening by itself is most appropriate for severely dysarthric patients. If a patient can produce a vowel or two and approximate a few consonants, muscle strengthening may be supplemented by direct work on speech production. Patients whose muscles do not have the strength, agility, or range of movement to talk but who can produce a few speech sounds will usually develop increased strength, agility, and range of movement in the muscle groups needed for speech as quickly (and more efficiently) if they are talking than if they are moving speech structures in nonspeech movement drills.

Modification of Muscle Tone Some dysarthric patients exhibit abnormalities in muscle tone that interfere with speech intelligibility. Some are *hypertonic*. Hypertonicity appears as *spasticity* when patients have upper motor neuron pathology, and as *rigidity* in Parkinson's disease. Both kinds of hypertonicity are constant over time and uniform across affected muscle groups. Hypertonicity also appears as a consequence of extrapyramidal diseases such as dystonia and chorea. In these disorders muscle tone tends to wax and wane within muscle groups and may move from muscle group to muscle group. Abnormally diminished muscle tone (hypotonicity) usually follows lower motor neuron or peripheral nervous system pathology. Hypotonicity is almost always constant over time and does not move from one muscle group to another.

A variety of procedures for relaxing hypertonic muscles have been reported in the literature. *Progressive relaxation* reduces the hypertonic patient's overall level of muscle tension. *Shaking* exercises (Froeschels, 1943) and *chewing exercises* (Froeschels, 1952) may help the patient relax muscle groups involved in speaking. Lying down while speaking may help some hypertonic patients by lowering their overall level of muscle tension. *Biofeedback,* in which the electrical activity in selected muscle groups is amplified and converted to auditory or visual signals that are monitored by the patient may help patients selectively relax the muscles (Netsell & Cleeland, 1973; Hand, Burns, & Ireland, 1979; Rubow, Rosenbek, Collins, & Celisia, 1984). When hypertonicity is caused by extrapyramidal pathology (such as Parkinson's disease) medications to reduce muscle tone may be more effective than behavioral treatment. In fact, hypertonicity caused by extrapyramidal disease usually is not responsive to behavioral treatment.

Hypotonicity (as in flaccid dysarthria), typically is treated by raising the patient's overall level of muscle tension. Simply asking the patient to increase his or her overall level of effort sometimes improves the intelligibility of patients with flaccid dysarthria (Rosenbek & LaPointe, 1985). If this approach is not effective, the patient's general level of muscle tension may be increased by asking them to push or pull against a stationary resistance while speaking. Pushing down on a table or on the arms of a chair or wheelchair, or clasping the hands together and pulling may increase overall muscle tone and improve the speech of hypotonic patients.

Posture and Speaking Position Modifying a dysarthric patient's posture and speaking position may sometimes improve his or her speech, especially when general muscle weakness is present, as in generalized neuropathies. Straightening the slouching patient's spine and neck and bringing his or her head to an upright position with braces or supports may improve the mechanical relationships among the structures involved in speech, with beneficial consequences for the quality of the patient's speech. Postural adjustments may help the patient compensate for weak muscles and stabilize the platform from which speech movements are carried out. Cervical collars, body braces, slings, and restraints, singly or in combination, may be used to get a weak patient into a more efficient position for speech and help the patient maintain that position. Posture and positioning are most often useful with weak or flaccid patients who have difficulty sitting up and keeping their head erect.

When the patient has been positioned in a better speaking posture, stabilization and support of selected muscle groups can enhance the intelligibility of the patient's speech. If a patient's neck muscles are weak, a cervical collar or neck brace may stabilize the patient's head. Girdles, stomach bands, or stomach boards (Rosenbek & LaPointe, 1985) may be used to stabilize and support weak abdominal muscles. Stomach boards are boards, usually fastened across the arms of a wheelchair, against which the patient can press her or his abdomen to compress it and generate greater expiratory pressure for speech. Girdles and stomach bands compress the abdomen, compensating for weak abdominal muscles and providing a firm base for exhalation during speech. Patients with movement disorders may wear cervical collars, neck braces, or body braces to limit involuntary movements.

Posturing, positioning, stabilization, and support should be carried out in collaboration with a physician, because changes in posture or bracing, banding, and belting may contribute to medical complications. For example, abdominal banding or girdling may restrict breathing and predispose patients to pneumonia. Cervical collars and neck braces may compress muscles and nerves in the patient's neck and shoulders.

Respiratory Capacity and Efficiency Respiratory capacity is most likely to be a problem for patients with generalized weakness, as in demyelinating disease, disease of the spinal cord, and disease affecting the neuromuscular junction. Increasing respiratory capacity may improve these patients' speech, but only if they can use the breath stream efficiently. In most cases, respiratory capacity is less important to speech than efficient use of the air stream. If a patient's glottal valving, velopharyngeal porting, and articulation are poor, increasing respiratory capacity will do little for the intelligibility of speech.

Treatment procedures for enhancing respiratory support take several forms. Postural adjustments, positioning, and stabilization may improve the mechanical background for respiration. Muscle strengthening activities may be directed toward the muscles of respiration.

Sometimes techniques for increasing muscle tone (such as pushing and bearing down) are employed to increase respiratory drive. Training in more efficient glottal valving and increasing articulatory precision may have indirect positive effects on respiratory support.

Exercises that deal directly with respiration also may be appropriate. Controlled exhalation, in which the patient slowly exhales a uniform stream of air over a period of time, may improve respiratory capacity and enhance control of exhalation. In most cases, direct treatment of respiration is an early phase of treatment, and the focus of treatment usually moves to speech production as soon as the patient achieves basic respiratory support for speech.

Direct Treatment Procedures

In direct treatment procedures, dysarthric patients produce speech under controlled conditions.* Treatment of dysarthric patients usually includes both indirect and direct procedures, and indirect procedures tend to fade into direct procedures, as, for example, when controlled exhalation leads into controlled phonation. Direct treatment procedures tend to overlap and merge one into another, as when controlled phonation progresses into articulation drills. Direct treatment procedures may address phonation, resonation, articulation, and prosody, either singly or in combination.

Phonation Speech activities to enhance phonation emphasize efficient laryngeal valving of the air stream and adjusting utterance length to the patient's respiratory capacity. Controlled phonation is the primary vehicle for increasing dysarthric patients' laryngeal efficiency. In the early stages of treatment, the patient may be asked to produce prolonged vowels and to gradually increase their duration. When vowel pro-

duction has stabilized, the patient is trained to produce strings of vowels or consonant-vowel syllables, with the length of the strings gradually increasing as the patient masters shorter ones. Gradual changes in intensity may then be superimposed on the strings to further enhance respiratory control. When the patient can say short phrases, treatment may incorporate the concept of *optimal breath group* (Linebaugh, 1983). The optimal breath group for a given patient is the number of syllables that he or she can produce comfortably on one breath. The optimal breath group approach entails determining the patient's optimal breath group, teaching the patient to keep the number of syllables per breath within the optimal breath group, then gradually increasing the length of the patient's optimal breath group by means of drills to enhance respiratory control and glottal valving.

When glottal valving is compromised by spastic laryngeal muscles, procedures for reducing laryngeal tension, including relaxation, massage of the larynx, or providing postural support may be combined with work on voice production. When laryngeal muscles are flaccid, pushing and bearing down during phonation may be incorporated into voice drills, and in some cases visual feedback, such as that provided by a VU meter or an oscilloscope tracing, may be used to help the patient control (and increase) the loudness of her or his phonation.

When loudness is a problem in dysarthria, it usually is a case of too little rather than too much. Dysarthric patients' speech may be made louder by improving respiratory support (teaching appropriate breath groups, positioning, bracing, banding, bearing down), by increasing the efficiency of phonation, or by speech exercises that directly target vocal intensity. *Contrastive stress drill* (Rosenbeck & LaPointe, 1985) is one way of giving dysarthric patients concentrated vocal intensity training. In contrastive stress drill, the clinician says a sentence, such as *Bob hit Bill* and then asks the patient questions such as ***WHO*** *hit*

---

* Technically, one cannot treat speech—one treats speech by changing the amplitude, speed, or accuracy of movements that generate speech. Consequently, even "direct" treatment procedures are indirect, in this sense.

Bill?, **WHAT** *did Bill do?*, and so on. The patient answers each question, putting emphatic stress on elements that answer the questions *(Bob hit **BILL**)*. If adequate vocal intensity cannot be obtained by means of behavioral treatment, a portable voice amplification system may be necessary. Portable amplification systems include either a throat-mounted or headset-mounted microphone connected to a small amplifier and speaker which can be worn in a pocket or on a strap or belt. However, as Rosenbek and La-Pointe (1985) caution, amplification is appropriate for patients with intelligible speech. Amplifying unintelligible speech only produces louder unintelligible speech.

Increasing *vocal pitch range* may be appropriate for some patients, particularly those with flaccid dysarthria. Techniques for increasing pitch range include phonation with gradually rising and falling pitch; counting, saying the alphabet, numbers, days of the week, or other sequences with gradually rising or falling pitch across the sequences; contrastive stress drill; asking questions (for rising pitch) and making assertions (for falling pitch) with exaggerated intonation. Control of *pitch changes* may be important for patients with ataxic dysarthria. Techniques for controlling pitch changes include continuous phonation while keeping pitch constant, and continuous phonation with slowly rising or falling pitch.

Resonance The resonance of speech is affected by the size and configuration of the oral cavity and the amount of communication between the oral and nasal cavities. Although aberrations in the shape of the oral cavity may change the resonance characteristics of speech, such changes are primarily cosmetic, affecting speech quality rather than speech intelligibility. (However, aberrations in the shape of the oral cavity are produced by abnormal positions of the articulators. For this reason, articulatory errors often are superimposed on the resonance abnormalities. The combination can sometimes destroy intelligibility.) By far the most important resonance aberration in dysarthria is hypernasality, caused by failure to close the velopharyngeal opening during denasalized segments of speech. This failure has two effects. It produces excessive nasal resonance. More importantly, it distorts or destroys sounds that require oral breath pressure, because the air required to produce them escapes through the nose.

Increasing velopharyngeal competence can create dramatic improvements in intelligibility for many hypernasal patients. Several behavioral techniques for controlling hypernasality have been described in the literature. They usually involve ear training to teach the patient to recognize hypernasality, and facilitating the movement of velopharyngeal muscles by having the patient push or bear down. Behavioral remediation of hypernasality usually is practical only when hypernasality is mild. If it is moderate or severe, prosthetic or surgical management usually is necessary.

Hypernasality caused by palatal insufficiency can sometimes be reduced by a palatal lift prosthesis. A palatal lift prosthesis is constructed by a prosthodontist, usually in collaboration with a speech pathologist. It consists of a plate that covers the hard palate. The plate is attached to the teeth by wires. The palatal lift is attached to the rear of the palate. The palatal lift is made of acrylic and is shaped to fit the patient's oropharynx. The lift mechanically pushes the patient's palate up and back, to help close the velopharyngeal port.

The literature (Netsell & Rosenbek, 1985; Rosenbek & LaPointe, 1985; Yorkston, Beukelman, & Bell, 1988) suggests that patients with the following characteristics are the best candidates for palatal lift prostheses.

- Patients who are extremely hypernasal, who cannot achieve velopharyngeal closure, and for whom behavioral intervention has been unsuccessful.

- Patients whose soft palates and pharyngeal muscles are not spastic. Spastic muscles resist displacement and may dislodge the prosthesis.

- Patients who have teeth to which the prosthesis can be anchored. Prostheses have been fitted to dentures, but the results usually are unsatisfactory.
- Patients who have reasonably good articulation and phonation. Hypernasal patients with severe articulatory or phonatory deficits will generally remain as unintelligible after the prosthesis is fitted as they were before.
- Patients who are likely to cooperate by wearing the lift and caring for it. Some severely involved patients may not tolerate the discomfort associated with wearing the prosthesis, and some unmotivated patients may not put up with the inconvenience of wearing the prosthesis and caring for it.
- Patients who do not have swallowing difficulties. Palatal prostheses sometimes interfere with swallowing.
- Patients without degenerative disease. Although fitting a prosthesis to such patients may provide temporarily increased intelligibility, the effects are likely to be transitory and eventually will be negated by the progression of the disease.

Articulation Improving dysarthric patients' articulation was for many years the core of treatment for dysarthria, because dysarthria was considered to be little more than defective articulation. However, as Rosenbek and LaPointe (1985) assert, "Articulation is being forced to share its popularity with other speech processes . . . and dysarthria is coming to mean speech—not articulation—deficit" (p. 294). Most dysarthric patients receive articulation treatment. However, few receive *only* articulation treatment.

Treatment procedures for improving articulation include *imitation, phonetic derivation* (deriving sounds that the patient cannot say from those that he or she can say), *phonetic placement* (physically adjusting or positioning the articulators), and *sequential repetition* of sounds, syllables, and words. In most cases, articulation exercises focus on speech movements (production of syllables or words), rather than on fixed positions (individual sounds). Only when a patient's dysarthria is severe is she or he likely to be drilled in producing fixed articulatory positions. When a patient's articulatory movements are imprecise, he or she may be taught to exaggerate them, making them more precise. Sometimes when a patient cannot produce an articulatory movement or position, a compensatory movement or substitute position may be taught. Work on articulatory precision often is combined with slowing the patient's speech rate. Slower speech rate allows the patient more time to make articulatory adjustments, and it allows the patient's listeners more time to decode what the patient is saying.

Prosody Activities for changing the prosodic characteristics of dysarthric patients' speech may focus on rate, loudness, or pitch (intonation). Changes in patients' *speech rate* can be produced by changes in articulation rate (the rate at which individual speech sounds are produced) or by increasing the number or duration of pauses in the patient's speech. Most dysarthric speakers have great difficulty changing articulation rate. Consequently, most rate manipulations are performed with pauses. If a patient is trained to produce optimal breath groups, pauses may occur automatically. However, the pauses are not likely to be at syntactic or semantic boundaries. It may help to teach these patients to mark the boundaries with pauses. Teaching a patient to put pauses at syntactic or semantic boundaries makes it easier for listeners to segment the patient's utterances into meaningful units.

There are several techniques for controlling dysarthric patients' speech rate. In most of them the patient speaks in unison with an external timing stimulus. The clinician may tap, gesture, or speak along with the patient. The patient may speak to the beat of a metronome or a flashing light. The patient may tap, drop beads in a cup, gesture, or produce other nonoral movements in unison with speaking. Teaching the patient to speak with exaggerated articulation and to exaggerate emphatic stress (contrastive stress drill) also may slow the patient's speech rate.

Environmental Control and Education

Most dysarthric speakers eventually discover that intelligibility in the speech clinic, where rooms are quiet and well-lighted and they are face-to-face with the clinician, is no guarantee of intelligibility in daily life, where rooms may be poorly lit and noisy, and where listeners may not always be nearby and/or looking. Skilled clinicians know this, and teach patients how to compensate for less-than-ideal speaking conditions. They also teach them how to control their speaking environment to be maximally intelligible. When a dysarthric speaker reaches reasonable levels of intelligibility in the controlled environment of the clinic, the clinician broadens the treatment program to maximize communication in less-than-ideal speaking situations. This usually requires both *environmental control* and *behavioral compensation.*

The patient can be taught ways to control the speaking environment to minimize adverse effects of environmental variables on speech intelligibility. The most effective controls relate to ambient noise, lighting, and the spatial relationships between the dysarthric speaker and his or her listener(s). Keeping ambient noise levels low is a primary requirement for the dysarthric speaker and those with whom the dysarthric speaker communicates. Turning the television set down or off and closing windows or doors to shut out outside noise are simple but effective ways to diminish ambient noise. Families can use the *mute* button on remote controls for television sets and install draperies or other acoustic treatments to control ambient noise levels in dysarthric speakers' homes.

Controlling lighting and the position of dysarthric speakers relative to their listeners may also enhance dysarthric speakers' communicative effectiveness. Lighting can be ad-

justed to illuminate the dysarthric speaker's face, and dysarthric speakers can routinely position themselves so that listeners can see their face.

Dysarthric speakers can be trained to monitor their listeners' comprehension by maintaining eye contact and, if necessary, asking listeners whether or not they understand. They also can be trained when (and how) to repeat, simplify, paraphrase, or exaggerate articulatory movements (especially when the patient perceives communication breakdown). Those around the dysarthric speaker can be taught to control the situational variables described above, to indicate (either gesturally or verbally) to the speaker when they do not understand, and to ask the dysarthric speaker to slow down, exaggerate articulatory movements, repeat, paraphrase, or simplify when the dysarthric speaker fails to communicate.

Medical and Surgical Treatment

Medical Treatment Some conditions causing dysarthria are medically treatable. When they are, medical treatment precedes behavioral intervention, and when medical treatment is successful, behavioral intervention may not be needed. Medically treatable conditions causing dysarthria include extrapyramidal diseases such as Parkinson's disease, irritative and inflammatory processes causing peripheral nerve dysfunction, and some metabolic and nutritional disturbances.

Parkinson's disease is caused by deficiencies in certain neurotransmitters (dopamines) and often responds well to medications such as levadopa (L-dopa) that replenish the missing neurotransmitters. These medications often diminish or eliminate the motor symptoms of the disease, including dysarthria. Movement disorders (such as chorea and dystonia) sometimes respond favorably to tranquilizers and related medications, although complete remission of symptoms with medication is unusual. Some facial paralyses are treatable with steroids. Neurologic diseases caused by abnormalities in central nervous system metabolism, such as Wilson's disease, may be medically treatable. When medical treatment of a dysarthric patient's neurologic disease is effective, his or her dysarthria often improves enough to make direct treatment of dysarthria unnecessary. However, medical treatment often decreases, but does not eliminate, a patient's dysarthria, so that behavioral treatment of the patient's dysarthria is necessary in conjunction with medical treatment.

Teflon Injections and Surgical Treatment
Sometimes surgical management is appropriate when structural abnormalities produce dysarthria. Velopharyngeal insufficiency can sometimes be reduced by surgical procedures or by injection of Teflon into the pharyngeal walls. Teflon may be injected into the posterior pharyngeal wall to remediate velopharyngeal insufficiency (Lewy, Cole, & Wepman, 1965; Bluestone, Musgrave, McWilliams, & Crozier, 1968). Teflon injections are most useful in cases of mild to moderate hypernasality when behavioral modification of hypernasality has not been successful. When dysphonia is caused by inability to adduct the vocal folds, injection of Teflon into the vocal folds may improve voice quality. These procedures often do not eliminate the patient's speech abnormalities, so that behavioral treatment of the patient's residual speech abnormalities may be necessary.

Surgical remediation of velopharyngeal insufficiency is helpful in some cases of severe velopharyngeal incompetence, although the general opinion seems to be that surgery is a last resort to be tried only after less dramatic approaches have failed. The most frequent surgical procedure for remediating velopharyngeal insufficiency is the *posterior pharyngeal flap.* In this procedure, bands of muscle tissue are surgically lifted from the posterior pharyngeal walls, and one end of each band is surgically attached to the soft palate. The bands shorten when the pharyngeal wall muscles contract, pulling the soft palate toward the pharyngeal walls.

Pharyngeal flap procedures are most common in management of palatal insufficiency for children with cleft palates. Their use to treat hypernasality in dysarthria is controversial. Gonzalez and Aronson (1970) assert that prosthetic management of velopharyngeal insufficiency usually produces better results than surgery. Hardy, Rembolt, Spriestersbach, and Jayapathy (1961) make a similar assertion regarding management of velopharyngeal insufficiency in children. Miniami, Kaplan, Wu, and Job (1975) did pharyngeal flaps on five dysarthric patients with "palatal paresis," and reported disappointing results. However, Johns (1985), after reviewing the literature and summarizing his own experience with surgical remediation of velopharyngeal insufficiency, concludes that surgical management "holds great promise for a large number of dysarthric patients" (p. 175).

Augmentative and Alternative Communication

Many severely dysarthric patients never regain enough intelligible speech to communicate even simple messages by talking. Nonspeech communication systems enable many of them to communicate. Nonspeech communication systems can be either *augmentative* or *alternative. Augmentative systems* supplement what the patient can say and permit the patient to communicate more elaborate messages or communicate simple messages with greater intelligibility. *Alternative systems* replace speech as a means of communication. Amplifiers are the most common augmentative systems for dysarthric speakers. There are four major categories of alternative (nonspeech) communication systems: (1) communication boards and communication books, (2) mechanical and electronic devices, (3) gesture and pantomime, and (4) sign language.

Selection of a nonspeech communication system for a dysarthric speaker requires consideration of her or his perceptual, motor, and linguistic abilities, because different systems require different abilities and different levels of skill within those abilities. Some systems require that the user point to symbols or operate a keyboard. Patients with poor manual dexterity may not be able to use such systems. Some systems require that the user spell, read, or arrange words into phrases or sentences. Patients with linguistic impairments may not be able to use them.

Communication Boards and Communication Books Communication boards and communication books are similar in content, but differ in form. A communication board is an array of symbols on a durable surface. A communication book is a collection of symbols arranged in book form. The symbols in either can be pictures, letters, words, phrases, or some combination of the four. To communicate, the patient points to the symbols, either singly or in sequence. Figure 10-4 shows examples of two kinds of communication boards. At the top is a simple board containing pictorial symbols and printed words. At the bottom is a more complex board containing letters, numerals, and words.

In general, communication boards and books containing letters, words, and phrases are best suited to patients without substantial linguistic impairments. The board shown at the top of Figure 10-4 would be usable by many linguistically impaired patients, because its symbols are nonverbal. The board shown at the bottom of Figure 10-4 would be inappropriate for linguistically impaired patients but would be appropriate for dysarthric patients without major linguistic impairment, as long as they have the motor ability to point to the symbols on the board.

Versions of communication boards that do not require the user to directly select symbols have been developed. The simplest is the *eye gaze board.* Eye gaze boards are used when speechless patients have good language abilities but cannot move their limbs to directly select symbols from a board (for example, patients who are quadriplegic following cervical spinal

cord injuries). Eye gaze boards allow such patients to indicate letters, words, phrases, or symbols by looking at them. Message recipients watch the patient's eye movements and say aloud what they believe the patient is looking at. The patient signals correct choices, usually by blinking. Because it is difficult for message recipients to tell exactly where a patient is looking, eye gaze boards have to be large, with large spaces between symbols. For this reason eye gaze boards cannot contain very many items. Most eye gaze boards contain an alphabet, numbers, and perhaps a few key words or phrases. Many are printed on transparent plastic sheets or have cutouts through which message recipients can monitor the patient's eye movements.

Mechanical and Electronic Devices Mechanical and electronic devices for augmenting or replacing speech differ in cost, complexity, portability, and output. They range in cost from less than one hundred dollars to several thousand dollars. They range in portability from small hand-held devices to large units that cannot be carried. The most common units are portable electronic devices that translate keyboard inputs into messages that are either displayed on electronic readouts, printed on paper tape, or translated into speech-like output. Some generate literal representations of what is entered on the keyboard, and what the auditor sees is what the user has entered. Other units translate codes entered by the user into programmed output messages; for example a three-digit code entered by the user might generate a five- or six-word phrase. Many (especially the hand-held devices) require finger dexterity and coordination to operate keyboards, and most require that the user read, spell, or remember codes, making them unsuitable for use with most aphasic patients, patients with moderate to severe cognitive impairments, or patients with poor motor control.

Gesture and Pantomime Some dysarthric patients may be taught gesture or pantomime to

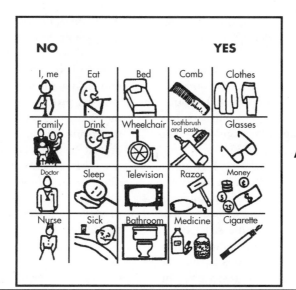

A

I CAN HEAR PERFECTLY	PLEASE REPEAT AS I TALK (THIS IS HOW I TALK BY SPELLING OUT THE WORDS)	WOULD YOU PLEASE CALL
A AN HE	AM ARE ASK BE BEEN BRING CAN	ABOUT ALL
HER I IT ME	COME COULD DID DO DOES DON'T	AND ALWAYS
MY HIM SHE	DRINK GET GIVE GO HAD HAS HAVE	ALMOST AS
THAT THE THESE	IS KEEP KNOW LET LIKE MAKE MAY	AT BECAUSE
THEY THIS WHOSE	PUT SAY SAID SEE SEEN SEND SHOULD	BUT FOR FROM
WHAT WHEN WHERE	TAKE TELL THINK THOUGHT WANT	HOW IF IN
WHICH WHO WHY	WAS WERE WILL WISH WON'T WOULD -ED	OF ON OR
YOU WE YOUR	-ER -EST -ING -LY -N'T -'S -TION	TO UP WITH
A B	C D E F G	AFTER AGAIN
H I	J K L M	ANY EVEN
N O	P Qu R S T	EVERY HERE
U V	W X Y Z	JUST MORE
1 2	3 4 5 6 7	ONLY SO
8 9	10 11 12 30	SOME SOON
		THERE VERY
SUN. MON. TUES. WED. THUR. FRI. SAT. BATHROOM	PLEASE THANK YOU GOING OUT	$¢½(SHHH!!)?
	MR. MRS. MISS START OVER MOTHER DAD DOCTOR END OF WORD	_____

B

Figure 10-4 ■ Communication boards. **(A)** A picture communication board suitable for a patient with moderate to severe language impairment. **(B)** A more complex board containing words and phrases that would be appropriate for a patient with good language abilities and sufficient finger and arm dexterity to point to letters and words at a reasonably fast rate.

augment speech, but usually other systems (communication boards, electronic devices) provide better communication.

Sign Languages Sign languages sometimes can be taught to patients who are not too aphasic to learn them. Sign languages that require spelling and syntactic abilities usually are less practical for brain-damaged persons than languages requiring less linguistic ability. *Amerind* (American Indian Sign; Skelly, 1979) contains signs that do not depend heavily on verbal skills. Consequently, they can be learned by some patients with linguistic impairments. Most Amerind signs are comprehensible to message recipients without extensive training. A major problem with most other sign languages is that the signs are not comprehensible to message recipients without training, so that patients who use them cannot communicate with untrained persons.

Other Considerations Silverman (1983) described several factors that clinicians should consider when one is choosing an alternative or augmentative system for a patient.

- The *cost* of the system is important when resources for purchasing it are limited.
- The amount of *training* needed for the patient to learn to use the system is important. If the system is to be a permanent replacement or augmentation for speech, then extensive training can be justified. If the system is for temporary use, or if an alternative means of communication is needed immediately, then systems requiring extensive training are not appropriate.
- *Interference* or the extent to which using the system interferes with other activities is important. A system that requires the patient to sit at a fixed terminal and use both hands to operate it is more disruptive than a portable system that can be operated with one hand.
- The *intelligibility* of the output of the augmentative or alternative system affect both the time required to make it functional and the generality with which it can be used by the patient. Systems that generate output that is intelligible to untrained message recipients require less time to become operational and will be useful in more different places than systems producing symbols whose meanings message recipients must be taught. Systems that print messages on paper tape or in liquid crystal displays cannot be used in the dark, over the telephone, or when patient and auditor are more than a few feet apart. Systems that generate messages on illuminated displays can be used in the dark, but not over the telephone or at a distance. Systems that generate speech-like output may be unintelligible in noisy environments and may not be intelligible over the telephone, depending on the fidelity of the augmentative or alternative system's output and the fidelity of the telephone system.
- The *acceptability* of the system to user and message recipients usually determines the extent to which it will be used in daily life. If the device or system is cumbersome, complicated, or unnatural, it may be discarded in favor of less cumbersome (and less effective) ways to communicate.

KEY CONCEPTS

- Dysarthria is a general label for a group of speech disorders caused by weakness, paralysis, sensory loss, or incoordination of muscle groups responsible for speech.
- Dysarthria may be caused by pathology affecting any of several parts of the nervous system, including the brain, corticobulbar tracts, the extrapyramidal system, the brainstem, the cerebellum, and, less often, the spinal cord or spinal nerves.
- Neuropathologies causing dysarthria may compromise articulation, phonation, velopharyngeal valving, or respiration, indi-

vidually or in combination. Consequently, evaluation of dysarthric patients requires that these mechanical/physiologic processes be assessed.

- Treatment of dysarthria usually involves a combination of direct treatment of phonation, resonation, articulation, and prosody by means of drills, together with indirect treatment procedures such as sensory stimulation, muscle strengthening, modification of muscle tone, modification of posture and speaking position, and enhancing respiratory support. Modifying the patient's daily life environment to enhance communicative success is an important adjunct to treatment for some dysarthric patients, and medical/surgical treatment may be appropriate for others.

- Augmentative or alternative communication systems may be appropriate for severely dysarthric patients who cannot produce intelligible speech.

Standard Medical Abbreviations

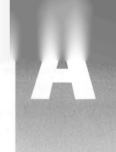

~	Approximately
△	Change
≃	Consistent with
†	Death
↘	Decrease
°	Degree
≤	Equal to or less than
>	Greater than
<	Less than
♀	Female
♂	Male
—	Negative
#	Number
%	Percent
%ile	Percentile
+	Positive
1°	Primary
2°	Secondary
∴	Therefore
c̄	With
ø	Without
AAROM	Active assisted range of motion
abn	Abnormal
a.c.	Before meals
ACA	Anterior communicating artery, anterior cerebral artery
ad lib	As desired
ADL	Activities of daily living
AK, AKA	Above the knee, above-knee amputation
alc, ETOH	Alcohol
AIDS	Acquired immunodeficiency syndrome

ALS	Amyotrophic lateral sclerosis
AMA	Against medical advice, American Medical Association
amb	Ambulatory
AMI	Acute myocardial infarction
ant	Anterior
angio	Angiogram
ante	Before
AODM	Adult onset diabetes mellitus
AP	Anterioposterior
ARD	Acute respiratory disease
ARF	Acute renal failure
ASA	Aspirin
ASAP	As soon as possible
ASCVD	Arteriosclerotic cardiovascular disease
ASHD	Arteriosclerotic heart disease
ASVD	Arteriosclerotic vascular disease
AV	Arteriovenous, atrioventricular
AVM	Arteriovenous malformation
b.i.d.	Twice a day
bil	Bilateral
BK	Below the knee
bm	Bowel movement
BM	Bone marrow
BMR	Basal metabolism rate
BP	Blood pressure
BRP	Bathroom privileges
bs	Bowel sounds
BS	Breath sounds
BUN	Blood urea nitrogen
bx	Biopsy

C	Celsius, centigrade	EENT	Eye, ear, nose, throat
CA	Cardiac arrest	EMG	Electromyogram
CA, ca	Carcinoma	ENT	Ear, nose, throat
Ca$^+$	Calcium	EOM	Extraocular movements
CAB	Coronary artery bypass	ER	Emergency room
CAD	Coronary artery disease	ETOH	Ethanol (alcohol)
cal	Calorie	exam	Examination
CAT	Computed axial tomography	ext	External, exterior
cath	Catheter	F	Fahrenheit
CBC	Complete blood count	FB	Foreign body
CBS	Chronic brain syndrome	FBS	Fasting blood sugar
CC	Chief complaint	FH	Family history
cc	Cubic centimeter	fib	Fibrillation
CHF	Congestive heart failure, chronic heart failure	fl, fld	Fluid
		FU	Follow-up
CHI	Closed head injury	FUO	Fever of unknown origin
cm	Centimeter	fx	Fracture
CMT	Continuing medication and treatment	GB	Gall bladder
		gen	General
CN	Cranial nerve	GI	Gastrointestinal
CNS	Central nervous system	gm	Gram
cont	Continue(d)	gr	Grain
COLD	Chronic obstructive lung disease	GSW	Gunshot wound
COPD	Chronic obstructive pulmonary disease	GTT	Glucose tolerance test
		GU	Genito-urinary
c/o	Complains of	GYN	Gynecology
CPR	Cardiopulmonary resuscitation	h, hr	Hour
CRF	Chronic renal failure	HA	Headache
CSF	Cerebrospinal fluid	HB	Heart block
CT	Computerized tomography	Hb	Hemoglobin
cu	Cubic	HBP	High blood pressure
CV	Cardiovascular	HCM	Health care maintenance
CVA	Cerebrovascular accident	HCVD	Hypertensive cardiovascular disease
CXR	Chest x-ray	HEENT	Head, eyes, ears, nose, throat
d	Day	Hg	Mercury
DNR	Do not resuscitate	Hg, Hgb	Hemoglobin
DNT	Did not test	HH	Homonymous hemianopsia
DOA	Dead on arrival	H/O	History of
DOE	Dyspnea (shortness of breath) on exertion	H&P	History and physical
		HPI	History of present illness
DT	Delirium tremens	HR	Heart rate
d/t	Due to	hs	Bedtime
DTR	Deep tendon reflex	HTN	Hypertension
DU	Diabetic urine	hx	History
Dx	Diagnosis	H_2O	Water
ECA	External carotid artery	I&O	Intake and output
ECG, EKG	Electrocardiogram	ICA	Internal carotid artery
ECT	Electroconvulsive therapy	ICP	Intracranial pressure
EEG	Electroencephalogram	ICU	Intensive care unit

IM	Intramuscular	OPD	Outpatient department
imp	Impression	OPT	Outpatient treatment
inc	Increase	OR	Operating room
inf	Inferior	OT	Occupational therapy
IU	International unit	oz.	Ounce
IV	Intravenous	p̱	Pulse
kg	Kilogram	p̄	After
KJ	Knee jerk	PA	Posteroanterior
L,l	Left	PAR	Postanesthesia recovery room
lab	Laboratory	path	Pathology
lat	Lateral	PC	Presenting complaint
LCA	Left coronary artery	p.c.	After meals
LE	Lower extremity	PCA	Posterior cerebral artery
liq	Liquid	PCN	Penicillin
LMD	Local medical doctor	PE	Physical examination
LOC	Loss of consciousness	PEG	Percutaneous endoscopic gastrostomy
LOM	Limitation of motion		
LOS	Length of stay	per	By
LP	Lumbar puncture (spinal tap)	PERRLA	Pupils equal, round, reactive to light and accommodation
LPN	Licensed practical nurse		
L&W	Living and well	PET	Positron emission tomography
MCA	Middle cerebral artery	PH	Past history
MH	Marital history	PI	Present illness
MI	Myocardial infarction	PMD	Personal medical doctor
ml	Milliliter	PMH	Past medical history
mm	Millimeter	PMR	Physical medicine and rehabili- tation
mHg	Millimeters of mercury		
MRI	Magnetic resonance image	p.o.	By mouth
MS	Multiple sclerosis	POD	Postoperative day
MVA	Motor vehicle accident	pos.	Positive
NA	Not applicable	post.	Posterior
NAD	No acute distress	PR	Pulse rate
neg	Negative	preop	Preoperative
neuro	Neurologic, neurology	prep	Preparation
NG	Nasogastric	prn, p.r.n.	As needed
NKA	No known allergies	PROM	Passive range of motion
no.	Number	Psych	Psychiatry
noc.	Night	Psychol	Psychology
NP	Neuropsychiatric	PT	Physical therapy
NPO, npo	Nothing by mouth	PTA	Prior to admission
N/S	Neurosurgery	pt	Patient
NSC	Not service connected	PX	Physical
N&V	Nausea and vomiting	q.a.m.	Every morning
OBS	Organic brain syndrome	q.d.	Every day
OD	Officer of the day	q.i.d.	Four times per day
OD	Overdose	q.h.	Every hour
OM	Otitis media	q.o.d.	Every other day
OOB, oob	Out of bed	R, r	Right
OP	Outpatient	RBC	Red blood cell

RIND	Reversible ischemic neurologic deficit	Sz	Seizure
		T	Temperature
RMS	Rehabilitation medicine service	TB, TBC	Tuberculosis
RN	Registered nurse	temp	Temperature
RND	Radical neck dissection	TIA	Transient ischemic attack
r/o	Rule out	TBI	Traumatic brain injury
ROM	Range of motion	t.i.d.	Three times per day
RR	Respiration rate	TPR	Temperature, pulse, respiration
Rt	Right	tx	Transplant
RT	Radiation therapy	Tx	Treatment
RT	Recreational therapy	UA	Urinalysis
RTC	Return to clinic	UCHD	Usual childhood diseases
Rx	Therapy	VD	Venereal disease
s, sec	Second	VDRL	Venereal Disease Research Laboratory Test (for VD)
s	Without		
SAB	Subarachnoid bleed	VF	Visual field
SAH	Subarachnoid hemorrhage	v fib	Ventricular fibrillations
SC	Service connected	VHD	Valvular heart disease
SCI	Spinal cord injury	VS	Vital signs
SH	Social history	W	White
SI	Seriously ill	w, wk	Week
SOB	Shortness of breath	WBC	White blood cells
s/p	Status post	WD	Well developed
spec	Specimen	WDWN	Well developed, well nourished
ss	One half	WNL	Within normal limits
SSN	Social security number	wt	Weight
stat	Immediately	w/u	Workup
surg	Surgery	Y/O	Year old
Sx	Symptoms	yrs	Years

Glossary

Acceleration Injury: Brain injury caused when the moving head strikes a stationary surface or the stationary head is struck by a moving object in a way that causes the head to move quickly from its resting position. *Linear acceleration injury* is caused by forces that propel the head on a linear path. *Angular acceleration injury* is caused by forces that propel the head at an angle from the path of the impact and cause it to rotate. See also *coup injury, contrecoup injury, diffuse axonal injury, translational trauma.*

Agnosia: Inability to recognize stimuli in a sensory modality in spite of intact sensation in the modality. Several varieties of agnosia have been described in the literature, including *auditory agnosia, visual agnosia, tactile agnosia,* and combinations such as *auditory-verbal agnosia* and *visual-verbal agnosia.*

Agrammatism: Speech in which content words (mainly nouns, verbs, adjectives) are present, but most function words (articles, prepositions, conjunctions) are missing. A common characteristic of the speech of adults with Broca's aphasia.

Agraphia (Dysgraphia): Impaired writing.

Alertness, Phasic: Rapidly occurring changes in receptivity to stimulation.

Alertness, Tonic: Ongoing receptivity to stimulation.

Alexia (Dyslexia): Impaired reading.

Alexia without Agraphia: A rare syndrome in which the patient cannot read, but can write. Usually caused by isolation of the visual cortices from Wernicke's area.

Alzheimer's Disease: A progressive neurologic disease characterized by increasing dementia and death.

Anesthesia: Complete loss of sensation.

Aneurysm: Balloon-like bulges in an artery caused by weakness in the arterial wall. Aneurysms are weaker than the arterial wall and are susceptible to hemorrhage.

Angiography (Arteriography): A laboratory procedure by which blood vessels can be visualized. A contrast medium is injected into the blood stream and a series of X-ray exposures is made to determine the condition of the patient's blood vessels.

Angular Gyrus: A prominent gyrus near the temporo-parietal-occipital junction, at the posterior end of the Sylvian (lateral) fissure. Damage in the region of the angular gyrus often causes problems with reading and arithmetic abilities.

Anosagnosia: Denial of illness. Often a symptom of right-hemisphere brain pathology.

Anterior Horn Cells: Spinal motor neurons located in the anterolateral part of the spinal cord.

Anton's Syndrome (Visual Anosagnosia): A condition in which a person is blind because of bilateral destruction of the visual cortex *(cortical blindness),* but denies being blind.

Aorta: The main artery from the heart.

Aphasia: A language impairment that crosses all input and output modalities. Can be divided into various syndromes.

Apraxia: Disruption of volitional movement sequences in the absence of sensory loss, weakness, paralysis, or incoordination of the muscles involved in the movements. Usually a consequence of damage in the premotor cortex. (See also *ideational apraxia, ideomotor apraxia, buccofacial apraxia, limb*

441

apraxia, verbal apraxia, dressing apraxia, and *constructional apraxia.*)

Arachnoid Villi: Sites at which cerebrospinal fluid is resorbed into the venous blood.

Arcuate Fasciculus: A major fiber tract that connects the temporal lobe with regions in the frontal lobe in each hemisphere. The arcuate fasciculus in the left hemisphere is considered the major pathway by which information from the language centers in the temporal lobe reach the frontal lobe for conversion into spoken or written output.

Arteriography: See *angiography.*

Arteriovenous Malformation (AVM): Convoluted collections of weak, thin-walled veins and arteries on the brain's surface or within the brain.

Association Cortex: Cortical areas that are adjacent to sensory or motor cortex. Association cortex is thought to play an important part in integrating motor or sensory information from adjacent cortical areas and input from other regions of the brain.

Astererognosis (Tactile Agnosia): Inability to recognize otherwise familiar objects by touch, even though the sense of touch is intact.

Astrocytoma: A common, relatively benign glioma.

Ataxia: Clumsiness and incoordination of movements caused by cerebellar damage.

Atherosclerosis (Arteriosclerosis): A disease process in which arterial walls become roughened and covered with fatty deposits. These deposits are called *atherosclerotic plaque.*

Athetosis: Slow, sinuous, writhing and uncontrollable muscle movements.

Atrophy: Shrinkage and wasting away of tissues.

Attention, Alternating: The ability to shift attention from one stimulus to another or from one aspect of a stimulus to another.

Attention, Divided: The ability to attend to more than one activity simultaneously.

Attention, Selective: The ability to maintain attention on selected stimuli in the presence of competing or distracting stimuli. Sometimes called *focused attention.*

Attention, Sustained: The ability to maintain attention on selected stimuli over time.

Auditory Cortex: A region of cortex on the top surface of each temporal lobe (the gyrus of Heschl). It has primary responsibility for auditory perception.

Axon: The conducting process of a nerve cell (neuron).

Ballism: See *chorea.*

Basal Ganglia: Several nuclei in the diencephalon, near the thalamus. They are responsible for regulation of major muscle groups that make postural adjustments and compensate for inertial forces during movement. They are a major component of the extrapyramidal system. Damage usually causes weakness, paralysis, sensory disruption, and the appearance of involuntary movements called *dyskinesia.* Depending on who is writing about them, the basal ganglia include the caudate nucleus, putamen, globus pallidus, subthalamic nucleus, and substantia nigra.

Basilar Artery: An artery that connects the two vertebral arteries to the posterior part of the circle of Willis. It progresses upward on the front surface of the pons and supplies blood to the pons.

Bell's Palsy: Ipsilateral paralysis of lower facial muscles caused by compression of the facial nerve (CN 7).

Binswanger's Disease: A rare disease caused by multiple infarcts in subcortical white matter.

Biopsy: Removal of a sample of tissue for laboratory analysis.

Brain Abscess: A cavity in the brain caused by infection with bacteria, fungi, or parasites.

Brainstem: A stalk-like structure at the base of the brain, atop the spinal cord. It contains centers that regulate some vital functions and contains most cranial nerve nuclei. Anatomists divide it into the midbrain (upper), pons (middle), and medulla (lower).

Broca's Area: A region of cortex just anterior to the lower end of the primary motor cortex. Damage in Broca's areas is said to cause *Broca's aphasia.*

Buccofacial Apraxia: Ideomotor apraxia of the oral musculature.

Calcarine Fissure: A deep groove in the occipital lobe of each hemisphere. It is important because the visual cortex is adjacent to it.

Caloric Testing: A diagnostic test in which cold or warm water is introduced into the external auditory canal. Patients with vestibular pathology respond with characteristic patterns of *nystagmus.*

Capgras Syndrome: The belief that friends, family, or acquaintances have been abducted and replaced by imposters.

Carotid Arteries: There are two external carotid arteries and two internal carotid arteries. The external carotid arteries supply blood to the face. The internal carotid arteries supply blood to the brain via the circle of Willis.

Catastrophic Reaction: A sudden and intense emotional outburst, usually anger, but sometimes crying, and rarely laughing. Catastrophic reactions usually are a brain-injured patient's response to being pushed beyond his or her limits.

Central Fissure: A deep groove that divides each brain hemisphere into roughly equal front and back halves. Sometimes it is called the *fissure of Rolando.*

Central Nervous System (CNS): The brain, brainstem, cerebellum, and spinal cord. The brain is responsible for perception and discrimination of external and internal stimuli, for regulation of vital body processes, for organization, regulation, and execution of behavior, and for mental processes. The brainstem contains motor and sensory fiber tracts, the cranial nerve nuclei, centers that regulate some aspects of respiration and heart rate, and structures that regulate level of consciousness. The cerebellum coordinates and modulates movements initiated elsewhere in the central nervous system. The spinal cord serves as a conduit for information going from the brain to muscles and glands and for sensory information going to the brain from sensory receptors.

Cerebellum: A structure that looks like a miniature brain, which lies beneath the posterior temporal lobes. It is important in integration and coordination of volitional movements.

Cerebral Aqueduct: A long narrow passageway between the third and fourth ventricles. Occlusion of the cerebral aqueduct is a common cause of hydrocephalus (enlarged ventricles). It is sometimes called the *aqueduct of Sylvius.*

Cerebral Arteries: There are three pairs, one set of three for each hemisphere called the *anterior, middle,* and *posterior cerebral arteries,* which serve the front, middle, and posterior parts of the hemisphere, respectively.

Cerebral Dominance: The belief that one hemisphere has primary responsibility for speech and language. (The left hemisphere in right-handed people.)

Cerebral Plasticity: The ability of the brain to reassign functions served by one area to a different area, usually in response to brain injury. Cerebral plasticity is greatest in infants and declines steadily with age.

Cerebrospinal Fluid (CSF): A clear, colorless fluid that fills the ventricles and surrounds the brain, brainstem, cerebellum, and spinal cord.

Cerebrovascular Accident (CVA): Temporary or permanent disruption of brain function due to interruption of its blood supply. Sometimes called *stroke.*

Cerebrum: What we usually think of as the brain. The two brain hemispheres.

Chorea: A disease that causes quick and forceful involuntary movements *(choreiform movements). Ballism* is an extreme form of chorea, in which the limbs are flung wildly about by the involuntary movements.

Choreoathetosis: A combination of choreiform and athetoid movements. (See *chorea* and *athetosis.*)

Circle of Willis: A heptagonal arrangement of arteries at the base of the brain that connects the internal carotid arteries and the basilar artery to the cerebral arteries. It is thought to serve as a "safety valve" for occlusions below the circle of Willis.

Circumduction: A characteristic gait of patients with hemiplegia *(circumducted gait).* The patient swings the leg outward from the hip in a semicircular movement without flexing the knee.

Circumlocution: Literally, *talking around* words that an individual is unable to say. Patients with conduction or Wernicke's aphasia often use circumlocution to communicate the sense of words they cannot retrieve.

Cistern: A cavity or space for storage of fluids.

Clasp-knife Phenomenon: The tendency of spastic muscles to resist stretching when the examiner first moves the patient's limb and to gradually become less resistant as the examiner continues to move the patient's limb at a constant rate.

Coagulation Time: The time it takes for blood to clot. Laboratory tests of coagulation time are useful in treating patients with occlusive vascular disease.

Coherence: The overall unity or point of discourse.

Cohesion: The degree to which words in discourse relate to one another. A product of *cohesive ties.*

Coma: Prolonged loss of consciousness.

Commissural Fibers (Commissures): Nerve fiber tracts that cross between the brain hemispheres. The corpus callosum is the major commissure in the brain. The anterior and posterior commissures are minor ones.

Commissurotomy: Surgically cutting the corpus callosum.

Computed Tomography (CT Scanning): A radiologic test in which a computer constructs cross-sectional images of internal body structures by analyzing information from a series of X-ray exposures made at consecutive horizontal levels of a body part.

Concreteness: Failure to appreciate abstract, indirect, nonliteral meanings of messages, events, or situations.

Confrontation Naming: Naming objects, pictures, and color swatches, etc.

Constructional Apraxia: A misnomer. Inability to copy geometric shapes, usually a disorder of visuospatial perception and integration, rather than a motor-planning disorder.

Contralateral: On the other side. In neurology, the term usually means *on the other side of the body from the nervous system disease.*

Contrast: Any of several fluids that may be introduced into internal spaces (usually blood vessels) or tissues to make structures easier to see in laboratory imaging studies.

Contrastive Stress Drill: A treatment for dysarthria and apraxia of speech in which the patient is coached to produce utterances with exaggerated emphatic stress on certain words, as in "Bob hit **Bill.**"

Contrecoup Injury: Brain injury on the opposite side of the brain from the impact.

Corpus Callosum: The major commissure connecting the brain hemispheres. Almost all neural communication between the hemispheres goes via the corpus callosum.

Cortex: The neuron-rich outer layer of the brain hemispheres. Cortex makes "higher mental processes" (thinking, reasoning, calculating, and so on) possible.

Corticobulbar: Going between the cortex and the brain stem.

Corticopontine: Going between the cortex and the pons.

Corticospinal: Going between the cortex and the spinal cord.

Coup Injury: Brain injury at the site of impact.

Cranial Nerves: Peripheral nerves that serve muscles and sensory receptors in the head and neck. Most connect with the central nervous system in the brain stem.

Cranial Vault: The inside of the skull. It contains the brain and cerebellum. It is divided into compartments by sheets of dura. The two major ones are the falx cerebri and the tentorium cerebelli.

Decomposition of Movement: Movements that have a jerky, segmented quality often seen following cerebellar damage. A component of *ataxia.*

Decussate: Cross the midline. Refers to the crossing of pyramidal tracts from one side of the central nervous system to the other at the medulla.

Dementia: Diffuse impairment of intellect and cognition caused by any of several diseases and conditions.

Dementia, Cortical: Dementia caused by pathology that affects the cerebral cortex.

Dementia, Mixed: Dementia caused by a combination of cortical and subcortical pathology.

Dementia, Subcortical: Dementia caused by pathology affecting the basal ganglia, thalamus, and brain stem.

Dendrite: Short, hair-like receptive processes of a nerve cell (neuron).

Dermatome: A region of skin innervated by a cranial or spinal sensory nerve.

Diagnosis: The act of assigning a label to a disease or condition.

Diaschisis: Disruption of brain function in areas remote from an area of injury, but connected to it by nerve pathways.

Diencephalon: A deep central region within the brain hemispheres. It contains the thalamus and basal ganglia. It plays an important part in the regulation and integration of motor activity and sensory experience.

Differential Diagnosis: Discriminating a disease or condition from others that may resemble it.

Diffuse Axonal Injury: Disseminated damage to nerve cell axons caused by *angular acceleration.*

Diplopia: Double vision often caused by weakness or paralysis of muscles responsible for moving one eyeball, which prevents the two eyes from fixating on the same point.

Disability: The effects of a structural or functional abnormality on a skill or ability. (For example, poor ambulation, caused by paralysis. See *impairment, handicap.*)

Disconnection Syndrome: A unique pattern of impairments caused by interruption of fibers in the corpus callosum that connect the hemispheres, which isolates the language-competent hemisphere from the language-incompetent hemisphere. Patients with disconnection syndrome cannot name, describe, or talk about stimuli directed exclusively to the language-incompetent hemisphere, because the information cannot get across the corpus callosum to the language-competent hemisphere.

Double Simultaneous Stimulation: Simultaneously stimulating sensory receptors at symmetrical points on both sides of the body. Patients with subtle sensory impairments report stimulation only on the unaffected side.

Dressing Apraxia: A misnomer. Dressing apraxia is not a true apraxia. It usually is seen in patients with nondominant-hemisphere pathology and is caused by disruptions of body schema, impaired appreciation of the relationship of the body to surrounding space, and, sometimes, neglect.

Dysarthria: Any of several speech abnormalities caused by nervous system damage that affects movement or sensation within body parts involved in speech.

Dyskinesia: Abnormal and involuntary muscle movements often seen as a consequence of extrapyramidal disease. (See also *tremor, chorea, ballism, dystonia, myoclonus, fasciculations, fibrillations,* and *tics.*)

Dyslexia, Deep: A reading impairment in which the individual cannot analyze words phonologically, but must depend on whole-word reading to recognize words.

Dyslexia, Surface: A reading impairment in which the individual cannot make use of whole-word recognition in reading, but must depend on phonologic analysis to recognize words.

Dysmetria: Slow and awkward movements. A component of *ataxia.*

Dystonia: Persisting involuntary contractions of muscles, sometimes called *torsion spasm.*

Echolalia: A tendency to repeat back what is said. A common characteristic of patients with *posterior isolation syndrome.*

Edema: Swelling.

Effectiveness: Whether or not treatment causes a meaningful change in patients' daily life adequacy.

Efficacy: Whether or not treatment causes a significant change in patients' performance on one or more objective measures.

Egocentrism: Inability to view events and situations from another's point of view.

Electroencephalography (EEG): A laboratory test in which the electrical activity of the brain cortex is measured and converted to a pen tracing on a moving strip of paper.

Electromyography (EMG): A procedure in which fine needle electrodes are inserted into muscles and the electrical activity in the muscles is recorded.

Ellipsoidal Deformation: Deformation of the restrained skull caused by the impact of a slow-moving object having a large surface area.

Embolus: A fragment that travels through a blood vessel. If it lodges and occludes an artery it causes an embolic stroke.

Emotional Lability: Exaggerated emotional responses to stimuli. Unusually wide swings in emotional tone.

Empty Speech: Speech that is syntactically correct but conveys little or no overall meaning. Often a result of substituting general words such as *thing* or *stuff* for more specific words.

Epidural: Between the dura mater and the skull.

Evoked Cortical Potentials: A laboratory procedure in which a computer averages the electrical activity of the brain cortex from many sites on the skull and produces a record of systematic changes in the electrical activity that occur with presentation of auditory, visual, or tactile stimuli.

Falx Cerebri: A rigid sheet of dura mater that goes from front to back within the longitudinal cerebral fissure. It often is called the *falx* for efficiency.

Familial: Diseases that have a greater-than-normal occurrence in families but do not have a known genetic inheritance pattern. The exact probability that offspring of parents who have the disease will inherit the disease cannot be calculated. (See also *hereditary.*)

Fasciculus: A fiber tract that connects regions in different lobes of the brain. The three major fasciculi are the arcuate fasciculus, the uncinate fasciculus, and the cingulum. The arcuate fasciculus plays a major part in speech and language.

Feedback: Information provided contingent on responses. *Incentive feedback* depends on response consequences that have primary reinforcing (or punishing) power. Incentive feedback can increase or maintain responses that have no other purpose than obtaining (or avoiding) the feedback (e.g., money, praise, electric shock). *Information feedback* has no intrinsic reinforcing or punishing power but provides information to an individual about the closeness of responses to a target. See *reinforcement, punishment.*

Festinating Gait: Short, rapid steps. A common consequence of Parkinson's disease.

Fibrillations: Contractions of a single muscle fiber or small group of fibers too small to be seen but detectable with sensitive instruments.

Fissure: A deep sulcus.

Fluency: When used to classify adults with aphasia, fluency refers to the prosodic or melodic characteristics of speech. Adults with fluent aphasia speak with essentially normal rate, intonation, pauses, and emphatic stress patterns. Adults with nonfluent aphasia speak slowly, with diminished intonation, abnormally placed and excessively long pauses, and diminished variation in emphatic stress. Fluent aphasia is associated with postcentral damage, and nonfluent aphasia is associated with precentral damage.

Focal: Affecting a limited region within the nervous system. The opposite of *diffuse.*

Foramen: An opening. There are several foramina in the skull, through which blood vessels and nerves pass. The major one is the *foramen magnum,* through which the brain stem passes. There are many foramina in the spinal cord, between the vertebrae, through which nerves and blood vessels pass (the intervertebral foramina).

Frontal Lobes: They make up approximately the anterior one third of the brain and are important for providing the initial impetus for overt behavior.

Fugue State: A period of disturbed consciousness, lasting from minutes to days, in which the patient goes about regular activities of daily living but has no subsequent memory for what happened during the period.

Functional Communication: Communication in daily life.

Gag Reflex: Coughing or choking when the posterior tongue or pharyngeal walls are touched.

Generalization: Transfer of learned skills, behaviors, or responses from one setting to another.

Generative Naming (Word Fluency): Providing names according to a category suggested by the examiner. For example, *"Tell me all the words you can think of that begin with the letter F,"* or *"Tell me all the vegetables you can think of."* (Usually limited to a 1-minute interval.)

Geographic Disorientation: Inability to identify one's geographic location even though one recognizes one's personal surroundings. An occasional consequence of right-hemisphere brain damage.

Glial Cells: Form the supporting tissue of the brain, which is called *glia.* Most of the cells in the brain are glial cells.

Glioblastoma Multiforme: A common, very malignant tumor of glial cells.

Glioma: A tumor that arises in brain glia.

Granulovacuolar Degeneration: Neuronal abnormalities seen in Alzheimer's disease, other neurologic diseases, and in some normal elderly. Small fluid-filled cavities appear within nerve cells and nerve cell function is adversely affected.

Gyrus: A "hill" on the surface of the brain. (Plural = gyri.)

Gyrus of Heschl: A strip of cortex on the top surface of each temporal lobe. Also known as the *primary auditory cortex.*

Handicap: The effects of a structural or functional abnormality on an individual's ability to carry out daily life roles and responsibilities. (For example, diminished ability to earn a living as a consequence of hemiplegia. See *impairment, disability.*)

Hematoma: Accumulation of blood from a hemorrhage.

Hemianopsia (Hemianopia): Blindness in one half of the visual field. *Homonymous hemianopsia* is blindness in the same (right or left) half of the visual field in each eye. *Heteronymous hemianopsia* is blindness in different halves of the visual field in each eye.

Hemiplegia: Paralysis of arm and a leg on one side of the body.

Hemorrhage: Bleeding. Accumulation of blood from a hemorrhage is called a *hematoma.*

Hereditary: Diseases that have a known genetic inheritance pattern. The probability that offspring of parents who have the disease will inherit the disease can be calculated, and "family trees" showing inheritance patterns can be constructed.

Herniation: Displacement of brain tissue by swelling or space-occupying lesions such as tumors or brain abscesses.

Heuristic Processes: "Top-down" comprehension processes, in which listeners and readers use general knowledge, intuition, and guessing to arrive at the meaning of spoken or printed verbal materials.

Huntington's Disease: A hereditary neurologic disease characterized by progressive chorea and dementia.

Hydrocephalus: Enlargement of the cerebral ventricles. Hydrocephalus usually is caused by obstruction of an intraventricular passageway but can also be a result of brain atrophy. The former is called obstructive hydrocephalus and the latter is called nonobstructive hydrocephalus.

Hyperesthesia: Abnormal sensitivity to stimulation.

Hypertonia: Abnormally high levels of tension in resting muscles.

Hypesthesia (Hypoesthesia): Diminished sensation.

Hypoperfusion: Diminished blood supply to the brain caused by insufficient blood volume or pressure.

Hypotonia: Abnormally low levels of tension in resting muscles.

Ideational Apraxia: Inability to carry out movement sequences because of loss of the concept, knowledge, or idea of what the movements are intended to accomplish.

Ideomotor Apraxia: Inability to carry out movement sequences because of loss of the ability to organize the motor plans or patterns for the movements.

Impairment: A structural or functional abnormality within an individual. (For example, paralysis. See *disability, handicap.*)

Infarct: Death of tissue caused by loss of blood supply.

Insula: A patch of cortex folded into the lateral fissure, sometimes called the *island of Reil.* The operculum surrounds it.

Internal capsule: The section of a dense band of nerve fibers going between the cortex and lower centers that lies within the basal ganglia.

Intersystemic Reorganization: A treatment for apraxia of speech in which patients are taught to execute nonspeech movements simultaneously with speech (e.g., gesturing the act of drinking from a glass while saying *"Drink some water"*).

Intracerebral: Within the brain.

Intrasystemic Reorganization: A treatment for apraxia of speech in which the locus of control of speech movements is shifted to another part of the system used to produce speech (e.g., speaking slowly and with exaggerated articulation.)

Intraventricular Foramen: A short passageway between each lateral ventricle and the third ventricle for movement of cerebrospinal fluid, sometimes called the *foramen of Munro.*

Ipsilateral: On the same side. (See also *contralateral.*)

Ischemia: Compromised blood supply.

Isolation Syndrome: An aphasia syndrome caused by isolation of the central region of the language-dominant hemisphere from the rest of the brain. Patients with *anterior isolation syndrome* have sparse speech output, intact comprehension, and good repetition. Patients with *posterior isolation syndrome* have fluent but echolalic speech output, impaired comprehension, and good repetition.

Jargon: Nonsensical utterances, such as *"There's a navy dog flying in the hoghouse this morning,"* in which words are uttered in syntactically legitimate strings but which have no overall meaning. The strings may contain *neologisms.*

Lacunar State: A progressive neurologic disease caused by successive small infarcts in the midbrain and brain stem.

Lateral Apertures: Two openings from the fourth ventricle into the subarachnoid space, sometimes called the *foramina of Luschka.*

Lateral Cerebral Fissure: A deep groove that separates the temporal lobe in each hemisphere from the frontal and parietal lobes, sometimes called the *fissure of Sylvius* or the *frontotemporoparietal fissure.* The primary auditory cortex is located on the floor of the lateral cerebral fissure.

Lenticular Nucleus: The putamen and globus pallidus (basal ganglia).

Limb Apraxia: Ideomotor apraxia of the arm and hand. Limb apraxias usually are more severe distally (away from the trunk) than proximally (near the trunk).

Localization: An approach to understanding the functional architecture of the nervous system by relating neurologically damaged patients' symptoms to damaged regions of the nervous system. When damage in a given part of the nervous system consistently causes certain impairments, the impaired function is attributed to the damaged part.

Logorrhea: See *press of speech.*

Longitudinal Cerebral Fissure: The deep groove at the apex of the cerebrum that separates the hemispheres. (Sometimes it is called the *superior longitudinal fissure* or *interhemispheric fissure.*)

Loose Training: Generalization training in which stimulus conditions, response requirements and reinforcement contingencies are permitted to vary to increase generalization from the training environment to other environments.

Lower Motor Neuron: Another name for the peripheral nervous system.

Lumbar Puncture (Spinal Tap): A procedure in which a needle is inserted into the spinal column, and a sample of cerebrospinal fluid is removed and analyzed for the presence of bacteria, viruses, parasites, or abnormalities in its chemical composition.

Lumen: The open passageway in a blood vessel.

Macular Sparing: The presence of a small region of intact vision near the center of a visual field in which a person is otherwise blind. Macular sparing is common when visual field blindness is caused by destruction of the visual cortex in one brain hemisphere.

Magnetic Resonance Imaging (MRI Scanning): A laboratory test that uses a strong magnetic field and a computer to create images of internal structures based on differences in the chemical composition of body tissues.

Manometer: An instrument for measuring breath pressure.

Masked Facies: Rigidity of facial muscles, causing fixed, unchanging facial expression. A prominent characteristic of Parkinson's disease.

Median Apertures: Two openings from the fourth ventricle into the subarachnoid space, sometimes called the *foramina of Magendi.*

Mediation: Elicitation of one response by another (usually internal) response (e.g., saying the names of letters to oneself while writing complex words).

Medulla: The bottom third of the brain stem. Contains five cranial nerve nuclei plus some centers concerned with hearing and balance. Pyramidal tract fibers decussate (cross the midline) here.

Melodic Intonation Therapy (MIT): A treatment procedure for patients with severe speech production impairments in which melody and exaggerated intonation are used to facilitate speech.

Memory, Episodic: Memory for personally experienced events.

Memory, Long Term: Sometimes called *secondary memory.* The third stage in some models of memory. It has large (perhaps infinite) capacity, information in it decays slowly if at all, and is considered a repository for our knowledge and sense of self.

Memory, Procedural: What we know about how to do things (make coffee, paint a picture, etc.)

Memory, Prospective: The ability to remember to do things at certain points in time (remembering to remember).

Memory, Retrospective: Memory for past experiences and for knowledge acquired in the past.

Memory, Semantic: Stored general knowledge.

Memory, Sensory: Sometimes called *sensory register.* The first stage in some models of memory, in which the traces of stimuli are briefly stored. The traces decay quickly and cannot be maintained by rehearsal.

Memory, Short-Term: Sometimes called *primary memory.* The second stage in some models of memory, in which information can be maintained by re-

hearsal. Without rehearsal, information decays within a few minutes. Short-term memory has limited capacity; only a few items of information can be stored there at one time.

Memory, Working: A mental space in which processing of information coming from short-term memory or retrieved from long-term memory takes place.

Memory Loss, Pretraumatic: Loss of memory for events immediately preceding brain injury. (Sometimes called *retrograde amnesia.*)

Memory Loss, Posttraumatic: Loss of memory for a period of time following brain injury. (Sometimes called *anterograde amnesia.*)

Memory, Declarative: What we know about things (names, faces, places, situations, etc.).

Meninges: The membranes between the skull and the brain. The toughest one lines the skull and is called the *dura mater.* (Think of DURable. Also, remember that if protection is the key, it makes sense that nature would put the toughest one on the outside.) The web-like one is the arachnoid (think spider). The one on the surface of the brain is the pia mater. To keep them in order, think PAD (for *p*ia, *a*rachnoid, *d*ura).

Meningioma: A tumor in the meninges.

Mesencephalon (Midbrain): A deep brain region that makes up the upper third of the brain stem. It contains several nuclei, including those for cranial nerves that move the eyes.

Metastasis: The process by which a tumor appears at a secondary site from the location of the original tumor.

Monoplegia: Paralysis of one limb.

Motor Cortex: A strip of cortex just ahead of the central fissure. It is responsible for initiating most volitional motor activity.

Myasthenia Gravis: A neurologic disease caused by damage to the acetylcholine receptors on muscle cells. Characterized by abnormally rapid muscle fatigue with use.

Myelogram: A laboratory procedure that permits visualization of the spinal cord. Contrast medium is injected into the subarachnoid space around the spinal cord and a series of X-ray exposures is made to visualize the structure of the spinal cord and surrounding tissues.

Myoclonus: Fine, rapid, irregular twitching movements caused by contractions of groups of muscle fibers. Usually observable as dimpling or rippling of the skin over the muscle fibers.

Myopathy: Disease of muscle.

Neglect: Inattention to some part of surrounding space that is most often seen as inattention to one half of surrounding space *(hemispatial neglect)*. A common consequence of nondominant-hemisphere pathology.

Neologisms: Nonword utterances that follow the phonologic conventions of the language. Neologisms often are heard in the speech of adults with severe Wernicke's aphasia or global aphasia.

Neuralgia: Pain caused by inflammation of a nerve.

Neuritic Plaques: Neuronal abnormalities seen in Alzheimer's disease, other neurologic diseases, and in some normal elderly people. Neuritic plaques are small areas of nerve cell degeneration, primarily occurring in cortical and subcortical brain regions.

Neurofibrillary Tangles: Neuronal abnormalities seen in Alzheimer's disease, other neurologic diseases, and in some normal elderly people. Neurofibrillary tangles are filamentous bodies seen in the nerve cell body, dendrites, axon, and sometimes in synaptic endings.

Neuron: A nerve cell.

Neurotransmitter: Any of several chemical compounds that are involved in transmission of nerve impulses between nerve cells.

Nonacceleration Injury: Brain injury caused when the stationary head is struck by a moving object.

Norms: Any of several statistics that summarize the test performance of a sample of individuals representing a population to which the norms apply. Sample means and standard deviations are the minimum normative statistics needed to relate the performance of an individual to a norm group.

Nystagmus: Rhythmic oscillation of the eyes, sometimes caused by weakness in the muscles that move the eyes, and sometimes caused by disturbances of balance and equilibrium.

Occipital Lobes: The rearmost portions of the brain hemispheres. The visual cortices are located in the occipital lobes.

Olfactory Cortex: A region of cortex on the inferior surface of each frontal lobe. It has principal responsibility for the sense of smell.

Operculum: The patch of cortex surrounding the insula.

Optic Chiasm: The point at which the crossing fibers in the human visual system cross. It is located at the base of the brain near the pituitary gland.

Orientation: Awareness of one's surroundings. Orientation is customarily subdivided into orientation for *person, place,* and *time.*

Outcome: The long-term (final) result of treatment.

Palmar Reflex: Sometimes called the *grasp reflex.* A pathologic reflex elicited by stroking the palm of the hand. The hand closes involuntarily and the fingers grasp the object used to stroke the palm.

Palsy: Another word for *paralysis.*

Papilledema: Swelling of the optic disk in the back of the eye, suggesting increased intracranial pressure, inflammation of the optic disk, or ischemia of the optic disk.

Paraphasia: Paraphasias are errors in speaking made by aphasic persons. There are two kinds: (1) *Literal (phonemic) paraphasias* are errors in which a speaker substitutes one sound in a word for another, such as saying *"spomb"* for *"comb."* (2) *Verbal (semantic) paraphasias* are errors in which a speaker substitutes one word for another, such as saying *"cup"* for *"glass."*

Paraplegia: Paralysis of both legs.

Paresis: Muscle weakness.

Paresthesia: Abnormal sensations (such as tingling, burning) in the absence of stimulation.

Parietal Lobes: The part of the brain hemispheres behind the central fissure and above the lateral fissure. The parietal cortex is important for somesthetic sensation (skin, muscle, joint, and tendon sensation).

Parkinson's Disease: A degenerative disease affecting neurons in the midbrain and brain stem.

Passage Dependency: The degree to which answering questions that test comprehension of discourse depends on having read or heard the discourse.

Patellar Reflex: A normal reflex elicited by tapping the patellar tendon just below the kneecap. The lower leg jerks upward when the patellar tendon is tapped. Diminished patellar reflexes may be a sign of peripheral nerve damage or muscle weakness; exaggerated patellar reflexes may be a sign of upper motor neuron damage.

Percentile: A score that represents the percent of individuals in a norm group that fall above or below the score. For example, a score that places an individual at the 95th percentile means that 94% of the norm group received lower scores.

Perimetry: A procedure for testing vision in all quadrants of the visual fields with a specialized instrument called a *perimeter.*

Peripheral Nervous System (PNS): Consists of the cranial nerves and spinal nerves. The peripheral nervous system is sometimes called the *lower motor neuron.* Cranial nerves and spinal nerves conduct efferent information (motor commands) from the central nervous system to muscles and glands and conduct afferent information (sensory input) from the sensory receptors to the central nervous system. The peripheral nervous system can be divided into autonomic and somatic subsystems. The autonomic system regulates vital functions (breathing, etc.) and the somatic system participates in conscious sensory perception and volitional motor activity.

Perseveration: Repetition of a response when it is no longer appropriate, as when a patient calls a *"comb"* a *"comb"* but continues to call subsequent objects *"comb."*

Persistent Vegetative State: A condition in which the individual has sleep-wake cycles but makes no purposeful responses to the environment.

Phonetic Dissolution: Distortion of speech sounds caused by articulatory breakdown. It sometimes resembles literal paraphasia, but literal paraphasia typically is characterized by substitution of one correctly articulated sound for another, whereas phonetic dissolution is characterized by distortions of sounds.

Pick's Disease: A progressive degenerative disease affecting the brain cortex. It is characterized by the presence of *Pick bodies* (dense globular formations within nerve cells) and *enlarged neurons* in the brain. Pick's disease is an important cause of (cortical) dementia.

Plantar Reflex: Sometimes called the *plantar extensor* or *Babinski* reflex. A pathologic reflex elicited by forcefully stroking the sole of the foot, causing the toes to bend upward and fan out. The *plantar flexor* reflex, in which the toes bend downward and do not fan, is the normal response to this stimulation.

Plaque (Arteriosclerotic Plaque, Atherosclerotic Plaque): Fatty deposits on the inner walls of arteries.

-plegia: A suffix denoting *paralysis.*

Pons: The middle third of the brain stem that contains three cranial nerve nuclei, plus some nuclei concerned with balance and hearing.

Positron Emission Tomography (PET): A laboratory procedure in which the metabolic activity of the brain is measured by introducing a metabolically active compound (usually glucose) tagged with a mildly radioactive element and measuring the regions in which the compound concentrates.

Posterior Horn Cells: Spinal sensory nerves located in the posterolateral part of the spinal cord.

Posttraumatic Memory Loss: See *memory loss, posttraumatic.*

Press of Speech (Logorrhea): Excessive verbosity. Patients with mild-to-moderate Wernicke's or conduction aphasia are most likely to exhibit press of speech.

Pretraumatic Memory Loss: See *memory loss, pretraumatic.*

Progressive Supranuclear Palsy (PSP): A progressive disease characterized by degeneration of brain stem neurons, causing increasingly severe motor impairments, especially in muscles served by cranial nerves.

Projection Fibers: Nerve fiber tracts that connect the brain, brain stem, and spinal cord. They can be either motor (efferent) or sensory (afferent).

Proprioception: The ability to tell the position of the head and limbs without seeing them.

Prosopagnosia: Inability to recognize faces.

Prospective Research: Research in which the design is established prior to subject intake, and subject intake and experimental procedures are defined in advance.

Pseudobulbar Affect: Exaggerated emotional responses to minimally emotional stimuli that is often an early, but usually transitory, consequence of brain damage.

Pure Word Deafness: An auditory impairment in which the individual loses the ability to comprehend spoken verbal materials in spite of intact hearing but retains the ability to recognize nonverbal auditory stimuli.

Pyramidal System: The neural system that is responsible for initiating most volitional movement. It is made up of the motor neurons in the motor cortex together with projection fibers, which connect the motor cortex to the brain stem and spinal cord. It is sometimes called the *upper motor neuron.*

Quadrantanopsia: Blindness in less than half of the visual field in each eye. (See also *hemianopsia.*)

Quadriplegia: Paralysis of both arms and both legs.

Reduplicative Paramnesia: The belief that two or more identical persons, places, or things exist in different locations. An occasional consequence of right-hemisphere brain damage.

Reflex: A spontaneous and uncontrollable movement in response to stimulation. The two major categories of reflexes are *superficial reflexes,* which are elicited by touching, stroking, or brushing the surface of body parts and *deep reflexes,* which are elicited by tapping or suddenly stretching muscles or tendons. (See also *gag reflex, swallow reflex, plantar reflex, palmar reflex, sucking reflex,* and *patellar reflex.*)

Regional Cerebral Blood Flow (rCBF): A laboratory procedure for measuring blood flow by introducing mildly radioactive substances into the blood stream and analyzing their concentration by means of sensitive detectors and a computer.

Reinforcement: *Positive reinforcement* is delivering positive consequences following desired behaviors in order to increase their frequency. *Negative reinforcement* is removing negative consequences following desired behaviors in order to increase their frequency.

Responsive Naming: Providing names in response to questions such as *"What do you drink coffee from?"* or requests such as *"Tell me what you use for digging a hole."*

Retention Span: The amount of information that can be held in primary memory at one time (from four to ten items for most normal adults).

Reticular Formation: Structures in the central core of the brain stem that regulate the individual's overall level of consciousness.

Retrospective Research: Research in which information about subjects is gathered from preexisting records.

Rigidity: Resistance of muscles to movement in any direction. A prominent characteristic of Parkinson's disease.

Scripts: Sometimes called *schemata.* Mental representations of familiar daily life routines or situations, such as eating in a restaurant, going to a party, or shopping for groceries.

Sedimentation Rate: The rate at which blood cells sink in a liquid. Sedimentation rate is an indicator of clotting potential.

Seizure: Episodes of disturbed consciousness caused by abnormal patterns of neuronal discharge in the brain. In *generalized seizures (convulsions, gran mal seizures),* the patient loses consciousness, with spasmodic contractions of most muscle groups. In *partial seizures (focal seizures),* the patient does not lose consciousness, and only some muscle groups are affected by spasmodic contractions. In *absence seizures (petit mal seizures),* the patient does not lose consciousness and does not experience spasmodic muscle contractions but does not respond purposefully to stimulation.

Sequential Modification: Generalization training in which stimulus conditions, response requirements, and reinforcement contingencies are gradually changed to resemble a target environment to increase generalization from the training environment to the target environment.

Sign: An objective indicator of illness or disease observed by an examiner (see *symptom*).

Social Validation: A procedure for evaluating the clinical significance of changes created by a treatment program, in which the effects of treatment on an individual's daily life performance are evaluated.

Somatosensory Cortex: A strip of cortex just behind the central fissure. It is responsible for skin, muscle, joint, and tendon sensation.

Somesthetic Sensation: Sensation from the skin, muscles, joints, and tendons.

Spastic Catch: A sudden increase in muscle tension when spastic muscles are quickly stretched by the examiner.

Spasticity: Abnormally high levels of tension in resting muscles caused by upper motor neuron damage.

Spinal Nerves: Peripheral nerves that supply muscles and sensory receptors in the trunk and limbs. Motor nerves have their cell bodies in the anterolateral part of the spinal cord (anterior horn cells), and sensory nerves have their cell bodies in the posterolateral part (posterior horn cells).

Stenosis: Narrowing, as of an artery.

Steppage Gait: A characteristic gait of patients with paralysis of muscles in the front of the lower leg, causing the foot to hang down as the patient walks. The patient lifts the legs abnormally high so that the toes clear the ground.

Stereognosis: The ability to identify objects by touch.

Stereotypies, Verbal: Repetitive, noncommunicative utterances made by brain-injured patients (*"me-me-me, wuna-wuna-wuna,"* etc.). They are often one indicator of severe aphasia.

Stroke: Temporary or permanent disruption of brain function due to interruption of its blood supply. Sometimes called *cerebrovascular accident (CVA).*

Subarachnoid: Between the arachnoid and the pia mater.

Subclavian Arteries: Two large arteries that branch off from the aorta. The vertebral arteries originate at the subclavian arteries.

Subdural: Between the dura mater and the arachnoid.

Sucking Reflex: A pathologic reflex elicited by touching or stroking on or near the lips, causing the lips to make involuntary sucking movements.

Sulcus: A "valley" on the surface of the brain. (Plural = sulci.) See also *fissure.*

Swallow Reflex: Swallowing when the posterior tongue or pharyngeal walls are touched.

Symptom: Indicators of illness or disease experienced by the patient (see *sign*).

Synapse: The point at which an axon of one nerve cell meets the dendrite of another and where transmission of nerve impulses takes place by means of chemicals called *neurotransmitters.*

Syncope: Fainting.

Telegraphic Speech: Speech in which function words are left out (see *agrammatism*).

Temporal Lobes: They make up approximately the bottom third of each hemisphere beneath the lateral cerebral fissure. The left temporal lobe plays an important role in language and audition.

Tentorium Cerebelli: A rigid sheet of dura that separates the cerebellum from the base of the brain. It is often called *the tentorium* for efficiency. Neurologists sometimes use the terms *supratentorial* and *subtentorial* to describe vertical locations in the cranial vault.

Testing the Limits: Deviating from standard test procedures to determine the underlying reasons for a patient's deficient performance on a test.

Thalamus: A pair of egg-shaped nuclei in the diencephalon. They are important for integration of sensory information, for regulating motor behavior, and they may regulate the overall activity of the cortex.

Thrombosis: Accumulation of a plug of material at a specific site in a blood vessel. If it grows large enough to occlude a cerebral artery, it causes a thrombotic stroke.

Tics: Stereotypic repetitive movements such as blinking, coughing, or sniffing. Tics usually are not related to nervous-system pathology.

Topographic Impairment (Topological Disorientation): A state of confusion regarding surrounding space and how one relates to it. A frequent consequence of right-hemisphere brain damage.

Torsion Spasm: See *dystonia.*

Toxemia: Inflammation or poisoning of brain tissue by foreign substances.

Transcranial Doppler Ultrasound: A laboratory test in which sound waves are transmitted into the head, and a computer measures blood pressure and flow by analyzing changes in the frequency of the reflected sound waves.

Transient Ischemic Attack (TIA): A temporary disruption of cerebral circulation, which causes a transient disturbance of motor, sensory, or mental functions.

Translational Trauma: Brain damage caused by acceleration of the head by outside forces.

Tremor: Cyclic, small amplitude involuntary movements, usually more severe in distal (away from the trunk) muscles than in proximal (near the trunk) muscles.

Trismus: Excessive and uncontrollable contraction of the muscles of mastication.

Upper Motor Neuron: Another name for the pyramidal system.

Validity: The degree to which a test actually measures what it purports to measure. *Content validity* is an indicator of how well the items in a test represent the domain of concern. *Construct validity* is an indicator of how well the content of a test relates to an established model, theory, or concept of the skill, process, or structure to which the test relates.

Vasospasm: Constriction of arteries by contraction of muscles in the arterial wall.

Ventricles (Cerebral Ventricles): Fluid-filled cavities within the brain. There are four of them: two lateral ventricles, a third ventricle, and a fourth ventricle. The passageways connecting them are the intraventricular foramina and the cerebral aqueduct.

Verbal Apraxia (Apraxia of Speech): Disruption of the motor plans for speech articulation. Verbal apraxia often accompanies Broca's aphasia (also see *apraxia, aquawmatism*).

Vertebral Arteries: Two arteries that begin at the subclavian arteries and progress upward on the front side of the medulla. They supply blood to the medulla and, via the basilar artery, to the posterior part of the circle of Willis.

Vestibular-reticular System: A diffuse neural system. It is responsible for balance and orientation of the body in space and for general states of attention and alertness.

Visual Cortex: A region of cortex in each occipital lobe. It has principal responsibility for visual perception.

Wernicke's Encephalopathy: A neurologic disease caused by thiamine deficiency. Usually associated with alcoholism.

Wernicke's Area: A region of cortex in the vicinity of the temporo-parietal-occipital junction. Damage in Wernicke's areas is said to cause *Wernicke's aphasia*.

Word Fluency: See *generative naming*.

Bibliography

Adamovich B: *A comparison of FIM evaluations by nurses and speech pathologists.* Paper presented at the Clinical Aphasiology Conference, Santa Fe, NM, June, 1990.

Adamovich BB, Brooks RA: A diagnostic protocol to assess the communication deficits of patients with right hemisphere damage. In Brookshire R, ed: *Clinical aphasiology conference proceedings,* Minneapolis, 1981, BRK, pp 244-253.

Adamovich BB, Henderson J: *Scales of cognitive ability for traumatic brain injury,* Chicago, 1992, Riverside.

Adams JH, Graham DI, Scott G and associates: Brain damage in fatal nonmissile head injury, *J Clin Pathol* 33:1132-1145, 1980.

Adams MJ, Collins A: A schema-theoretic view of reading. In Freedle RO, ed: *New directions in discourse processing,* Norwood, NJ, 1979, Ablex.

Adams RD, Victor M: *Principles of neurology,* ed 2, New York, 1981, McGraw-Hill.

Alberico AM, Ward JD, Choi SC and associates: Outcome after severe head injury: relationship to mass lesion, diffuse injury, and ICP course in pediatric and adult patients, *J Neurosurg* 67:648-656, 1987.

Albert ML, Feldman RG, Willis AL: The "subcortical dementia" of progressive supranuclear palsy, *J Neurol, Neurosurg, Psychiatry* 37:121-130, 1974.

Albert ML: A simple test of visual neglect, *Neurology* 23:658-664, 1973.

Albert ML and associates: *Clinical aspects of dysphasia,* New York, 1981, Springer-Verlag.

Alexander MP, Lo Verme SR: Aphasia after left hemisphere intracerebral hemorrhage, *Neurology* 30:1993-1202, 1980.

Alexander MP, Loverso FL: A specific treatment for global aphasia, *Clinical Aphasiology* 21:277-289, 1993.

Alexander MP, Naeser MA, Palumbo C: Correlations of subcortical CT lesion sites and aphasia profiles, *Brain* 110:961-991, 1987.

Alfano DP: Recovery of function following brain injury. In Finlayson MAJ, Garner SH, eds.: *Brain injury rehabilitation: clinical considerations,* Baltimore, 1994, Williams & Wilkins, pp 34-56.

American Psychiatric Association: *Diagnostic and statistical manual of mental disorders,* ed 3 (revised). Washington DC, 1987, American Psychiatric Press.

American Speech-Language-Hearing Association: *Functional assessment of communication skills for adults:* project update, Bethesda, Md, 1994, American Speech-Language-Hearing Association.

Anderson T, Boureston N, Greenberg F: *Rehabilitation predictors in completed stroke,* Minneapolis, 1971, Sister Kenny Rehabilitation Institute.

Andrews PJD and associates: Secondary insults during intrahospital transport of head injured patients, *Lancet* 1:327-330, 1990.

Annegers JF and associates: Seizures after head trauma: a population study, *Neurology* 30:683-689, 1980.

Appell J, Kertesz A, Fishman M: A study of language functioning in Alzheimer patients, *Brain Lang* 17:73-81, 1982.

Arguin M, Bub D: Modulation of the directional attention deficit in visual neglect by hemispatial factors, *Brain Cogn* 22:148-160, 1993.

Armus SR, Brookshire RH, Nicholas LE: Aphasic and non–brain-damaged adults' knowledge of scripts for common situations, *Brain Lang* 36:518-528, 1989.

Arthur G: *A point scale of intelligence tests,* New York 1947, The Psychological Corporation.

Aten JL, Lyon J: Measures of PICA subtest variance: a preliminary assessment of their value as predictors of language recovery in aphasia. In Brookshire RH, ed: *Clinical aphasiology conference proceedings,* Minneapolis, 1978, BRK, pp 106-116.

Baddeley AD: *Working memory,* London, 1986, Oxford University Press.

Baddeley A and associates: Closed head injury and memory. In Levin HS, Grafman J, Eisenberg HM, eds: *Neurobehavioral recovery from head injury.* New York, 1987, Oxford University Press, pp 295-317.

Barber JB, Webster JC: Head injuries: a review of 150 cases, *J Natl Med Assoc* 66:201-204, 1974.

Barco DP and associates: Training awareness and compensation in postacute head injury rehabilitation. In Kreutzer JS, Wehman PH, eds:, *Cognitive rehabilitation for persons with traumatic brain injury: a functional approach,* Baltimore, 1991, Paul H. Brookes, pp 129-146.

Barlow DH, Herson M: *Single-case experimental designs: strategies for studying behavior change,* ed 2, New York 1984, Pergamon Press.

Barton M, Maruszewski M, Urrea D: Variation of stimulus context and its effect on word finding ability in aphasics, *Cortex* 5:351-365, 1969.

Basso A, Capitani E, Vignolo LA: Influence of rehabilitation on language skills in aphasic patients: a controlled study, *Arch Neurol* 36:190-196, 1979.

Basso A: Anatomo-clinical correlations of the aphasias as defined through computerized tomography: exceptions, *Brain Lang* 26:201-229, 1985.

Bayles KA: Management of neurogenic communication disorders associated with dementia. In Chapey R, ed: *Language intervention strategies in adult aphasia, ed 3,* Baltimore, 1994, Williams & Wilkins, pp 535-545.

Bayles KA, Kaszniak AW, Tomoeda C: *Communication and cognition in normal aging and dementia,* Boston, 1987, College-Hill.

Bayles KA, Tomoeda C: *Arizona battery for communication disorders of dementia, res ed,* Tuscon, 1991, Canyonlands.

Benson DF: Aphasia. In Heilman KM, Valenstein E, eds: *Clinical neuropsychology,* New York, 1979, Oxford University Press, pp 22-58.

Benton AL: *The revised visual retention test, ed 4,* New York, 1974, Psychological Corporation.

Benton AL, Smith KC, Lang M: Stimulus characteristics and object naming in aphasic patients, *J Commun Disord* 5:19-24, 1972.

Bever TG, Garrett MF, Hurtig R: The interaction of perceptual processes and ambiguous sentences, *Memory and Cognition* 1:277-286, 1973.

Bisiach E: Perceptual factors in the pathogenesis of anomia, *Cortex* 2:90-95, 1966.

Blonder LX, Bowers D, Heilman KM: The role of the right hemisphere in emotional communication, *Brain* 114:1115-1127, 1991.

Bloom RL and associates: Impact of emotional content on discourse production in patients with unilateral brain damage, *Brain Lang* 42:153-164, 1992.

Bluestone CD and associates: Teflon injection pharyngoplasty, *Cleft Palate Journal* 5:19-26, 1968.

Boll TJ: Neurologically impaired adults. In Miltersen MM, Turner SM, eds.: *Diagnostic interviewing, ed 2,* New York, 1994, Plenum, pp 345-372.

Bond MR: Assessment of the psychosocial outcome of severe head injury, *Acta Neurochir* 34:57-70, 1976.

Bonin G von: Anatomical asymmetries of the cerebral hemisphere. In Mountcastle VB, ed: *Interhemispheric relationships and cerebral dominance,* Baltimore, Md, 1962, Johns Hopkins Press, pp 122-135.

Boning RA: *Specific skill series, ed 4,* New York, 1990, Macmillan/McGraw-Hill.

Borkowski JG, Benton AL, Spreen O: Word fluency and brain damage, *Neuropsychologia* 5:135-140, 1967.

Bower GH, Black JB, Turner TJ: Scripts in memory for texts, *Cognitive Psychology* 11:177-220, 1979.

Bowers SA, Marshall LF: Outcome in 200 consecutive cases of severe head injury treated in San Diego County: a prospective analysis, *Neurosurgery* 6:237-242, 1980.

Breyden MP, Ley RG: Right hemispheric involvement in imagery. In Perecman E, ed: *Cognitive processing in the right hemisphere,* New York, 1983, Academic Press, pp 111-123.

Brismar B, Engstrom A, Rydberg U: Head injury and intoxication: a diagnostic and therapeutic dilemma, *Acta Chirurgica Scandinavica* 149:11-14, 1983.

Brooks DN: Cognitive deficits after head injury. In Brooks DN, ed: *Closed head injury: psychological, social, and family consequences,* New York, 1984, Oxford University Press, pp 44-73.

Brooks N: Closed head trauma: assessing the common cognitive processes. In Lezak M, ed: *Assessment of the behavioral consequences of head trauma,* New York, 1989, A.R. Liss, pp 61-86.

Brookshire RH: Effects of task difficulty on naming performance of aphasic subjects, *J Speech Hear Res* 15:551-558, 1972.

Brookshire RH: Consequences in speech pathology: incentive and feedback functions, *J Commun Disord* 6:1-5, 1973.

Brookshire RH: Differences in responding to auditory verbal materials among aphasic patients, *Acta Symbolica* 3:1-17, 1974.

Brookshire RH: Effects of prompting on spontaneous naming of pictures by aphasic subjects, *J Can Speech Hear Assoc* 63-71, Autumn 1975.

Brookshire RH: Effects of task difficulty on sentence comprehension performance of aphasic subjects, *J Commun Disord* 9:167-173, 1976.

Brookshire RH: Auditory comprehension and aphasia. In Johns DF, ed: *Clinical management of neurogenic communicative disorders,* Boston, 1978, Little-Brown, pp 103-128.

Brookshire RH: *An introduction to neurogenic communication disorders, ed 4,* St Louis, 1992, Mosby.

Brookshire RH, Krueger K, Nicholas L, Cicciarelli A: Analysis of clinician-patient interactions in aphasia treatment. In Brookshire RH, ed: *Clinical aphasiology conference proceedings,* Minneapolis, 1977, BRK, pp 181-187.

Brookshire RH, Lommel M: Perception of sequences of visual temporal and auditory spatial stimuli by aphasic, right-hemisphere-damaged, and non–brain-damaged subjects, *J Commun Disord* 7:155-169, 1974.

Brookshire RH, Nicholas LE: Comprehension of directly and indirectly stated main ideas and details in discourse by brain-damaged and non–brain-damaged listeners, *Brain Lang* 21:21-36, 1984a.

Brookshire RH, Nicholas LE: Consistency of the effects of rate of speech on brain-damaged subjects' comprehension of information in narrative discourse. In Brookshire RH, ed: *Clinical Aphasiology,* Vol 15, Minneapolis, 1985, BRK, pp 262-271.

Brookshire RH, Nicholas LE: *The discourse comprehension test.* Minneapolis, 1993, BRK.

Brookshire RH, Nicholas LE: Performance deviations in the connected speech of adults with no brain damage and adults with aphasia, *Am J Speech-Lang Path* 4:118-123, 1995.

Brookshire RH, Nicholas LE, Krueger KM: Sampling of speech pathology treatment activities: an evaluation of momentary and interval sampling procedures, *J Speech Hear Res* 21:652-667, 1978.

Brookshire R and associates: Effects of clinician behaviors on acceptability of patients' responses in aphasia treatment sessions, *J Commun Disord* 12:369-384, 1979.

Brown JW: *Aphasia, apraxia, and agnosia: clinical and theoretical aspects,* Springfield, Ill, 1972, Charles C. Thomas.

Brown JI, Bennett JM, Hanna G: *The Nelson-Denny reading test,* Chicago, 1981, Riverside.

Brownell HH: The neuropsychology of narrative comprehension, *Aphasiology,* 2:247-250, 1988.

Brownell H and associates: Influence of deficits in right-brain–damaged patients, *Brain Lang* 27:310-321, 1986.

Brust JC and associates: Aphasia in acute stroke, *Stroke* 7:167-174, 1976.

Bryan KL: *The right hemisphere language battery,* Leicester, 1989, Far Communications.

Buckingham HW: Explanation in apraxia with consequences for the concept of apraxia of speech, *Brain Lang* 8:202-226, 1979.

Burns MS, Halper AS, Mogil SI: *Clinical management of right hemisphere dysfunction,* Rockville, Md, 1985, Aspen.

Busch C, Brookshire RH: Aphasic adults' auditory comprehension of yes-no questions, Unpublished manuscript, 1982.

Butfield E, Zangwill OL: Re-education in aphasia: a review of 70 cases, *J Neurol Neurosurg Psychiatry* 9:75-79, 1946.

Cancelliere AEB, Kertesz A: Lesion localization in acquired deficits of emotional expression and comprehension, *Brain Cogn* 13:133-147, 1990.

Candelise L and associates: Prognostic significance of hyperglycemia in acute stroke, *Arch Neurol* 42:409-426, 1985.

Canter GJ: Dysarthria, apraxia of speech, and literal paraphasia: three distinct varieties of articulatory behaviors in the adult with brain damage. Paper presented at the annual convention of the American Speech and Hearing Association, Detroit, 1973.

Caplan D: *Neurolinguistics and linguistic aphasiology.* New York, 1987, Cambridge University Press.

Caplan LR: *Stroke,* CIBA Clinical Symposia, Summit, NJ, 1988, CIBA Pharmaceutical Company.

Caplan LR: *Stroke: a clinical approach,* Boston, 1993, Butterworth-Heinemann.

Cappa SF and associates: Subcortical aphasia: two clinical CT-scan correlation studies, *Cortex* 19:227-242, 1983.

Cappa SF, Cavalotti G, Vignolo L: Phonemic and lexical errors in fluent aphasia: correlation with lesion site, *Neuropsychologia,* 19:171-177, 1981.

Cappa SF, Vignolo LA: "Transcortical" features of aphasia following left thalamic hemorrhage, *Cortex* 15:121-130, 1979.

Carlsson GS, Svardsudd K, Welin L: Long term effects of head injuries sustained during life in three male populations, *J Neuropsy* 67:197-205, 1987.

Caramazza A, Zurif EB: Dissociation of algorithmic and heuristic processes in language comprehension: evidence from aphasia, *Brain Lang* 3:572-582, 1976.

Caronna J, Levy D: Clinical predictors of outcome in ischemic stroke. In Barnett HJM, ed: *Neurologic clinics: cerebrovascular disease,* Philadelphia, 1983, W.B. Saunders, pp 103-117.

Carroll JB, Davies P, Richman B: *The American Heritage word frequency book,* New York, 1971, American Heritage.

Carrow-Woodfolk E: *Test for auditory comprehension of language,* Allen, Tex, 1984, DLM Teaching Resources.

Carver RP: Reading as reasoning: implications for measurement. In MacGinitie WH, ed: *Assessment problems in reading,* Newark, Del, 1973, International Reading Association, pp 173-195.

Celesia GG, Wanamaker WM: Psychiatric disturbances in Parkinson's disease, *Diseases of the Nervous System* 33:577-583, 1972.

Cermak LS: Imagery as an aid to retrieval in alcoholic Korsakoff's patients, *Cortex* 11:163-169, 1975.

Chall JS: *Stages of reading development,* New York, 1983, McGraw-Hill.

Chapey R: The assessment of language disorders in adults. In Chapey R, ed: *Language intervention strategies in adult aphasia, ed 2*, Baltimore, 1986, Williams & Wilkins, pp 81-140.

Chapey R: *Language intervention strategies in adult aphasia, ed 3*, Baltimore, 1994, Williams & Wilkins.

Cherney LR, Halper AS, Miller TK: Treatment of Communication Problems. In Halper AS, Cherney LR, Miller TK, eds: *Clinical management of communication problems in adults with traumatic brain injury*, Gaithersbury, Md, 1991, Aspen, pp 57-131.

Cicone M, Wapner W, Gardner H: Sensitivity to emotional expressions and situations in organic patients, *Brain Lang* 16:145-158, 1980.

Clark HH, Haviland SE: Comprehension and the given-new contract. In Freedle RO, ed: *Discourse comprehension and production*, Norwood, NJ, 1977, Ablex, pp 1-40.

Cohn R, Neumann, MS, Wood NH: Prosopagnosia: a clinicopathological study, *Ann Neurol* 1:177-182, 1977.

Collins M: *Global aphasia*, San Diego, 1991, College-Hill Press.

Colsher PL, Cooper WE, Graff-Radford N: Intonational variability in the speech of right-hemisphere damaged patients, *Brain Lang* 32:379-383, 1987.

Connell PJ, Thompson CJ: Flexibility of single-subject experimental designs. Part III: using flexibility to design or modify experiments. *J Speech Hear Disord* 51:214-225, 1986.

Corlew MM, Nation JE: Characteristics of visual stimuli and naming performance in aphasic adults, *Cortex* 11:186-191, 1975.

Corkin SH and associates: Consequences of penetrating and nonpenetrating head injury: posttraumatic amnesia, and lasting effects on cognition. In Levin HS, Grafman J, Eisenberg HM, eds: *Neurobehavioral recovery from head injury*, New York, 1987, Oxford University Press, pp 318-329.

Correia L, Brookshire RH, Nicholas LE: Aphasic and non–brain-damaged adults' descriptions of aphasia test pictures and gender-biased pictures, *J Speech Hear Disord* 55:713-720, 1990.

Craik FI, Lockhart RS: Levels of processing: a framework for memory research, *J Verbal Learn Verbal Behav* 11:671-684, 1972.

Crary MA, Haak MJ, Malinsky AE: Preliminary psychometric evaluation of an acute aphasia screening protocol, *Aphasiology* 2:67-78, 1989.

Croft CB, Shprintzen RJ, Rakoff SJ: Patterns of velopharyngeal valving in normal and cleft palate subjects: a multiview videofluoroscopic and nasendoscopic study, *Laryngoscope* 91:265-271, 1981.

Culton GL: Spontaneous recovery from aphasia, *J Speech Hear Res* 12:825-832, 1969.

Cummings JL: Cortical Dementias. In Benson DF, Blumer D, eds: *Psychiatric aspects of neurologic disease*, New York, 1983, Grune & Stratton.

Cummings JL: Clinical diagnosis of Alzheimer's disease. In Cummings JL, Miller BL, eds.: *Alzheimer's disease: treatment and long-term management*, New York, 1990, Dekker, pp 3-20.

Cummings JL, Benson DF: *Dementia: a clinical approach*, Boston, 1983, Butterworths.

Cummings JL, Benson DF: *Dementia: a clinical approach, ed 2*, Boston, 1992, Butterworth-Heinemann.

Dabul B, Bollier B, Therapeutic approaches to apraxia, *J Speech Hear Disord* 41:268-276, 1976.

Dale E, Chall JS: A formula for predicting readability, *Educational Research Bulletin* 27:11-20, 1948.

Damasio AR: Disorders of complex visual processing: agnosias, achromatopsia, Baliut's syndrome, and related difficulties of orientation and construction. In Mesulum MM, ed: *Principles of behavioral neurology*, Philadelphia, 1985, FA Davis, pp 259-288.

Damasio AR, Damasio H: Localization of lesions in achormatopsia and prosopognosia. In Kertesz A, ed: *Localization in neuropsychology*, New York, 1983, Academic Press, pp 417-428.

Darley FL: The classification of output disturbance in neurologic communication disorders. Paper presented at the American Speech and Hearing Association Convention, Chicago, 1969.

Darley FL: *Aphasia*, Philadelphia, 1982, WB Saunders.

Darley FL, Aronson AE, Brown JR: *Motor speech disorders*, Philadelphia, 1975, WB Saunders.

Davis GA: *A survey of adult aphasia and related language disorders, ed 2*, Englewood Cliffs, NJ, 1993, Prentice-Hall.

Davis GA, Wilcox MJ: *Adult aphasia rehabilitation: language pragmatics*, San Diego, 1985, College-Hill.

Deal JL, Deal LA: Efficacy of aphasia rehabilitation: preliminary results. In Brookshire RH, ed: *Clinical aphasiology conference proceedings*, Minneapolis, 1978, BRK Publishers, pp 66-77.

Deaton AV: Group interventions for cognitive rehabilitation: increasing the challenges. In Kreutzer JS, Wehman PH, eds: *Cognitive rehabilitation for persons with traumatic brain injury: a functional approach*, Baltimore, 1991, Paul H. Brookes.

DeKosky ST and associates: Recognition and discrimination of emotional faces and pictures, *Brain Lang* 9:206-214, 1980.

Delis DC and associates: *The California verbal learning test: adult version*, San Antonio, Tex, 1987, The Psychological Corporation.

Delis DC, Kramer J, Kaplan E: *California proverb test*, Lexington, Mass, 1988, Boston Neuropsychological Foundation.

DeRenzi E, Ferrari C: *The reporter's test:* a sensitive test to detect expressive disturbances in aphasics, *Cortex* 14:279-283, 1978.

DeRenzi E, Vignolo LA: *The token test:* a sensitive test to detect receptive disturbances in aphasics, *Brain* 85:665-678, 1962.

Deutsch SE: Oral form identification as a measure of cortical sensory dysfunction in apraxia of speech and aphasia, *J Commun Disord* 14:65-71, 1981.

Dewitt LD and associates: MRI and the study of aphasia, *Neurology* 35:861-865, 1985.

Diggs CC, Basili AG: Verbal expression of right CVA patients, *Brain Lang* 30:130-147, 1987.

Diller L, Weinberg J: Differential aspects of attention in brain-damaged persons, *Percept Mot Skills* 35:71-81, 1977.

Doyle P, Goldstein H, Bourgeois M: Experimental analysis of syntax training in Broca's aphasia: a generalization and social validation study, *J Speech Hear Disord* 52:143-155, 1987.

Duffy JR: Boston diagnostic aphasia examination. In Darley FL, ed: *Evaluation and appraisal techniques in speech and language pathology,* Reading, Mass, 1979, Addison-Wesley, pp 198-202.

Duffy JR: Slowly progressive aphasia. In Brookshire RH, ed: *Clinical aphasiology,* Minneapolis, 1987, BRK, pp 349-356.

Duffy JR: *Motor speech disorders: substrates, differential diagnosis, and management,* St Louis, 1995, Mosby.

Duffy JR and associates: Performance of normal (non–brain-injured) adults on the Porch Index of Communicative Ability. In Brookshire RH, ed: *Clinical aphasiology conference proceedings,* Minneapolis, 1976, BRK, pp 32-42.

Dunlop JM, Marquardt TP: Linguistic and articulatory aspects of single word production in apraxia of speech, *Cortex* 13:17-29, 1977.

Dunn LM, Dunn LM: *Peabody picture vocabulary test—Revised,* Circle Pines, Minn, 1981, American Guidence Service.

Dunn LM, Markwardt FC: *Peabody individual achievement test,* Circle Pines, Minn, 1970, American Guidance Service.

Dworkin JP, Johns DF: Management of velopharyngeal incompetence in dysarthria: a review, *Clinical Otolaryngology* 5:61-74, 1980.

Eastwood MR, Lautenschlaeger E, Corbin S: A comparison of clinical methods for assessing dementia, *J Am Geriatr Soc* 31:342-347, 1983.

Efron R: Temporal perception, aphasia, and dejavu, *Brain* 86:403-424, 1963.

Eisenberg HM, Weiner RL: Input variables: how information from the acute injury can be used to characterize groups of patients for studies of outcome. In Levin HS, Grafman J, Eisenberg HM, eds: *Neurobehavioral recovery from head injury,* New York, 1987, Oxford University Press, pp 13-29.

Eisenson J: *Examining for aphasia,* New York, 1954, The Psychological Corporation.

Eisenson J: *Adult aphasia: assessment and treatment,* New York, 1973, Appleton-Century-Crofts.

Eisenson J: Aphasia: a point of view as to the nature of the disorder and factors that determine prognosis for recovery, *Neurology* 4:287-295, 1964.

Elman RJ, Bernstein-Ellis E: What is functional? Paper presented at the Clinical Aphasiology Conference, Sunriver, Ore, June, 1995.

Erlich JS, Sipes AL: Group treatment of communication skills for head trauma patients, *Cognitive Rehab* 3:32-37, 1985.

Evans RW, Palsane MN, Carrere S: Type A behavior and occupational stress: a cross-cultural study of blue-collar workers, *J Pers Soc Psychol* 36:1213-1220, 1987.

Ewert J and associates: Procedural memory during posttraumatic amnesia in survivors of severe closed head injury, *Arch Neurol* 46:911-916, 1989.

Faber MM, Aten FL: Verbal performance in aphasic patients in response to intact and altered pictorial stimuli. In Brookshire RH, ed: *Clinical aphasiology conference proceedings* Minneapolis, 1979, BRK, pp 177-186.

Filley CM and associates: Neurobehavioral outcome after closed head injury in childhood and adolescence, *Arch Neurol* 44:194-198, 1987.

Finlayson MAJ, Garner SH: Challenges in rehabilitation of individuals with acquired brain injury. In Finlayson MAJ, Garner SH, eds: *Brain injury rehabilitation: clinical considerations,* Baltimore, 1994, Williams & Wilkins, pp 3-10.

Fitch-West J, Sands ES: *Bedside evaluation screening test,* Rockville, Md, 1987, Aspen.

Folstein MF, Folstein SE, McHugh PR: "Mini-mental state," *J Psychiatr Res* 12:189-198, 1975.

Foss DJ, Jenkins CM: Some affects of context on the comprehension of ambiguous sentences, *J Verbal Learn Verbal Behav* 12:577-589, 1973.

Friedman WA: *Head injuries,* CIBA Clinical Symposia, Summit, NJ, 1983, CIBA Pharmaceutical Company.

Friedman A, Polson MC: The hemispheres as independent processing systems: limited capacity processing and cerebral specialization, *J Experimental Psychol: Human Percep Perform* 7:1031-1058, 1981.

Froeschels E: A contribution to pathology and therapy of dysarthria due to certain cortical lesions, *J Speech Hear Disord* 8:301-321, 1943.

Froeschels E: Chewing method as therapy, *Arch of Otolaryngol* 61:427-435, 1952.

Fromm D, Holland AL: Functional communication in Alzheimer's disease, *J Speech Hear Disord* 54:535-540, 1989.

Gaddes WH, Crockett DJ: The *Spreen-Benton aphasia test:* normative data as a measure of normal language development, Victoria, BC, 1973, Research monograph #25, Neuropsychology Laboratory, University of Victoria.

Gates WH: *Gates-MacGinitie reading tests,* Chicago, 1978, Riverside.

Gainotti G: Frontal lobe damage and disorders of affect and personality. In Swash M, Oxbury J, eds: *Clinical Neurology,* Edinburgh, 1991, Churchill-Livingstone, pp 71-81.

Gainotti G, Tiacci C: Patterns of drawing disability in left and right hemisphere patients, *Neuropsychologia* 8:379-384, 1970.

Gardiner BJ, Brookshire RH: Effects of unisensory and multisensory presentation of stimuli upon naming by aphasic subjects, *Lang Speech* 15:342-357, 1972.

Gardner H, Albert ML, Weintraub S: Comprehending a word: the influence of speed and redundancy on auditory comprehension in aphasia, *Cortex* 11:155-162, 1975.

Gardner H and associates: Missing the point: the role of right hemisphere in the processing of complex linguistic materials. In Perecman E, ed: *Cognitive processing in the right hemisphere,* New York, 1983, Academic Press, pp 169-192.

Garner SH, Valadka AB: Medical management and principles of head injury rehabilitation. In Finlayson MAJ, Garner SH, eds: *Brain injury rehabilitation: clinical considerations,* Baltimore, 1994, Williams & Wilkins, pp 83-101.

Gauthier L, Dehaut F, Joanette Y: The Bells test: a quantitative and qualitative test for visual neglect, *Intern J Clin Neuropsychol* 11:49-54, 1989.

Gernsbacher MA: Resolving twenty years of inconsistent interactions between lexical familiarity and orthography, completeness, and polysemy, *J Exp Psychol: Gen* 113:256-280, 1978.

Geschwind N, Quadfasel FA, Segarra J: Isolation of the speech area, *Neuropsychologia* 6:327-340, 1968.

Gilchrist E, Wilkinson M: Some factors determining prognosis in young people with severe head injuries, *Arch Neurol* 36:355-359, 1979.

Giles GM, Clark-Wilson J: *Brain injury rehabilitation: a neurofunctional approach,* London, 1993, Chapman & Hall.

Gleason JB and associates: The retrieval of syntax in Broca's aphasia, *Brain Lang* 2:451-471, 1975.

Glisky EL, Schacter DL: Remediation of organic memory disorders: current status and future prospects, *J Head Trauma Rehab* 1:54-63, 1986.

Gloag D: Rehabilitation after head injury: cognitive problems, *British Med J* 290:834-837, 1985.

Glonig I and associates: Comparison of verbal behavior in right-handed and non-right-handed patients with anatomically verified lesion of one hemisphere, *Cortex* 5:43-52, 1969.

Glonig K and associates: Prognosis and speech therapy in aphasia. In Lebrun Y, Hoops R, Eds: *Recovery in aphasics,* Atlantic Highlands NJ, 1976, Humanities Press.

Glosser G, Deser T: Patterns of discourse production among neurological patients with fluent language disorders, *Brain Lang* 40:67-88, 1990.

Glosser G, Goodglass H: Disorders in executive control functions among aphasic and other brain-damaged patients, *J Clin Exp Neuropsychol* 12:485-501, 1990.

Glosser G, Wiener M, Kaplan E: Variations in aphasic language behaviors, *J Speech Hear Res* 53:115-124, 1988.

Godfrey H, Knight R: Cognitive rehabilitation of memory functioning in amnesic alcoholics, *J Consult Clin Psychol* 43:555-557, 1985.

Goldman-Eisler F: *Psycholingustics: experiments in spontaneous speech,* New York, 1968, Academic Press.

Goldstein K: *Language and language disturbances,* New York, 1948, Grune & Stratton.

Golper LAC and associates: Connected language sampling: an expanded index of aphasic language behavior. In Brookshire R.H. ed: *Clinical aphasiology: conference proceedings,* Minneapolis, 1980, BRK Publishers, pp 174-186.

Gonzalez J, Aronson A: Palatal lift prosthesis for treatment of anatomic and neurologic palatopharyngeal insufficiency, *Cleft Palate J* 7:91-104, 1970.

Goodglass H: *Understanding aphasia,* San Diego, 1993, Academic Press.

Goodglass H and associates: The effect of syntactic encoding on sentence comprehension in aphasia, *Brain Lang* 7:201-209, 1979.

Goodglass H, Kaplan E: *The assessment of aphasia and related disorders,* ed 2, Philadelphia, 1983, Lea & Febiger.

Goodglass H, Kaplan E: *The Boston diagnostic aphasia examination,* Philadelphia, 1972, 1983, Lea & Febiger.

Goodglass H and associates: The tip of the tongue phenomenon in aphasia, *Cortex* 12:145-153, 1976.

Goodglass H and associates: Specific semantic word categories in aphasia, *Cortex* 2:74-89, 1966.

Goodglass H, Quadfasel F: Language laterality in left-handed aphasics, *Brain* 77:523-528, 1954.

Goodglass H, Stuss DT: Naming to picture versus description in three aphasia subgroups, *Cortex* 15:199-211, 1979.

Gordon WA and associates: *Evaluation of the deficits associated with right brain damage: normative data on the Institute of Rehabilitation Medicine test battery,* 1984, Department of Behavioral Sciences, NYU Medical Center.

Gorham DR: A Proverbs test for clinical and experimental use, *Psychol Rep* 2:1-12, 1956.

Graham DI, Adams JH, Doyle D: Ischemic brain damage in fatal non-missile head injuries, *J Neurol Sci* 39:213, 1978.

Graham RK, Kendall BS: *The memory for designs test: Revised general manual. Percept Mot Skills Suppl* 11:147-188, 1960.

Grant DA, Berg EA: A behavioral analysis of degree of reinforcement and ease of shifting to new responses in a Weigl-type card sorting problem, *Journal of Experimental Psychology* 38:404-411, 1948.

Gray L, Hoyt P, Mogil S and associates: A comparison of clinical tests of yes/no questions in aphasia, In Brookshire RH, ed: *Clinical aphasiology conference proceedings,* Minneapolis, 1977, BRK, pp 265-268.

Greenberg DA, Aminoff MJ, Simon RP: *Clinical neurology, ed 2,* Norwalk, Conn, 1993, Appleton & Lange.

Gronwall DMA: Paced auditory serial addition task: a measure of recovery from concussion, *Percept Mot Skills* 44:367-373, 1977.

Guilford AM, Hawk AM: A comparative study of form identification in neurologically impaired and normal subjects, *Speech and Hearing Science Research Reports,* Ann Arbor, Mich, 1968, University of Michigan.

Gunning R: *The technique of clear writing,* New York, 1952, McGraw-Hill.

Haas J, Cope DN, Hall K: Premorbid prevalence of poor academic performance in severe head injury, *J Neurol Neurosurg Psychiatry* 50:52-56, 1987.

Hachinsky VC, Iliff LD, Zilhka E and associates: Cerebral blood flow in dementia, *Archives Neurol* 32:632-637, 1975.

Hagen C, Malkamus D: Interaction strategies for language disorders secondary to head trauma. Paper presented at the annual convention of the American Speech-Language-Hearing Association, Atlanta, Ga, 1979.

Halliday MAK, Hasan R: *Cohesion in English,* New York, 1976, Longman.

Halpern H: Effect of stimulus variables on dysphasic verbal errors, *Percept Mot Skills* 21:291-298, 1965.

Hammill DD: *Detroit test of learning aptitudes,* Austin, Tex, 1985, Pro-Ed.

Hand CR, Burns MO, Ireland E: Treatment of hypertonicity in muscles of lip retraction, *Biofeedback Self Regul* 4:171-176, 1979.

Hanna G, Schell LM, Schreiner R: *The Nelson reading skills test,* Chicago, 1977, Riverside.

Hannay HJ, Levin HS, Grossman RG: Impaired recognition memory after head injury, *Cortex* 15:269-283, 1979.

Hardy JC and associates: Surgical management of palatal paresis and speech problems in cerebral palsy, *J Speech Hear Disord* 26:320-327, 1961.

Hart T, Hayden ME: The ecological validity of neuropsychological assessment and remediation. In Uzzell BP, Gross Y, eds: *Clinical neuropsychology of intervention,* Boston, 1986, Martinus Nijhoff, pp 21-50.

Harvey AM and associates: *The Principles and practice of medicine,* ed 19, Norwalk, Conn, 1988, Appleton & Lange.

Haskins S: A treatment procedure for writing disorders. In Brookshire RH, ed: *Clinical aphasiology conference proceedings,* Minneapolis, 1976, BRK, pp 192-199.

Hayes DP: Speaking and writing: distinct patterns of word choice, *J Mem Lang* 27, 572-578, 1988.

Hayes DP: *Guide to the lexical analysis of texts.* Technical Report Seriec 89-96. Ithaca, NY, 1989, Cornell University Department of Sociology.

Heath PD, Kennedy P, Kapur N: Slowly progressive aphasia without generalized dementia. *Ann Neurol* 13:687-688, 1983.

Hecaen H, Assal G: A comparison of constructive deficits following left and right hemisphere lesions, *Neuropsychologia* 8:289-303, 1970.

Heilman KM, Schwartz HD, Watson RT: Hypo-arousal in patients with the neglect syndrome and emotional indifference, *Neurology* 28:229-232, 1978.

Helm NA, Barresi B: Voluntary control of involuntary utterances: a treatment approach for severe aphasia. In Brookshire RH, ed: *Clinical aphasiology conference proceedings,* Minneapolis, 1980, BRK.

Helm-Estabrooks NA: "Show me the . . . whatever": some variables affecting auditory comprehension scores of aphasic patients. In Brookshire RH, ed: *Clinical aphasiology conference proceedings,* Minneapolis, 1981, BRK, pp 105-107.

Helm-Estabrooks N, Barresi B: Voluntary control of involuntary utterances: a treatment approach for severe aphasia. In Brookshire R, ed: *Clinical aphasiology conference proceedings,* Minneapolis, 1980, BRK, pp 308-315.

Helm-Estabrooks N, Fitzpatrick PM, Barresi B: Visual action therapy for global aphasia, *J Speech Hear Disord* 47:385-389, 1982.

Helm-Estabrooks N, Hotz G: *Brief test of head injury,* Chicago, 1991, Riverside.

Hier D, Hagenlocker K, Shindler AG: Language disintegration in dementia: effects of etiology and severity, *Brain Lang* 25:117-133, 1985.

Hillbom M, Holm L: Contribution of traumatic head injury to neuropsychological deficits in alcoholics, *J Neurol Neurosurg Psychiatry* 49:1348-1353, 1986.

Hixon TJ: *Respiratory function in speech and song,* San Diego, 1987, College-Hill.

Hixon TJ, Hawley JL, Wilson JL: An around-the-house device for the clinical determination of respiratory driving pressure, *J Speech Hear Disord* 47:413-415, 1982.

Holland AL: Some practical considerations in aphasia rehabilitation. In Sullivan M, and Kommers MS, eds: *Rationale for adult aphasia therapy,* Lincoln, 1977, University of Nebraska Medical Center, pp 167-180.

Holland AL: *Communicative abilities in daily living,* Baltimore, 1980, University Park Press.

Hooper HE: *The Hooper visual organization test,* Los Angeles, 1983, Western Psychological Services.

Horner J and associates: Task-dependent neglect: computed tomography size and locus correlations, *J Neurolog Rehab* 3:7-13, 1989.

Howard D, Hatfield FM: *Aphasia therapy: historical and contemporary issues.* Hillsdale, NJ, 1987, Lawrence Erlbaum.

Humphrey M, Oddy M: Return to work after head injury. A review of postwar studies, *Injury* 12:107-114, 1981.

Jastak S, Wilkinson GS: *Wide Range Achievement Test-*Revised. Wilmington, Del, 1984, Jastak Associates.

Jennett B: Assessment of the severity of head injury, *Journal of Neurol Neurosurg Psychiatry* 39:647-655, 1976.

Jennett B, Bond M: Assessment of outcome after severe brain damage: a practical scale, *Lancet* 1:480-484, 1975.

Jennett B, Teasdale G: *Management of Head Injuries.* Philadelphia, 1981, FA Davis Company.

Jennett B and associates: Predicting outcome in individual patients after severe head injury, *Lancet* 1:878-881, 1976.

Jennett B and associates: Prognosis of patients with severe head injury, *Neurosurgery* 4:283-289, 1979.

Jennett B, Teasdale G, Galbraith S and associates: Severe head injuries in three countries, *Journal of Neurol Neurosurg Psychiatry* 40:291-298, 1977.

Jerger J and associates: Bilateral lesions of the temporal lobe: a case study, *Acta Otolaryngol* 258:1-51, 1969.

Joanette Y and associates: Language in right-handers with right-hemisphere lesions: a preliminary study including anatomical, genetic, and social factors, *Brain Lang* 20:217-248, 1983.

Johns D, ed: *Clinical management of neurogenic communication disorders,* Boston, 1985, Little-Brown.

Johns DF, Darley FL: Phonemic variability in apraxia of speech, *J Speech Hear Res* 13:556-583, 1970.

Jorm AF, Korten AE, Henderson AS: The prevalence of dementia: a quantitative integration of the literature, *Acta Psychologica Scandinavia* 76:465-479, 1987.

Kahneman D: *Attention and effort,* Englewood Cliffs, NJ, 1973, Prentice-Hall.

Kaplan E, Goodglass H, Weintraub S: *The Boston naming test,* Philadelphia, 1983, Lea & Febiger.

Katsuki-Nakamura J, Brookshire RH, Nicholas LE: Comprehension of monologues and dialogues by aphasic listeners, *J Speech Hear Res* 53:408-415, 1988.

Katz DI: Recovery following severe head injuries, *J Head Trauma Rehab,* 7:1-15, 1992.

Katz DI, Alexander MP: Traumatic brain injury. In Good DC, Couch JR, eds: *Handbook of neurorehabilitation,* New York, 1994, Dekker, pp 493-549.

Katz RC, Tong Nagy V: A computerized approach for improving word recognition in chronic aphasic adults. In Brookshire RH, ed: *Clinical aphasiology conference proceedings,* Minneapolis, 1983, BRK, pp 65-72.

Kay T, Silver SM: Closed head trauma: assessment for rehabilitation. In Lezak M, ed: *Assessment of the behavioral consequences of head trauma,* New York, 1989, A.R. Liss, pp 145-170.

Kazdin AE: *Single-case research designs: methods for clinical and applied settings,* New York, 1982, Oxford University Press.

Kearns KP: Flexibility of single-subject experimental designs. Part II: design selection and arrangement of experimental phases, *J Speech Hear Disord* 51:204-214, 1986.

Kearns K, Hubbard DJ: A comparison of auditory comprehension tasks in aphasia. In Brookshire RH, ed: *Clinical aphasiology conference proceedings,* Minneapolis, 1977, BRK, pp 32-45.

Kearns KP, Salmon SJ: An experimental analysis of auxiliary and copula verb generalization in aphasia, *J Speech Hear Disord* 49:152-163, 1984.

Kearns KP, Simmons NN: Group therapy for aphasia: A survey of V.A. medical centers. In Brookshire RH, ed: *Clinical aphasiology conference proceedings,* Minneapolis, 1985, BRK Publishers.

Kearns KP, Simmons NN: Motor speech disorders: the dysarthrias and apraxia of speech. In Lass NJ, McReynolds LV, Northern JL, Yoder DE, eds: *Handbook of speech-language pathology and audiology,* Philadelphia, 1988, BC Decker, pp 434-448.

Keenan JS, Brassell EG: *Aphasia language performance scales,* Murfreesboro, Tenn, 1975, Pinnacle Press.

Kennedy M and associates: Analysis of first-encounter conversations of right-hemisphere-damaged adults, *Clin Aphasiol* 22:67-80, 1994.

Kertesz A: *Aphasia and associated disorders: taxonomy, localization, and recovery,* New York, 1979, Grune and Stratton.

Kertesz A: *Western aphasia battery,* New York, 1982, Grune & Stratton.

Kertesz A, McCabe P: Recovery patterns and prognosis in aphasia, *Brain* 100:1-18, 1977.

Kimelman MDZ, McNeil MR: An investigation of emphatic stress comprehension in aphasia: a replication, *J Speech Hear Res* 30:295-300, 1987.

Kimura D: Right temporal lobe damage, *Arch Neurol* 8:264-271, 1963.

Kintsch W: *The representation of meaning in memory,* Hillsdale, NJ, 1974, Lawrence Erlbaum.

Kirshner HS and associates: Progressive aphasia without dementia: two cases with focal spongiform degeneration, *Ann Neurol* 22:527-533, 1987.

Klare GR: Readability. In Pearson PD, ed: *Handbook of reading research,* New York, 1984, Longman, pp 681-744.

Knopman DS and associates: Recovery of naming in aphasia: relationship to fluency, comprehension, and CT findings, *Neurology* 34:1461-1470, 1984.

Knopman D and associates: A longitudinal study of speech fluency in aphasia: CT correlates of recovery and persistent nonfluency, *Neurology* (Cleveland), 33:1170-1178, 1983.

Kratchowill TR: *Single-subject research: strategies for evaluating change*, New York, 1978, Academic Press.

Kreindler A, Gheorghita N, Voinescu I: Analysis of verbal reception of a complex order with three elements in aphasics, *Brain* 94:375-386, 1971.

Kremin H: Therapeutic approaches to naming disorders. In Paradis M, ed: *Foundations of aphasia rehabilitation*, New York, 1993, Pergamon, pp 261-292.

Kreutzer JS, Wehman PH, eds: *Cognitive rehabilitation for persons with traumatic brain injury: a functional approach*, Baltimore, 1991, Brookes.

Lackner JR, Garrett MF: Resolving ambiguity: effects of biasing context in the unattended ear, *Cognition* 1:359-372, 1972.

Lambrecht K, Marshall R: Comprehension in severe aphasia: a second look. In Brookshire RH, ed: *Clinical aphasiology conference proceedings*, Minneapolis, 1983, BRK, pp 186-192.

Langfitt TW: Measuring outcome from head injuries, *J Neurosurg* 48:673-678, 1978.

LaPointe LL: Base-10 programmed stimulation: task specification, scoring, and plotting performance in aphasia therapy, *J Speech Hear Disord* 42:90-105, 1977.

LaPointe LL, Johns DF: Some phonemic characteristics in apraxia of speech, *J Commun Disord* 8:259-269, 1975.

LaPointe LL, Holtzapple P, Graham LF: The relationship among two measures of auditory comprehension and daily living communication skills. In Brookshire RH, ed: *Clinical aphasiology conference proceedings* Minneapolis, 1985, BRK pp, 38-46.

LaPointe LL, Horner J: *Reading comprehension battery for aphasia*, Tigard, Ore, 1979, CC Publications.

Larimore HW: Some verbal and nonverbal factors associated with apraxia of speech. Doctoral dissertation, University of Denver, 1970.

Lee L: *Northwestern syntax screening test*, Evanston, Ill, 1971, The Northwestern University Press.

Lenneberg E: *Biological foundations of language*, New York, 1967, Wiley.

Lesser R: Verbal and non-verbal memory components in the token test, *Neuropsychologia* 14:79-85, 1976.

Levin HS, Benton AL, Grossman RG: *Neurobehavioral consequences of closed head injury*, New York, 1982, Oxford University Press.

Levin HS and associates: Long-term neuropsychological outcome of closed head injury, *Journal of Neurosurgery* 50:412-422, 1979.

Levin HS, O'Donnell VM, Grossman RG: The Galveston orientation and amnesia test: a practical scale to assess cognition after head injury, *J Nerv Ment Dis* 167:675-684, 1979.

Lewinsohn PM, Danaher BG, Kikel S: Visual imagery as a mnemonic aid for brain-injured persons, *J Consult Clin Psychol* 45:717-723, 1977.

Lewy R, Cole R, Wepman J: Teflon injection in the correction of velopharyngeal insufficiency, *Ann Otol Rhinol Laryngol* 78:874, 1965.

Ley RG, Bryden MP: Hemispheric differences in processing emotions and faces, *Brain Lang* 7:127-138, 1979.

Lezak MD: *Neuropsychological assessment*, ed 2, New York, 1983, Oxford University Press.

Lezak MD: *Neuropsychological assessment*, ed 3, New York, 1995, Oxford University Press.

Li EC, Williams SE: The effects of grammatical class and cue type on cueing responsiveness in aphasia, *Brain Lang* 38:48-60, 1990.

Lichtheim L: On aphasia, *Brain* 7:433-484, 1884.

Liepmann H: Das Krankheitsbild der Apraxia, *Monatsschr Psychiatrie Neuroligie* 7:11-18, 1900.

Liles BZ, Brookshire RH: The effects of pause time on auditory comprehension of aphasic subjects, *J Commun Disord* 8:221-236, 1975.

Lincoln NB and associates: Effectiveness of speech therapy for aphasic stroke patients: a randomized controlled trial, *Lancet* 1197-1200, June, 1984.

Linebaugh CW: Treatment of anomic aphasia. In Perkins WH, ed: *Language handicaps in adults* New York, 1983, Thieme-Stratton, pp 35-43.

Linebaugh C, Lehner L: Cueing hierarchies and word retrieval: a therapy program. In Brookshire RH, ed: *Clinical aphasiology conference proceedings*, Minneapolis, 1977, BRK, pp 19-31.

Livingstone MG, Livingstone HM: The Glasgow Assessment Schedule: clinical and research assessment of head injury outcome, *International Rehabilitation Medicine* 7:145-149, 1985.

Lomas J and associates: The communicative effectiveness index: development and psychometric evaluation of a functional communication measure for adult aphasia, *J Speech Hear Disor* 54:113-124, 1989.

Longstreth WT and associates: Prognosis: keystone of clinical neurology. In Evans RW, Baskin DS, Yatsu FM, eds: *Prognosis of neurological disorders*, New York, 1992, Oxford University Press, pp 19-44.

Love RJ, Webb WJ: The efficacy of cueing techniques in Broca's aphasia, *J Speech Hear Disord* 42:170-178, 1977.

Luria AR: Neuropsychological analysis of focal brain lesions. In Wolman BB, ed: *Handbook of clinical psychology* New York, 1965, McGraw-Hill, pp 42-58.

Luria AR: *Human brain and psychological processes*, New York, 1966, Harper & Row.

Luria AR: *Traumatic aphasia*, The Hague, Netherlands, 1970, Mouton.

Mackay DG: To end ambiguous sentences, *Perception and Psychophysics* 1:426-436, 1966.

Macniven E: Factors affecting head injury rehabilitation outcome: premorbid and clinical parameters. In Finlayson MAJ, Garner SH, eds: *Brain injury rehabilitation: clinical considerations,* Baltimore, 1994, Williams & Wilkins, pp 57-82.

Mahurin RK, Pirozzolo FJ: Chronometric analysis: clinical applications in aging and dementia, *Developmental Neuropsychol* 2:345-362, 1986.

Major BJ, Wilson KJ: *Computerized reading for aphasics,* San Diego, 1985, College-Hill.

Markwardt FC, Jr: *The Peabody individual achievement test-revised,* Circle Pines, 1989, American Guidance Service.

Marshall RC: Word retrieval behavior of aphasic adults, *J Speech Hear Disord* 41:444-451, 1976.

Marshall RC, King PS: Effects of fatigue produced by isokinetic exercise upon the communication ability of aphasic adults. In Wertz RT, Collins M, eds: *Clinical aphasiology: conference proceedings,* Madison, Wis, 1972, Veterans Administration Medical Center.

Marshall JC, Newcombe F: Patterns of paralexia: a psycholinguistic approach, *J Psycholinguist Res* 2:175-199, 1973.

Marshall RC, Phillips DS: Prognosis for improved verbal communication in aphasic stroke patients, *Archives Phys Med Rehabil* 64:597-600, 1983.

Martin R, Feher E: The consequences of reduced memory span for the comprehension of semantic versus syntactic information, *Brain Lang* 38:1-20, 1990.

Martino AA, Pizzamiglio L, Razzano C: A new version of the token test for aphasics: a concrete objects form, *J Commun Disord* 9:1-5, 1976.

Massengill R and associates: Therapeutic exercise and pharyngeal flap, *Cleft Palate J* 5:44-52, 1968.

McDonald S: Viewing the brain sideways? Frontal versus right hemisphere explanations of nonaphasic language disorders, *Aphasiology* 7:535-549, 1993.

McFie J, Zangwill OL: Visual construction disabilities associated with lesions of the left cerebral hemisphere, *Brain* 83:243-260, 1960.

McNeil MR, Prescott TE: *Revised token test,* Baltimore, 1978, University Park Press.

McNeil MR, Kimelman MDZ: Toward an integrative information-processing structure of auditory comprehension and processing in adult aphasia, *Seminars in Speech and Language* 7:123-146, 1986.

McNeil M, Odell K, Tseng CH: Toward the integration of resource allocation into a general model of aphasia. In Prescott T, ed: *Clinical Aphasiology,* Austin, Tex, 1990, Pro-Ed, pp 21-39.

McKeever WF, Dixon MF: Right-hemisphere superiority for discriminating memorized from unmemorized faces: affective imagery, sex, and perceived emotionality effects, *Brain Lang* 12:246-260, 1981.

McReynolds LV, Kearns KP: *Single-subject experimental designs in communicative disorders,* Baltimore, 1983, University Park Press.

McReynolds LV, Kearns KP: Flexibility of single-subject experimental designs, Part I: review of the basics of single-subject designs, *Journal of Speech and Hearing Disorders* 51:194-203, 1986.

Meadows JC: The anatomical basis of prosopagnosia, *J Neurol Neurosurg Psychiatry* 37:489-501, 1974.

Mesulam MM: A cortical network for directed attention and unilateral neglect, *Ann Neurol* 10:309-325, 1982.

Metter EJ and associates: Correlations of glucose metabolism and structural damage to language function in aphasia, *Brain Lang* 21:187-207, 1984.

Metter EJ and associates: Comparisons of metabolic rates, language and memory in subcortical aphasias, *Brain Lang* 19:33-47, 1983.

Meyer BJF: *The organization of prose and its effects on memory,* Amsterdam, 1975, North-Holland.

Meyer BJF, McConkie GW: What is recalled after hearing a passage? *J Educational Psychol,* 65:109-117, 1973.

Miceli G and associates: Patterns of dissociation in comprehension and production of nouns and verbs, *Aphasiology,* 2:351-358, 1988.

Miller JD and associates: Early insults in the injured brain, *JAMA* 240:439-442, 1978.

Mills RH and associates: Cognitive loci of impairments of picture naming by aphasic subjects, *J Speech Hear Res* 22:73-87, 1979.

Milner B: Interhemispheric differences in the localization of psychological processes in man, *Br Med Bull* 27:272-277, 1971. Reported in Lezak, 1995.

Milner B: Psychological aspects of focal epilepsy and its neurosurgical management, *Adv Neurol* 8:299-321, 1975.

Miniami RT and associates: Velopharyngeal incompetency without overt cleft palate, *Plastic and Reconstructive Surgery* 55:573-587, 1975.

Mohr JP: Broca aphasia: pathologic and clinical aspects, *Neurology* 28:311-324, 1978.

Mohr JP, Walters WC, Duncan GW: Thalamic hemorrhage and aphasia, *Brain Lang* 2:3-17, 1975.

Moll KL: Speech characteristics of individuals with cleft lip and palate. In Spriesterbach DC, Sherman D, eds: *Cleft palate and communication,* New York, 1968, Academic Press.

Murdoch BE: *Acquired speech and language disorders,* New York, 1990, Chapman & Hall.

Murray J and associates: Differential diagnosis of aphasia and dementia from aphasia test battery scores, *J Neurolog Comm Disord,* 1:33-39, 1984.

Myers PS: Profiles of communication deficits in patients with right cerebral hemisphere damage: implications for diagnosis and treatment. In Brookshire RH, ed: *Clinical aphasiology conference proceedings,* Minneapolis, 1979, BRK Publishers, pp 38-46.

Myers PS: Inference failure: the underlying impairment in right hemisphere communication disorders. In Prescott

TE, ed: *Clinical Aphasiology: Volume 20,* Austin, Tex, 1991, Pro-Ed, pp 167-180.

Myers PS: Communication disorders associated with right-hemisphere brain damage. In Chapey R, ed: *Language intervention strategies in adult aphasia, ed 3,* Baltimore, 1994, Williams & Wilkins, pp 513-534.

Myers PS, Mackisack EL: Right hemisphere syndrome, In LaPointe LL, ed: *Aphasia and related neurogenic language disorders,* New York, 1990, Thieme, pp 177-195.

Naeser MA and associates: Aphasia with predominantly subcortical lesion sites: description of three capsular putamenal aphasia syndromes, *Arch Neurol* 39:2-14, 1982.

Naeser MA, Borod JC: Aphasia in left-handers, *Neurology* 36:471-488, 1986.

Naeser MA and associates: Quantitative CT scan studies in aphasia: I. Infarct size and CT numbers, *Brain Lang* 12:140-164, 1981.

Naeser MA and associates: Quantitative CT scan studies in aphasia: II. Comparison of right and left hemispheres. *Brain Lang* 12:165-189, 1981.

Naeser MA and associates: Severe nonfluency in aphasia: role of the medial subcallosal fasciculus and other white matter pathways in recovery of spontaneous speech, *Brain* 112:1-38, 1989.

Navia BA, Jordan BD, Price RW: The AIDS dementia complex: clinical features, *Ann Neurol* 19:517-524, 1986.

Netsell R, Cleeland C: Modification of lip hypotonia in dysarthria using EMG feedback, *J Speech Hear Disord* 38:131-140, 1973.

Netsell R, Hixon TJ: A noninvasive method for clinically estimating subglottal air pressure, *J Speech and Hear Disord* 43:326-330, 1978.

Netsell R, Rosenbek JC: Treating the dysarthrias. In Darby J, ed: *Speech and language evaluation in neurology: adult disorders,* New York, 1985, Grune & Stratton, pp 87-101.

Newcombe F: *Missle wounds of the brain,* London, 1969, Oxford University Press.

Nicholas LE, Brookshire RH: Effects of pictures and picturability on sentence verification by aphasic and nonaphasic subjects, *J Speech Hear Res* 24:292-298, 1981.

Nicholas LE, Brookshire RH: Syntactic simplification and context: effects on sentence comprehension by aphasic adults. In Brookshire RH, ed: *Clinical aphasiology conference proceedings,* Minneapolis, 1983, BRK pp 166-172.

Nicholas LE, Brookshire RH: Consistency of the effects of rate of speech on brain-damaged adults' comprehension of narrative discourse, *J Speech Hear Res* 29:462-470, 1986.

Nicholas LE, Brookshire RH: Error analysis and passage dependency of test items from a standardized test of multiple-sentence reading comprehension for aphasic and non-brain-damaged adults, *J Speech Hear Disord* 52:358-366, 1987.

Nicholas LE, Brookshire RH: A system for quantifying the informativeness and efficiency of the connected speech of adults with aphasia, *J Speech Hear Res* 36:338-350, 1993.

Nicholas LE, Brookshire RH: Presence, completeness, and accuracy of main concepts in the connected speech of non-brain-damaged adults and adults with aphasia, *J Speech Hear Res* 38:145-156, 1995a.

Nicholas LE, Brookshire RH: (1995b). Comprehension of spoken narrative discourse by adults with aphasia, right-hemisphere brain damage, or taumatic brain injury, *Am J Speech-Lang Path* 4:69-81, 1995b.

Nicholas LE and associates: Revised administration and scoring procedures for the Boston Naming Test and norms for non–brain-damaged adults, *Aphasiology* 3:569-580, 1989.

Nicholas LE, MacLennan DL, Brookshire RH: Validity of multiple-sentence reading comprehension tests for aphasic adults, *J Speech Hear Disord* 51:82-87, 1986.

Nicholas M and associates: Empty speech in Alzheimer's disease and fluent aphasia, *J Speech Hear Res* 28:405-410, 1985.

Noll DJ, Lass ND: Use of the Token Test with children: two contrasting socioeconomic groups. Paper presented at the American Speech and Hearing Association Convention, San Francisco, November, 1972.

Nolte J: *The Human Brain,* ed 3, St Louis, 1993, Mosby.

Norman DA, Bobrow DG: On data-limited and resource-limited processes, *Cognitive Psychol* 7:44-64, 1975.

Ojemann GA: Language and the thalamus: object naming and recall during and after thalamic stimulation, *Brain Lang* 2:101-120, 1975.

Ommaya AK, Grubb RL, Naumann RA: Coup and contre-coup injury: observations on the mechanics of visible brain injuries in the rhesus monkey, *J Neurosurg* 35:503-507, 1971.

Orgass B, Poeck K: Clinical validation of a new test for aphasia: an experimental study of the *Token Test, Cortex* 2:222-243, 1966.

Osgood C, Miron M: *Approaches to the study of aphasia,* Chicago, 1963, University Park Press.

Pang D: Physics and pathophysiology of closed head injury. In Lezak M, ed: *Assessment of the behavioral consequences of head trauma,* New York, 1989, A.R. Liss, pp 1-19.

Parente R, DiCesare A: Retraining memory: theory, evaluation, and applications. In Kreutzer JS, Wehman PH, eds: *Cognitive rehabilitation for persons with traumatic brain injury: a functional approach,* Baltimore, 1991, Brookes, pp 147-162.

Parkin HJ: Residual learning capability in organic amnesia, *Cortex* 18:417-440, 1982.

Parkhurst BG: The effects of time altered speech stimuli on the performance of right hemiplegic adult aphasics. Paper presented at the annual convention of the American Speech and Hearing Association, New York, 1970.

Parr S: Everyday reading and writing practices of normal adults: implications for aphasia assessment, *Aphasiology* 6:273-283, 1992.

Pashek GV, Brookshire RH: Effects of rate of speech and linguistic stress on auditory paragraph comprehension by aphasic individuals, *J Speech Hear Res* 25:377-382, 1982.

Pasternak KF, LaPointe LL: Aphasic-nonaphasic performance on the Reading Comprehension Battery for Aphasia (RCBA). Paper presented to the annual convention of the American Speech Language and Hearing Association, Toronto, 1982.

Pease DM, Goodglass H: The effects of cueing on picture naming in aphasia, *Cortex* 14:178-189, 1978.

Podraza BL, Darley FL: Effect of auditory prestimulation on naming in aphasia, *J Speech Hear Res* 20:669-683, 1977.

Poeck K: What do we mean by "aphasic syndromes?" A neurologist's view, *Brain Lang* 20:79-89, 1983.

Poeck K, Huber W, Willmes K: Outcome of intensive language rehabilitation in aphasia, *J Speech Hear Disord* 54:471-479, 1989.

Polinko PR: Working with the family: The acute phase. In Ylvisaker M, ed: *Head injury rehabilitation: children and adolescents,* San Diego, 1985, College-Hill, pp 87-101.

Poppelreuter W: *Die Psychischen Schodigringendurch Kopfschuss im Kriege,* 1914/1916, Leipzig, 1917, Verlag von Leopold Voss.

Porch BE: Treatment of aphasia subsequent to the Porch Index of Communicative Ability (PICA). In Chapey R, ed: *Language intervention strategies in adult aphasia, ed 3,* Baltimore, 1994, Williams & Wilkins, pp 175-183.

Porch BE: *Porch Index of Communicative Ability,* Palo Alto, Calif, 1967, 1981a, Consulting Psychologists Press.

Porch BE: Therapy subsequent to the PICA. In Chapey R, ed: *Language intervention strategies in adult aphasia, ed 2,* Baltimore, 1981b, Williams & Wilkins, pp 283-296.

Porch BE: Treatment of aphasia subsequent to the Porch Index of Communicative Ability. In Chapey R, ed: *Language intervention strategies in adult aphasia,* ed 3, Baltimore, 1994, Williams & Wilkens, pp 175-183.

Porch BE: Treatment of aphasia subsequent to the Porch Index of Communicative Ability (PICA). In Chapey R, ed: *Language intervention strategies in adult aphasia, ed 3,* Baltimore, 1994, Williams & Wilkins, pp 178-183.

Porch BE, Callaghan S: Making predictions about recovery: is there HOAP? In Brookshire RH, ed: *Clinical aphasiology conference proceedings,* Minneapolis, 1981, BRK, pp 187-200.

Porch BE and associates: Statistical prediction of change in aphasia, *J Speech Hear Res* 12:312-321, 1980.

Posner MI and associates: How do the parietal lobes direct covert attention? *Neuropsychologia* 25:135-145, 1987.

Powell J, Martindale A, Kulp S: An evaluation of time-

sampling measures of behavior, *J Appl Behav Anal* 8: 463-469, 1975.

Powers GL, Starr CD: The effects of muscle exercise on velopharyngeal gap and nasality, *Cleft Palate J* 11:28-40, 1974.

Prigitano G and associates: Neuropsychological rehabilitation after closed head injury in young adults, *J Neurol Neurosurg Psychiatry* 47:505-513, 1984.

Prins RS, Snow CE, Wagenaar E: Recovery from aphasia: spontaneous speech versus language comprehension, *Brain Lang* 6:192-211, 1978.

Prutting CA, Kirchner DM: A clinical appraisal of the pragmatic aspects of language, *J Speech Hear Disord* 52:105-119, 1987.

Rabins PV, Mace NL, Lucas MJ: The impact of dementia on the family, *JAMA* 248:333-336, 1982.

Raven JC: *The standard progressive matrices,* New York, 1960, The Psychological Corporation.

Raven JC: *The coloured progressive matrices,* New York, 1965, The Psychological Corporation.

Reisberg B and associates: The global deterioration scale for assessment of primary degenerative dementia, *Am J Psychiatry* 139:1136-1139, 1982.

Reitan RM, Wolfson D: *The Halstead-Reitan neuropsychological test battery: theory and clinical interpretation,* Tucson, 1993, Neuropsychology Press.

Repp AC and associates: Differences among common methods for calculating interobserver agreement, *J Appl Behav Anal* 9:109-113, 1973.

Rey A: Psychological examination of traumatic encephalopathy, *Archives de Psycholgie* 28: 286-340; sections translated by Corwin J, Bylsma FW, *The Clinical Neuropsychologist,* 1993, pp 4-9.

Rey A: *L'examen clinque en psychologie,* Paris, 1964, Presses Universitaires de France. Reported in Lezak, 1995.

Rivers DL, Love RJ: Language performance on visual processing tasks in right hemisphere lesion cases, *Brain Lang* 10:348-366, 1980.

Rizzo M, Robin DA: Simultanagnosia: a defect of sustained attention yields insights on visual information processing, *Neurology* 40:447-455, 1990.

Robertson I: Does computerized cognitive rehabilitation work? A review, *Aphasiology* 4:381-405, 1990.

Robin D, Scheinberg S: Subcortical lesions and aphasia, *J Speech Hear Disord* 55:90-100, 1990.

Robin DA, Tranel D, Damasio H: Auditory perception of temporal and spectral events in patients with focal left and right cerebral lesions, *Brain Lang* 39:539-555, 1990.

Rochford G, Williams M: Studies in the development and breakdown in the use of names, IV: the effects of word frequency, *J Neurol Neurosurg Psychiatry* 28:407-413, 1965.

Rosenbek JC: Treating apraxia of speech. In Johns DF, ed: *Clinical management of neurogenic communication disorders,* Boston, 1978, Little-Brown, pp 191-241.

Rosenbek JC, Collins MJ, Wertz RT: Intersystemic reorganization for apraxia of speech. In Brookshire RH, ed: *Clinical aphasiology conference proceedings,* Minneapolis, 1976, BRK, pp 255-260.

Rosenbek JC, LaPointe LL: The dysarthrias: description, diagnosis, and treatment. In Johns DF, ed: *Clinical management of neurogenic communication disorders,* Boston, 1978, Little-Brown, pp 251-310.

Rosenbek JC, LaPointe LL: The dysarthrias: description, diagnosis, and treatment. In Johns DF, ed: *Clinical management of neurogenic communication disorders,* ed 2, Boston, 1985, Little-Brown and Company, pp 97-152.

Rosenbek JC, LaPointe LL, Wertz RT: *Aphasia: a clinical approach,* Boston, 1989, Little-Brown.

Rosenbek JC and associates: A treatment for apraxia of speech in adults, J Speech Hear Disord 38:462-472, 1973.

Rosenbek JC, Wertz RT: Treatment of apraxia of speech in adults. In Wertz RT, Collins M, eds: *Clinical aphasiology conference proceedings,* Madison, Wis, 1972, Veterans Administration Medical Center, pp 191-198.

Rosenbek JC, Wertz RT, Darley FL: Oral sensation and perception in apraxia of speech and aphasia, *J Speech Hear Res* 16:22-36, 1973.

Rosenshine BV: Skill hierarchies in reading comprehension. In Spino RJ, Bruce BC, Brewer WF, eds: *Theoretical issues in reading comprehension,* Hillsdale, NJ, 1980, Lawrence Erlbaum.

Rosenthal M and associates: *Rehabilitation of the adult and child with traumatic brain injury,* Philadelphia, 1990, FA Davis.

Ross DG: *Ross Information Processing Assessment,* Austin, Tex, 1986, Pro-Ed.

Rubens AB: Aphasia with infarction in the territory of the anterior cerebral artery, *Cortex* 11:239-250, 1975.

Rubens AB: The role of changes within the central nervous system during recovery from aphasia. In Sullivan M, Kommers MS, eds: *Rationale for adult aphasia therapy* Lincoln, Neb, 1977, University of Nebraska Medical Center, pp 28-43.

Rubow RT and associates: Reduction of hemifacial spasm in dysarthria following EMG feedback, *J Speech Hear Disord* 49:26-33, 1984.

Ruesch J: Intellectual impairment in head injuries, *Am J Psychiatry* 100:480-496, 1944.

Russell EW: A multiple scoring method for the assessment of complex memory functions, *J Consult Clin Psychol* 43:800-809, 1975.

Russell WR: *The traumatic amnesias,* New York, 1971, Oxford University Press.

Russell WR, Espir MLE: *Traumatic aphasia,* London, 1961, Oxford University Press.

Russell WR, Nathan PW: Traumatic amnesia, *Brain* 69:183-187, 1946.

Rutherford WH: Diagnosis of alcohol ingestion in mild head injuries, *The Lancet* 1:1021-1023, 1977.

Rutter M: Psychological sequelae of brain damage in children, *Am J Psychiatry* 183:1533-1549, 1981.

Saint-Cyr JA, Taylor AE: The mobilization of procedural learning: the "key signature" of the basal ganglia. In Squire LR, Butters N, eds: *Neuropsychology of Memory,* ed 2, New York, 1992, Guilford Press.

Salvatore AP, Strait M, Brookshire RH: Effects of patient characteristics on delivery of *Token Test* commands by experienced and inexperienced examiners, *J Commun Disord* 11:325-334, 1978.

Salvatore AP, Thompson C, Treatment of global aphasia. In Chapey R, Ed: *Language intervention strategies in adult aphasia,* ed 2, Baltimore, 1986, Williams & Wilkins, pp 402-419.

Sands E, Sarno MT, Shankweiler D: Long term assessment of language function in aphasia due to stroke, *Arch Phy Med Rehabil* 50:202-207, 1969.

Sarno MT: *The functional communication profile,* New York, 1969, NYU Medical Center Monograph Department.

Sarno MT, Silverman M, Sands E: Speech therapy and language recovery in severe aphasia. *J Speech Hear Res* 13:607-623, 1970.

Sbordone RJ: Overcoming obstacles in cognitive rehabilitation of persons with severe traumatic brain injury. In Kreutzer JS, Wehman PH, eds: *Cognitive rehabilitation for persons with traumatic brain injury: a functional approach,* Baltimore, 1991, Brookes, pp 105-115.

Schacter DL, Glisky EL: Memory remediation: restorations, alleviation, and the acquisition of domain-specific knowledge. In Gross Y, Uzzell BP, eds: *Clinical neuropsychology of intervention* Boston, 1986, Martinus Nijhoff, pp 257-282.

Schacter D, Rich S, Stampp A: Remediation of memory disorders: experimental evaluation of the spaced-retrieval technique, *J Clin Exp Neuropsychol* 7:79-96, 1985.

Schuell HM: A short examination for aphasia. *Neurology* 7:625-634, 1957.

Schuell HM: *The Minnesota test for differential diagnosis of aphasia,* Minneapolis, 1965, 1972, University of Minnesota Press.

Schuell HM, Jenkins JJ: Reduction of vocabulary in aphasia, *Brain* 84:243-261, 1961.

Schuell HM, Jenkins JJ, Jimenez-Pabon E: *Aphasia in adults,* New York, 1965, Harper and Row.

Schuell HM, Jenkins JJ, Landis L: Relationship between auditory comprehension and word frequency in aphasia, *J Speech Hear Res* 4:30-36, 1961.

Selnes OA and associates: Computed tomographic scan correlates of auditory comprehension deficits in aphasia: a prospective recovery study, *Ann Neurol* 13:558-566, 1983.

Selnes OA and associates: The critical role of Wernicke's area in sentence repetition, *Ann Neurol* 17:549-557, 1985.

Shallice T: Specific impairments of planning, *Philos Trans R Soc Lond* 298:199-209, 1982.

Shallice T, Warrington EK: Independent functioning of the verbal memory stores: a neuropsychological study, *Q J Exp Psychol* 22:261-273, 1970.

Shankweiler D, Harris KS: An experimental approach to the problem of articulation in aphasia, *Cortex* 2:277-292, 1966.

Shapiro BE, Danly M: The role of the right hemisphere in the control of speech prosody in propositional and affective contexts, *Brain Lang* 25:19-36, 1985.

Shewan CM: *The auditory comprehension test for sentences,* Chicago, 1979, Biolinguistics Clinical Institutes.

Shewan CM: The Shewan spontaneous language analysis system (SSLA) for aphasic adults: description, reliability, and validity, *J Commun Disord* 21:103-138, 1988.

Shewan CM, Canter GJ: Effects of vocabulary, syntax, and sentence length on auditory comprehension in aphasic patients, *Cortex* 7:209-226, 1971.

Shewan CM, Kertesz A: Reliability and validity characteristics of the Western Aphasia Battery (WAB), *J Speech Hear Disord* 45:308-324, 1980.

Shewan CM, Kertesz A: Effects of speech and language treatment on recovery from aphasia, *Brain Lang* 23:272-299, 1984.

Silverman FH: Dysarthria: communication augmentation systems for adults without speech. In Perkins WH, ed: *Dysarthria and apraxia,* New York, 1983, Thieme-Stratton, pp 115-121.

Skelly M: *Amer-Ind gestural code,* New York, 1979, Elsevier.

Sklar M: *The Sklar aphasia scale.* Los Angeles, 1973, Western Psychological Services.

Smith A: Diagnosis, intelligence, and rehabilitation of chronic aphasics. Final Report. Ann Arbor, Mich, 1972, University of Michigan Press.

Snow P, Douglas J, Ponsford J: Discourse assessment following traumatic brain injury: a pilot study examining some demographic and methodological issues, *Aphasiology* 9:365-380, 1995.

Sohlberg MM, Mateer CA: *Introduction to cognitive rehabilitation: theory and practice,* New York, 1989, Gulford.

Sparks R, Helm NA, Albert ML, Aphasia rehabilitation resulting from melodic intonation therapy, *Cortex* 10:303-316, 1974.

Sparks R, Holland AL: Method: melodic intonation therapy for aphasia, *J Speech Hear Disord* 41:287-297, 1976.

Spreen O, Benton AL: *Neurosensory center comprehensive examination for aphasia,* Victoria, BC, 1977, Neuropsychology Laboratory, University of Victoria.

Square PA, Weidner WE: Oral sensory perception in adults demonstrating apraxia of speech. Paper presented to the American Speech and Hearing Association, Houston, Tex, 1976.

St Louis KO, Ruscello DM: *Oral speech mechanism screening examination,* Austin, Tex, 1987, Pro-Ed.

Stachowiak FJ and associates: Text comprehension in aphasia, *Brain Lang* 4:177-195, 1977.

Stanczak DE and associates: Assessment of level of consciousness following severe neurological insult, *J Neurosurg* 60:955-60, 1984.

Stanton K and associates: Language utilization in teaching reading to left neglect patients. In Brookshire RH, ed: *Clinical aphasiology conference proceedings,* Minneapolis, 1981, BRK, pp 262-271.

State University of New York at Buffalo Research Foundation *Guide for the use of the uniform data set for medical rehabilitation: functional independence measure,* Buffalo, 1993, State University of New York.

Stedman's Medical Dictionary, Baltimore, 1990, Williams & Wilkins.

Steele RD and associates: Computer-based visual communication in aphasia, *Neuropsychologia* 27:409-426, 1989.

Stimley MA, Noll JD: The effects of semantic and phonemic prestimulation cues on picture naming in aphasia, *Brain Lang* 41:496-509, 1991.

Stoicheff ML: Motivating instructions and language performance of dysphasic subjects, *J Speech Hear Res* 3:75-85, 1960.

Stokes TF, Baer DM: An implied technology of generalization, *J Appl Behav Anal* 10:349-367, 1977.

Swindell CS, Holland AL, Fromm D: Classification of aphasia: WAB type versus clinical impression. In Brookshire RH, ed, *Clinical aphasiology conference proceedings,* Minneapolis, 1984, BRK, pp 48-54.

Teasdale G, Jennett B: Assessment of coma and impaired consciousness, *Lancet, ii,* 81-84, 1974.

Teasdale G, Jennett B: Assessment and prognosis of coma after head injury, *Acta Neurochir* 34:45-55, 1976.

Teasdale G, Mendelow D, Pathophysiology of head injuries. In Brooks DN, ed: *Closed head injury: psychological, social, and family consequences,* Oxford, 1984, Oxford University Press.

Terman LM, Merrill MA: *Stanford-Binet intelligence scale,* Boston, 1973, Houghton-Mifflin.

Thompson C, Byrne M: Across setting generalization of social conventions in aphasia. In Brookshire RH, ed: *Clinical aphasiology conference proceedings,* Minneapolis, 1984, BRK, pp 132-144.

Thompson C, Holmberg M, Baer DM: A brief report on a comparison of two time-sampling methods, *J Appl Behav Anal* 7:623-626, 1974.

Thompson RS, Rivara FP, Thompson DC: A case control study of the effectiveness of bicycle safety ahlmets, *New England Journal of Medicine* 320:1362-1367, 1989.

Thurstone LL: *A factorial study of perception,* Chicago, 1944, University of Chicago Press.

Tomlinson BE, Henderson G: Some quantitative cerebral findings in normal and demented old people. In Terry R, Gerskor S, eds: *Neurobiology of aging,* New York, 1976, Raven.

Tompkins CA: *Right hemisphere communication disorders: theory and management,* San Diego, Calif, 1995, Singular Publishing Group.

Tompkins CA, Flowers CR: Perception of emotional intonation by brain-damaged adults: the influence of task processing levels, *J Speech Hear Res* 28:527-538, 1985.

Tow PM: *Personality changes following forntal leucotomy,* London, 1955, Oxford University Press.

Trost JE, Canter GJ: Apraxia of speech in patients with Broca's aphasia: a study of phoneme production accuracy and error patterns, *Brain Lang* 1:63-79, 1974.

Trupe EH: Reliability of rating spontaneous speech in the western aphasia battery: implications for classification. In Brookshire RH, ed: *Clinical aphasiology conference proceedings,* Minneapolis, 1984, BRK, pp 55-69.

Tuiman JJ: Determining the passage dependency of comprehension test questions on five major tests, *Reading Research Quarterly* 2:206-233, 1974.

Tulving E: Episodic and semantic memory. In Tulving E, Donaldson W, eds: Organization of memory, New York, 1972, Academic Press.

Tulving E: Elements of episodic memory, Oxford, 1983, Clarendon Press.

Tweedy JR, Shulman PD: Toward a functional classification of naming impairments, *Brain Lang* 15:193-206, 1982.

Ulatowska HK and associates: Production of procedural discourse in aphasia, *Brain Lang* 18:315-341, 1983.

Uzzell BP and associates: Influence of lesions detected by computed tomography on outcome and neuropsychological recovery after severe head injury, *Neurosurgery* 20:396-402, 1987.

Vallar G, Baddeley AD: Phonological short-term store, phonological processing, and sentence processing: a neuropsychological case study, *Cognitive Neuropsychol* 1:121-142, 1984.

Van Buskirk C: Prognostic value of sensory deficit in rehabilitation of hemiplegics, *Neurology* 6:407-411, 1955.

Van Houten R and associates: Prevention of brain injuries by improving safety-related behaviors. In Finlayson MAJ, Garner SH, eds: *Brain injury rehabilitation: clinical considerations,* Baltimore, 1994, Williams & Wilkins, pp 313-331.

Van Zomeren AH, Brouwer WH, Deelman BG: Attentional deficits: the riddles of selectivity, speed, and alertness. In Brooks N, ed: *Closed head injury: psychological, social, and family consequences* Oxford, 1984, Oxford University Press, pp 74-107.

Verfaelli M, Bauer RH, Bowers D: Autonomic and behavioral evidence of implicit memory in amnesia, *Brain Cogn* 15:10-25, 1991.

Veterans Administration: Veterans Administration cooperative study group on antihypertensive agents: effects of treatment on morbidity in hypertension III: Influence of age, diastolic pressure, and prior cardiovascular disease; further analysis of side effects, *Circulation* 45:991-1004, 1972.

Vignolo LA: Evolution of aphasia and language rehabilitation: a retrospective study, *Cortex* 1:344-367, 1964.

Vignola LA and associates: Unexpected CT scan findings in global aphasia, *Cortex* 22:55-70, 1986.

Von Bonin G: Anatomical asymmetries of the cerebral hemispheres. In Mountcastle VB, ed: *Interhemispheric relations and cerebral dominance* Baltimore, 1962, Johns Hopkins Press, pp 1-11.

Wagenaar E, Snow CE, Prins RS: Spontaneous speech of aphasic patients: a psycholinguistic analysis, *Brain Lang* 2:281-303, 1975.

Waller MR, Darley FL: The influence of context on the auditory comprehension of paragraphs in aphasic subjects, *J Speech Hear Res* 21:732-745, 1978.

Walsh KW: *Understanding brain damage,* Edinburgh, 1985, Churchill-Livingstone.

Warren RL: Functional outcome: an introduction, *Clin Aphasiol* 21:59-65, 1992.

Warrington EK, James M: Disorders of visual perception in patients with localized cerebral lesions, *Neuropsychologica* 5:253-266, 1967.

Warrington EK, Shallice T: The selective impairment of auditory-verbal short-term memory, *Brain* 92:885-896, 1969.

Watson RT, Heilman KM: Thalamic neglect, *Neurology* 29:690-694, 1979.

Webb WG: Acquired dyslexias. In LaPointe LL, ed: *Aphasia and related language disorders.* New York, 1990, Thieme, pp 130-146.

Wechsler D: *Wechsler adult intelligence scale-revised,* New York, 1981, Psychological Corporation.

Wechsler D: *Wechsler memory scale—revised manual,* San Antonio, Tex, 1987, The Psychological Corporation.

Wegner ML, Brookshire RH, Nicholas LE: Comprehension of main ideas and details in coherent and noncoherent discourse by aphasic and nonaphasic listeners, *Brain Lang* 21:37-51, 1984.

Weidner WE, Jinks AF: The effects of single versus combined cue presentations on picture naming by aphasic adults, *J Speech Hear Disord* 16:111-121, 1983.

Weigl E: On the problem of cortical syndromes: experimental studies. In ML Simmell, ed: *The reach of mind,* New York, 1968, Springer, pp 143-159.

Weiner F: *Aphasia I: noun association,* Baltimore, 1983, University Park Press.

Weisenburg TH, McBride KE: *Aphasia,* New York, 1935, Commonwealth Fund.

Wener DL, Duffy JR: An investigation of the sensitivity of the reporter's test to expressive language disturbances (abstract). In Brookshire RH, ed: *Clinical aphasiology conference proceedings,* Minneapolis, 1983, BRK, pp 15-17.

Wepman JM: *Recovery from aphasia,* New York, 1951, Ronald Press.

Wertz RT and associates: Veterans Administration cooperative study on aphasia: a comparison of individual and group treatment, *J Speech Hear Res* 24:580-594, 1981.

Wertz RT and associates: A comparison of clinic, home, and deferred language treatment for aphasia: a VA cooperative study, *Arch Neurol* 43:653-658, 1986.

Wertz RT, Deal JL, Robinson AJ: Classifying the aphasias: a comparison of the Boston Diagnostic Aphasia Examination and the Western Aphasia Battery. In Brookshire RH, ed: *Clinical aphasiology conference proceedings,* Minneapolis, 1984, BRK, pp 40-47.

Wertz RT, Dronkers NF, Hume JL: PICA intrasubtests variability and prognosis for improvement in aphasia. In Lemme ML, ed: *Clin Aphasiol* 31:207-211, 1993.

Wertz RT, Keith RL, Custer DD: Normal and aphasic behavior on a measure of auditory input and a measure of verbal output. Paper presented at the annual convention of the American Speech and Hearing Association, Chicago, 1971.

Wertz RT, LaPointe LL, Rosenbek JC: *Apraxia of speech in adults: the disorder and its management,* Orlando, Fla, 1984, Grune & Stratton.

West JF: Auditory comprehension in aphasic adults: improvement through training, *Arch Phys Med Rehabil* 54:78-86, 1973.

West JF, Kaufman GA: Some effects of redundancy on the auditory comprehension of adult aphasics. Paper presented at the annual convention of the American Speech and Hearing Association, San Francisco, 1972.

Whitely AM, Warrington EK, Prosopagnosia: a clinical, psychological, and anatomical study of three patients, *J Neurol Neurosurg Psychiatry* 40:395-403, 1977.

Willanger R, Danielson UT, Ankerhaus J: Visual neglect in right-sided apoplectic lesions, *Acta Neurol Scand* 64:310-326, 1981.

Williams SE, Canter GJ: The influence of situational context on naming performance in aphasic syndromes, *Brain Lang* 17:92-106, 1982.

Wilson B: Teaching a patient to remember people's names after removal of a left temporal tumor, *Behavioral Psychotherapy* 9:338-344, 1981.

Wilson B: Success and failure in memory training following a cerebral vascular accident, *Cortex* 18:582-594, 1982.

Wilson BA, Cockburn J, Halligan P: *Behavioral Inattention Test,* Suffolk, England, 1987, Thames Valley Test Company.

Wilson JA and associates: The functional effects of head injury in the elderly, *Brain Injury* 1:183-188, 1987.

Woodcock RW, Johnson MB: Woodcock-Johnson Psychoeducational Battery-Revised, Allen, Tex, 1989, DLM Teaching Resources.

World Health Organization: *International classification of impairments, disabilities, and handicaps,* Geneva, 1980, World Health Organization.

Wyke M, Holgate D: Colour naming defects in dysphasic patients: a qualitative analysis, *Neurolopsychologia* 11:451-461, 1973.

Ylvisaker MS, Holland AL: Coaching, self-coaching, and rehabilitation of head injury. In Johns DF, ed: *Clinical management of neurogenic communication disorders,* Boston, 1985, Little-Brown, pp 243-257.

Ylvisaker M, Urbanczyk B: Assessment and treatment of speech, swallowing, and communication disorders following traumatic brain injury. In Finlayson MAJ, Garner SH, eds: *Brain injury rehabilitation: clinical considerations,* Baltimore, 1994, Williams & Wilkins.

Yorkston KM: Treatment of right hemisphere damaged patients: a panel presentation. In Brookshire RH, ed. *Clinical aphasiology conference proceedings,* Minneapolis, 1981, BRK, pp 281-283.

Yorkston KM, Beukelman DR: An analysis of connected speech samples of aphasic and normal speakers, *J Speech Hear Disord* 45:27-36, 1980.

Yorkston KM, Beukelman DR: *Assessment of Intelligibility of Dysarthric Speech,* Tigard, Ore, 1981, CC Publications.

Yorkston KM, Beulkelman DR, Bell KR: *Clinical management of dysarthric speakers,* San Diego, 1988 College-Hill.

Yorkston KM and associates: A Phoneme identification task as a measure of perceived articulatory adequacy. Paper presented at the third biennial Clinical Dysarthria Conference, Tuscon, Ariz, 1986.

Yorkston KM, Marshall RC, Butler M: Imposed delay of response: effects on aphasics' auditory comprehension of visually and nonvisually cued material, *Perceptual and Motor Skills* 44:647-655, 1977.

Yules RB, Chase RA: A training method for reduction of hypernasality in speech, *Plast Reconstr Surg* 43:180-185, 1969.

Index

Italic page numbers indicate illustrations; *t* indicates table.